MEDICAL PARASITOLOGY

MEDICAL PARASITOLOGY

[Approved for the undergraduate and postgraduate students of Zoology, Entomology, Protozoology, Helminthology, Medicine (Allopathy, Homoeopathy and Ayurveda), Microbiology and Pathology]

T K Dey

MBBS (Cal), MIAP (Washington), MD, D Bact (Manchester), FISD (New York), FRSM (London)

Author of *A Textbook of Bacteriology, A Textbook of Pathology, A Handbook of Practical Pathology and Microbiology, Medical Bacteriology, Medical Mycology, Skin Diseases in the Tropics,* etc.

New Central Book Agency (P) Ltd

LONDON

HYDERABAD ERNAKULAM BHUBANESWAR

DELHI KOLKATA PUNE GUWAHATI

NCBA

REGD OFFICE
8/1 Chintamoni Das Lane, Kolkata 700 009, India
email: ncbapvtltd@eth.net

OVERSEAS
NCBA (UK) Ltd, 149 Park Avenue North, Northampton, NN3 2HY, UK

EXPORT
NCBA Exports Pvt. Ltd, 212 Shahpur Jat, New Delhi 110 049
email: ncbaexp@ncbapvtltd.com

BRANCHES

212 Shahpur Jat
New Delhi 110 049
email: ncbadel@ncbapvtltd.com

Shop Nos. 3 & 4, Vinayak Towers
681/B Budhwar Peth, Appa Balwant Chowk
Pune 411 002
email: ncbapune@ncbapvtltd.com

Shop No. 15, Bharati Towers, Ground Floor
Forest Park, **Bhubaneswar** 751 001
email: ncbabub@ncbapvtltd.com

House No. 3-1-315, 1st Floor
Nimboliadda, Kachiguda, **Hyderabad** 500 027
email: ncbahydb@ncbapvtltd.com

GSS Shopping Complex, 1st Floor
Opposite College Post Office, Convent Road
Ernakulam 682 035
email: ncbaernk@ncbapvtltd.com

Radhamayee Complex (Second Floor)
Opp. SBI, Panbazar, Jaswanta Road
Guwahati 781 001
email: ncbaguwahati@ncbapvtltd.com

Medical Parasitology • T K Dey

Revised and Enlarged Tenth Edition: 1991
Eleventh Edition: 2010
Reprinted: 2014

PUBLISHER AND TYPESETTER
New Central Book Agency (P) Ltd
8/1 Chintamoni Das Lane, Kolkata 700 009

PRINTER
New Central Book Agency (P) Ltd
Web-Offset Division, Dhulagarh, Sankrail, Howrah

COVER DESIGNER
Soumen Paul

COVER PRINTER
Biswanath Studio, Kolkata

TECHNICAL EDITOR
Dipan Roy

PROJECT COORDINATORS
Suman Dutta, Prabhat Jas

ISBN: 978 81 7381 117 3

Price ₹ 385.00

CONTENTS

PREFACE TO THE ELEVENTH EDITION

The book has been thoroughly revised and totally recast. Amongst many other changes notable additions are in the chapter PNEUMOCYSTIC CARINII which has been thought to be under the classification of fungi; the chapter has been totally recast and practically rewritten.

A new chapter has been incorporated that deals with Toxoplasmosis, Cryptosporidiosis, Microsporidiosis and others. The new chapter has been named MICROSPORIDA.

Names of different more species have been added wherever required. New modern drugs and chemotherapeutics have been recorded for different infections and they have been listed appropriately under the heading of different infections in APPENDIX III.

A detailed INDEX has been appended to save the searching time of the readers.

This unbeaten book has become highly popular, and has been approved and recommended in India and also in foreign countries like Canada.

I am sure that this eleventh edition shall be a golden treasure to the teachers and students of MICROBIOLOGY, ZOOLOGY, ENTOMOLOGY and MEDICINE and will pave their way to new heights to learn and have a thorough grasp on the subject.

I wish cordially an all-round success to the readers.

Kolkata
January 2010

T. K. DEY
Professor N. C. Dey Memorial
Diagnostic & Research Centre

PREFACE TO THE TENTH EDITION

There has not been any marked change in the subject during the last one year except for some minor immunological aspects of diseases. Some recently developed drugs and their doses with special reference to anti-malarial drugs and management of the patients have, however, been discussed in the present edition of the book. Steps have also been taken to provide ready references to the modern drugs and treatment of Protozoal and Helminthic episodes, as far as possible.

I do hope that this volume will be helpful to the students and practitioners in the field as regards the parasitic diseases caused by Protozoa and Helminths.

My cordial thanks are due to Mrs. S. Dey, who has taken keen interest and meticulously looked after the volume during its preparation.

Calcutta
1991

T. K. Dey

CHAPTER

1 INTRODUCTION

Parasitology is the science that deals with parasites and their pathogenic effects.

Parasites of animal kingdom are divided into three main groups, namely, Protozoa, Helminths or Arthropods and, accordingly, Parasitology may be divided into three sections : I. Protozoology, II. Helminthology and III. Entomology.

Parasites of man belonging to the animal kingdom may be divided as in Table 1.1.

Terms and Terminologies of Parasitology

Parasite. A living organism which receives nourishment and shelter from another organism; the latter is host.

Host. An organism which harbours the parasite.

Association of living objects. An association which is formed between animals of different species may be divided as follows:

SYMBIOSIS. An association in which both are so dependent upon each other that one cannot live without the help of the other.

COMMENSALISM. An association in which the parasite only is benefitted without causing injury to its host.

PARASITISM. An association in which the parasite derives benefit and the host gets nothing in return and always suffers some injury.

Zoonosis. Infection or infestation shared in nature by human and lower vertebrates.

TABLE 1.1

KINGDOM :	ANIMALIA		
PHYLUM :	**Protozoa** (First animals)		**Metazoa** (After-animals)
SUB PHYLUM :	I. Sarcomastigophora	II. Sporozoa	III. Cilliophora
CLASS :	Rhizopodea Zoomastigophorea	Telosporea	Ciliatea
PHYLUM	Platyhelminthes	Aschelminthes	Arthropoda
CLASS :	1. Cestoda (Tapeworms) 2. Trematoda (Flukes)	Nematoda Nematomorpha	Insecta

Types of Parasites

Ecto-parasite (Ectozoa): Lives outside on the external surface of the body of the host.

Endo-parasite (Entozoa): Lives inside the body of the host.

Facultative parasite: Lives a parasitic life when opportunity occurs.

Obligatory parasite: Cannot exist without a parasitic life in some host.

Occasional or Accidental parasite: Parasite which attacks an unusual host.

Temporary parasite : Visits a host for a short period.

Permanent parasite : Leads a parasitic life all through its life.

Wandering or *Aberrant parasite* : Parasite reaches a place where it cannot live.

Types of Hosts

Alternate host: When two hosts harbour the same parasite, either is called an alternate host.

Definitive host: Host harbours the adult or sexual stage of the parasite,

Intermediate host: Harbours the larval (asexual) stages of the parasite.

Paratenic host (A carrier or transport host) : Where the parasite remains viable without further development.

ORDER FOLLOWED IN A PARASITOLOGICAL STUDY

1. History of discovery
2. Geographical distribution
3. Habitat inside the host (human)
4. Morphology (staining, culture), and Life cycle
5. Modes of infection : Reservoir host, sources, portal of entry, transmission
6. Effect of the parasite : Pathologic lesions, clinical manifestations, complications
7. Immunology
8. Methods for diagnosis
9. Prophylaxis
10. Therapy
11. Prognosis.

The study of animal parasites infecting man and producing clinical manifestations should include the following:

History. The year in which the parasite was first identified and any important discovery and study regarding it.

Geographical Distribution. Environmental factors, social customs and habits of the person concerned greatly influence the distribution of parasites and, accordingly, each parasite has got a specific distribution.

Morphology and Life Cycle

The morphological structure of a parasite and its various stages through which it passes its life are important. The parasite may complete its life cycle in one host or it may change its host (see Definitive and Intermediate hosts).

Sources and Modes of Infection

Parasitic transmission form one host to other is caused by certain stages called infective forms. Ways by which infective agents are transferred from one host to another and the path through which they enter the human host is important. In an endemic area, parasitic infection occurs continuously by the presence of hosts acting as reservoirs of infection; such hosts may be either animals or man. Where an insect intermediate host (vector) plays a part in dissemination of diseases, bionomic of the vector should be studied carefully.

Sources of infection and Portal of Entry

(See Table 1.2)

Infective stage of the parasite reaches the body in the ways shown in Table 1.2.

I. Contamination of Food and Drink—gain entrance to digestive tract

1. Cysts of *E. histolytica* and ova of *A. lumbricoides* contaminate food or drink.
2. The infective forms remain in the flesh of intermediate hosts, which, when taken as food, may infect:
   (a) Beef: ***T. saginata*** (***Cysticercus bovis***)
   (b) Pork: ***T. solium*** (***Cysticercus cellulosae***) and ***T. spiralis***
   (c) Fish containing plerocercoid larvae of ***D. latum*** and metacercariae of ***C. sinensis***
   (d) Crabs or crayfish containing metacercarial forms of ***P. westermani***.
3. Intermediate host harbouring the infective form may be eaten as a whole, like cyclops infected with the larval forms of D. medinensis are ingested with water.
4. The infective forms emerge from its intermediate host and encyst in aquatic plants, which is

taken as food e.g., metacercariae or *F. hepatica* in watercress.

II. Contamination of Skin or Mucous Membrane

1. Filariform larvae of *A. duodenale*, *N. americanus* and *S. stercoralis* from damp soil penetrate the unbroken skin.
2. Cercarial forms of *S. haematobium, S. mansonii* and *S. japonicum* in infected water may penetrate the skin.

III. Agency of Insect Host

An infected blood-sucking arthropod introduces the organism directly into blood or into skin or skin layers during a blood-meal, like Malarial parasites by anopheline mosquitoes, trypanosoma by Tsetse flies, Leishmania by sandflies and Wuchereria by Culicline mosquitoes.

PATHOLOGY

In protozoal infections, the lesions depend on proliferation, multiplication and metastasis of the organism. Trophozoites of *E. histolytica* secrete a powerful histolytic toxin which causes destruction of the tissues, while malarial parasite causes destruction of erythrocytes.

In the majority of helminthic infections, the adult parasites are found inside the human body and no multiplication occurs except in cases of hymenolepiasis and strongyloidiasis. It is the dose—i.e., the number of invading organisms gaining entrance during primary infection and reinfection—that constitutes the most important factor in the pathogenesis of helminthiasis. Pathogenic effects depend on the sites of attack, the site and pattern of laying ova and larva. In certain helminthic infections the secretions and excretions of the growing larvae and the liberated products of dead parasites may behave like an antigen producing allergic state in helminthic infections which may be diagnosed by immunological skin tests with specific antigens.

SOME IMPORTANT PATHOGENIC EFFECTS

Pathological changes produced by parasites are sometimes as a result of immunological response, e.g., Pernicious malaria may cause Blackwater fever, and Malaria can also cause idiopathic tropical splenomegaly and nephrotic syndrome. Granuloma formation resulting in fibrosis which occurs in schistosomiasis is proved to be due to cell-mediated immunological response. Occult filariasis is also an immunological response against filaria parasite.

Some helminthic infections, like trichinelliasis, strongyloidosis, ascariasis, etc., may carry viruses and bacteria to blood and other tissue during their larval migration from the bowel.

Sometimes parasitic infections producing an immunosuppressive state may allow bacterial infections, e.g., Malaria, Kala-azar (agranulocytosis), Trypanosomiasis. Also such an immunosuppression may result in fulminant parasitaemia by multiplication in tissue and blood (heavy parasitic load), e.g., Pernicious Malaria, and may cause opportunistic infections. e.g., Toxoplasmosis, or may cause massive invasion of tissue, e.g., Strongyloidosis.

Parasitic infections may contribute to the formation of a tumour, such as, Burkitt's lymphoma—a sequellae of chronic malaria, Adenocarcinoma of the bile duct in fascioliasis, Primary hepatoma in clonorchiasis, and hepatic, vesical, colonic and rectal carcinoma may follow schistosomiasis.

Immunology. Two chief types of immunity is encountered (1) Innate and Acquired *Immunity*. It is not dependent upon previous exposure to infection and is not the result of specific responses of immunocompetent cells. Probably it is related to the genetic make-up of the host. The example of genetic innate immunity of man to "human" parasitic infection is seen amongst West Africans who are more resistant than White Americans to hookworm infection and B. T. malaria. Also African children carrying the sickle-cell trait shows relative resistance to *P. falciparum* infection. (2) *Acquired immunity* may be gradually built after a natural infection, or induced artificially, as in cutaneous leishmaniasis. This is *active immunity*. Immune bodies IgG fraction 7S may be passively transferred to the foetus in utero *via* placenta and *via* milk of an immune breast-feeder.

IMMUNITY

As a result of parasitic infection, the following conditions of immunity may develop in the host:

Natural Immunity

Human beings are immune to infection by avian and most of the simian plasmodia.

Acquired immunity to malaria results from antigenic stimulation by the parasites or other products.

Active immunity is acquired by the host himself often after acquiring a disease. It may be *concomittant*, i.e., immunity is present when there is parasitaemia; or it may be residual, persisting after eradication of the parasite. This is differentiated from *tolerant immunity*.

TABLE 1.2

SOURCES AND SPREAD OF INFECTION

Source	Infective Stage in	Portal of Entry	Infective Parasite	Disease
ARTHROPODS Crabs/Cray fish/Cyclops	Metacercariae in crabs or cray fish	G. I. Tract	*P. westermani*	Paragonimiasis
	(i) Larvae inside body cavity of cyclops	G. I. Tract	*D. medinensis*	Dracunculosis or Dracontiasis
	(ii) Procercoid larvae in the body of cyclops	G. I. Tract	Spirometra (Sparganum) Plerocercoid larva in fish (Secondary intermediate host)	Sparganosis of Fish
Reduvid bug	Metacyclic form in hindgut	Skin contamination and subsequent inoculation	*T. cruzi*	Chagas' disease
House fly	Cysts in alimentary canal	G. I. Tract	*E. histolytica*	Amoebiasis
Sand fly	Promastigotes in buccal cavity and pharynx	Skin inoculation	*L. donovani*	Kala-azar
		,, ,,	*L. tropica*	Oriental sore
		,, ,,	*L. brasiliensis*	Espundia
Tsetse fly	Metacyclic forms of Trypomastigotes in salivary gland	Skin inoculation	*T. brucei* Subgroup	Sleeping sickness
Anopheles Mosquito	Sporozoites in salivary glands	Skin inoculation	Plasmodia species	Malaria
Culex Mosquito	Larve in proboscis	Skin inoculation	*W. bancrofti*	Bancroft's filariasis
Mansonioides	,, ,,	,, ,,	*Br. malayi*	Malayan filariasis
Chrysops	,, ,,	,, ,,	*L. loa*	Loasis
Simulium	,, ,,	,, ,,	*O. volvulus*	Onchocerciasis
MOLLUSCS	Cercariae encysted in aquatic vegetation, water chestnut. etc.	G. I. Tract	*F. hepatica*	Fascioliasis
,,	Cercariae liberated in water	Skin penetration	*Fp. buski* Schistosoma species	Fasciolopsiasis Schistosomiasis or Bilharziasis
FISHES	Plerocercoid larvae in fish flesh	G. I. Tract	*D. latum*	Diphyllobothriasis
,,	Metacercariae in fish flesh	G. I. Tract	*C. sinensis*	Clonorchiasis
,,			*H. heterophyes*	Heterophyasis
,,			*M. yokogawai*	Metagonimiasis

(*Contd.*)

(*Contd.*)

Source	Infective Stage in	Portal of Entry	Infective Parasite	Disease
MAMMALS				
Cow	*Cysticercus bovis* in muscles	G. I. Tract	*T. saginata*	Taeniasis saginata
Pig	*Cysticercus cellulosse* in muscles	G. I. Tract	*T. solium*	Taeniasis solium
Pig	Encysted larvae in muscles	G. I. Tract	*Tr. spiralis*	Trichinelliasis
Pig or humen	*Bal. coli* in faeces	G. I. Tract	*Balantidium coli*	Balantidial dysentery or Balantidiasis
Dog	Ova of *Ech. granulosus*	G. I. Tract	*E. granulosus*	Echinococcosis or Hydatid disease
	Ova of Toxocara canis	G. I. Tract	*T. canis* (VLM)	Viscaral Larva Migrans
Cat	Oocysts in faeces	G. I. Tract	*T. gondii*	Toxoplasmosis
HUMAN	Ova of Oxyuris	G. I. Tract	*O. vermicularis*	Oxyuriasis (Enterobiasis)
	Ova of Hymenolepis species	G. I. Tract	*H. nana* & *H. diminuta*	Hymenolepiasis
	Ova of *T. saginata* & *T. solium*	G. I. Tract	*T. saginata* *T. solium*	Taeniasis
	Cysts of *Bal. coli*	G. I. Tract	*Bal. coli*	Balantidiasis
SOIL	Cysts of *E. histolytica*	G. I. Tract	*E. histolytica*	Amoebiasis
A. Polluted with human faeces :	Fertilised ova of Ascaris	G. I. Tract	*A. lumbricoides*	Ascariasis
	Ova of Trichuris	G. I. Tract	*T. trichuria*	Trichuriasis
	Filariform larvae of: (i) *Hookworm species*	Skin penetration	*A. duodenale* *N. americanus*	Ankylostomiasis Necatriasis
	(ii) *Strongyloides stercoralis*	Skin penetration	*S. stercoralis*	Strongyloidiasis or Strongylosis
B. Polluted with faeces of dogs and cats	Fertilised ova of *Toxocara canis* & *T. cati*	G. I. Tract	*T. canis* & *T. cati*	Visceral larva migrans (VLM)
	Filariform larvae of A. *caninum* A. *btaziliense*	Skin penetration	*A. caninum* (CLM) *A. braziliense* (CLM)	Cutaneous Larva Migrans (CLM)
WATER	From Snail, Schistosome Cercariae free in water	Skin penetration	*Schistosoma species*	Schistosomiasis
	Dracunculus larvae in cyclops	G. I. Tract	*D. medinensis*	Dracunculosis

Tolerant Immunity (Tolerance)

It is the immunity that lessens the effect of the disease on the host for a given quantum of parasite. In other words, a larger quantum of parasites is necessary to produce infection. Subjects with tolerance may have symptomless parasitaemia.

Premunition (Tolerant Immunity)

It is a state of incomplete immunity which exists as long as the host harbours the parasite and it tends to disappear soon after the host is cured of the parasite. It is seen in malarial infection in which the parasites may disappear from the peripheral blood but it persists in organs. *viz.*, the spleen, liver and bone marrow. During this period the subject is relatively refractory to reinfection.

Passive immunity in infants is due to the transfer of antibodies from the mother to the child through the placenta or the first milk. Administration of antisera or gamma-globulins isolated from man also confers passive immunity.

In hyperendemic infectious areas, infants born of naturally immuned mothers may thus be protected for the first 3 to 6 months of life against infection. As child suffers from infection, acquired immunity is gradually built up, and, as the child grows up, it becomes tolerant to reinfection. It is a balance between infection and resistance. This often occurs in case of *P. falciparum* infection.

Basis of humoral immunity

It occurs by synthesis of specific immunoglobulins. Macrophages take up and process the antigens. They pass the processed antigen to the immunocompetent cells or immunocytes in the lymphoreticular systems—mainly in the spleen and lymph nodes. Immunocytes are the lymphocytes and plasma cells taking part in the synthesis of antibody. The bursa-equivalent follicular lymphocytes are the chief cells which code for the synthesis of immunoglobulins concerned with humoral antibodies. There are 5 classes of immunoglobulins—IgG, IgM, IgA, IgD and IgE—the former 2 classes are most important. In parasitic infections and infestations, the specific immunoglobulin level rises which may offer a protective function and helps recovery from infections.

Some precipitating and complement fixing antibodies (immunoglobulins) are also manufactured.

Non-specific IgM level in blood is markedly raised in trypanosomal infection. There is marked increase of serum antibodies in kala-azar. In malaria infection, marked rise in IgG level is specific (antiplasmodial), while rise in IgM is responsible only for phagocytosis. Protective antibodies indeed develop in helminthic infections, like ascariasis, strongyloidiasis, hookworm disease, etc., which lower the burden of the worm.

Basis of cellular immunity. DEVELOPMENT OF SPECIFIC CELL-MEDIATED IMMUNITY. The thymus-derived or the thymic-dependent lymphocytes present in the spleen and lymph nodes are responsible for conferring cell-mediated immunity. These lymphocytes become sensitised by the antigen of parasites. They play a dominant role in eliminating them (exteriorisation). The cell-mediated immunity can be transferred by lymphoid cells only, and not by serum. This type of immunity can be suppressed by immuno-suppressive agents, like corticosteroids. In case of cell-mediated immunity, certain type of antibodies are produced by certain antigens which usually produce delayed hypersensitivity. The antibodies are not readily released but remain firmly bound to the cells. They act as specific antigen-recognising system and immunologically react accordingly, e.g., Casoni's test in hydatid disease, also in case of trichinelliasis, schistosomiasis, oriental sore, etc.

Autoimmunity. This is a state of raised antibody level against 'self'–antigen of one's own body-tissue. Auto-antibody develops against RBCs in malaria and kala-azar, which is responsible for causing anaemia in malaria and kala-azar.

Allergy. It is a condition of hypersensitive state produced by an antigen. By introduction of the same or similar antigen intracutaneously into the sensitised host, the allergic state can be demonstrated, e.g., *Montenegro's reaction* in leishmaniasis, *Casoni's test* in hydatid disease; *Fairley's test* in schistosomiasis. Dracunculus antigen in dracontiasis and dirofilaria antigen in filariasis is also used.

Anaphylaxis. In this the host becomes hypersensitive to the protein of the parasite or its body fluid and introduction or escape of the parasitic protein (antigen) into tissue may produce severe anaphylactic shock. Anaphylaxis has been observed in : (a) hydatid disease as a result of escape of hydatid fluid into the peritoneal cavity. (b) the nephrotic syndrome that occurs in quartan malaria.

Prophylactic immunisation is a failure except in Oriental sore.

LABORATORY DIAGNOSIS

DIRECT METHODS

It depends on the nature of infection.

I. Blood examination

Peripheral blood film examination when the parasite circulates in blood stream:

(a) Malaria parasites in R. B. C.

(b) L-D bodies in monocytes in Kala-azar.

(c) Trypomastigotes in plasma in Sleeping sickness, Chagas' disease, microfilariae in Filariasis.

II. Stool Examination

Stool examination: In intestinal infections and biliary tract localisation, parasites dicharge ova into the intestine.

Trophozoites are found in acute stage and cysts in chronic stage of amoebiasis, giardiasis and balantidiasis.

In helminthic infections of the intestine, adult worms or their ova may be found in the stool, such as :

(a) Adult worms
Segments of adult taenia

(b) Larvae in strongyloidiasis

(c) Ova in ascariasis, ankylostomiasis, clonorchiasis, diphyllobothriasis, dipylidiasis fascioliasis, fasciolopsiasis, hymenolepiasis. Intestinal schistosomiasis, taeniasis, trichuriasis

(d) Ova of oxyuris.

III. Urine

(a) In Vesical schistosomiasis, terminal-spined ova of *S. hematobium* in urine

(b) Microfilariae of *W. bancrofti* are found in urine (chyluria).

IV. Sputum

(a) Trophozoites, cysts of *E. histolytica*, ova or larvae may be detected. Trophozoites of *E. histolytica* in amoebic lung abscess

(b) Hooklets and scolices of *Ech. granulosus* after rupture of hydatid cyst

(c) Ova of *P. westermani* in paragonimiasis (lung fluke disease).

V. Biopsy Material

(a) **Aspiration (Biopsy)**

(i) Hydatid fluid in Hydatic disease.

(ii) Liver in Amoebic liver abscess.

(iii) Hydrocele fluid for microfilaria, Liver for Trophozoites of *E. histolytica, hydatid fluid for* scolex of *E. granulosus.*

(b) **Bone-marrow puncture**: In Kala-azar, African trypanosomiasis

(c) **Liver puncture**: In Kala-azar, visceral schistosomiasis

(d) **Lumbar puncture**: In African trypanosomiasis (CSF)

(e) **Lymph node puncture**: In African trypanosomiasis, Filariasis, kala-azar

(f) **Muscle biopsy**: In Chagas' disease, Cysticercosis, Trichinelliasis

(g) **Rectal biopsy**: In Intestinal cysticercosis

(h) **Skin biopsy**: In Dermal leishmanoid espundia, Onchocerciasis.

(i) **Spleen puncture**: In Kala-azar.

INDIRECT METHODS

1. CYTOLOGICAL CHANGES

Peripheral Blood Smear

(i) Anaemia—In Malaria, Kala-azar, hookworm infection

(ii) Eosinophilia—In Helminthic infections during tissue invasion

(iii) Leucopenia—In Kala-azar

(iv) Polymorphonuclear (neutrophilic) leucocytosis—In amoebic liver abscess.

2. BIOCHEMICAL CHANGES

Hypergammaglobulinaemia with reverse A : G ratio occurs in African trypanosomiasis, Kala-azar, Schistosomiasis, Visceral larva migrans can be detected by biochemical analysis of blood. On the other hand, only hypergammaglobulinaemia can be detected serologically by Napier's aldehyde (formol gel) test, or Precipitation test of Sia, or Brahmachari, or Chopra's antimony test.

3. SEROLOGICAL REACTIONS

(i) **Specific Complement Fixation Tests** in amoebiasis Chagas' disease, Kala-azar, Toxoplasmosis, and Clonorchiasis, Filariasis, Hydatid disease, Schistosomiasis, Trichinelliasis, etc.

(ii) **Nonspecific Complement Fixation Test** by W.K.K. (Tubercle-bacilli) antigen in Kala-azar, Strongyloidosis (cross reaction with filarial antigen).

(iii) **Specific Precipitation Tests** in Amoebiasis, Hydatid disease, Schistosomiasis.

(iv) **Specific Flocculation Test** in Hydatid disease, Trichinelliasis, etc.

(v) **Immunofluorescent Test** with fluorescein isothiocyanate-labelled (tagged) homologous antibody in Amoebiasis, Kala-azar, Malaria, Toxoplasmosis, etc., and Onchocerciasis, Schistosomiasis, Trichinosis.

(vi) **Immobilisation Test** in Amoebiasis.

(vii) **Intradermal (Allergic) Reactions**

(Immunological skin reactions). In protozoal infections, like Amoebiasis, Chagas' disease,

Espundia, Oriental sore, Toxoplasmosis, etc., and in helminthiasis, like Ascariasis (Ascaron), Filariasis (Filarin), Hydatid disease (Casoni's), Schistosomiasis (Fairley's) and Trichinosis, such a test is done.

PROPHYLAXIS

1. Therapeutic Prophylaxis

Prevention of dissemination of infectious agent by attacking the parasites in host.

2. Drug Prophylaxis

Chemotherapeutic specific drug therapy is called drug or clinical or chemo (chemical) prophylaxis or suppressive therapy malaria. It prevents spread of disease and formation of disease and formation of gametocytes.

3. Personal Prophylaxis

Measures taken by a susceptible individual against disease prevention and spread.

4. Bio-Prophylaxis or Diseases Control Destruction of

(i) Less important intermediary hosts

(ii) Free-existing infective agents outside human hosts

(iii) Eradication of infection in reservoirs.

Example : Control of mosquitoes—Malaria
" " sand flies—Kala-azar

TREATMENT

Most of the protozoal diseases are successfully cured by specific drugs. Intestinal helminthic infections are also curable by orally administered drugs.

HOST-PARASITE RELATIONSHIPS

Major portions of the host-parasite relationship have been covered in definition of terms, like the facultative and obligate parasites, the 'ecto' and the endoparasites. The commensals and the pathogens; the different types of hosts, the definitive, intermediate, vertebrate, invertebrate, the primary and the secondary hosts, etc., the free-living state or form of parasites as in the case of *Strongyloides stercoralis* (*S. stercoralis*) which are also called *spurious parasites*—isolated either in the living or dead state from human excreta; the various types of infections, such as the superinfection (see *S. stercoralis*), autoinfection and reinfection (see *Oxyuris vermicularis, E. histolytica*); the difference between infection and infestation; the various immunities and premunition; the predilection of parasites for particular tissues; the by-pass organs, or the organs involved in helping in the development of larvae of various parasites (see helminths); all these discussions should be included in discussing the subject "Host-Parasite relationship". Also, the toxicity and pathogenicity, the pathogenesis and an outline of organic pathology may be stated while discussing the subject.

TAXONOMY AND NOMENCLATURE

The animal parasites are divided into three main groups:

(i) Phylum Protozoa—*Medical Protozoology*

(ii) Phylum Platyhelminthes and Phylum Axchelminthes—*Medical Helminthology*

(iii) Phylum Arthropoda—*Medical Entomology.*

Linnaeus' (1758) ***binomial nomenclature*** for animals—universally followed for nomenclature and classification.

Accordingly, Order ends in *ida*; Suborder ends in *idea*; Superfamily ends in *oidea*; Family ends in *idae*; Subfamily ends in *inae*, and the Tribe ends in *ini*.

The genus is written with an initial capital letter and the species following it in small letters. The generic name, accompanying the genus and species is expressed in italics. Males are indicated by Mars ♂ and females by Venus ♀.

A ***parasitic disease*** is often named after the parasite which produces the disease. □

Phylum ⟶ Subphylum ⟶ Superclass ⟶ Superfamily
↓ ↓ ↓
Phylum ⟶ Subphylum ⟶ Class ⟶ Order ⟶ Family ⟶ Genus ⟶ Species
↓ ↓ ↓
Subclass Suborder Subfamily ⟶ " ⟶ "

CHAPTER 2

Section I: PROTOZOAL CELL

PROTOZOOLOGY

The science of the study of the protozoa is known as protozoology (*protos*—first, primitive; *zoon*—living animal). Protozoa are primitive unicellular living units in the lowest state of evolution of animal kingdom, complete morphologically and functionally with powers of digestion, nutrition and reproduction, etc.

DEFINITIONS OF TERMS USE FOR PROTOZOA

AXOSTYLE. This is the axial rod of a flagellate acting as its support, e.g., *Giardia lamblia*.

BLEPHAROPLAST. It is a chromatin dot (DNA) from which the flagellum arises and functions as a part of the nucleus which is stained readily due to its staining affinity.

CHROMATOID BODY. It is a refractile extranuclear body composed of or stained like chromatin and contained within the cytoplasm of a mature cyst, but it is not a part of cytoplasm.

CYST. It is a non-motile resting stage protected by a cyst wall and the protozoon may be readily transmitted to a new host by ingestion of a mature cyst.

CYTOSTOME. It corresponds to the mouth part of a ciliate.

CYTOPYGE. It is the excretory or anal opening of a ciliate.

ENCYSTATION. It is the transformation of a trophozoite into a cyst, forming a tough cyst wall. In ENCYSTMENT, protozoa—like *Entamoeba histolytica, Giardia lamblia, Balantidium coli* may show a resting phase, when they enclose themselves within a resistant membranous wall and are called cysts. Cysts are non-motile and resist unfavourable environmental conditions better than the trophozoite form. Cysts like those of *E. histolytica, Bal. coli* are infective to man. Encystment serves double functions of protection and reproduction.

EXCYSTATION. It is the dissolution of the cyst with liberation of a motile metacystic trophozoite in the case of *E. histolytica*.

FLAGELLUM. It is a long, hair-like process attached to a protozoal cell.

KARYOSOME. It is a dot or mass of chromatin within the nucleus.

TABLE 2.1

DIFFERENCES BETWEEN PROTOZOA AND METAZOA

	PROTOZOA	METAZOA
Morphology	Unicellular A single cell forming "Unit of life"	Multicellular A number of cells, making up a complex individual
Physiology	A single cell performs all the functions—respiration, digestion, excretion, reproduction, etc.	Each special type of cell performs a particular function

TROPHOZOITE. This is the vegetative, motile stage of a protozoon which feeds, multiplies and forms colonies in the host.

GEOGRAPHICAL DISTRIBUTION

Intestinal protozoa of man are cosmopolitan in their distribution, known to occur in human beings in all parts of the world, where they have been investigated. Haemoflagellates and haemosporozoa have restricted endemic areas in relation to humidity, temperature, altitude, etc.

MORPHOLOGY

The structure of a protozoal "cell" is composed of (1) Cytoplasmic body and (2) Nucleus.

CYTOPLASM. Divided into two parts

(a) *Ectoplasm.* The external hyaline portion; function is locomotive, protective and sensory.

(b) *Endoplasm.* The internal granular portion; function is nutritive and reproductive.

STRUCTURES DEVELOPED FROM ECTOPLASM

1. *Organelles of Locomotion.*

(a) PSEUDOPODIA. Prolongation of temporary ectoplasmic process, as in Rhizopodea. Locomotory speed 0.2 to 3.0 microns/second.

(b) FLAGELLA. Long, thin, thread-like filaments seen in Zoomastigophorea. Locomotory speed 15-30 microns/second.

(c) In SPOROZOAS, the organisms in the motile stage (when present) move by PSEUDOPODIA and not by any special external locomotive organs. In the sexual cycle, exflagellation takes place in male gametes. They are motile.

2. *Contractile vacuoles.* Situated inside the endoplasm; excretory function.
3. *Rudimentary digestive organ.* Cytostome ("cell mouth") and Cytopharynx, as in *Bal. coli.*
4. *Cyst-wall.* A thickened resistant wall, seen in the cystic stage (see earlier *Encystation*; see later—*Encystment*).

Ectoplasm is the external hyaline part of the cell and is chiefly concerned with

(a) *Locomotion*, by production of pseudopodia, flagella or cilia.

(b) *Response* to stimulus, besides acting as a sensory organ and helping in capture of food. In some protozoa, there are distinct organs called *peristome* and *cytostome* corresponding to the mouth and oesophagus, respectively.

(c) *Excretion*, effected through contractile vacuoles present in the ectoplasm. It is absent in *Entamoeba histolytica*, *parasitic* Mastigophora and are not developed in Sporozoa but is seen in *Balantidium coli*.

(d) *Protection*, by secretion of substances to form a thick cyst wall.

Functions of ectoplasm are, therefore: locomotive, sensory and nutritive, excretory, and protective.

ENDOPLASM is the internal granular portion of the cell and contains

(a) Food vacuoles which help in the digestion of food (digestive ferments are secreted by them).

(b) Various granules, like glycogen, fat globules, protein (chromatoidal bodies), bacteria, pigment, etc., depending on the species.

(c) Mitochondria, easily demonstrated in the endoplasm.

NUCLEUS. It is the initiator and director of all cell-activities. It controls the various functions and regulates reproduction. Situated in the endoplasm its structure comprises:

(a) Bounded externally by a well-defined nuclear membrane.

(b) Made up of a lining network in the nuclear sap.

(c) Chromatin granules line the inner side of the nuclear membrane and appear as condensation on lining threads. They are supposedly genes.

(d) Karyosome (plastin) situated inside the nucleus—either centrally or peripherally.

Nucleus may be one or more and is chiefly concerned with nutrition and reproduction. It consists of achromatic substance and chromatin.

Achromatic substances have no special affinity for stains. It comprises:

(i) Nuclear membrane. (ii) Nuclear sap or karyolymph. (iii) Nuclear reticulum. (iv) Nuclear plastin, often in masses called nucleoli.

Chromatin stains purple with Leishman's and jet black with iron haematoxylin stain. A mass of chromatin substance which is often central in position and has special affinity for stain is known as *Karyosome*.

Extranuclear chromatin substance is called *chromatoid body*, or *chromidia* and found in the cysts of *Entamoeba histolytica*. They are supposed to be protein food material.

Types of nucleus. The nucleus may be vesicular with a central karyosome, or granular with chromatin grains. The number of nuclei may help in identification of the organism.

Micronucleus and Macronucleus

One nucleus found in most protozoa. In Ciliatea two nuclei are present, a small micronucleus and a large macronucleus.

KINETOPLAST

In addition to nucleus, Trypanosomatid Flagellates show a non-nuclear DNA-containing body called *Kinetoplast*, near which flagellum originates; there is a small body at the point of origin of the flagellum known as the *basal body*.

CENTROSOME. It is generally situated just outside the nucleus singly or in pair as in metazoa, or it may even be in the centre of the karyosome when it is called a *Centriole*.

NUTRITION. Nutrition occurs by osmosis (holophytic) or by ingestion (holozoic). Mastigophora are holophytic and are believed to be more primitive. Cytoplasm consists of food vacuoles which may contain solid food engulfed by them.

EXCRETION. The products left after digestion pass out in the medium in which the organism lives. Excretion of waste products occurs by means of contractile vacuoles or through osmosis.

RESPIRATION. Respiration occurs by osmosis.

MOVEMENT. Some protozoa are less motile than others, as, in the case of malarial parasite inside the red blood corpuscle, they are sluggish; whereas Trypanosomes and other flagellates and ciliates are actively motile and possess definite organs of locomotion (flagella or cilia). Amoebae move by cytoplasmic processes called pseudopodia; Leishmania, on the other hand, have no movement except in the leptomonad (promastigote) form.

REPRODUCTION. The life cycle in some protozoa is often complete in two stages—asexual and sexual.

(A) ASEXUAL. (i) *Binary fission*. This is a process of simple cell division, where cells divide into two; division of the kinetoplast (if present) and the nucleus is followed by division of cytoplasm. Binary fission may occur either in the transverse axis of the cell as in *E. histolytica* and *L. donovani*, or in the longitudinal axis as in Trypanosoma (Fig. 2.1).

(ii) *Sporulation*. In this the nucleus undergoes successive division in series with an equal number of cytoplasmic aggregations around the nuclear substance followed by division, e.g., schizogony in malarial parasites.

(B) SEXUAL. (i) *Conjugation* (*Isogamy*). In this, two similar individuals unite temporarily and interchange of nuclear material takes place. After the union, the individuals separate, each being rejuvenated (Ciliates).

(ii) *Syngamy*. The union of sexually differentiated cells is known as syngamy.

Encystment. (CYST FORMATION). The Protozoal parasite possesses the property of being transformed from active (trophozoite) to an inactive stage, losing its motility. Trophozoite encloses itself within a tough wall (Cyst wall). The protoplasmic body enclosed in cyst wall formed—is called a *cyst*. Parasite also loses its power of growth and multiplication and motility. This is a resting protective phase under adverse environmental circumstances.

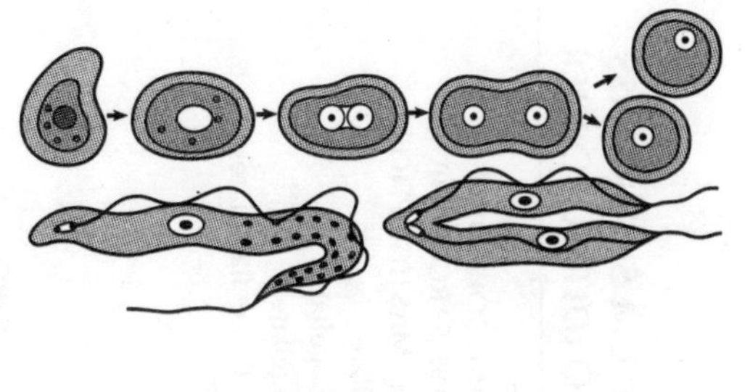

Fig. 2.1 Binary fission in protozoa
Upper—*E. histolytica*. Lower—Trypanosoma

TABLE 2.2

PROTOZOAL PARASITES PATHOGENIC TO HUMAN

SUBPHYLUM SUPERCLASS CLASS, ORDER/SUBORDER	GENUS	SPECIES	HABITAT	PATHOGENIC EFFECTS
Subphylum SARCOMASTIGOPHORA SUPERCLASS SARCODINA	Entamoeba	*E. histolytica*	Large intestine	Dysentery, hepatitis, liver abscess
Subphylum: MASTIGOPHORA				
Oral flagellate	Trichomonas	*T. ranax*		
Intestinal flagellate	Giardia	*G. intestinalis*	Small intestine	Diarrhoea
Genital flagellate	Trichomonas	*T. vaginalis*	Vaginal canal	Vaginitis
Blood and tissue flagellates	Trypanosoma	*T. brucer Sub group*	Blood, Lymph node C N S	African trypanosomiasis (Sleeping sickness)
		T. cruzi	Heart, Nervous system	South American trypanosomiasis (Chagas' disease)
	Leishmanie	*L. donovani*	R. E. system	Kala-azar and Dermal leishmanoid
		L. tropica	Skin	Oriental sore
		L. brasiliensis	Oro-nasal mucous membrane	Espundia
Subphylum: SPOROZOA CLASS TELOSPOREA ORDER EUCOCCIDA SUBORDER: 1. HAEMOSPORINAE		*P. falciparum*	R. B. C	Malignant tertian malaria and Pernicious malaria
		P. malariae	R B C	Quartan malaria
		P. ovale	R B C	*P. ovale* tertian malaria
		P. vivax	R B C	Benign tertian malaria
Suborder : II Eimeriinae	Isospora (Not described in this book)	*I. hominis*	Intestinal epithelia	Diarrhoea
		I. belli	Intestinal epithelia	Diarrhoea
	Toxoplasma	*T. gondii*	R E system, parenchyma cells of Nervous system, eyes, lungs, liver, spleen, bone marrow, lymph nodes, heart and skeletal muscles	Encephalomyelitis, choroidoretinitis, etc.
Subphylum : CILIPHORA CLASS : CILIATEA	Balantidium	*Bal. coli*	Large intestine	Dysentery
PROTOZOA OF UNCERTAIN CLASSIFICATION (See Chapter 7)	Pneumocystis	*P. carinli*	Lungs, Parotid ducts	Interstitial pneumonia

TABLE 2.3

SYSTEMIC CLASSIFICATION OF PROTOZOA

PHYLUM PROTOZOA

SUBPHYLUM :	PLASMODROMA	SARCOMASTIGOPHORA			SPOROZOA		CILIPHORA
CLASS	RHIZOPODA	MASTIGOPHORA			TELOSPOREA		CILIATEA
SUBCLASS :					COCCIDIA		
ORDER :	Amoebida	Protomonadida		Dlplomonadida	Eucoccidiida		
SUBORDER :		Intestinal/ Oral cavity	In blood and tissues	In intestine	Eimerine	Haemosporina	
GENUS SPECIES	Entamoeba *E. histolytica*	Chilomastix *C. mesnili*	Trypanosoma *T. Brucei* subgroup	Giardia *G. Intestinalis*	Toxoplasma *T. gondii*	Plasmodium *P. vivax*	Balantidium *Bal. coli*
,,	*E. coli*	GENUS : Trichomonas				*P. falciparum*	
,,	*E. gingivalis*	*Tr. hominis* (Syn. *Tr. intes tinalis*)	*T. cruzi*			*P. malariae*	
,,	GENUS Endolimax *E. nana*	*Tr. vaginalis* *Tr. tenax*				*P. ovale*	
		GENUS Enteromonas *E. hominis*	GENUS Leishmanla *L. donovani*				
	Iodamoeba *I. butschlii*						
GENUS : Dientamoeba *D. fragilis*		GENUS : Embadomonas *G. intestinalis*	*L. tropica* *L. brasiliensis*				

The *cyst* is resistant to inimicals and is infective to man and so required to be transferred by a carrier or intermediaries (house flies) to food and drink. Taking in of such substances contaminated with the cysts infect man. In the intestine, as in case of amoeba. the organism leaves the cyst (EXCYSTATION) and continues its life in trophozoite stage. So, ENCYSTMENT is not a reproductive process but a means of the species from extinction. However, in case of amoeba, multiplication occurs within cyst as evidenced by nuclear fission into 2, 4 or 8 daughter nuclei. Complete division of cell occurs when the organism leaves the cyst and a number of organisms are liberated free.

LIFE CYCLE. Protozoa can multiply by (i) asexual method for a long time. It may switch on to (ii) sexual method of reproduction, or undergoes (iii) cystic change to change its host. Sexual reproduction occurs in a different host and not in the same used for asexual reproduction. This process is known as ALTERNATION OF GENERATION along with alternation of host, e.g., Plasmodia.

LIFE CYCLE ONLY IN ONE HOST. Amoebae, intestinal flagellates, *Bal. coli,* etc. need one host for their Life cycles. The parasites may adopt in a different host as well and transfer themselves passively in cystic stage.

LIFE CYCLE IN TWO HOSTS. Leishmania, Trypanosoma and Plasmodia require two hosts to complete their life cycle. In Leishmaniasis, sandfly is the intermediate host and man is the definitive host; in Trypanosomiasis, Tsetse fly is the intermediate host and man is the definitive host. In Plasmodia (malaria) infection, man is the intermediate host but mosquito is the definitive host.

Rhizopodes. (*Rhiza*—root; *pod*—foot). Organisms of this class move by producing pseudopodia. They multiply by binary fission and form cysts, e.g., *E. histolytica*.

Mastigophores. (*Mastig*—whip; *phoros*—bearing). They move by means of flagella; binary fission occurs by longitudinal division, as in *Trypanosoma*, *Leptomonad*, etc.

Sporozoas. (*Sporos*—seed; *zoon*—living animal). They have no organ of locomotion and move by amoeboid movement with change in form and position. They multiply asexually by sporulation (schizogony) within the vertebrate host and sexually (sporogony) by reduction division. Fusion gametes is followed by sporozoite formation in a sporocyst as in the invertebrate host, e.g., anopheline mosquito in human malaria caused by *Plasmodium vivax*, *P. falciparum*, *P. malaria* and *P. ovale*.

Ciliates. They move by cilia and multiply by transverse division of the body. They also produce cysts. Only species pathogenic is *Balantidium coli*. □

TABLE 2.4

PROTOZOA NON—PATHOGENIC TO HUMAN

SUBPHYLUM	CLASS	GENUS	SPECIES	HABITAT
I. Sarcomastigophora	Rhizopodea	Entamoeba	*E. gingivalis*	Mouth
			E. coli	Large intestine
		Endolimax	*End. nana*	Large intestine
		Diantamoeba	*E. fragilis*	Large intestine
II. Mastigophora	Zoomastigophorea	Chilomastix	*C. mesnili*	Caecum
		Trichomonas	*Tr. hominis*	Iliocaecal region
			Tr. tenax	Teeth and gum
		Enteromonas	*Ent. hominis*	Large intestine
		Embadomonas	*Embd. intestinalis*	Large intestine
		Trypanosoma	*T. rangeli*	Blood

CHAPTER

3

SUBPHYLUM : SARCOMASTIGOPHORA
SUPERCLASS : SARCODINA

Class I : RHIZOPODEA

ORDER : AMOEBIDA
AMOEBAE

Protozoal parasites of this class move by pseudopodia. Their nuclear character for identification is considered (**Fig. 3.1**). Six amoebae found in man belong to 4 Genera and distinguished as in Table 3.1.

ENTAMOEBA HISTOLYTICA

(Schaudinn, 1930)

(The causative organism of amoebic dysentery)

Incidence. 7 to 11 per cent population in the tropics were said to suffer from infection with *E. histolytica*. On routine examination of 1,544 patients in Kolkata and Midnapur area, 60 per cent were found to be infected by *E. histolytica* (Dey, 1974). Further, he found *E. histolytica* during routine examination of stool in 94 per cent cases in Gaya area (Dey, 1976).

Geographical distribution. cosmopolitan; tropics and subtropics.

Habitat. Trophozoite form is in amoebic ulcers of large gut wall of metastatic abscess in liver, lung, etc.

MORPHOLOGY

Two morphological forms, large (infective) and small race, Studied in

(i) *Unstained (saline)*,

(ii) *Stained iodine preparation*, and

(iii) *Iron-haemotoxylin permanent*, or

(iv) *M-R stained preparation.*

3 phases of Morphology in life cycle.

I. TROPHOZOITE (VEGETATIVE) FORM

(Growing or feeding stage).

Slow *gliding movement* is seen.

Ectoplasm shows jerky movement to eject out pseudopodia, and flowing in of the granular endoplasm is seen.

Shape: Indefinite due to constant change of form (See **Fig. 3.2**)

Size: Average 20-30 micrometres (μm.).

Cytoplasm : Divided into

(i) Translucent *ectoplasm*,

(ii) Granular *endoplasm* containing RBC, or tissue debris.

Nucleus: Spherical 4-6 μm.

It is eccentric; Staining clearly shows

(i) Nuclear membrane,

(ii) Linin network,

(iii) Karyosome (see before for differences in genus and species).

Glycogen mass, absent in trophozoites.

II. Precystic form. Organism is smaller 10-20 μ m. round to ovoid with blunt, roundish pseudopodia with no RBC. Characteristic nuclear structure is soon.

III. Cystic form. During encystment cyst develops; parasite becomes rounded; surrounded by a highly refractile tough membrane, the *Cyst Wall*. It is 7-9 μ (small race), and 12-15 μ (large race), uninucleate. Binucleate phase is very short and unseen. As it matures if becomes tetranucleate.

An uninucleate cyst divides to become binucleate (*binary fission*), which becomes tetranucleate by fission. The single nucleus ultimately divides into 4 daughter nuclei of reduced size 2 μm, in diameter (**Fig. 3.3**). Immature cysts, when passed in stool matures outside the body, which remains alive for 10 days in moisture; thermal death point is 50°C. Chlorination of water cannot kill the cysts. Weak eosin solution stains only dead cysts.

In early stage of development of a cyst, the cytoplasm shows certain features

(i) Chromatoid or chromidial bars.

They are 1-2 highly *refractile* extranuclear bodies unstained by iodine but *jet black with iron-haematoxylin*.

(ii) Glycogen vacuole in cysts stain brown with iodine.

PREPARATIONS

Morphology under (coverslip) Saline preparation. Trophozoites: Look slaty grey (Endoplasm). Pseudopodial movement seen in outer 1/3rd clear ectoplasm. RBC seen in food vacuole with active churning movement. Nucleus not visible (**Fig. 3.2**).

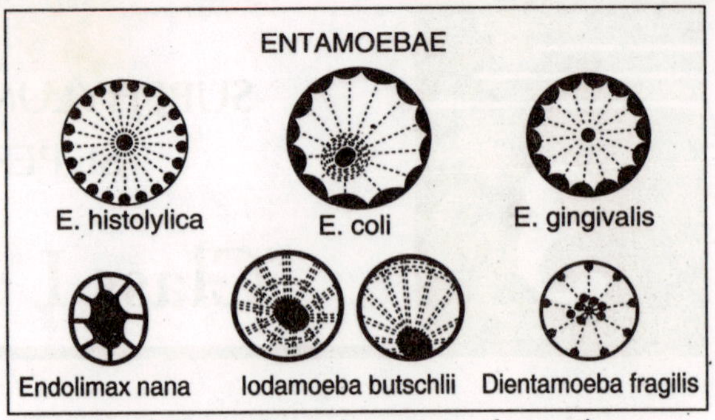

Fig. 3.1 Nuclear characters of amoebae found in human

Cyst: Smooth cyst wall, highly refractile (12-15μ), Chromatoid bars (rounded ends), No visible glycogen mass (**Fig. 3.2**).

IODINE STAINED PREPARATION

Trophozoite: Yellow with clear Nuclear detail dark brown Glycogen Nucleus; "*histolytica type*" central karyosome.

Cyst: Smooth and hyaline. Nucleus clearly seen (1 to 4) with central karyosome "*histolytica type*" Chromatoid bars unstained. Glycogen mass deep brown.

TABLE 3.1
CHARACTERISTICS OF AMOEBAE

GENERA	ORGANISM	PATHOGENIC	NON-PATHOGENIC COMMENSAL	HABITAT INTESTINAL/ ATRIAL
1. ENTAMOEBA	*E. histolytica*	Yes	...	Intestine
Nuclear membrane lined by chromatin granules	*E. coli*	...	Yes	Intestine
Karyosome Central or eccentric usually with a halo around it	*E. gingivalis*	...	Found more in unhealthy gums and teeth, but less so in healthy ones	Mouth
2. ENDOLIMAX Large mass of karyosome at periphery connected with a small mass	*End. nana*	...	Yes	Intestine
3. IODAMOEBA Large circular mass of karyosome surrounded by refractile globules	*I. buschlii*	...	Yes	Intestine
4. DIENTAMOEBA 6 chromatin granules in karyosome, and 2 nuclei	*D. fragilis*	...	Yes	Intestine

PLATE 3.1
LIFE CYCLE OF *ENTAMOEBA HISTOLYTICA*

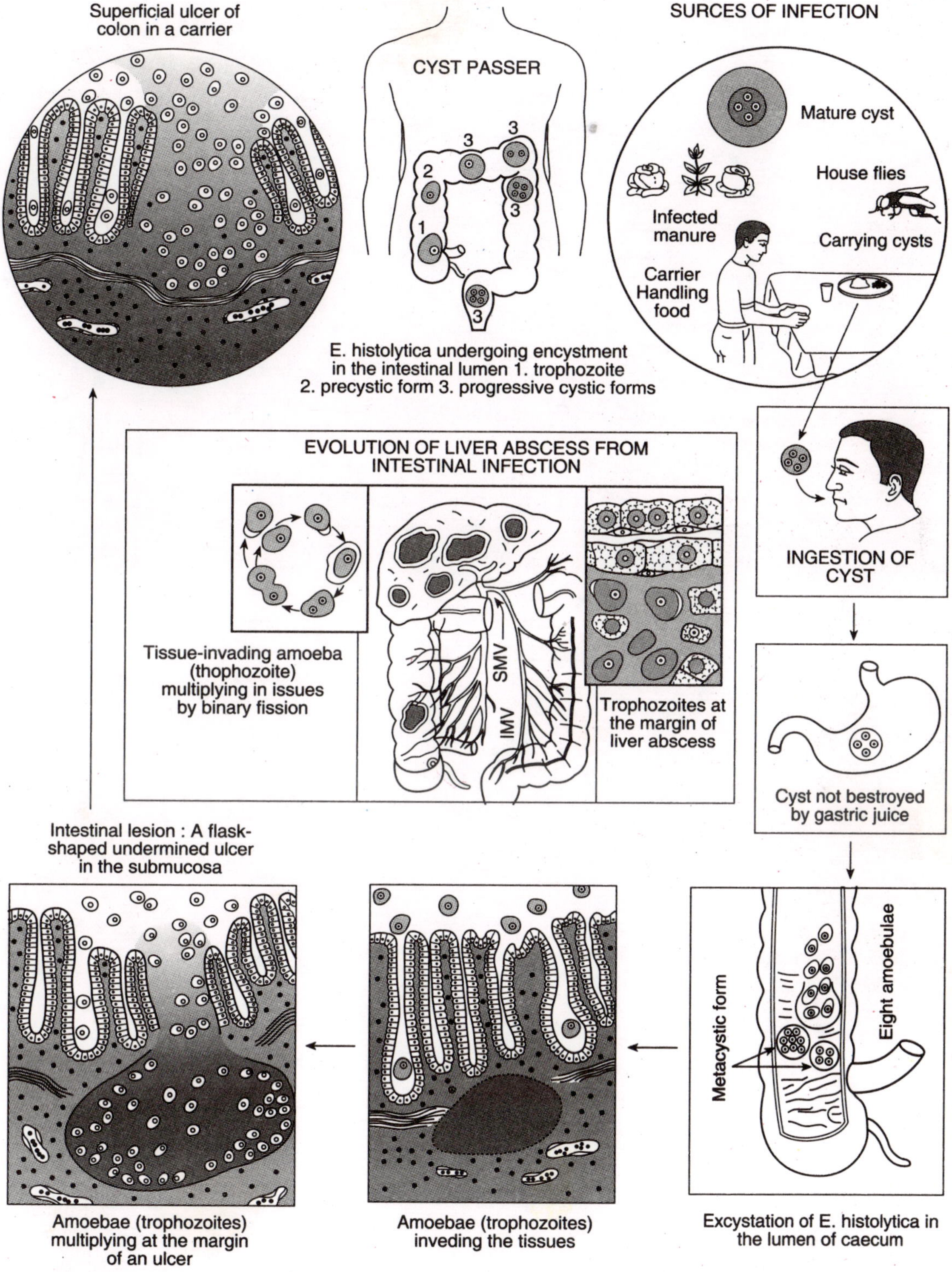

Showing mode of infection, evolution in hosts and carriers, and various pathologic lesions

PERMANENT PREPARATION WITH IRON-HAEMATOXYLIN

Trophozoite: Nuclear membrane delicate, inner surface with a layer chromatin dots. Karyosome minute in the centre of nucleus. Chromatin invisible; RBC present.

Cyst: 6-20 μ, spherical, cytoplasm homogeneous vacuolated. jet black chromatoid bars. 1 to 4 nuclei with chromatin granules, central karyosome as a dot ***"histolytica type"*** **(Fig. 3.2)**.

Permanent preparation with M-R (Mukherjee-Ray) Stain

It stains permanently in 10 minutes.

In Cyst, Cytoplasm stains light pink, chromatoid bodies bluish green and nuclear chromatin greenish purple.

CULTIVATION

1. GENERAL CULTURE

(a) It is generally cultivated in serum agar slope to which Ringer's solution and starch powder are added. Also nonpathogenic enteric bacteria, and *T. cruzi* from culture may be added in culture medium.

(b) It is also being grown in a medium containing thioglycollate and "Penicillin-inhibited living streptobacilli" which have stopped multiplying.

2. MICRO-CULTURE: These are made from single washed amoebae in micro-tubes containing medium of thioglycollate, horse serum and an overlay of rich culture of *T. cruzi* (PHILIPS' MEDIUM).

ANIMAL PATHOGENICITY

(Susceptible Animals)

Kittens are best for observing sloughing and ulceration of colonic mucosa and they die in 2 to 3 days. No encystment seen. Dog's intestinal lesion is smaller than that of human and they survive longer.

IMMUNOLOGY

Specific *immune bodies* are recognized in patients who have suffered more from amoebic hepatitis than dysentery, but this antibody does not protect against re-infection (non-protective).

Immunological Reactions

They are: *Precipitation* test by capillary tube method, *gel diffusion* method and *fluorescent antibody* test, helpful for characterization of invasive *E. histolytica* antigen **Appendix I**).

Serological Reactions

Complement fixing antibodies develop, which react with antigen from culture.

LIFE CYCLE

Life cycle is completed on one host (Human). Four phases of development seen : **(PL. 3.I)**

I. CYSTIC (INFECTIVE) STAGE

II. METACYSTIC STAGE (IN BOWEL)

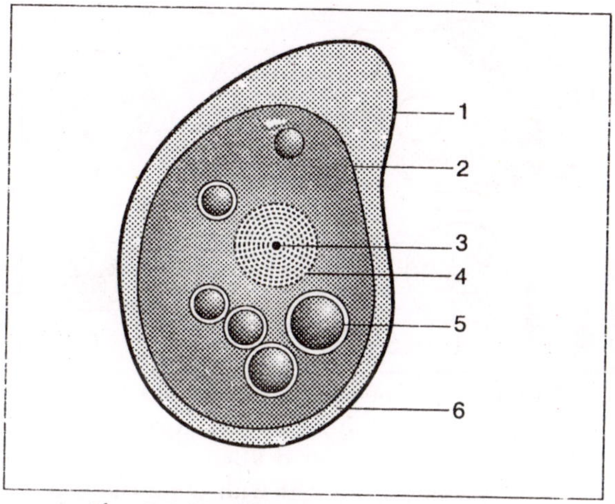

Fig. 3.2 Trophozoite of *E. histolytica*
1. Pseudopodium; 2. Endoplasm;
3. Karyosome; 4. Nuclear membrane;
5. Ingested red blood cells; 6. Ectoplasm

III. TROPHOZOITE STAGE **(Figs. 3.2, 3.3** and **3.4)**

IV. SHORT TRANSITORY PRECYSTIC STAGE (IN BOWEL). From this cysts develop.

I. INFECTIVE (CYSTIC) STAGE: The mature qudrinucleate cysts are INFECTIVE (See **Fig. 3.4**).

II. METACYSTIC STAGE: Quadrinucleate cysts are swallowed with contaminated food and drink. No change in stomach. In intestine, trypsin dissolves cyst wall.

EXCYSTATION: Occurs in lower part of intestine (weakly alkaline medium).

Cytoplasmic body retracts and loosens from cyst wall, little cytoplasmic mass escapes by vigorous amoeboid movement and then whole body comes out containing TETRANUCLEATE CYTOPLASMIC

MASS. Similarly nuclear division occurs in each, forming *octanucleate* (8 nucleate) body.

METACYSTIC FORM (BODY). With cytoplasmic fission 8 amoebulae develop. These amoebulas are METACYSTIC TROPHOZOITES.

III. TROPHOZOITE STAGE: They are actively motile and invade tissues, lodge in submucosa of large gut. They grow and form adult trophozoites. Trophozoites multiply by binary fission and by their histolytic enzyme form characteristic ulcers and flourish there (see intestinal lesions and AMOEBIC ULCER). They obtain nourishment through absorption of tissue juices and wander from necrosed ulcerated area to healthy sites and enter deeper layers and reach up to serous coat and radicles of portal vein to reach the liver. In liver, progress is often arrested and trophozoites grow and multiply there *without cyst formation*.

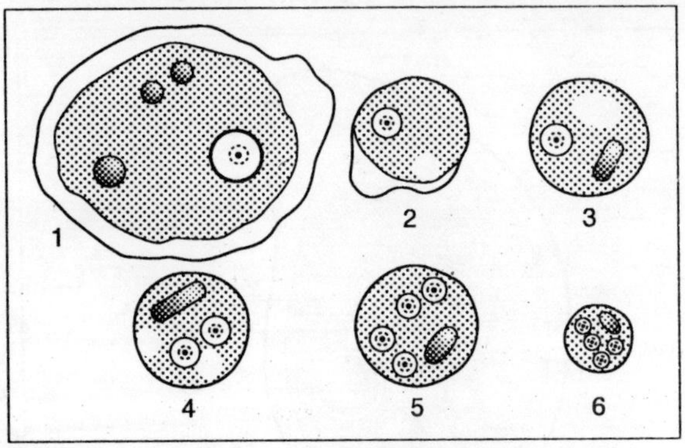

Fig. 3.3 *Entamoeba histolytica* 2000 (Iron haematoxylin). 1–Active trophozoite with pseudopodia and ingested RBCs. 2–Precystic amoeba. 3–Uninucleate cyst with chromatoid bar and a glycogen vacuole. 4–Binucleate cyst with chromatoid body and glycogen vacuoles. 5–Mature four nucleate cyst. 6–Mature four-nucleate cyst of small race with chromatoid body

IV. PRECYSTIC STAGE AND CYST FORMATION: In the intestine many trophozoites are discharged into the lumen from the bowel wall and transformed into transient small *precystic form* from which *cysts* develop (***PL. 3.II***). Cysts are passed in stool. Auto-ingestion can occur.

In resistant host, injury by the parasite is minimal.

Mature quadrinucleate cysts are resistant and cysts require transferance to another host where they grow and continue the life cycle to prevent species extinction.

EPIDEMIOLOGY

RESERVOIR OF INFECTION: Human is the commonest source of infection. Monkeys and dogs may be infected. In kittens, no encystment is seen *in vivo*.

PATHOGENESIS OF AMOEBIASIS

MODE OF INFECTION: Infection occurs through ingestion of mature quadrinucleate cysts with faecal contamination of water, raw vegetables, fruits and food.

CARRIERS: Food handlers, cysts—passers are called carriers. There may be "contact" and "convalescent" carrier who are not suffering from amoebiasis.

The trophozoites live for a few hours and is not source of infection. They are digested by gastric juice while cysts are not.

HOUSE-FLIES: They convey the infection by carrying cysts as they fly from faeces to unprotected food stuffs; so also droppings of cockroaches So 3 F's are important:

i) Finger ii) Faeces iii) Fly.

PATHOLOGIC LESIONS

1. PRIMARY OR INTESTINAL LESIONS: Limited to large intestine.

2. SECONDARY OR METASTATIC LESIONS: Extra-intestinal areas where the trophozoite (vegetative) form can migrate producing lesions which mainly include:

(a) Liver, (b) Lungs, etc. (also see later **PLs. VII, VIII**)

DEVELOPMENT OF PRIMARY INTESTINAL LESIONS

(Figs. 3.5, 3.6 and 3.7)

Metacystic trophozoite forms of *E. histolytica* are liberated after excystation. They enter the crypt of Leiberkühn of large intestine (caecum) by penetrating columnar epithelial calls of the **mucous membrane** by then amoeboid activity and also by dissolving there with secreted proteolytic ferment (**cytolysin or histolysin**). They pass to **submucosa** by continuous lysis and also by amoebic *movement*.

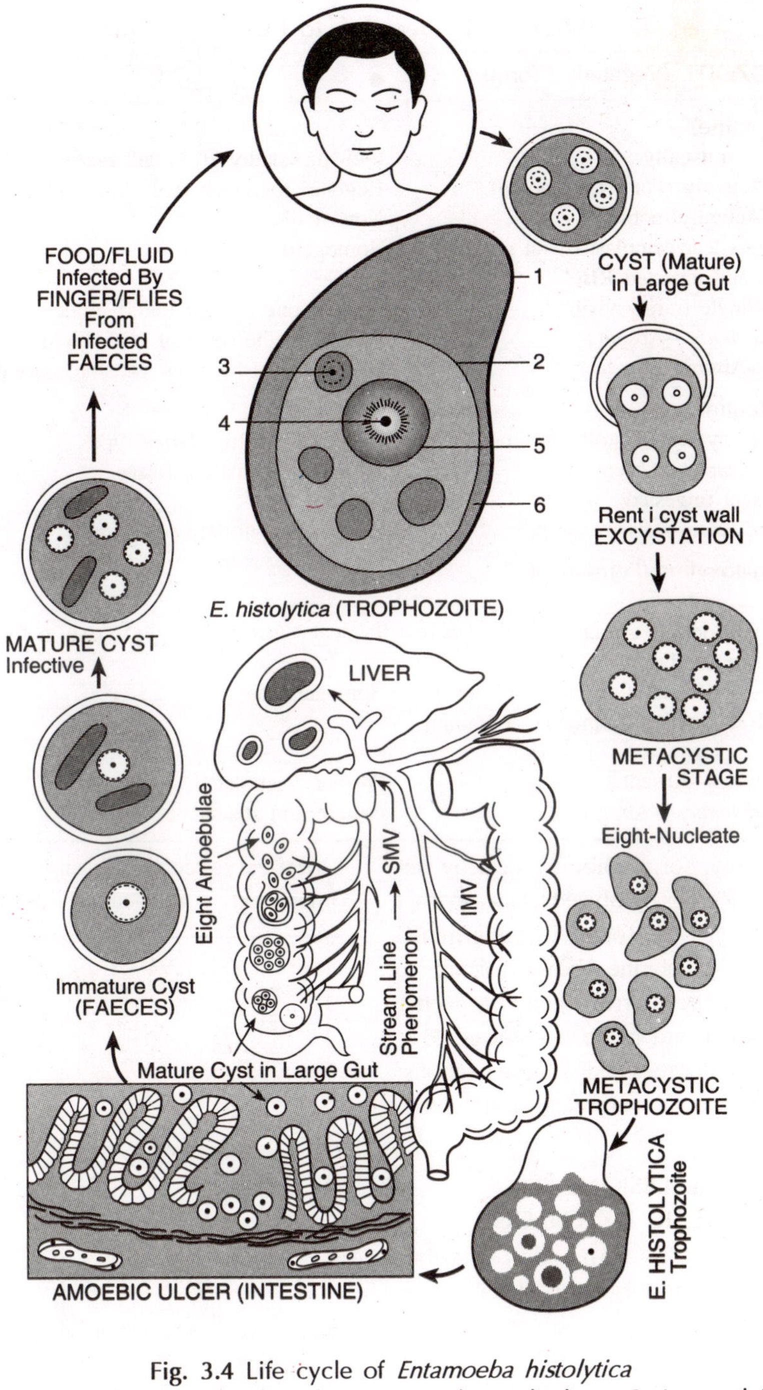

Fig. 3.4 Life cycle of *Entamoeba histolytica*

1. Ectoplasm forming pseudopodia, 2. Granular endoplasm. 3. Ingested RBCs. 4. Karyosome in the nucleus. 5. Nucleus. 6. Ectoplasm

TABLE 3.2

DIFFERENCES BETWEEN TROPHOZOITE AND CYSTIC FORMS OF *E. HISTOLYTICA* (See Ref. to PL. 3.IV & 3.IX)

TROPHOZOITE (Vegetative form)	Cyst
I. In saline: (Routine)	
(a) *Size*—10-30 μ usually	6-18 μ, usually 10 (small race) and 14 μ (large race)
(b) *Outline*—Actively (For pseudopodia)	Regular, round or oval with double cyst wall
(c) *Motility*—Actively motile	Non-motile
(d) *Cytoplasm*—Clear ectoplasm with granular endoplasm and ingested RBC	Homogeneous
(e) *Nucleus*—Single (rarely visible)	Usually one or four (short binucleate phase)
(f) *Chromatoid body*—Absent	Present in the form of bars, highly refractile
(g) *Glycogen*—Absent	Glycogen washed, but vacuole present
II. In Iodine: (Routine)	
(a) *Nucleus*—1; Typical (histolytica type)	1-4; Typical (histolytica type)
(b) *Glycogen vacuole*—Absent	Present in immature forms
(c) *RBC*—Present (ingested)	Absent
(d) *Chromatoid body*—Absent	Present, but ill-defined
III. In Iron haematoxylin: (Permanent preparation)	
(a) *Nucleus*—Full details available, "*histolytica type*", one in number	Typical "*histolytica type*", one to four
(b) *Cytoplasm*—Differentiation of ectoplasm (clear) and endoplasm (granular), containing RBCs	Homogeneous
(c) *Glycogen mass*—Absent	Present, vacuolated
(d) *Chromatoid bodies*—Absent	Present and stained jet black

They rapidly multiply, form colonies, destroy tissues in vicinity and absorbs cytolysed tissues extract as food. These changes are found in undermined area of the mucous membrane above (forming a shape of a glass flask). they burrow their way deeper down the muscle layer and reach the serous coat. The destroyed area undergoes coagulative necrosis. When the necrosed mucous membrane sloughs out, ulcer is formed.

INTESTINAL LESIONS IN ACUTE AMOEBIC DYSENTERY

GROSS PATHOLOGY (Morbid Anatomy) Distribution of Ulcers: confined to large gut—localised or generalised.

(A) LOCALISED LESIONS

(i) Ileo-caecal region—and ascending colon are twice as frequently involved as the sigmoid or rectum **(Fig. 3.8)**.

(ii) Pelvi-rectal region—Sigmoid and rectum comes next to ileo-caecal region.

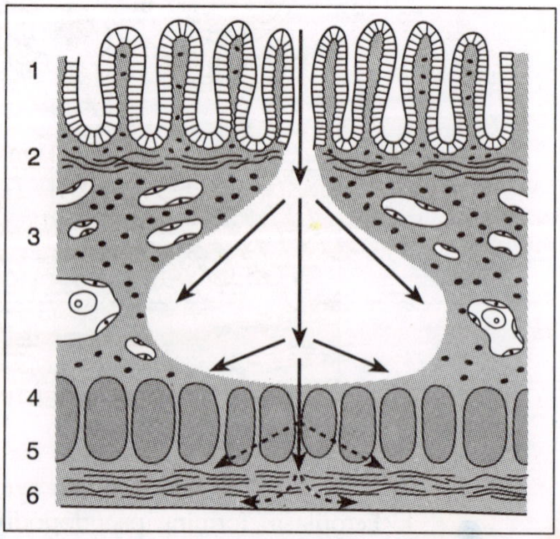

Fig. 3.5 Invasion of *E. histolytica* through the intestinal wall

PLATE 3.II

REPRODUCTION OF *ENTAMOEBA HISTOLYTICA*

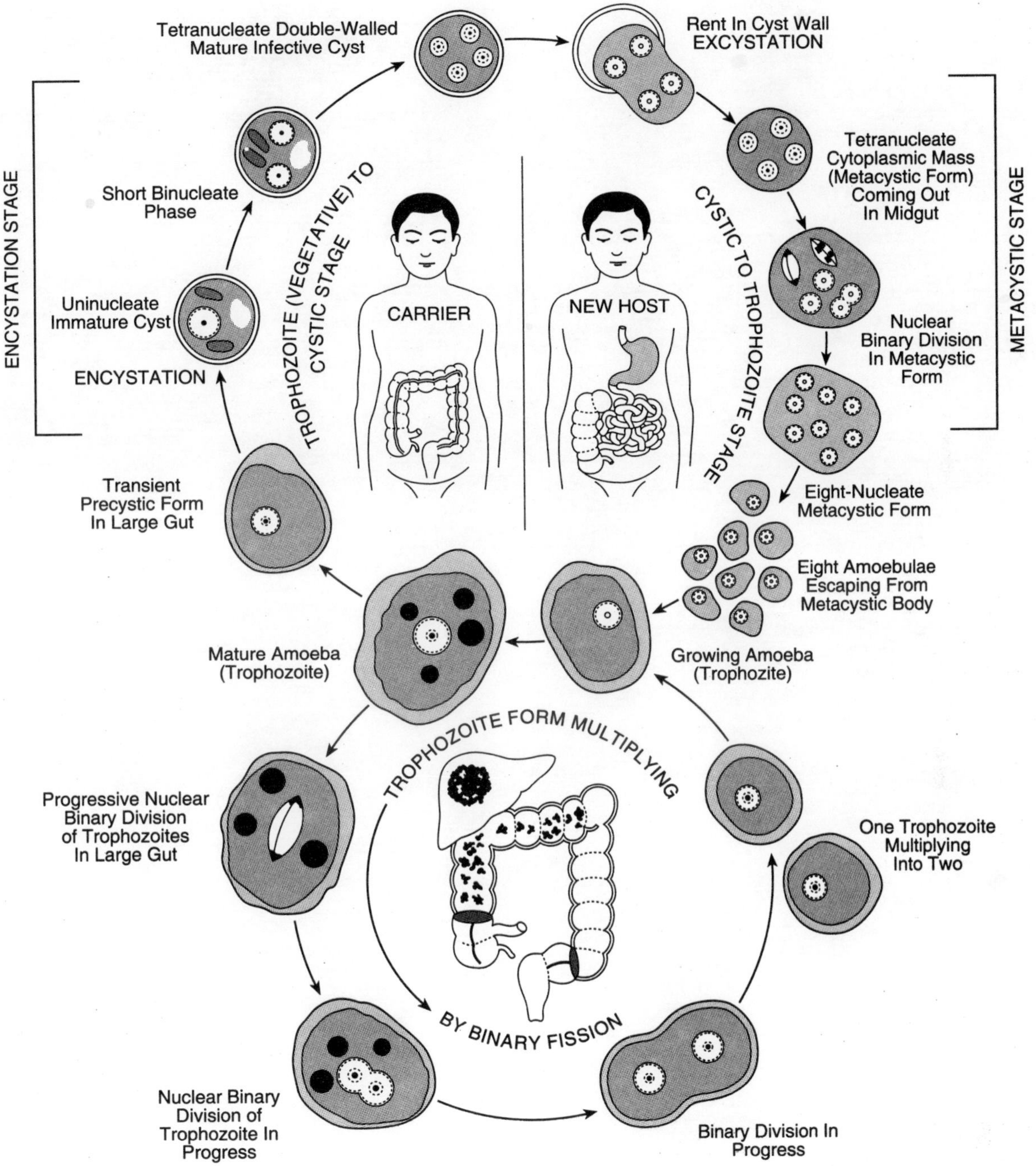

Showing developmental stages of *E. histolytica* in a carrier and a new host

PLATE 3.III
INTESTINAL LESIONS IN AMOEBIC DYSENTERY

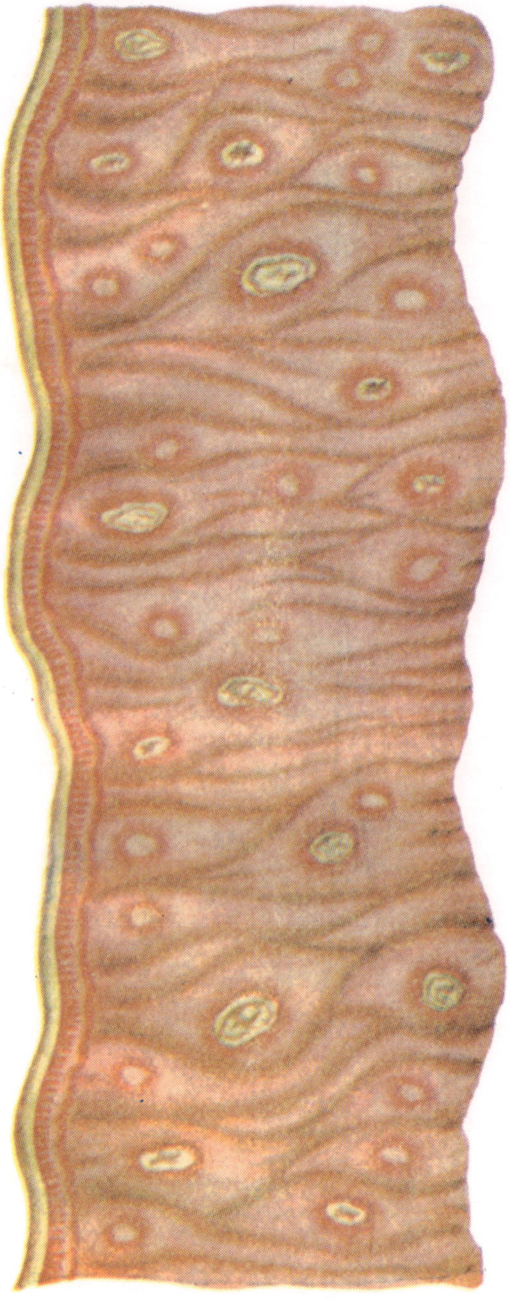

Fig. A Early lesions of the large intestine in acute amoebic dysentery showing nodular elevations, and acute and subacute ulcerations with areas of marked congestion around ulcers

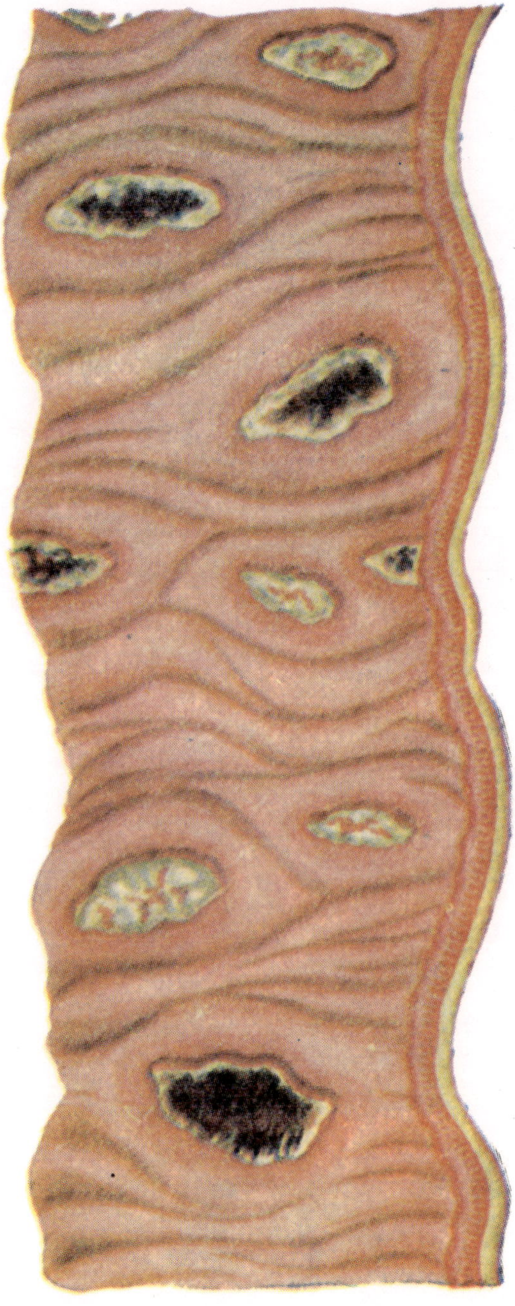

Fig. B Advanced lesions of the large intestine in amoebic colitis showing chronic amoebic ulcers with brownish black slough having shaggy appearance within. Moderate congestion is seen round the ulcers

(B) GENERAL LESIONS

Whole of large gut from ceacum to anal sphincter is involved where pathology remains the same as localised lesion.

CHARACTER OF ULCERS: Ulcers are best seen from mucous surface, as they are undermined, discrete. Healthy mucous membrane intervenes between

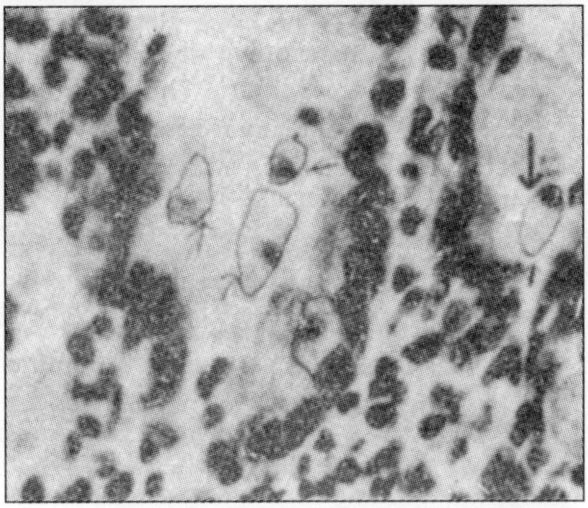

Fig. 3.6 Section from the margin of an amoebic ulcer of the caecum showing a collection of *E. histolytica* (trophozoite form) lying along interglandular spaces

ulcers even when extensive (undermined "flask shaped" ulcers). The earliest lesion is a small hemispherical module with erythema; varies from pinhead to a pea. Subsequently, there are scattered areas of small nodules. By pressure and cytolysin nodules undergo gelatinous necrosis, on cutting through brownish yellow material of necrotic tissue bulges out, containing *trophozoites*.

DESCRIPTION OF ULCER

SIZE: Pinhead to the size of 1″ or more.

SHAPE: Round or oval; large ulcers are transversely distributed.

MARGIN: Ragged and undermined, by overhanging mucosa. Vertical section shows an appearance of a GLASS FLASK (**Fig. 3.5, 3.6** and **3.7**).

FLOOR: Ulcers are shallow superficial; usually does not extend beyond muscular coat. Floor is formed by submucous coat with adherent sloughs.

BASE: Formed by muscular layer, filled up with the yellowish blackish slough (Fig. 3.9 and PL. 3.IV.)

INTERVENING AREA: In longitudinal cut section, Undermining excaration of mucosa gives the appearance of a glass flask (Fig. 3.5. PL. 3.III).

EXTENSION. Superficial ulcers are limited to submucosa. In deep ulcers cytolysis and necrosis is progressive extending deeper to peritoneal coat giving rise to complications, like local peritonitis,

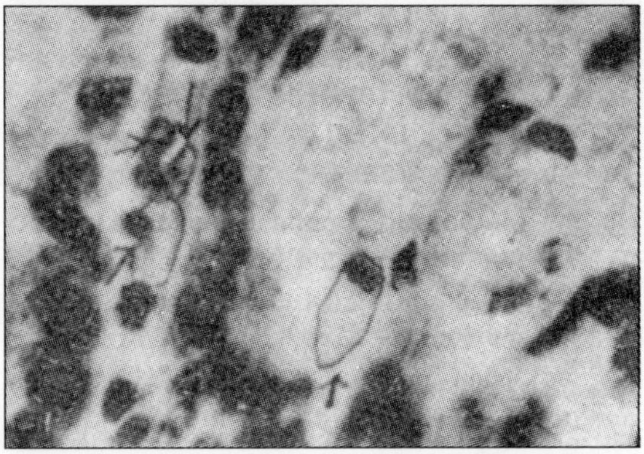

Fig. 3.7 An early amoebic ulcer of the caecum showing trophozoites of *E. histolytica* creeping along the crypts of Lieberkuhn (intact and destroyed), eroding the basement membrane of the epithelial lining and penetrating deeper into the tissue (a trophozoite is seen passing the barrier at the bottom)

haemorrhage, pericolic abscess, pericolitis, perforation, sloughing and gangrene of the large gut. *Pericolitis*, when occurs, is fatal with complications associated with secondary bacterial infection and requires immediate and urgent treatment in a few

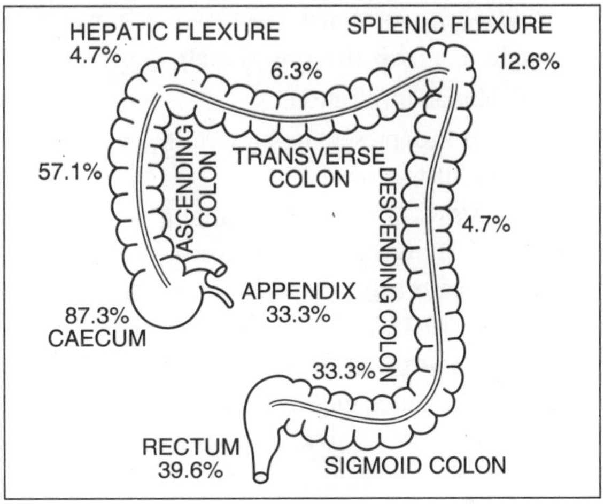

Fig. 3.8 Regional distribution of amoebic ulcers of large intestine (after Clerk)

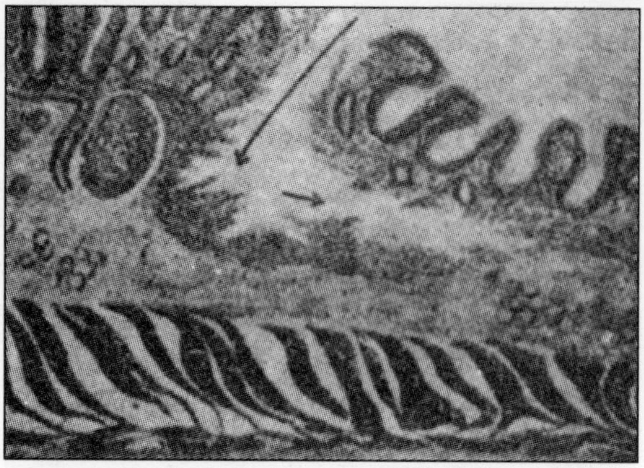

Fig. 3.9 Histopathological appearance of an amoebic (flask-shaped) ulcer

minutes, otherwise death occurs from shock and collapse.

In advanced cases, ulcers are larger with haemorrhage due to erosion of blood vessels at the base.

In *advanced acute cases*, ulcers show frayed (moth-eaten) black sloughs hanging from the bowel wall, called "*dyak-hair sloughs*" (Figs. 3.10, 3.11 and PL.3.III).

MICROSCOPIC PATHOLOGY

1. Absence of mucosa over ulcerated area. Early ulcers are limited to Muscularis.
2. Tissue in various stages of degeneration—organism IS NOT FOUND AT THE CENTRE (area necrosed and degenerated).
3. *E. histolytica* IS FOUND AT THE PERIPHERY in single or group (healthy tissue).
4. No cellular infiltration.
5. Trophozoites present in–between scars and gland causing histolysis.

IN ADVANCED STAGE, epithelia of crypts of Lieberkuhn show varying degrees of necrosis with basement membrane damage. Trophozoites penetrate deep (**Figs. 10/11**).

IN ADVANCED LESION of acute amoebic dysentery, trophozoites migrate down from ulcer sites, invade intermuscular spaces and progress to serous layer. Amoebae burrow into small venules or lying within lumina of venous radicles causing haemorrhage. Endothelial cells of many small blood vessels undergo hyperplasia causing thrombosis containing Trophozoites surrounded by autolysed tissue (Fig. 3.12).

INTESTINAL LESIONS IN CHRONIC AMOEBIASIS

The lesions are same as acute, with variation in degree. The course depends on host resistance. Lesions are characterised by following changes:

1. Small ulcers of the mucosa (from surface upto peritoneal coat).
2. Hyperaemia in superficial ulcers.
3. Marked scarring with THINNING, DILATATION and SACCULATION of intestinal wall.
4. Adhesions with neighbouring viscera.
5. Localised and generalised palpable THICKENING of the large intestinal wall with occasional narrowing of bowel.
6. Amoebic infection of appendix with *chronic appendicitis* with significant presence of *E. histolytica*.
7. Formation of AMOEBIC GRANULOMA or *amoeboma* (Fig. 3.11).
8. Ulcers extending up to peritoneal layer may cause PERICOLIC ABSCESS AND PERFORATION.

HEALING: Small ulcers heal by restoration of mucous membrane (regeneration). Big and deep ulcers heal by fibrosis (secondary union by granulation tissue) and no epithelia grow on the surface. The healed ulcers show pigmented, slate-coloured,

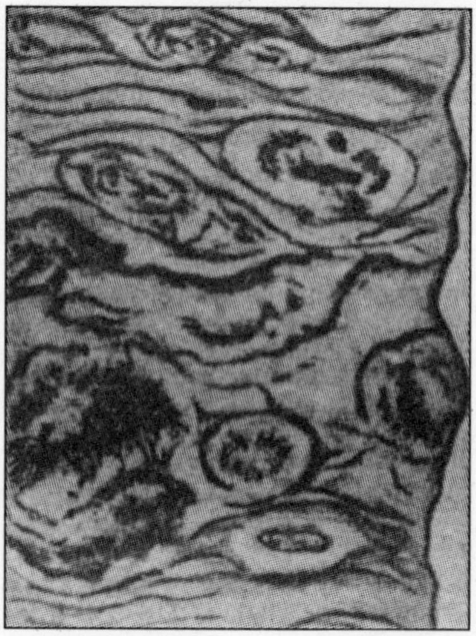

Fig. 3.10 Amoebic ulcer of the colon

depressed scars of parchment type, resulting in cicatrix formation (cicatricial contracture) generalised thickening, and sacculation of large gut. Adhesions between the proximal loops of the colon or between the peritoneal coat and the omentum, or adhesion of the gut to the spleen, liver or other viscera may occur. Polypoid condition results from *papillomatous* proliferation of the mucosa. A gangrenous destruction of the mucosa as a result of secondary infection is often a terminal condition.

CARRIER STAGE. This results from symbiosis between the host and the parasite but an acute exacerbation often occurs due to lowering of resistance of the host. The individual may not show any symptom of dysentery, but often passes cysts of *E. histolytica* in the stools. The symptoms of chronic amoebiasis are present in carriers.

Complications of amoebic infection are pericaecal or pericolic abscess, haemorrhage, perforation, fistula, etc.

CLINICAL FEATURES (Symptomatology).

AMOEBIASIS is caused by *E. histolytica*, *Amoebic dysentery* signifies primary infection of the large bowel and *chronic amoebic dysentery* means either chronicity of the primary lesion, or the secondary large intestinal lesions with passage of mucus and or blood in stool. Amoebiasis is named after the respective organs involved, like intestinal amoebiasis, pulmonary amoebiasis, etc.

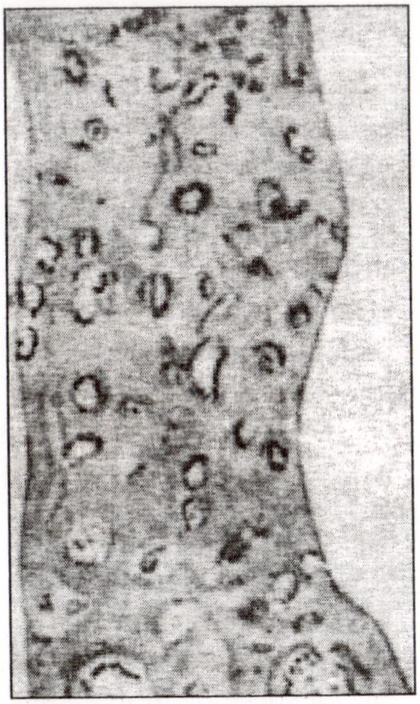

Fig. 3.11 Amoebic ulcer of the rectum

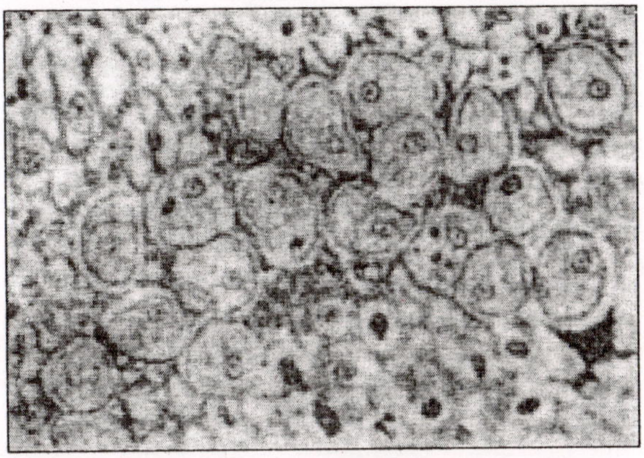

Fig. 3.12 Microscopic picture of the margin of the amoebic ulcer of colon with no cellular infiltration. Amoebae are lying surrounded by autolysed tissues around each of them (after Dobell and O'Connor, 1921); × 450.

SYMPTOMATOLOGY

ACUTE AMOEBIC DYSENTERY

Number of motions—6-8 times in 24 hours, Passage of loose stools with mucus and little blood. Occasional pus cells are present in stool specimen.

Fever—Almost nil. Toxaemia—Nil.

Pain—Over the caecum or colon according to the site of affection. (In bacillary dysentery, pain is around umbilicus).

Tenesmus—Much less.

Dehydration—Absent.

Prognosis—Not bad. Faecal matter present in faeces.

CHRONIC AMOEBIC DYSENTERY

Constipation alternating with diarrhoea occurs. Spasm of large bowel in places of ulcers. (Flatulence, acidity and heart burn—duodenal ulcer).

Dyspepsia—Anorexia, heaviness, gas of abdomen

Typhlitis—Amoebic typhlitis (caecal affection). Thickening and tenderness—of large bowel—according to site of affection.

Hypersonic resonance occurs on percussion of the abdomen (due to flatulence).

Visceroptosis and extensive adhesions occur.

Neurasthenia—Present.

Malnutrition—Present, resembling sprue or vitamin deficiency.

LABORATORY DIAGNOSIS OF INTESTINAL AMOEBIASIS

1. Stool. Collected and examined as fresh as possible after saline purgative to demonstrate trophozoite and cystic forms of *E. histolytica*. Examination of stool helps to establish the diagnosis to differentiate from Bacillary dysentery (**Table 3.3**).

2. Cultural Examination. Stools which are microscopically negative may often show positive growth of *E. histolytica* (for details see **Appendix II**).

3. Serological Reaction. *Complement fixation test*. It is of value in intestinal amoebiasis when the parasite cannot be demonstrated by repeated examination of stools (see **App. II**).

4. Immunologic Diagnosis. This is done by *immunofluorescent technique*. Bright immunofluorescence can be demonstrated in amoebae exposed to fluorescent tagged homologous (same species) antiserum.

5. *Immobilization* of *E. histolytica* from culture can be demonstrated by hyperimmune rabbit antisera.

6. Animal Inoculation. In a kitten should be finally undertaken (see **App. II**).

7. Sigmoidoscopic Examination. Character of the ulcer may be determined by endoscope microscopic attachment with **illumination**.

Course. It runs a chronic course with frequent intermissions and relapses—patients with chronic infection complain of diarrhoea rather than dysentery.

AMOEBIC HEPATITIS AND AMOEBIC LIVER ABSCESS

Syn. Hepatic Amoebiasis; Amoebic liver abscess; Tropical liver abscess; Solitary liver Abscess.

Amoebic liver abscess is caused by Trophozoite (Vegetative) form of *E. histolytica* from intestinal amoebiasis.

INCIDENCE: 2% to 10% occurs as a hepatic complication of intestinal amoebiasis. It is common in man. History of amoebiasis is obtained in 50% of cases. It occurs when intestinal symptoms subside. Earliest abscess occurs anytime after 3 months of dysentery. Fatal cases occur.

PATHOGENESIS: Amoebic liver abscess is produced secondary to intestinal amoebiasis.

SITE: Usually upper surface of the right lobe.

NUMBER: Usually single (70%).

ORGANISM: Trophozoites in *abscess wall*.

From the base of the intestinal ulcers (in the large gut) *E. histolytica* trophozoites penetrate the wall of portal vein radicles. There is endothelial cell hyperplasia, a thrombus is formed, and the amoebae ride on the thrombus. They are carried in blood stream to reach the liver as emboli through branches of portal vein. *Parasites settle at the Right lobe of the liver* for the following causes:

(i) In the portal vein their is no ADMIXTURE OF BLOOD OF THE LEFT AND RIGHT SIDE. Blood drains from the Right part of the intestine (caecum) through the superior mesenteric vein and *via* Right branch of portal vein to the right lobe of the liver. So parasites most easily reach the Right lobe of the liver.

(ii) Sometimes amoeba may ENTER THE INFERIOR SURFACE OF THE right lobe of the LIVER DIRECTLY, when the intestinal ulcer is situated near RIGHT FLEXOR OF THE COLON (HEPATIC FLEXOR). Thus amoeba will enter the Right lobe of the liver. In the liver the PORTAL VEIN RAMIFIES INTO SMALLER BRANCHES and, ultimately, capillaries are formed. The amoeba are arrested in the capiliary flow and settle there (See **Fig. 3.13**).

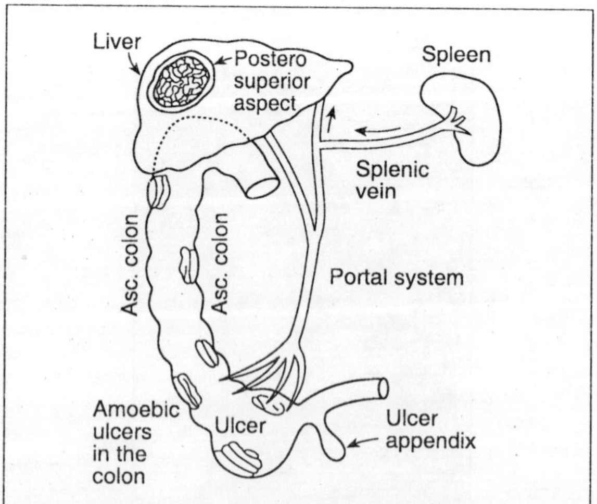

Fig. 3.13 Showing path of infection from Large Intestine to Liver through superior mesenteric vein *via* Portal vein. For better understanding Anatomical plan of diagram is modified

PLATE 3.IV

MICROSCOPIC FEATURES OF STOOL

AMOEBIC DYSENTERY

BACILLARY DYSENTERY

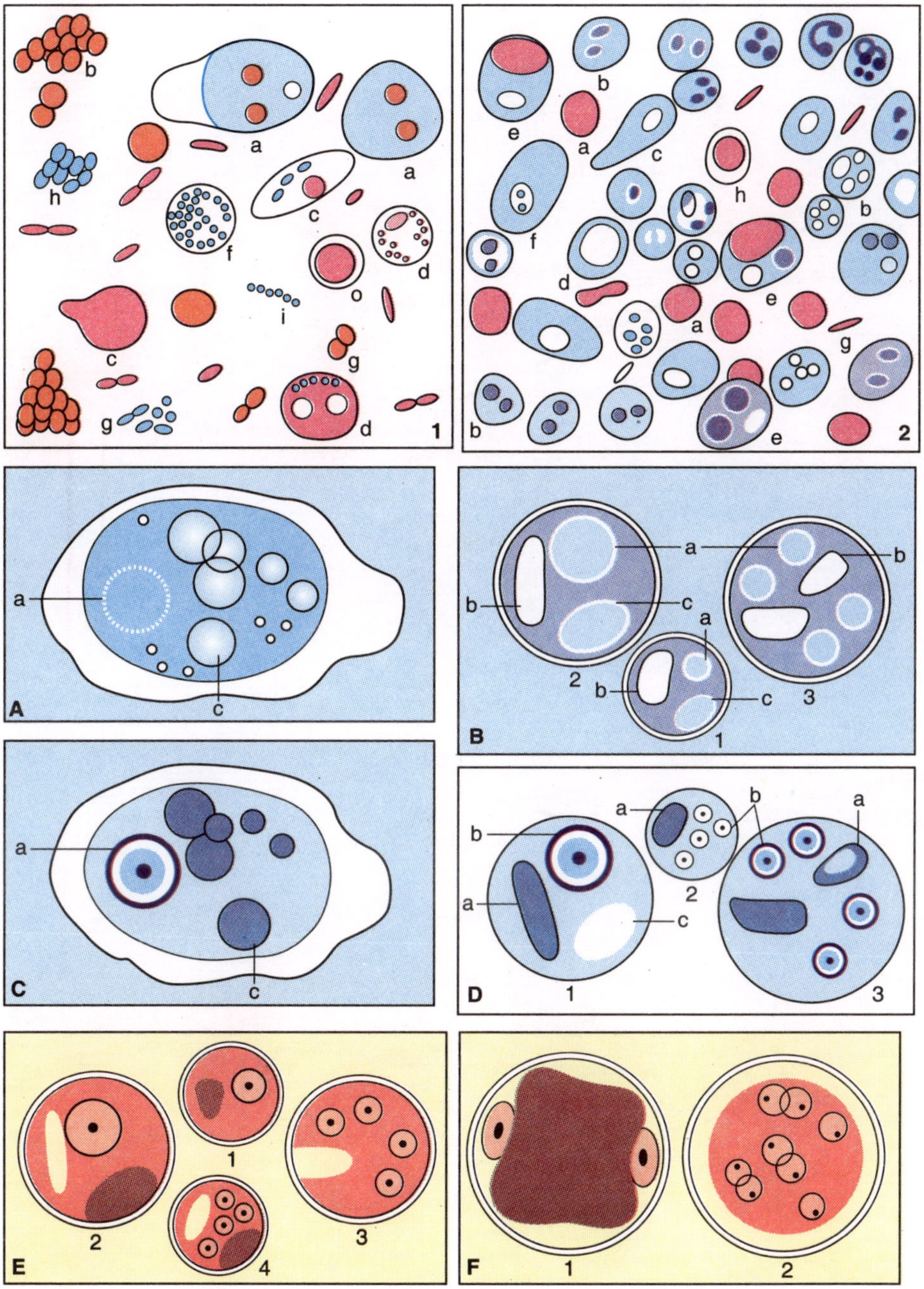

CYSTS OF *E. HISTOLYTICA*

CYSTS OF *E. COLI*

IODINE PREPARATION

TABLE 3.3 (PL. 3.IV & 3.VII)

DIFFERENCES BETWEEN THE CHARACTERS OF STOOLS IN AMOEBIC AND BACILLARY DYSENTERY (Cellular exudats)

	AMOEBIC DYSENTERY	BACILLARY DYSENTERY
Number	6 to 8 motions a day	Over 10 motions a day
Macroscopic		
Amount	Relatively copious	Small
Nature	Blood and mucus mixed with faeces	Blood and mucus, no faeces
Colour of Blood	Dark red (altered blood)	Bright red (fresh blood)
Consistency	Liquid or formed; mucus not adherent to the container	Viscid; mucus adherent to the container
Odour	Offensive	Odourless
Chemical		
Reaction	Acid	Alkaline (for fresh blood)
Microscopic		
Exudate		
(a) RBC	In clumps; reddish-yellow in colour	Discrete or in rouleaux, bright red in colour
(b) Pus Cells	Scanty	Numerous
(c) Macrophages	Very few	Large and numerous, many of them contain RBC; hence mistaken for *E. histolytica*
Pyknotic Bodies (Pyknotic nuclear residues)	Very common	Nil
Ghost Cells (Degenerated macrophages)	Nil	Numerous
Eosinophils	Present	Absent
Charcot-Leyden Crystals (rhomboid crystals; degenerated eosinophils 5 to 50 μ in length; highly refractile)	Present	Absent
Parasite	Trophozoites or cysts of *E. histolytica* present	Absent
Bacteria	Numerous (motile *Esch. coli* and other Enterobacteria)	Scanty, non-motile (Shigella group or Klebsiella)
Culture	*E. histolytica* grown (B-D medium)	Shigella grown (MacConkey medium)

POSTERO-SUPERIOR ASPECT OF RIGHT LOBE OF THE LIVER IS THE COMMON SITE.

The causes are

(i) Right lobe is bigger in size. (ii) More blood is drained in the right lobe. (iii) Due to a peculiar STREAMLINE PHENOMENON of blood stream from the right side (caecum, ascending colon) *via* superior mesenteric vein in the right portal stream line (See **Fig. 3.13**).

AMOEBIC HEPATITIS

In this stage the liver is enlarged and congested but no abscess is formed. This stage is known as AMOEBIC HEPATITIS.

As the capillaries are blocked, the liver cells do

not get any nutrition and undergo ischaemic necrosis. In the necrosed tissue the capillaries lose their support and damaged by anoxia. The capillaries rupture and the amoebae come out of the capillary and affect the liver cells. The multiply in large numbers and start destruction of liver cells by CYTOLYSIN. Thus minute abscesses are formed which join to form a big abscess.

Macroscopically (PL. 3.V)

1. The liver is enlarged and the right lobe affected more than the left lobe, which also enlarges due to compensatory hypertrophy in late stage.
2. Liver may be congested.
3. There is presence of a big abscess.

The features of the abscess are:

(a) Site: Right lobe (Postero-superior).

(b) Size: May be very big and may contain a litre of pus.

(c) Number: Usually single, multiple abscesses surround the main abscess. The liver shows moth-eaten appearance.

(d) Wall: Irregular and ragged. In long-standing cases the wall may be smooth due to fibrosis.

(e) Content: Pus is known as "ANCHOVY SAUCE PUS□□. It is bacteriologically sterile. In Secondary bacterial infection (*Streptococcus haemolyticus*, or *Escherichia coli*), the content becomes purulent.

(f) The surrounding area: A congested zone will be present in-between the abscess cavity and healthy part.

Microscopically: In an early abscess it reveals central area of necrosed tissue, few leucocytes, RBCs, oedematous connective tissue and debris. Trophozoites appear late in the collected pus—about 4 to 5 days later after evacuation of the abscess. Trophozoites are not present in freshly aspirated pus.

In an advanced case, when a section is made through the margin of a liver abscess, three (3) zones are seen from the centre to periphery as follows: (PL. 3.VI)

CENTRAL ZONE: (i) Necrosed granular material in the centre, but no TROPHOZOITE.

INTERMEDIATE ZONE: Degenerated liver cells, RBCs, some leucocytes, fibroblasts and occasionally trophozoites of *E. histolytica*.

PERIPHERAL ZONE: Congested capillaries with the varying degrees of necrotic liver cells and large number of trophozoites.

In an abscess of long-standing the peripheral zone comprises:

Actively proliferating fibroblasts and mononuclear cells, (Lymphocytes, Plasma cells, Histiocytes). The scraping of abscess wall shows trophozoites.

In multiple (miliary) abscesses, the liver cells may show fatty change.

ANCHOVY SAUCE PUS

This is one of the complications of amoebic liver abscess. This is not a true pus but formed by the destruction of liver cells. It is expectorated with the sputum giving rise to haemoptysis ***when abscess ruptures in the lung*** (***through diaphragm*** by a fistulous connection). It is chocolate brown in colour and is known as ANCHOVY SAUCE PUS. It consists of:

(i) Necrosed liver cells

(ii) Lecithine crystals

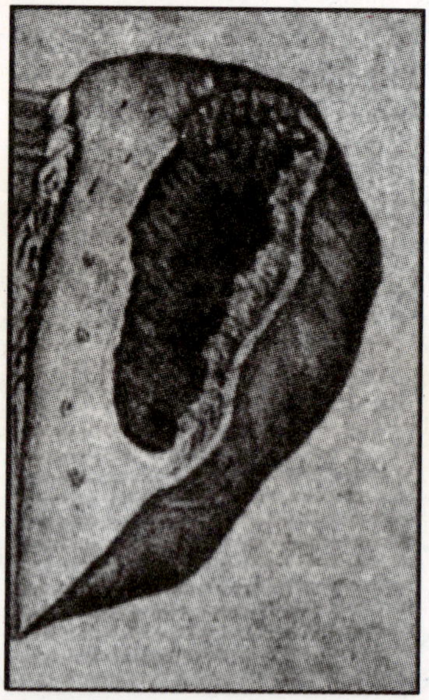

Fig. 3.14 Amoebic liver abscess which has destroyed the liver tissue giving a shaggy appearance

PLATE 3.V
TROPICAL (AMOEBIC) LIVER ABSCESS

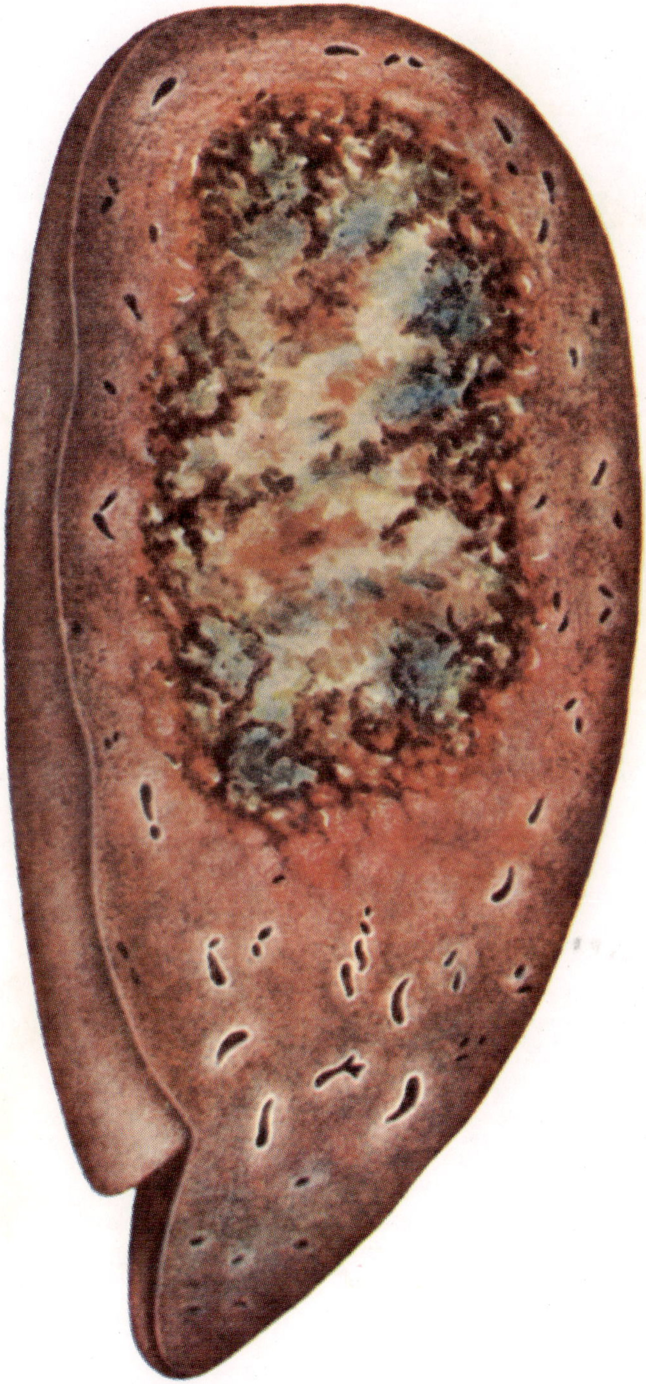

Liver showing big solitary area of necrosis (Histolysis).
Trophozoites are exclusively found in the abscess wall scrapings

PLATE 3.VI
AMOEBIC LIVER ABSCESS

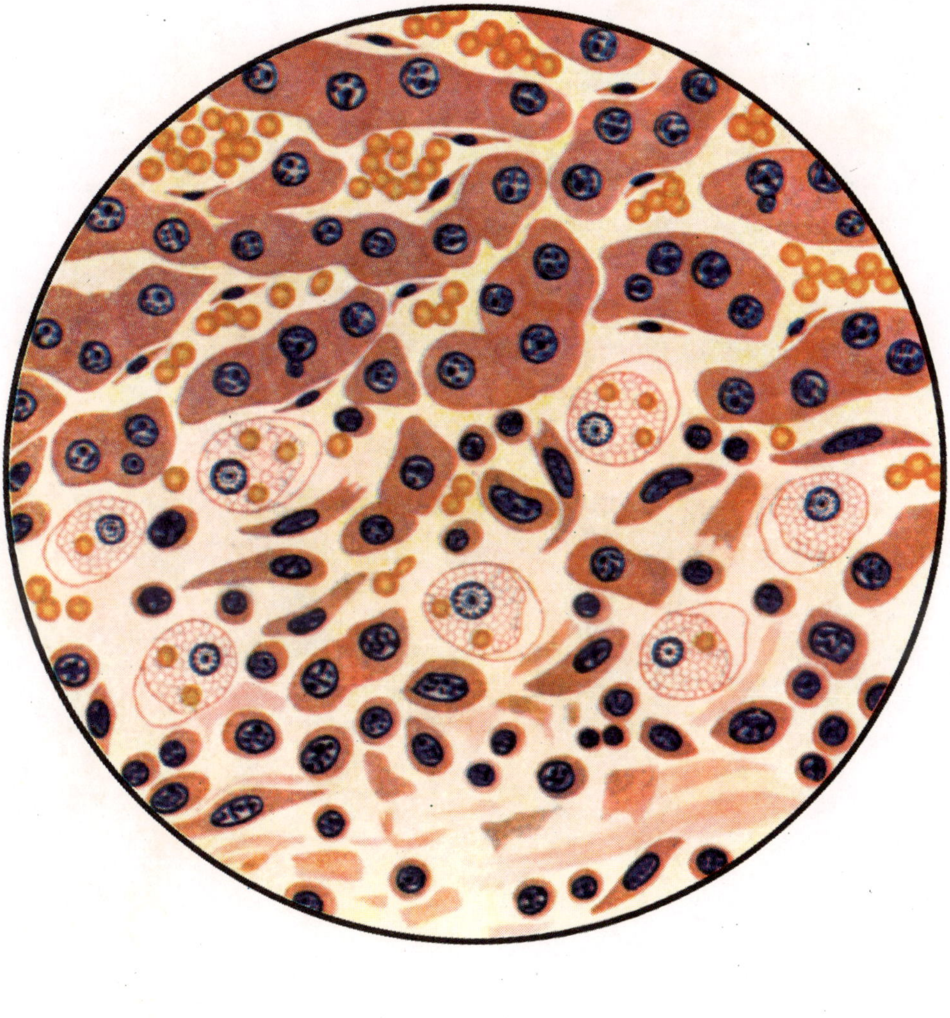

Solitary/Micro-histologic appearance of solitary/tropical/amoebic liver abscess. Necrosed liver cells (eosinophilic without nuclei) and seven trophozoite amoebae are seen in the abscess margin in the lower half of the diagram. Healthy liver cells are seen at the upper part with RBCs in the sinusoidal and capillary spaces. Phagocytosed RBCs are seen in the trophozoites. (H & E) ×600

(iii) Charcot-Leyden crystals (**Fig. 3.16**)
(iv) Cholesterol crystals
(v) RBCs
(vi) Pyknotic bodies (nuclear residues).

COMPLICATIONS, FATE (COURSE AND TERMINATION) OF AMOEBIC LIVER ABSCESS

1. If the abscess is small, it may heal by fibrosis and calcification, and the content is dried up.
2. A chronic abscess can be formed with thickening of its wall (by compression of surrounding liver tissue).
3. If the abscess is big, it can rupture into the neighbouring organs or structures through which the contents are discharged.

A. RIGHT-SIDED LIVER ABSCESS MAY RUPTURE AS FOLLOWS:

(a) *Through skin.* Spontaneous rupture through the parietal peritoneum and skin. The skin may be secondarily infected with trophozoites forming a *granuloma* AMOEBIASIS CUTIS.

(b) *Into the Lungs.* The "pus" is expectorated with sputum giving rise to haemoptysis. (a viscid "Anchovy Sauce Pus"). *Microscopically*, liver cells and trophozoites of *E. histolytica* may be recognised.

(c) *Into the Right sided Pleural Cavity.* Leading to EMPYEMA THORACIS (right side).

(d) *Below the Diaphragm.* Producing sub-diaphragmatic (subphrenic) abscess.

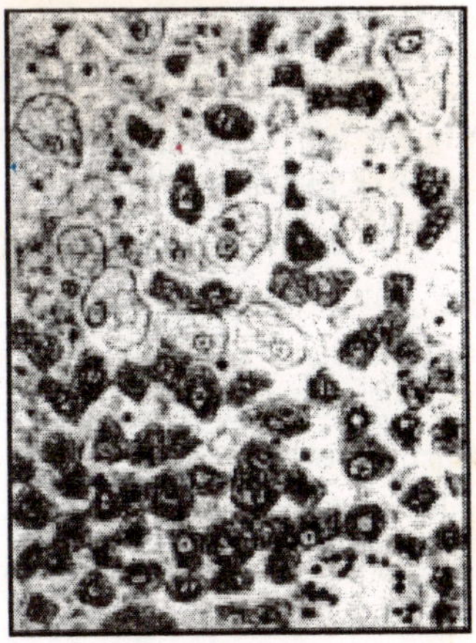

Fig. 3.15 The trophozoite form of *E. histolytica* at the margin of an amoebic liver abscess (after Dobell and O'Connor, 1921)

(e) *Into the Peritoneal Cavity.* Producing generalised peritonitis. This is usually not fatal.

B. LEFT-SIDED LIVER ADSCESS MAY RUPTURE AS FOLLOWS:

(a) *Externally*, through epigastric region causing AMOEBIASIS CUTIS.

(b) *Stomach.* Anchovy Sauce Pus is vomited out with haematemesis.

(c) *Pericardial Cavity.* Causing Pyopericardium ending fatally.

(d) *Left sided Pleural Cavity.* Causing EMPYEMA THORACIS of the left side.

C. An Abscess on the inferior surface may rupture into

(a) *Peritoneal Cavity.* Causing fatal peritonitis.

(b) *Bowel : Duodenum or Transverse Colon.* Causing diarrhoea "pus" discharge.

D. An abscess situated on the posterior surface may rupture into

Inferior Vena Cava: which is very rare but invariably fatal.

OTHER COMPLICATIONS: PL.3.VIII.

I. Brain may be affected very rarely as a complication of hepatic or pulmonary abscess. The abscess is small, single and usually fatal and affect the cerebral hemisphere. Death occurs in 10 days.

II. SKIN

1. Leucoderma.
2. Allergic amoebic dermatosis, Anal pruritus, Urticaria, Acne rosacea, etc.
3. Amoebiasis cutis and Amoeboma.

Amoeboma. It is an ulcerating granuloma of colon or rectum from gut wall invasion by *E. histolytica*. This results in a mass of pseudoepitheliomatous granulation tissue, projecting into the lumen of the gut as an ulcerating fungating mass or as an annular constructing band. It contains the trophozoites seen even in Biopsy material. Commonest sites are caecum, flexures of colon, rectosigmoid junction, causing signs of obstruction. Amoeboma around a fistulous opening in the skin also occurs.

IV. Urogenital tract. *E. histolytica* may involve the urogenital tract through a *rectovesical or rectovaginal fistula* producing *cystitis or vaginitis*.

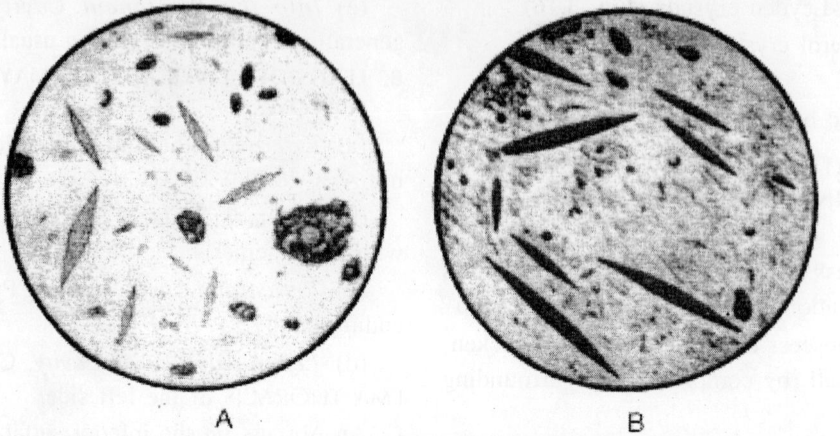

Fig. 3.16. Charcot-Leyden crystals
A. Unstained as seen under saline preparation (After Acton and Knowles).
B. As stained by iron haematoxylin (After Thomson and Robertson, 1921)

INTESTINAL LESIONS WHEN AMOEBIC LIVER ABSCESS IS DETECTED

Primary focus of all lesions of metastatic amoebic affection is the large intestine.

AUTOPSY Finding

1. Superficial ulcers with thickening of the large gut.
2. A latent ulcer in the caecum.
3. Heated areas of scarring of large gut.
4. Extensive ulcers are not found usually in amoebic hepatitis or liver abscess.

SYMPTOMATOLOGY OF AMOEBIC LIVER ABSCESS

Pain and tenderness in the right hypochondrium stretching of Glisson's capsule referred to acromial tip phrenic nerve (irritation under diaphragm-shoulder pain) causing dry cough. Pain may be referred to right iliac region or lower abdomen.

SYMPTOMS

Onest is gradual and insidious.

Fever. Low remittent (evening) or hectic or quotidian (pyrogenic effect of necrosis).

General health. Emaciated.

Jaundice. Unusual occurrence.

SIGNS

Tender, palpable liver below the costal margin. Movement of right chest diminished. Liver dullness extends upwards. Right rectus is rigid (Muscle guard).

Liver. Left lobe may be palpable (compensatory hypertrophy). When the abscess points, parietes may bulgde out.

Lungs. Base of right lung collapsed (pressure effect). Pleural collection present.

Heart. Apical impulse displaced laterally and upwards by a big abscess.

Intestine. Thickening and tenderness.

STOOL EXAMINATION : USUAL FINDINGS

(a) *E. histolytica*—Trophozoite liquid stool.

(b) Cysts in solid stool.

Absence of them does not exclude diagnosis.

CLINICAL DIAGNOSIS OF LIVER ABSCESS SYMPTOMS

1. **Fever** (38°–39°C) in 60% with chill or rigor, goes away with sweating.
2. **Pain** and Heaviness in Right Hypochondrium (90%); Dull ache (early); later throbbing/stabbing in inspiration/coughing/sneezing; radiates in right shoulder or scapula.
3. **Weakness**, anorexia, cough, hiccough, odema feet; rarely jaundice.
4. **Haemoptysis** or haematemesis associated with Anchovy Sauce Pus.

PLATE 3.VII

MICROSCOPIC APPEARANCES OF CELLULAR EXUDATE IN AMOEBIC AND BACILLARY DYSENTERY

(Fresh Preparations)

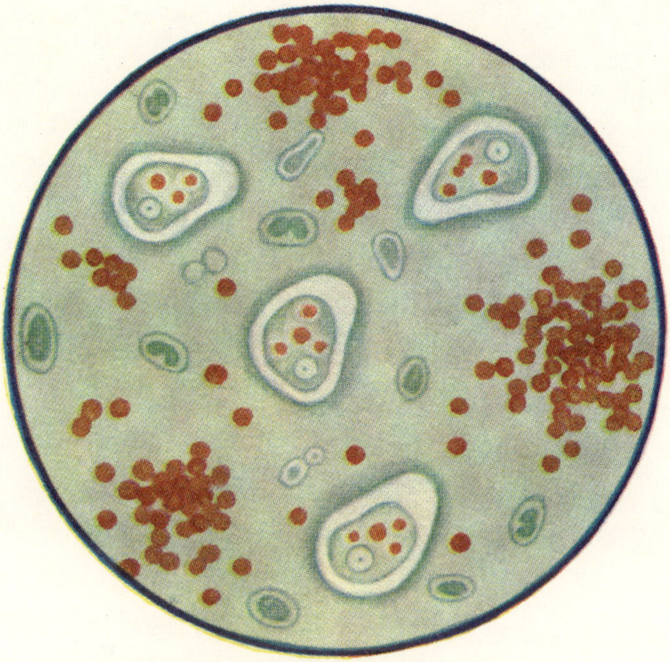

A. Microscopic appearance of stools of amoebic dysentery showing occasional (few) pus cells, conglomerated red blood cells and four *E. histolytica* with ingested red cells.

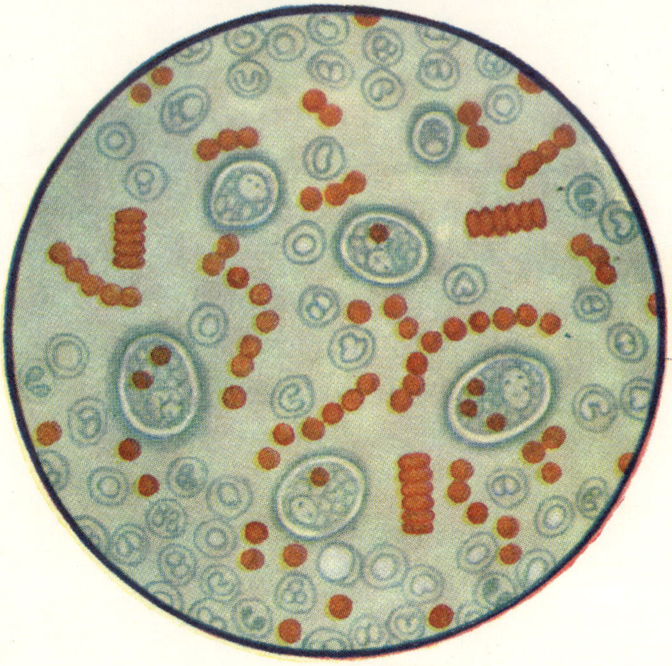

B. Microscopic appearance of stools of bacillary dysentery showing typical cellular exudate comprising a large number of pus cells with fatty change, discrete red cells, and macrophages with ingested red blood cells.

PLATE 3.VIII

ENUMERATION OF PATHOLOGICAL LESIONS CAUSED BY *E. HISTOLYTICA*

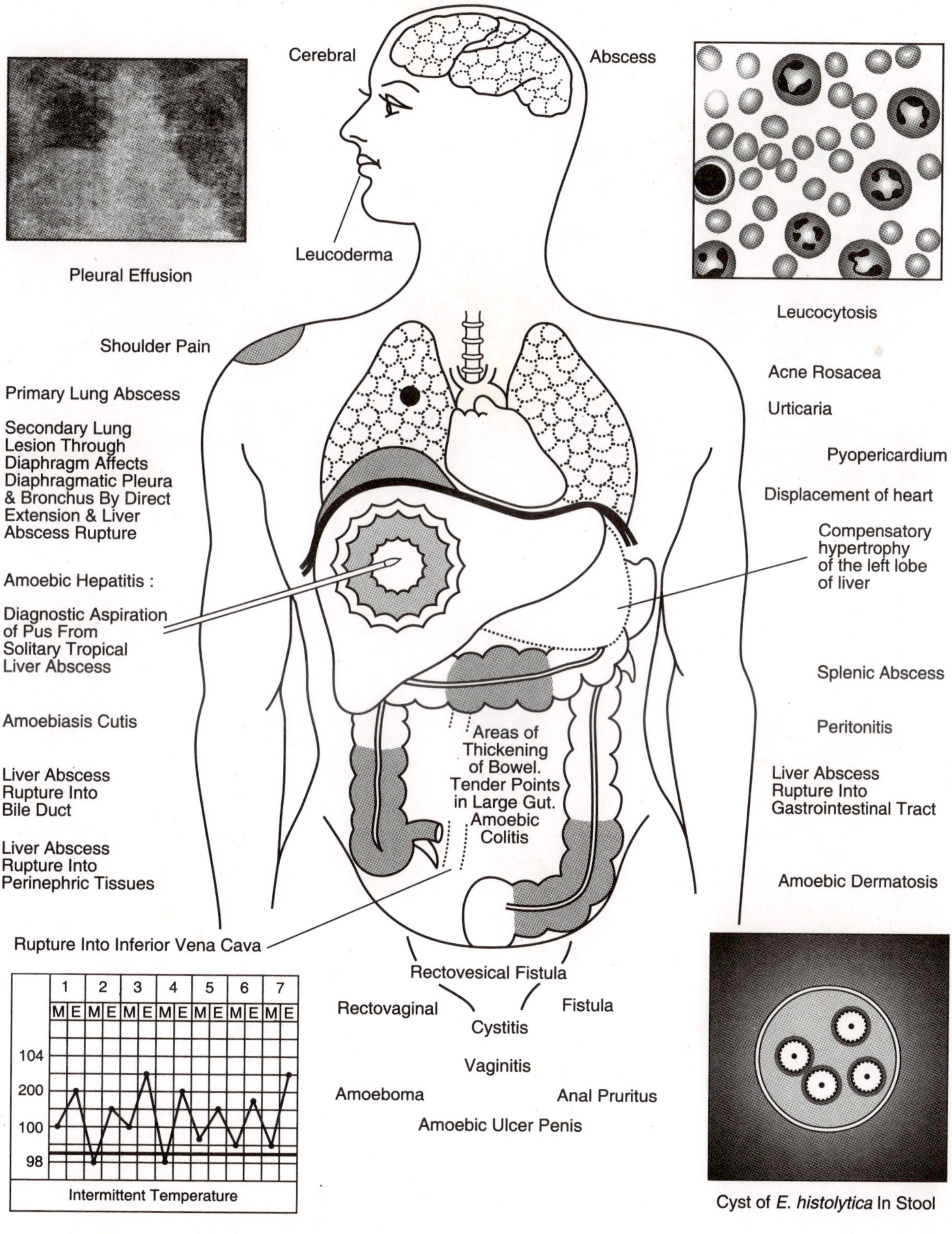

SIGNS

1. General health—Emaciated.
2. Fever.
3. Tongue—Dry, anaemic.
4. Liver—Enlarged, tender, palpable, soft, with irregular lower margin *HEPATIC rub* on auscultation.
5. Intestine—Thickened, tender rapid fatal.
6. Lungs—Dullness at right base (collapse by growing liver abscess).

   Crepitations signifies intrahepatic suppuration. ← Breath sound diminished. *Pleural rub*/frank signs of *effusion*.
7. Heart—Dullness *Pericardial rub* → (pericarditis), Apex beat lateral up.

LABORATORY DIAGNOSIS OF LIVER ABSCESS

1. *Blood Examination*: Leucocytosis (15,000 to 20,000) Neutrophils rarely above 80% (secondary infection).
2. *Examination of Stool* : Cystic *E. histolytica* (over 50% cases) in liquid stools after saline purgative. **PL.IX.**
3. *Liver* (Needle) biopsy : Trophozoite *E. histolytica* is seen when abscess wall comes out. **PL.3.IV.**
4. *Diagnostic Aspiration* : (Exploratory puncture to confirm the diagnosis). In aspirated "*Anchovy Sauce Pus*" is seen trophozoite *E. histolytica.*
5. *Serological Tests* (Immunologic Diagnosis) : They positivity depend on specific serum antibody :
   1. **C.F. Test:** is replaced by other tests.
   2. **Indirect Haemagglutination Test:** Positive in invasive amoebiasis.
   3. **Immobilisation Test**: Specific antisera mixed with living culture of *E. histolytica* causes immobilisation of parasites.
   4. **Passive Cutaneous Anaphylaxis Test (PCA)** done in guinea pigs.
   5. **Precipitin Test** done with pt. serum by Agar gel Double Diffusion technic (Ouchterlony).
   6. **Goldman's Test** (1953, 1962) : done by fluorescein tagged antibody with specimen of stool. *E. histolytica* emits bright light.

      Amoebic antigen: derived from trophozoites of *E. histolytica* culture in axenic media.
6. *Intradermal Test* : In an infected individual injection of 0.1 ml antigen produces erythema after 3 hours, maximum after 24 hours (10 cm diameter), disappearing in another 48 hours.

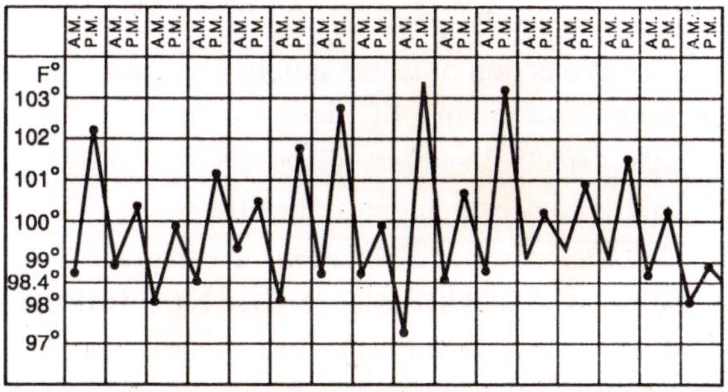

Fig. 3.17 Temperature chart in amoebic abscess of the liver

DIAGNOSIS OF PULMONARY AMOEBIASIS

Radiological Examination: The right dome of the diaphragm (higher level), the commonest site of Liver Abscess (Postero-superior surface), shows "tenting"—indicating basal pleurisy.

1. Finding of trophozoites of *E. histolytica* in the sputum.
2. Various Immunological tests.

Expectorated Anchovy Sauce Pus shows motile forms of *E. histolytica* (trophozoites).

TREATMENT OF AMOEBIASIS

I. LUMINAL AMOEBICIDES

A. Directly acting luminal amoebicides called contact amoebicides.

1. **Halogenated hydroxyquinolines**
   (i) Di-iodohydroxyquinoline (diodoquin)
   (ii) Iodochloro hydroxyquinoline (clioquinol)
2. **Dichloracetamide Group**
   (i) Chlorophenoxamide (mebinol)
   (ii) Diloxamide (entamide)
   (iii) Chlorbetamide (mantomide)
3. **Oral emetine**
   (i) Emitine bismuth iodide (EBI)
   (ii) Dehydroemetine bismuth iodide
4. **Pentavalent Arsenicals:** not used.
5. **Antibiotics:** Paromomycin (humatin)

B. Indirectly acting luminal amoebicides by reducing bacterial flora (inhibition of Symbiosis): Broad–spectrum Antibiotics.

II. Tissue Amoebicides : They act on trophozoites in tissues.

A. Acting in the intestinal wall, liver and other metastatic areas. Emetine and or dihydroemetine (DHE) parenterally administered.

B. In the liver and lungs: 4-aminoquinoline derivative (Chloroquine or Resochin).

III. Both Luminal and Tissue Amoebicides

They act on cysts and trophozoites

1. Niridazole (Ambilhar)
2. Metronidazole (Metrogyl) of *E. histolytica*.

PROPHYLAXIS OF AMOEBIC INFECTION

1. Personal Prophylaxis

(i) Use of boiled drinking water.

(ii) Protection of food and drink from flies, cockroaches and rats.

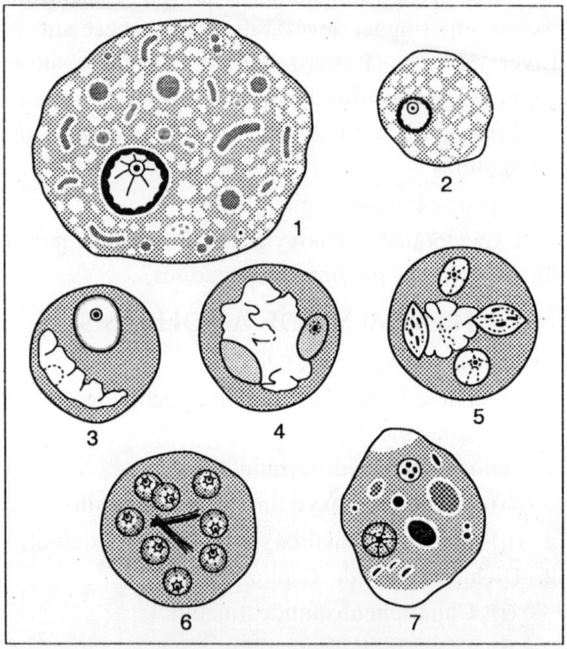

Fig. 3.18 *Entamoeba coli* and *E. gingivalis*. x1500. 1-6-*E. coli* from human faeces. I–Trophozoite with ingested bacteria, etc. 2–Precystic form. 3-6–Cysts. 3–One-nucleate cyst with glycogen vacuole. 4–Two nucleate form with a large glycogen vacuole. 5–Four-nucleate form (2 nuclei dividing). 6–Eight-nucleate form (mature) with filamentous chromatin. 7–*Entamoeba gingivalis* cyst with glycogen vacuole. 4 Two nucleate form oral cavity with central (sometimes eccentric) karyosome and various cytoplasmic inclusions. (Adapted from Dobell, 1919; and Dobell and O'Connor, 1921)

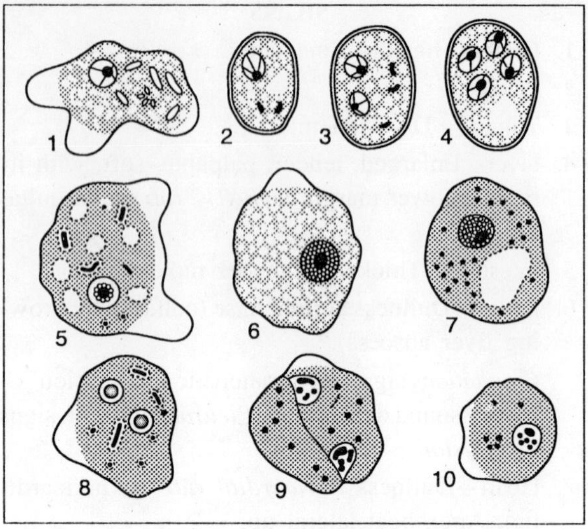

Fig. 3.19 Nonpathogenic amoebae from human faeces. Adapted from Dobell and O'Connor, 1921 and Wenyon. 1923.

(-4) *Endolimax nana*. (1) Trophozoite form with food vacuoles, ingested food particles and nuclear structures; (2-4)-Cysts. at the uninucleate, binucleate and tetranucleate phases. They show volutin and chromatoid granules (5-7)–*Iodamoeba butschlii* (5)–Trophozoite form with finger-like pseudopodia and food vacuoles containing bacteria. Note nucleus with a zone of chromatin granules around it. These are less intensely stained. (6)–Precystic form. (7)–Cystic form with a large glycogen vacuole and volutin granules. Nucleus is near the nuclear membrane (basket pattern) and nuclear granules accumulating near the nuclear membrane. (8-10)–*Dientamoeba fragilis* (only the trophozoite form). (8)–Form with two nuclei. The nucleus contains a number of chromatin granules. (9)–Same with two nuclei connected with centrodesmus. (10)–Uninucleate form

(iii) Avoid raw fruits and vegetables.

(iv) Following of hygienic cleanliness.

2. Community Prophylaxis

(i) Protection of water supply lines from faecal pollution and control of flies.

(ii) Effective sanitary disposals.

(iii) Avoid excrement as fertilisers.

(iv) Detection and isolation of carriers.

PRIMARY AMOEBIC MENINGO-ENCEPHALITIS

Caused by free-living amoebae genera Naegleria and Hartmannella in fresh water, mud, moist soil, distinct from *E. histolytica*. They have smaller TROPHOZOITE FORM and a FLAGELLATE PHASE.

PLATE 3.IX(1)
SALINE PREPARATION

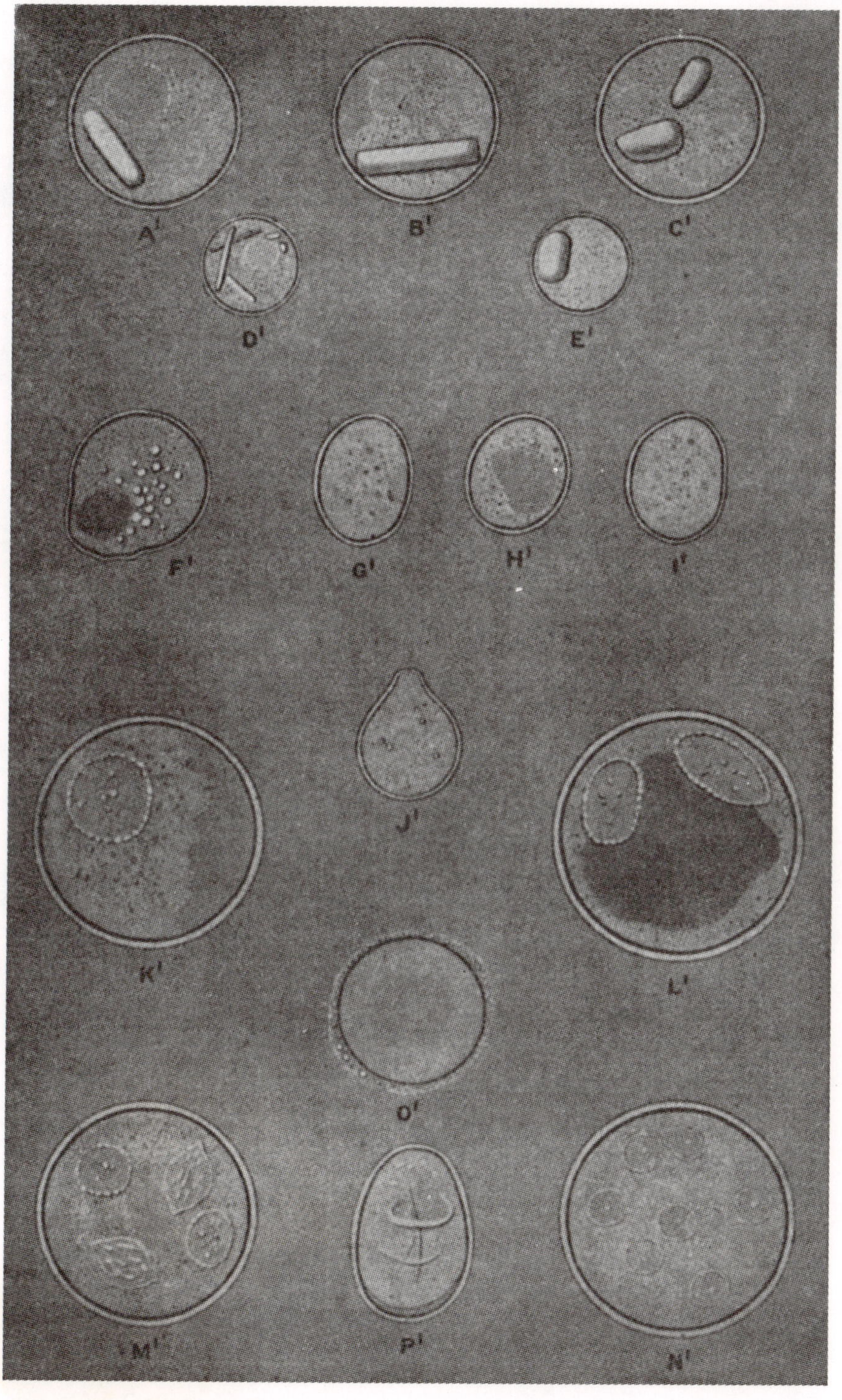

Cysts of Chief Intestinal Protozoa of Man

PLATE 3.IX(2)
IODINE PREPERATION

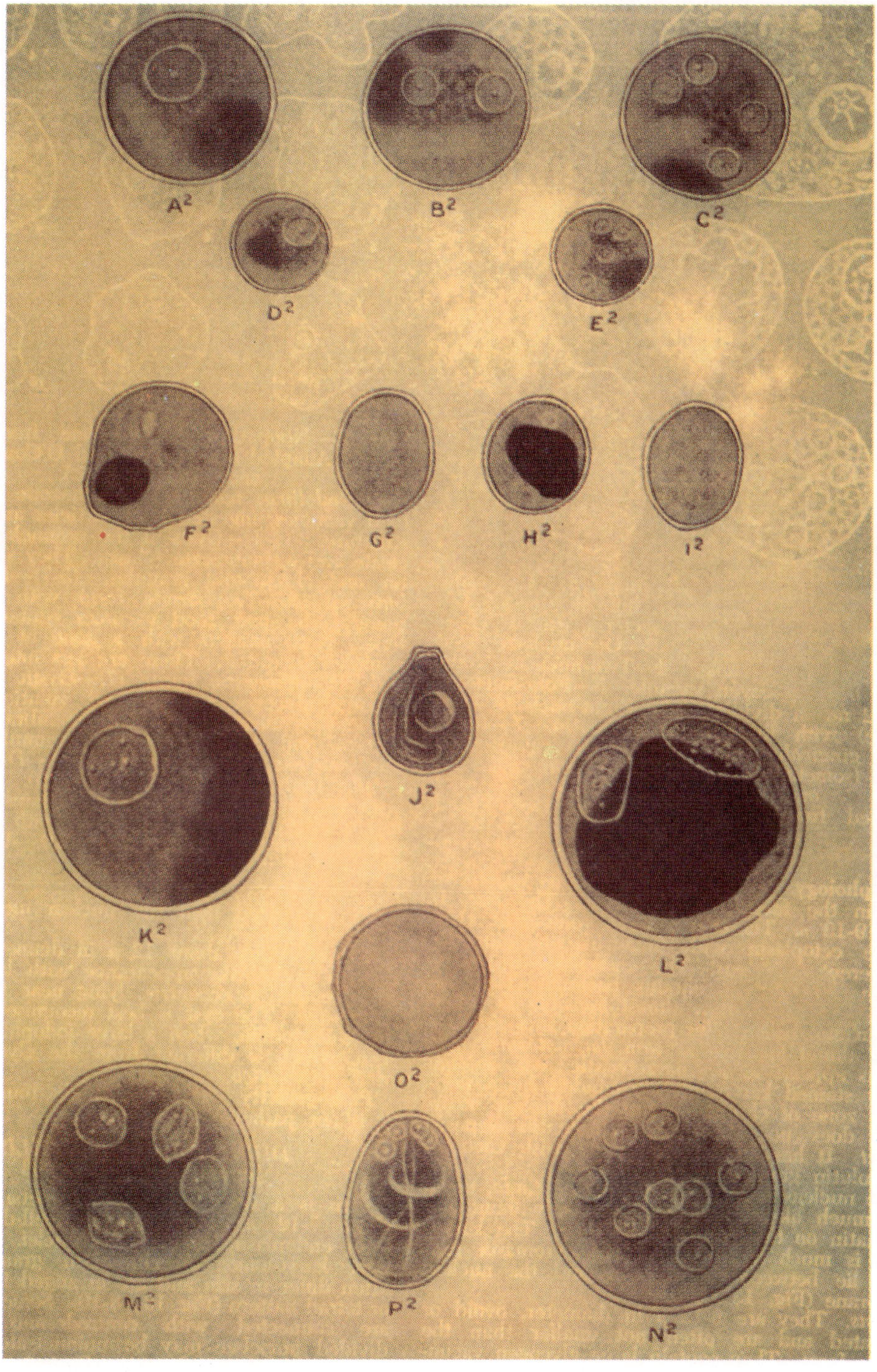

Cysts of Chief Intestinal Protozoa of Man.

PLATE 3.IX(3)
IRON-HAEMATOXYLIN STAIN

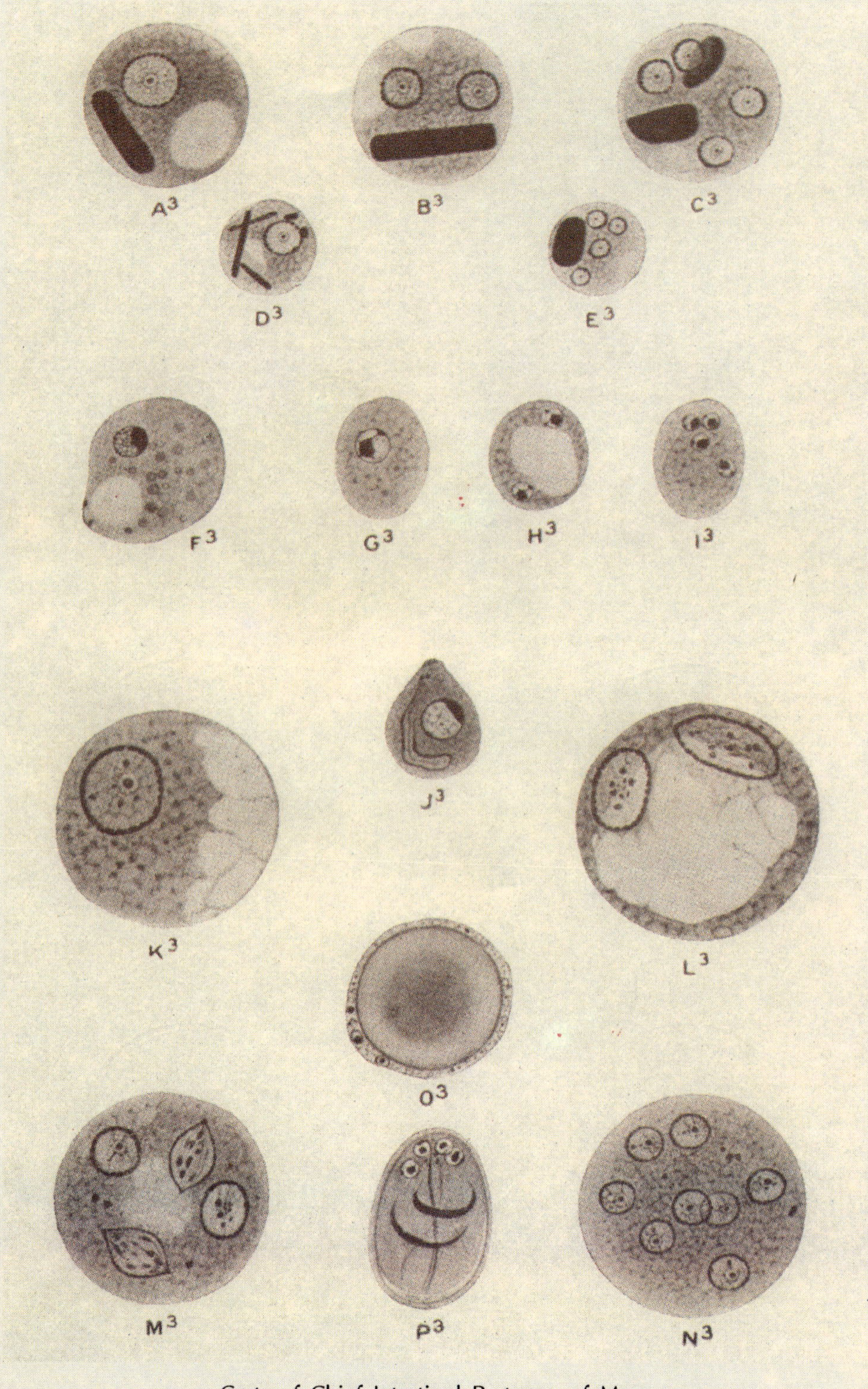

Cysts of Chief Intestinal Protozoa of Man.

TABLE 3.4

DIFFERENCE BETWEEN *E. HISTOLYTICA* AND *E. COLI* PL.III.IV

E. HISTOLYTICA	*E. COLI*
A. Trophozoite	
OCCURRENCE: Fairly abundant in amoebic dysentery stools	Not abundant in stools (see pathogenicity)
SIZE: 10 to 30 μ	20 to 40 μ
OUTLINE: Shows finger-like pseudopodia when fresh	Pseudopodia not prominent
MOTILITY: Actively motile	Sluggishly motile
Cytoplasm	
ECTOPLASM: Prominent	Not prominent
ENDOPLASM: Finely granular with ingested RBCs	Coarsely granular loaded with bacteria, yeasts, etc., but never with RBCs
VACUOLES: Scanty, spherical and defined	Often numerous, clefts and cracks are seen
Nucleus	
SALINE PREPARATION: Indistinct and small	Distinct and large
STAINED: Nuclear membrane uniformly studded with chromatin; karyosome is central	Nuclear membrane shows chromatin irregularly stained; karyosome eccentric
B. Precystic Stage	
SIZE: 5 to 15 μ	12 to 17 μ
C. Cyst	
SIZE: 6 to 18 μ	10 to 30 μ
CHROMATOID BODY: Present with rounded ends; they are bar-like	Absent; pointed, needle-like or like splintered glass with square-cut or pointed ends
NUMBER OF NUCLEI: Usually one or four	Usually two or eight
NUCLEUS: Not visible when unstained	Visible when unstained
Kiodophilic vacuole: Prominent in uninucleate phase	Largest in two-nucleate phase

FEATURES OF AMOEBA (Naegleria)

Size: 6μ to 15μ in diameter

Shape: Slug-shaped with a broad and a pointed end ("LIMAX" FORM)

Nucleus: Large, single 2μ with a nucleolus and delicate nuclear membrane.

Cysts: Uninucleate with double cyst-wall.

Intranasal inoculation into mice caused meningo-encephalitis; animals died in 5 days.

Human Infections: These occur from nasopharyngeal contamination while swimming in heavily infected water. I.p. is 7 days. Organisms are neurotropic. Cerebral invasion occurs through olfactory nerves. Exudate maximum in subarachnoid basal cistern (neutrophils 50%, macrophages 50% and amoebae). CSF protein and sugar is higher than in pyogenic meningitis.

Diagnosis: Unstained preparations show typical amoebae.

Differential Diagnosis: Acute pyogenic meningitis.

Prognosis: Illness is 108 hours; rapid fatal if untreated.

TREATMENT

1. Large doses of sulphadiazine along with amphotericin B are helpful.

METASTATIC AMOEBIC LESIONS PL.III.VII.

(See complications of Amoebic Liver Abscess)

Cerebral Amoebiasis. rare complication of liver/lung abscess. Abscess is single; affect one hemisphere.

Pulmonary Amoebiasis. This is rarely primary, or secondary, as a complication of liver abscess, a solitary abscess at right lung base.

Cutaneous Amoebiasis. See "Amoeboma".

Splenic Abscess. Occurs by transmission of trophozoite adherent splenic flexure.

Enumeration of Pathological Lesions of *E. histolytica* According to Sites

A. Intestinal Amoebiasis (of Large gut).

1. Acute Amoebiasis Dysentery: Multiple, deep extensive ulcers.

2. Chronic Intestinal Amoebiasis (Amoebic Dysentery).
   - (a) Single caecal or sigmoidal ulcer.
   - (b) Multiple, small superficial ulcers or healed ulcers may be pigmented throughout the large bowel.
   - (c) Thickened caecum or colon; (Cicatrix).

B. Extra-Intestinal Amoebiasis

1. **Hepatic Amoebiasis**
   - (i) Multiple miliary abscesses.
   - (ii) Solitary large abscess in the postero-superior surface of the right lobe.
2. **Pulmonary Amoebiasis**
   - (i) *Primary lesion*: Multiple, small abscesses.
   - (ii) *Secondary lesion*: Solitary abscess (variable size) Right lower lobe.
3. **Skin:** Amoebic granuloma (Amoeboma) commonly occurs in perianal region.
4. **Urogenital System:** Recto-vesical or recto-vaginal fistula. Direct abscess causing amoebic vaginitis and penile ulcer.
5. **Spleen:** Splenic abscess; rare.
6. **Brain:** Small, solitary abscess. para-

NON-PATHOGENIC AMOEBAE

ENTAMOEBA COLI (Grassi, 1879) Hickson, 1909

Habitat. large gut, does not invade tissue.

Morphology (Fig 3.18).

(a) **Trophozoite Form**. 20 to 40μ in diameter, narrow zone of ectoplasm (not prominent); *endoplasm* more opaque contains nucleus. *Karyosome* in nucleus is eccentric. *Cytoplasm* contains food particles in food vacuoles but no *RBC* against.

(b) **Cyst**. 17μ, has eight nuclei, with *Iodine* nuclei and glycogen massess well marked in two-nucleate phase (PL.III.VF).

Pathogenicity. It is non-pathogenic.

Very high population of *E. coli* in human gut is associated with (a) *leucoplakia* of buccal mucosa or tongue, (b) *dyspepsia*, (c) hyperacidity and gastritis.

For differentiating points see Table 3.4.

ENTAMOEBA GINGIVALIS (Gros, 1894) Brumpt, 1913

Habitat. The tartar of teeth, pus pockets of pyorrhoea alveolaris.

Morphology. (Fig 3.18, 7). *Trophozoite* is 10 to 20μ, characters are like *E. coli*. The ectoplasm is clear with rapid pseudopodial activity. It is a voracious feeder, ingesting bacteria.

The nucleus is ring type with characteristics of the genus Entamoeba, clearly visible in saline as a refractile ring, a large central or eccentric karysome. Chromatin uniformly distributed in nuclear membrane. Cystic form unknown.

Pathogenesis. It is present in pyorrhoea alveolaris and supposed to cause pyorrhoea.

ENDOLIMAX NANA (Wenyon and O'Connor, 1917) Brug, 1918

Habitat. Commonest amoeba of Intestine.

Morphology. (Fig. 3.19: 1-4) *Trophozoite* is 5 to 15μ, ectoplasm, fairly differentiated movement sluggish, trace of ectoplasm with pseudopodia, granular endoplasm. Greenish, Nucleus inconspicuous with Chromatin and prominent karyosome.

Cysts are oval—5 to 14μ and contain one, two or four nuclei. Karyosome comparatively large, eccentric chromatoid body may be absent, present in filamentous forms in four-nucleate cysts.

Pathogenicity. It is nonpathogenic.

IODAMOEBA BUTSCHLII (Prowazek, 1912) Dobell, 1919

Habitat. Colon; never invades tissues.

Morphology. Rarely seen in its vegetative form *Trophozoite*. 9-13μ. *Precyst*. one-nucleate body with vacuoles, volutin granules, nucleus big, karyosome large, small chromatin granules between nucleus and nuclear membrane (Fig. 3.19 : 5-7).

Cysts. 9-12μ, refractile, glycogen vacuole stain deep with Iodine. Nucleus pushed near nuclear membrane in matured cysts, cysts produce basket-like appearance with large eccentric, karyosome which lies near the nuclear membrane.

Pathogenicity. Not pathogenic to men.

DIENTAMOEBA FRAGILIS (Jepps and Dobell, 1918)

Small active amoeba, 7-12μ connected with centrodesums. Recently divided amoebae are uni-nucleate with centrodesmus, quickly disintegrates in faeces, Cyst not known, nonpathogenic.

EXPLANATIONS OF PLATE 3.IX(1), 3.IX(2) AND 3.IX(3)

Semidiagrammatic figures of cysts of *Chief Intestinal Protozoa of Man* for aid to diagnosis (Drawn from actual specimens; × 2000 diameters throughout. (From *Intestinal Protozoa of Man by* Dobell and O'Connor, 1921; reproduced by kind permission of Staples Printers Ltd., London, successors to John Bale, Sons and Danielsson, Ltd.)

Plate 3.IX (1). Saline preparation, unstained—labelled as A, B, C, etc.

Plate 3.IX (2). Iodine preparation, stained—labelled as A2, B2, C2, etc.

Plate 3.IX (3). Stained with iron haemotoxylin—labelled as A3, B3, C3, etc.

Figs. A, B, C. 1-nucleate, 2-nucleate and 4-nucleate cysts, respectively, of *Entamoeba histolytica* ca* 12μ in diameter

Figs. D, E. 1-nucleate and 4-nucleate cysts of *E. histolytica*, a strain with small cysts, ca 7.5μ in diameter.

Fig. F. Mature 1-nucleate cysts of *Iodamoeba butschlii.*

Figs. G, H, I. 1-nucleate, -nucleate and 4-nucleate cyst respectively of *Endolimax nana*. (H is a cyst containing a lump of glycogen).

FIg. J. Mature 1-nucleate cyst of *Chilomastix mesnili.*

Figs. K, L, M, N. 1-nucleate, 2-nucleate, 4-nucleate and 8-nucleate cyst, respectively, of *Entamoeba coli.*

Fig. O. A specimen of *Blastocystis hominis* (for comparison).

Fig. P. A 4-nucleate cyst of *Giardia intestinalis.*

*ca means approximately

CHAPTER 4

SUBPHYLUM : SARCOMASTIGOPHORA

SUPERCLASS : MASTIGOPHORA (FLAGELLATES)

Class II : ZOOMASTIGOPHOREA

General characters. Movement of parasites of this group occurs by flagella.

According to infection site organisms of class Mastigophora (FLAGELLATES) are divided into 2 groups:

(A) INTESTINAL AND ANTRAL FLAGELLATES. In intestinal canal, antrum of oral cavity and genital tract. Few are nonpathogenic. They are classified into 2 orders: (a) Protomonadida characterised by 1 nucleus and flagella anteriorly (b) Diplomonadida has 2 nuclei and flagella, symmetrically distributed anteriorly.

(B) HAEMOFLAGELLATES in blood and invade body tissues remain either in intercellular fluid, Trypanosoma, or are engulfed by the RE cells and leucocytes as in Leishmania. Of 6 genera, pathogenic parasites belong to 2 genera under Trypanosomatide, family, e.g., Trypanosoma and Leishmania.

Classification. See Table 4.1.

TABLE 4.1

CLASSIFICATION OF PATHOGENIC FLAGELLATES OF THE CLASS ZOOMASTIGOPHOREA AND SUBCLASS ZOOMASTIGINA

ORDER	GENUS	SPECIES	HABITAT	PATHOGENICITY
Protomonadida	Enteromonas	*E. hominis*	Intestine	Doubtful
	Chilomastix	*C. mesnili*	Caecum	Not known
	Retortamonas	*R. intestinalis*	Intestine	Doubtful
	Trichomonas	*T. hominis*	Ileocaecal region	Doubtful
		T. vaginalis	Vagina	Vaginitis
		T. tenax	Teeth & Gum	Commensal
	Leishmania	*L. donovani*	Blood	Kala-azar and Dermal leishmanoid
		L. tropica	Skin	Oriental sore
		L. braziliensis	Mucocutaneous tissue	Espundia
	Trypanosoma	*T. gambiense*	Blood	African sleeping sickness
		T. rhodesiense	Blood	,, (acute)
		T. cruzi	Blood	Chagas' disease
Diplomonadida	Giardia	*G. intestinalis*	Duodenum and jejunum	Chronic diarrhoea

INTESTINAL AND ANTRAL FLAGELLATES

General characters. They have two phases in life cycle trophozoite and the cystic stages.

TROPHOZOITE STAGE is characterised by 2 to 5 flagella arising from a *blepharoplast*. An *undulating membrane* is supported by a basal fibre called *costa*, but costa is absent in some. In some species, an *axostyle*, a central supporting rod and a *cytostome* (rudimentary mouth) is present. Nuclear characters are distinctive. *Nucleus* contains a *nuclear membrane* and a central *karyosome*, 2 nuclei occur in trophozoite *Giardia intestinalis*. Cytoplasm contains volutin granules in certain species. *Reproduction* occurs by BINARY FISSION of the blepharoplast followed by *nuclear* division and cytoplasm resulting in longitudinal splitting of the body into two.

CYSTIC STAGE. It is a protective resting stage. Mature cysts, excreted in faeces, are infective.

Life cycle. The flagellates complete their life cycle in a single host, and a second host whom they infect is necessary for the continuation of species. Cysts when swallowed with contaminated food—liberate trophozoites in the intestine (excystation); which multiply.

Cultivation. Except *G. intestinalis*, other species are cultivated (*E. histolytica* medium-Appendix II).

CHILOMASTIX MESNILI (Wenyon, 1910) Alexeieff, 1912

This is a non-pathogenic flagellate found in cases of diarrhoea due to some other cause.

Morphology. (Fig. 1.1; 1 & 2). Trophozoite form. These are pear-shaped, motile organisms, 10 to 15μ by 5μ, tapering posteriorly.

Cysts are 7 to 10μ in length and appear as double contoured lemon-shaped bodies.

RETORTAMONAS INTESTINALIS (Wenyon and O'Conner, 1917) Wenrich, 1932

Synonym: *Embadomonas intestinalis*

There are rare commensals of the small or large intestine. The Trophozoites are small elongated bodies, 4-9μ by 3 to 4.5μ the CYSTS are pear-shaped. 4 to 5μ in length, containing a single nucleus; (Fig. 1.1 : 3-4).

ENTEROMONAS HOMINIS de Fonseca, 1915

It is a commensal of the small/large intestine of man. In the TROPHOZOITE form 8μ 4μ (Fig. 1.1; 5). The cysts are almost of the same size as the trophozoite (Fig. 1.1; 6-7). It is a harmless commensal.

FAMILY : *TRICHOMONADIDAE* Wenyon, 1926

GENUS : *TRICHOMONAS* Donne, 1837

They are seen in diarrhoeic stools, having only trophozoite form; cystic form is absent. They are actively motile, pear-shaped, 7-15μ long with anterior portion rounded, posterior portion tapering and a mouth-like cleft at the side. They have a nucleus single, ovoid at anterior end. They have 3-5 free anterior flagella, thicker one passes back along the side of the body forming undulating membrane and coming out free at the posterior end. The undulating membrane is supported at its base by a rod-like structure called *costs*. *Axostyle* runs posteriorly down the middle of the body ending in a pointed tail-like extremity.

Classification. I. INTESTINAL. 1. *Trichomonas hominis*, inhabiting ileoceacal region.

II. ANTRAL. 1. *Trichomonas vaginalis* inhabiting vagina and urinary tract (males and females). 2. *Trichomonas tenax*, in tartar and pyorrhoea sockets. of oral cavity.

TRICHOMONAS HOMINIS da Fonseca, 1915

Intestine commensal in diarrhoeic stool. It is of doubtful pathogenicity.

TRICHOMONAS VAGINALIS Donne, 1837

It causes trichomonas vaginitis closely related to *T. hominis*. present in leucorrhoeic discharge in females.

Diagnosis. In females *T. vaginalis* is present in sedimented urine, vaginal secretion or scraping, but in males in the urine or in prostatic secretion after prostatic massage.

Prophylaxis. Male and female partners are treated at the same time (contracted by sexual intercourse). Its control and prevention requires patience and discipline.

Treatment. Metronidazole (Flagyl, Metron)

Dose. 1 tablet 3 times daily for 3 weeks.

Topical therapy combined with oral medication gives satisfactory results. *Locally* suppositories containing iodohydroxyquinoline (di-iodoquine, vioform, etc.) or oxytet-

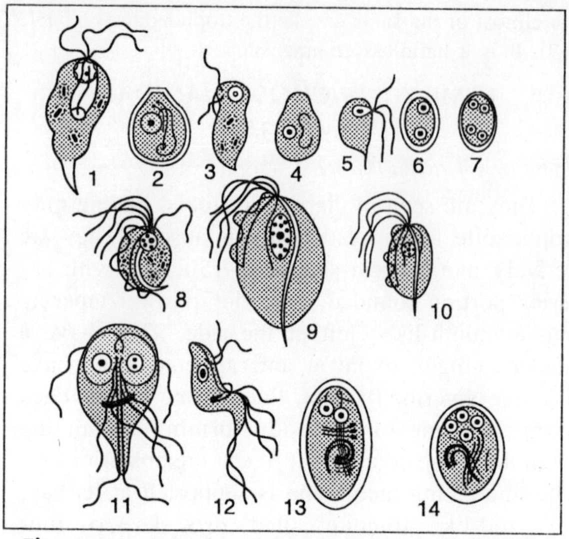

Fig. 4.1 Intestinal and antral flagellates, × 1000 approx

1 and 2 *Chilomastrix mesnili*; 1–Active flagellate and 2–Cyst. 3 and 4–*Retortamonas intestinalis*; 3–Active flagellate form; 4 Cyst. 5-7–*Enteromonas hominis*; 5–Active flagellate form; 6 and 7 Cyst. 8–*Trichomonas hominis*. 9–*T. vaginalis*, 10–*T. tenax*. 11-14–*Giardia lamblia*; 11 and 12–Active flagellate form; front and profile views; 13 and 14–Binucleate and tetranucleate cysts. Adapted from Dobell and O'Connor, 1921. Wenyon, 1922, and others.

racycline may be of use to kill the secondary organisms. Lactic acid solution douche, to alter *p*H to acid side. Cure is expected provided reinfection does not occur. In males, oxytetracycline ointment into urethra and irrigation; by antibiotic solution. Oral diodoquine or antibiotics may be helpful. Gynosan tablet push may be helpful.

TRICHOMONAS TENAX

(O. F. Muller, 1773)

Dobell, 1939

It is like *T. vaginalis* but smaller and more slender. (5-12μ) and has 4 free flagella; the fifth one is on the margin of the undulating membrane, which does not reach up to the posterior end. The *axostyle* is thick with granular cytoplasm. *Nucleus* is ovoid, vesicular, few chromatin granules. Cytostome is near anterior end opposite the undulating membrane. They are in pus of pyorrhoea alveolaris.

GIARDIA INTESTINALIS

(Lambl, 1859), Stiles, 1915

SYNONYM: Giardia lamblia, Lamblia intestinalis.

Morphology. It exists in 2 forms; trophozoite and cyst (Fig. 1.1; 11-14).

TROPHOZOITE FORM (Fig. 1.1; 11-12). These are on its own axis moving flagellates; live in upper small Intestine, appear in diarrhoeic stools. They are rocket-shaped when lying flat, 10 to 16μ by 7μ. In *profile* (side) view, pear-shaped, concave ventrally, and convex dorsally; ventral surface has a central sucking disc with a raised circumference by which they fix to Intestinal epithelium, 4 pair of *flagella* arising from anterior end. A pairs of rod-like *axostyle* runs down the centre of the body near ventral surface. In the anterior part paired nuclei are characteristic. Comma-shaped chromatoid bar (*parabasal body*) is near the middle across (dorsum to axostyle).

CYSTS (Fig. 1.1; 13-14). In *saline* preparations cysts are oval 12 μ by 8 μ. Containing 2 or 4 nuclei at the anterior end. Cysts show remains of flagella across axostyle (Fig. 1.1; 13-14; PL. III.IX, p[1], p[2], p[3]).

In *iodine* preparations (Pl. III.IX, p[2]) the structures appear more clearly defined.

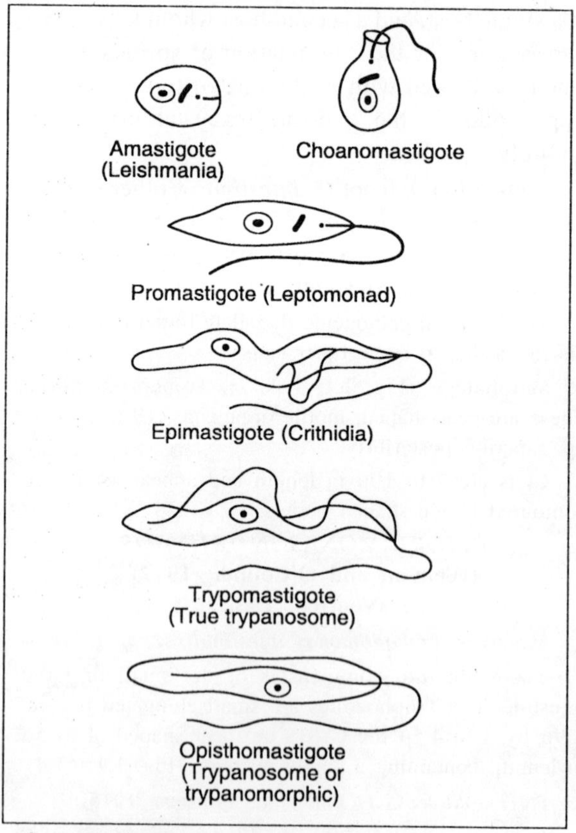

Fig. 4.2 Showing morphological forms of genera Leishmania and Trypanosoma

CULTIVATION: Successfully cultivated in a medium comprising of : 1. Chick Embryo Extract 2. Human Serum 3. Hottinger's Digest 4. Hank's Solution 5. Yeast organism "*Candida guiller-mondi*".

LIFE CYCLE

Parasite multiplies in small intestine by binary fission. Under unfavourable condition (*p*H) in duodenum, undergo cyst formation (encystment) in large gut, secrete a *thick resistant wall*; divide *into two* cysts and are excreted in stool.

Infection occurs by ingesting cysts. After $^1/_2$ hour, each cyst hatches out two trophozoites and each trophozoite by binary fission multiply in large number and remain in duodenum. To escape the high acidity which sometimes occur in the duodenum, they localise in biliary tract and gall bladder.

Pathogenicity. Doubtful; found in chronic intractable diarrhoea or dysentery.

By the sucking disc trophozoite attaches to the convex margin of intestinal epithelial cells leading to fat malabsorption, causing looseness of bowels, passage of yellowish greasy stool (mild steatorrhoea). Mucus may be present (enteritis and enterocolitis). Toxic allergic effects occur.

CLINICAL STYDY.

There may be following features:

1. Silent, symptomless giardiasis.
2. Acute enterocolitis.
3. Chronic enteritis (Steatorrhoeic).
4. With or without enteritis—Fever, Anaemia. and allergy may occur.
5. Chronic cholecystopathy.
6. TRIAD OF : (A) CHOLECYSTO-DUODENAL PAIN, (B) LOOSE FROTHY STOOL, (C) EMACIATION are characteristic features.

TABLE 4.2

DEVELOPMENTAL FORMS OF HAEMOFLAGELLATES IN DIFFERENT HOSTS

Haemoflagellates	Amastigote (Leishmania) form	Promastigote (Leptomonad) form	Epimastigote (Crithidial) form	Trypomastigote (Trypanosomal) form	
				Metacyclic	Mature
Leishmania					
L. donovani (Kala-Azar)	Human (blood and RE cells)	Mid-gut of sandflies and in culture	—	—	—
L. tropica (Oriental Sore)	**Skin** (RE cells)	"	—	—	—
L. braziliensis	**Mucocutaneous** (RE cells)	"	—	—	
Trypanosoma					
T. gambiense } *T. rhodesiense* } (Sleeping Sickness)	—	—	Salivary gland of the insect vector (Glossina) and culture	Salivary gland of the insect vector (transfer stage)	Human (Blood)
T. cruzi (Chagas' Disease)	Human (Intracellular macrophages of liver, spleen, lymph node, skin, brain, heart, etc.)	Human (Transitional stage only)	In the mid-gut of insect vector (triatomid bug)	Faeces of the triatomid bug, (the transfer stage in insect vector)	Human (Blood)

Immunology. No antibody.

Diagnosis. Cysts are present in the stool and these are often confused with cysts of *Chilomastix mesnili* which are pear-shaped and show only one nucleus instead of two or four (Cf. Fig. 1.1; 2).

Bile and Duodenal fluid sample (*duodenal intubation*) shows Trophozoites.

Treatment. Mepacrine hydrochloride or Atebrin (9-aminoacridine). Adult dose 0.1 gm T.D.P.C. for 5 days. For children $^1/_3$ or $^1/_2$ tablet (0.1 g) is administered according to age, thrice daily for 3 days. Orcamoquin (amodiaquine) hydrochloride 0.2 g B.D.P.C. for 5 days. The course is repeated, or Metronidazole 400 mg. Bi. D. for 21 days.

EVALUATION STAGES OF LEISHMANIA AND TRYPANOSOMATID FLAGELLATES

New terminologies have evolved. Leishmania and Trypanosomes on the basis of International Code of Zoological Nomenclature based on the characteristics of flagellates as well as at the point of emergence of flagella in relation to Kinetoplast. These are described as follows:

1. **Amastigote form:** Former *leishmania form.* Genera Leishmania, Trypanosomes, rounded forms; no *flagella* (Mastigos).
2. **Promastigote form:** Former leptomonad form having kinetoplast *antinuclear* flagellum arises from anterior part of body.
3. **Epimastigote form:** Former crithidial form having kinetoplast lying anterior and close to nucleus (*juxtanuclear*). Flagellum arises near kinetoplast from one side of body to run along a short undulating membrane.
4. **Trypomastigote form:** Former trypanosomal form (Trypanom = to bore; soma = body), having kinetoplast posterior to nucleus near posterior end (*postnuclear*). Flagellum arises near the kinetoplast and emerges from one side of the body to run along undulating membrane.
5. **Metacylic trypomastigote stage:** These are short, stumpy forms of trypomastigotes in late stage. This is the infective stage.

The other terminologies of not related to the genera of medical importance are, however, given below:

6. **Opisthomastigote form:** This terminology is restricted to genus '*Herpetomonas*'.

HAEMOFLAGELLATES

(*Flagellates of both blood and tissues*)
Family: *Trypanosomatidae*
Doffein, 1901

General Characters. It has elongated body, flattened and lancet-shaped, a single vesicular nucleus with Leishman, shows irregular granules and large central karyosome. Organ of locomotion is a single flagellum, from one end of the body to the opposite end along the outer margin forming a frilled outgrowth, the undulating membrane. The flagellum starts from a blepharoplast near parabasal body, disc-shaped rounded, or rod-shaped, Blepharoplast and parabasal body form *kinetoplast* which stains as chromatin.

Morphology. BODY is elongated, may be curved with a flagellum in the Trypanosomes (Trypomastigote). Leptomonad (Promastigote), Crithidia (Epimastigote), but non-flagellate and ovoid in Leishmania (Amastigote).

Nucleus, large, round or oval, central (on one side in Leishmania). It is concerned with nutritive function, called *trophonucleus*.

Kinetoplast (*blepharoplast and parabasal body*) is smaller than nucleus, elongated or rod-shaped, before or behind nucleus. (In *Trypomastigote* posterior, in *Epimastigote* and *Promastigote* anterior to nucleus. In *Promastigotes* near anterior pole).

FLAGELLUM is thin hair-like arising from belpharoplast and comes out from anterior end; absent in Leishmania.

UNDULATING MEMBRANE is flagellum, which curves and thrown into folds.

THE AXONEME or, RHIZOPLAST is the intracellular remnant of the flagellum.

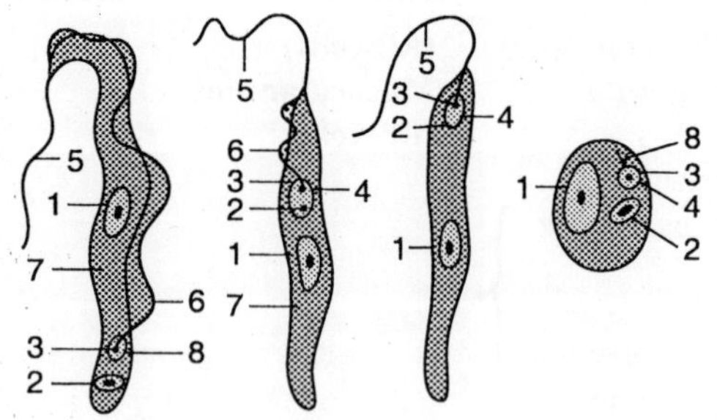

Fig. 4.3 Morphology of haemoflagellates
A. Trypomastigote (Trypanosome). B. Epimastigote (Crithidia). C. Promastigote (Leptomonad). D. Amastigote (Leishmania). 1. Nucleus. . Kinetoplast. 3. Basal granule or blepharoplast. 4. Vacuole 5. Flagellum. 6. Undulating membrane. 7. Volutin granules. 8. Axoneme

Multiplication. Longitudinal binary fission. Basal granule and kinetoplast divide into 2; 1 daughter kinetoplast retains old flagellum; form new flagellum in basal granule, accompanying the second kinetoplast. Nucleus divides. In trypanosome, longitudinal fission occurs from anterior end. 2 daughter trypanosomes separate. Sexual phenomenon not known.

Nutrition. Trypanosomes have no mouth. They absorb food by osmosis.

Life Cycle. Both Leishmania and Trypanosomes developing in two hosts, i.e., man/animal representing definitive/final host, a blood sucking insect vector is intermediate host, transmitting infection. In both hosts, stages of development occurs (1) *Trypomastigote* (*Trypanosome*) (2) *Epimastigote* (*Crithidial*) (3) *Promastigote* (*Leptomonad*) and (4) *Amastigote* (*Leishmania*) stages. All these are modifications of Trypanosomal form but amastigote (*Leishmania*) stage arises from any form by loss of flagellum and rounding up the body under unfavourable/degenerated condition. By developing flagellum and body elongation, amastigote develops into flagellate form.

Amastigote (*Leishmania*) form is a constant stage in Leishmania and *T. cruzi*.

In Genus Leishmania, 2 stages of development are seen : (a) *Amastigote* (Leishmania) in *human host*, and (b) *Promastigote* (Leptomonad) in insect *vector*, and *culture*, Members of trypanosoma genus assume all stages, in life cycle.

Classification. In Haemoflagellates out of 6 genera, 2 are Medically important; *Trypanosoma*, and *Leishmania*.

Morphological Forms (Fig. 4.2 & 4.3)

1. Amastigote (Leishmania) Form. 2 to 4μ long oval with a nucleus (trophonucleus), stains lightly. Deeply stained portion is *kinetoplast* and *axoneme*. The kinetoplast consists of parabasal body and Blepharoplast, Near the former a vacuole is found (Fig. 4.3-6). Parasite is intracellular, in tissues of *vertebrate* host (K-A) and *T. cruzi*.

(2) Promastigote (Leptomonad) Form. Body is elongated, contains volutin granules. Nucleus is near the middle and kinetoplast is in anterior portion and a vacuole near it. From the blepharoplast, a flagellum arises, passes through the anterior part of the body (Fig. 4.3-C). This form is found in invertebrate host and culture (of Leishmania).

(3) Epimastigote (Crithidia) Form. This is elongated form nucleus near middle; kinetoplast anterior to nucleus. From blepharoplast flagellum arises forming undulating membrane (Fig. 4.3-B). This form is in invertebrate host and culture.

(4) Trypomastigote (Trypanosomal) Form. Body is elongated, contain coarse volutin granules in the middle, kinetoplast is at posterior end. The flagellum and frill-like undulating membrane pass anteriorly (Fig. 4.3-A). This is in peripheral blood of vertebrate host.

METACYCLIC TRYPOMASTIGOTE (*Trypanosome*). This is the final stage of development of trypanosomes at the end of cyclic development in vector. This differs biologically and morphologically from other types. After ingestion of blood by Tsetse fly, in which cyclic development occurs, the trypanosome develops into crithidial form followed by metacyclic form resembling the mature form, infecting mammalian host, blood. It is shorter and more stumpy. This represents the infective stage, transmitted to new mammalian host. The *cyclic*

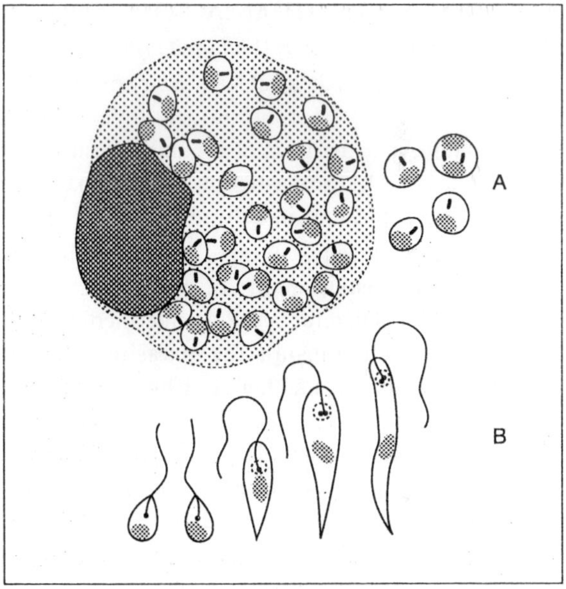

Fig. 4.4 Amastigote (Leishmania) and Promastigote (Leptomonad) forms of *L. donovani* ; × 1600 approx. A–L-D bodies in an endothelial cell and extracellular. B–Promastigote (Leptomonad) forms as seen in the sandfly and culture

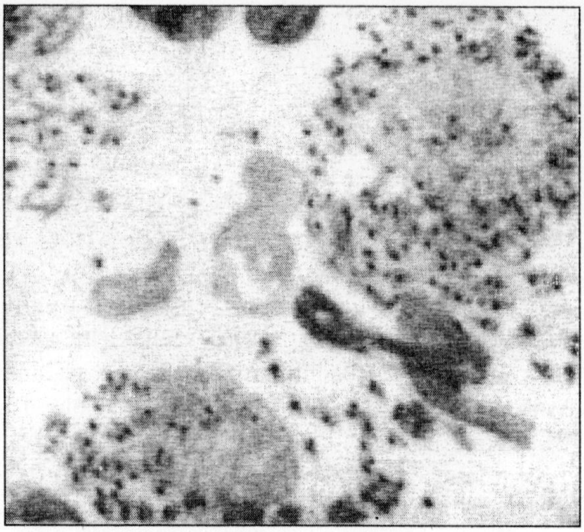

Fig. 4.5 *Leishmania donovani* in the endothelial cells which are distended with the parasite

method of transmission is differentiated from the *mechanical method* of transmission by the contaminated mouth part within a few hours without the development stage in the vector. Development forms —See Table 4.2.

GENUS : LEISHMANIA ROSS, 1903

(*named after Sir William Leishman*)

It includes parasites of Kala-azar, oriental sore and Espundia. 2 Morphological developmental stages. (a) Amastigote (Leishmania) form and in vertebrate host (b) Promastigote (Leptomonad) form in sandfly vector, and in culture (Figs. 4.4 & 4.5).

They are parasites of man, dog, gerbil, other rodents (final hosts); sandfly of genus Phlebotomus blood-sucking Diptera, serve as intermediate hosts (vectors) which transmit the parasite from one mammalian host to another. Leishmania produces 2 types of lesion, (1) *visceral leishmaniasis* (Kala-azar), (2) *cutaneous leishmaniasis* (Oriental sore) including variant of mucocutaneous leishmaniasis or Espundia in South America.

L. infantum of Mediterranean Kala-azar is synonymous with *L. donovani*.

Species differentiation of 3 leishmania is based on agglutination of cultured Promastigotes leishmania, parasitic with **hyperimmune rabbit sera** (rapid side agglutination technique).

LEISHMANIA DONOVANI

Ross, 1903

(Causative organism of Kala-azar)

Kala-azar or visceral leishmaniasis caused by *L. donovani* is characterised by irregular fever, progressive enlargement of spleen and liver. Cachexia skin pigmentation voracious perverted appetite, and complications, like epistaxis, cancrum oris, skin infection, pulmonary affections, diarrhoea, dysentery and oedema of the feet. Blood picture shows pancytopenia.

Geographical distribution. China, Sudan, Tropical Africa, S. America. In India, in Assam, Bengal, Bihar, Chennai, eastern U.P.

SPECIES PARASITIC TO HUMAN

Species	Disease produced
Leishmania donovani	Kala-azar (visceral leishmaniasis) and dermal leishmanoid
Leishmania tropica	Oriental sore
Leishmania braziliensis	Espundia in Central & South America

Habitat. (1) Amastigote parasite occurs in cells of RE system; spleen, liver, bone-marrow. (2) Promastigote (leptomonad) form occurs in gut of *Phlebotomus argentipes*.

MORPHOLOGY

I. PARASITE IN THE MAMMALIAN HOST. AMASTIGOTES (*Leishmania*) (Fig. 4.5) in mammalian host are small, ovoid 2.5-4.5 μ by 1.5-.5 μ, called Leishman-Donovan (L-D) bodies (Fig. 4.3-D, 4.4 and 4.5).

Parasite is biconvex, dorsal surface flatter than ventral one. *Nucleus* lies on the convex side of the parasite (ventrally). With Leishman (Romanowsky stain), 2 purple bodies are seen in it. The larger one, the nucleus, is more nucleus lightly stained and opposite to it is deeply stained *kinetoplast*. Rudimentary flagellum arising from blepharoplast (Fig. 4.3-D). Cytoplasm stains light blue with a vacuole between nucleus and kinetoplast, taking eosin stain in mature flagellate phase. Parasites multiply in endothelial (mononuclear), cells by binary fission (rosette formation seen with 4 to 12 parasites).

PROMASTIGOTE (*Leptomonad*) FORM (Fig. 4.4-C). Insects (sandflies) are intermediate hosts (vectors) females are blood-suckers.

When a sandfly vector feeds on a reservoir host (infected man, dog, wild rodent) amastigotes are taken with blood meal into mid-gut. *Promastigotes* multiply rapidly. By 3rd day, masses of flagellates are set free in the lumen from gut wall. They are numerous in anterior part (proventriculus) of mid-gut, and extend forward. By 5th day, they reach oesophagus and pharynx. By 7th day they block the passage. After a second feed, Promastigotes are found on 9th day in pharynx and biting parts.

Promastigotes have pyriform bodies with broad anterior (flagellum emerges) and a tapering posterior end. They are 10μ to 20μ by 2 to 3μ. Single flagellum is of the body length. Multiplication occurs by ***longitudinal binary fission***, flagellates form rosette. Nucleus is central, parabasal body lies transversely near anterior end, before which is the flagellum root and eosinophilic vacuole.

To summarise Morphology:

AMASTIGOTE FORM

In man Definitive Host; Parasites colonise in RE System (Bone marrow, Liver, Spleen, Lymph nodes). Found also in Dogs and Hamsters.

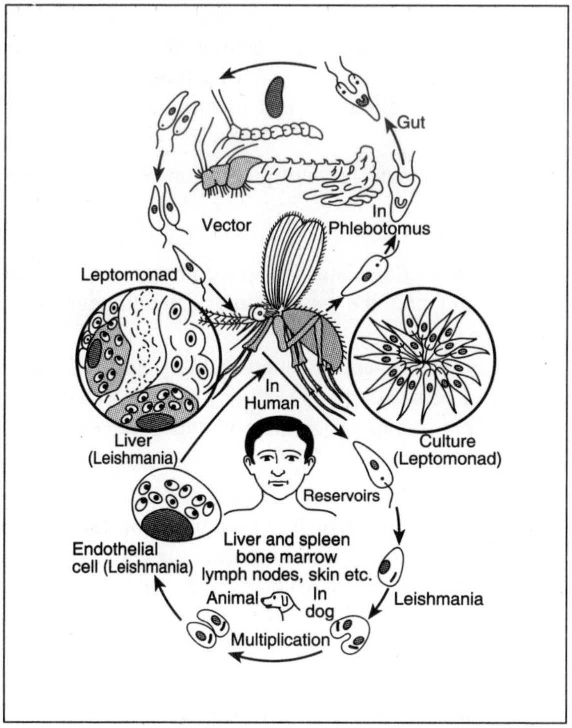

Fig. 4.6 Life cycle of *Leishmania donovani*

Size: 2–4μm.

Shape: Round to oval

Cell membrane: Delicate

Nucleus: 1μm in diameter alongside cell wall in the central part of the body.

Kinetoplast: At right angles or, tangentially to the nucleus; comprises mitochondrial structure or DNA.

Axoneme (Rhizoplast): Delicate filamentous structure from kinetoplast to body margin. It is the flagellar root.

Vaculole: A clear space alongside axoneme.

PROMASTIGOTE FORM

(Flagellar Form)
(In Sandllies, Intermediate Host; and In Culture)

Size: 5-10μm. 2-3μm. in early stage, 15-20μm. 1-2μm. in late stage.

Shape: Long, tapering, Slender leaf-like.

Nucleus: Centrally placed.

Kinetoplast: Transversely placed near anterior end.

Eosinophilic Vacuole: In front of kinetoplast (the root of flagellum).

Flagellum: Of the same length as the body or longer, from anterior end NO UNDULATING MEMBRANE.

Cultivation. The material obtained from peripheral blood, sternum, liver, spleen puncture (Appendix I) is inoculated into water of condensation of NNN (Novy, Mac Neal and Nicolle) Sanekjio's medium (*Ascorbic acid* and *haematin* favour growth). 4 culture tubes taken, each is examined weekly up to 4 weeks, incubated at 22°C to 28°C. In culture amastigotes change to large number of promastigotes, as actively multiply by longitudinal binary fission. For staining, see Appendix I.

Intracellular growth (*L. donovani*) stays in tissue culture (37°C) for a month.

Susceptible Animals: Dogs are naturally infected, Chinese hamsters (*Cricetulus* griseus) and ground squirrels are susceptible, the latter is reservoir, Mice are less, Rats and guinea-pigs are non-susceptible.

Immunology: Promastigotes enter the body by sandfly bites, change to Amastigotes, which cause

Cell-Mediated Immune Reaction. Mono-nuclear cells proliferate in *Spleen, Liver, Bone-marrow, Lymph nodes and Skin*.

Amastigotes (L-D bodies) enormously multiply in RE cells, which are destroyed by two processes:

(i) Cellular immunity reaction (cytotoxicity and cytolysis).

(ii) Spontaneous bursting of cells—enormous release of Amastigotes.

There is lack of humoral Immune response due to *Immuno-suppressive effect of parasites*. Cellular immunity and delayed hypersensitivity to Leishmania antigen *develops* only *WHEN INFECTION IS CONTROLLED*.

Hyper-gammaglobulinaemia which occurs is non-protective but *responsible for* Formal-Gel (Aldehyde) Test. Reversal of A : G ratio occurs (2.8 : 4.0).

Serological reactions:

1. CFT Positive in 3 weeks.
2. Antimony (Flocculent precipitation) Test–Positive after 6-8 weeks.
3. Aldehyde (Formol-Gel) Test: Positive after 3 months of infection.
4. Haemagglutination test (see later).
5. Fluorescent Antibody (Immuno-fluorescence) Test.

CFT & Formal Gel Test are popular. LIFE CYCLE OF *L. Donovani*.

Cycle occurs in stages in 2 hosts.

1. AMASTIGOTE (Leishmania) stage in man or dog (DEFINITIVE HOST).
2. PROMASTIGOTE (Leptomonad) in the Sandfly vector (INTERMEDIATE HOST).

IN HUMAN (Fig. 4.6). Flagellated PROMASTIGOTES enter the body through infected sandfly bite and events are as follows:

PATHOGENESIS

Parasites enter the Skin

↓

Engulfed by R.E. Cells

↓

Promastigotes develop into Amastigotes (L-D Bodies). In R.E. Cells.

↓

Amastigotes multiply by binary fission. R.E. Cells are packed with the parasites, enlarged, distended and burst (50 to 200 parasites are set free from each R.E. Cell).

↓

Free parasites pass to differant organs of the body and are engulfed by new R.E. Cells where they multiply and the cycle is repeated.

↓

In this way the entire Reticulo-endothelial system becomes progressively infected.

↓

A blood-sucking Sandfly draws Amastigotes (L-D BODIES) with its blood-meal (by bite of proboscis).

This occurs during the INCUBATION PERIOD of the disease, usually 2 to 4 months (but may be 10 days for heavy dose of promastigote inoculation).

Free parasites entering the circulation perchance are phagocytosed by neutrophils/monocytea macrophacea and destroyed.

IN SANDFLY (Fig. 4.7) : Amastigotes (L-D BODIES) taken with blood meal develop into Promastigote forms in the midgut of sandfly on the third day after blood meal.

↓

Promastigotes multiply by binary fission in enormous number.

↓

Multiplication takes place rapidly at 22°C–23°C and suitable humidity. On the 5th day the promastigotes gather round the proventricular end of the gut.

↓

Multiplication and forward propulsion continues till 7th day.

↓

Solid mass of flagellates fill up the proventricular end of the midgut and the oesophagus, extending up to the pharynx.

A heavy pharyngeal infection of the sandfly is usually observed between 6th and 9th day of its infected blood-meal. This is known as anterior station development.

↓

In certain sandflies heavy infection blocks the esophagus. Such sandflies at the time of sucking blood cause regurgitation of Promastigotes from their buccal cavity in the puncture by proboscis (biting organ) and infection results. Heavily infected sandflies also transmit the disease; their Salivary glands are never infected.

Epidemiology: 1. Transmission. Sandflies fed on fruit juice after an infective blood meal, developed heavy infection and were capable of infecting hamsters and mice exposed to bites of sandflies human volunteers exposed to bite of sandflies fed on raising after infective blood meal became infected. Thus, after 20 years, transmission of Kala-azar was finally proved.

2. **Vectors.** ***P. argentipes*** is the vector in India and ***P. major*** var. Chinensis in China, most prevalent in rural areas of low alluvial plains under 2000 ft. altitude. They do not fly far from the breeding place and seldom above the first floor. Life span is 2 weeks.

3. **Types of Disease.** Visceral leishmaniasis affect human and dogs. In man it is found in **4 different forms** :

(1) affects young adults (60 per cent) and children 2 to 15 years).
(2) **Infantile kala-azar** affects below 5 years.
(3) **Sudanese kala-azar** affects the same age group as Indian Kala-azar, affects skin, viscera and mucocutaneous area.
(4) Chinese type is like that found in India, parasites occur in lymph nodes.

4. Distribution of the Parasite:

RE CELLS of SPLEEN (Pulp Cells). LIVER (Kupffer Cells), BONE-MARROW (LITTORAL CELLS) and LYMPH NODES (pulp cells).

PATHOLOGY

L. donovani is parasite of RE CELLS. Parasites invade RE cells where they reside, multiply, and are distributed in LIVER, SPLEEN, BONE-MARROW, and LYMPH NODES. RE Cells proliferate to tackle parasites. So liver, spleen ENLARGE in size. In chronic cases, various biochemical changes are seen due to liver function derangement.

SPLEEN

Marcoscopical Appearance (PL. 4.I):

(i) Enormously enlarged.
(ii) Capsule stretched and thin; or thickened (Perisplenitis).
(iii) It is soft, friable cuts easily.
(iv) Cut surface–marked congestion and deep red. Alternate small areas of ELEVATIONS AND DEPRESSIONS (atrophy of lymphoid follicles). (proliferation of splenic pulp and RE Cells).

Microscopic Appearance (PL. 4.II):

(i) Marked dilatation and engorgement of blood sinuses.
(ii) The reticulum fibres and trabeculae are thin & atrophic.
(iii) Macrophages contain ingested blood cells (Hypersplenism).
(iv) Malpighian Corpuscles hyperplastic pulp tissue. Pressure atrophy by
(v) Plasma cells – Increased.

LIVER

Macroscopic Appearance:

(i) Enlarged, congested.
(ii) Cut surface Nutmeg appearance.

Microscopic Appearance (PL. 4.III):

(i) Kuffer's cells–Increased in size and number, packed with *L. donovani.*
(ii) Capillaries engorged dilated.
(iii) Liver cells–Atrophied by pressure of dilated sinusoids. *Parasites not found in liver cells,* but found in Kupffer cells (Fixed macrophages, very active).

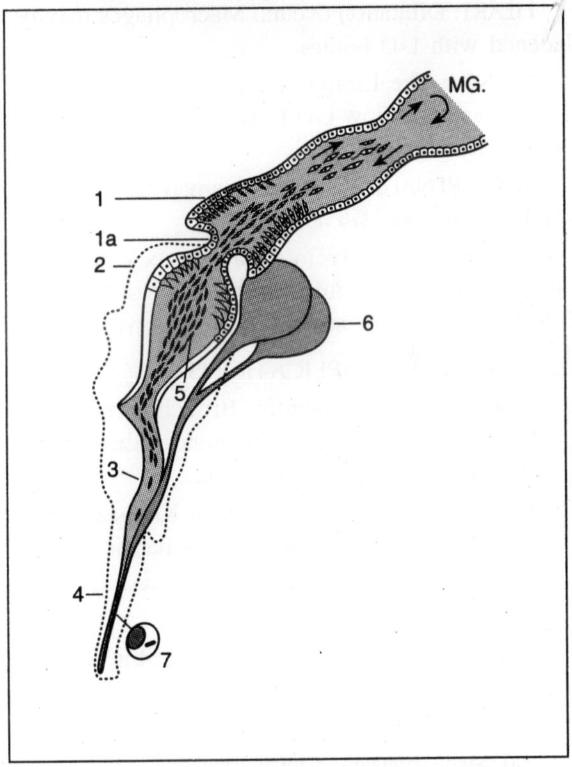

Fig. 4.7 Diagrammatic representation of the alimentary canal of sandfly where *L. donovani* develops into the promastigote (leptomonad) form in the midgut of the sandfly. P. argentipes on the 7th day after feeding (After Short. Barraud and Craighed. 1926)

BONE MARROW

Macroscopic Appearance:

(i) Extensive hyperplasia of RE cells, suppresses leucoblastic elements causing Neutropenia.

(ii) Bone marrow — Red (formative bone marrow Response), and soft.

(iii) In advanced cases, haemopoietic tissue replaced much by the RE cell proliferation.

Microscopic Appearance:

Macrophages packed with L-D bodies seen in a smear (PL. 4.IV).

OTHER ORGANS

LYMPH NODES. The positive finding depends on the proliferation of RE cells and parasitisation of macrophages.

SKIN: Leishmania-laden lining endothelial cells in arterioles around sweat glands.

HEART: Dilatation occurs. Macrophages may be ladened with L-D bodies.

KIDNEY: The Lining endothelial cells of renal capillaries may show L-D bodies. Tubular epithelia show fatty change.

SUPRARENALS: Parasites in small foci of macrophages in *zoria fasciculate.*

Intestine Dysentery in Kala-azar is caused by amoebic or bacillary infections due to low vitality. Intestinal ulcers are secondary infections.

COMPLICATIONS

1. Respiratory — Bronchitis, Bronchopneumonia, Pulmonary tuberculosis, Gangrene of Lung, Lung abscess, Pleurisy with effusion.
2. Skin — Scabies, Carbuncle, Post Kala-azar Dermal Leishmaniasis (PKDL), Dermatitis.
3. Alimentary — Gingivitis, Cancrum oris, Terminal dysentery.
4. Cardiovascular — Cardiac dilatation, Hypertension.
5. Blood — Anaemia, Agranulocytosis.
6. Other Complications — Epistaxis and in rercurrent infection.

ANAEMIA IN KALA-AZAR

Haemoglobin level 5 to 10 gm%

Causes of anaemia

(1) Marrow Hypoplasia of anemia (as thought in the past).

(2) Haemolyses (red cells sequestered and destroyed in the spleen; i.e., hypersplenic syndrome).

Types of Anaemia

(1) Macrocytic–Due to hepatic damage (Deranged assimilation)–and parenchymatous degeneration and fatty storage of Vitamin B 12.

(2) Microcytic–Occurs in 5% (lack of iron absorption from intestine).

(3) Aplastic Anaemia–Extensive multiplication of parasites in bone-marrow.

CLINICAL FEATURES

Onset–Three types

(a) Typhoid type — Continuous or high remittent temperature for 3-6 weeks.

(b) Malarial type — Fever with Chill and Rigor comes daily *Fastigium.*

(c) Insidious type — With irregular type of temperature, enlargement of spleen, liver, etc.

SYMPTOMS

(a) Fever: Early symptom, may be *continuous, remittent, or intermittent,* Double rise of tempera-

TABLE 4.3

RESERVOIRS OF INFECTION

Countries	Sources of infection
(a) Mediterraneans, China, Brazil	– Dog is the reservoir
(b) Endemic areas of India	– Human
(c) In Brazil	– Foxes are wild reservoirs
(d) Tadjikistan	– Jackals naturally infected
(e) In Sudan and East Africa	– Primarily a rodent infection
(f) Russia (rural areas)	– Jackals are reservoirs of infection

PLATE 4.1
SPLEEN IN KALA-AZAR

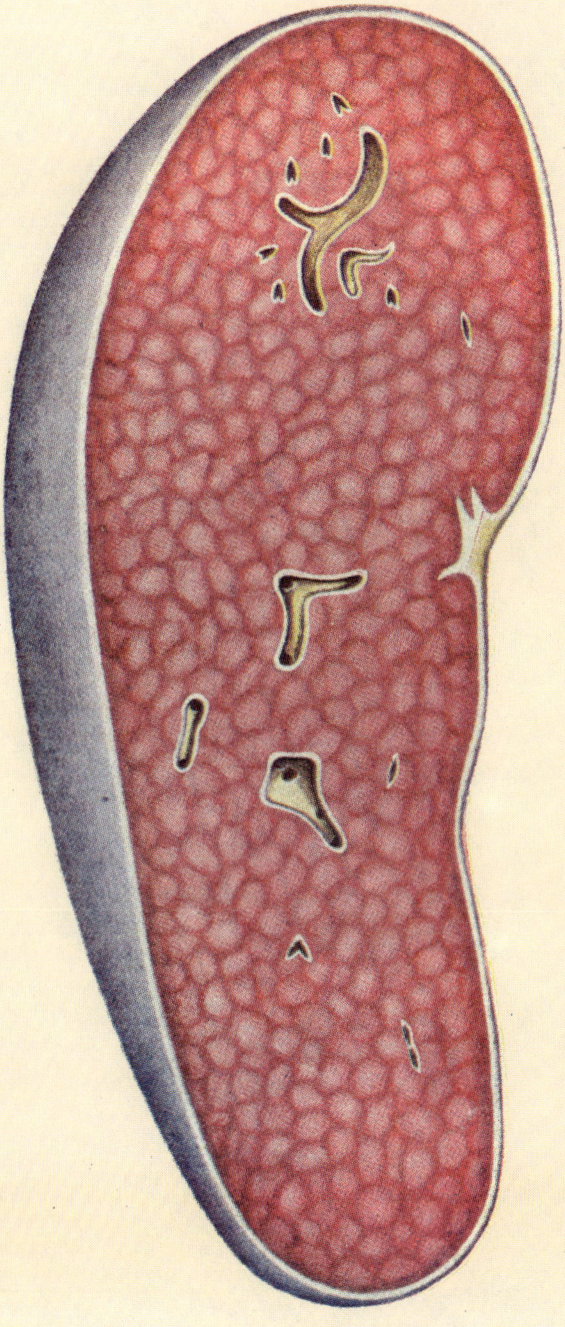

Macroscopic appearance of the spleen in kala-azar showing massive enlargement and intense congestion with areas of elevations and depressions seen on cut surface

PLATE 4.II

SPLEEN IN KALA-AZAR

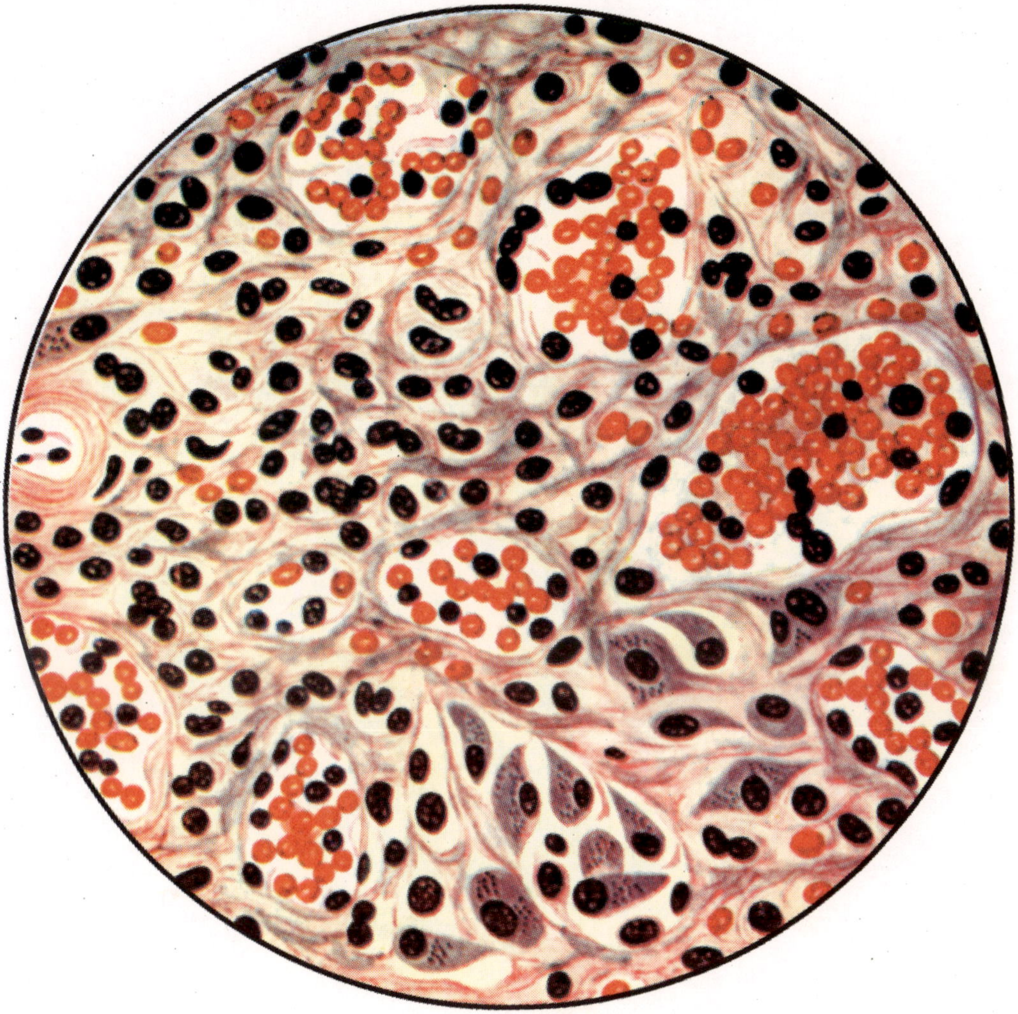

Histopathological appearance of the spleen in kala-azar showing proliferated RE cells containing dotted L-D bodies. Sinusoids are markedly dilated and congested (Iron-haematoxylin and Eosin; × 4000)

PLATE 4.III

LIVER IN KALA-AZAR

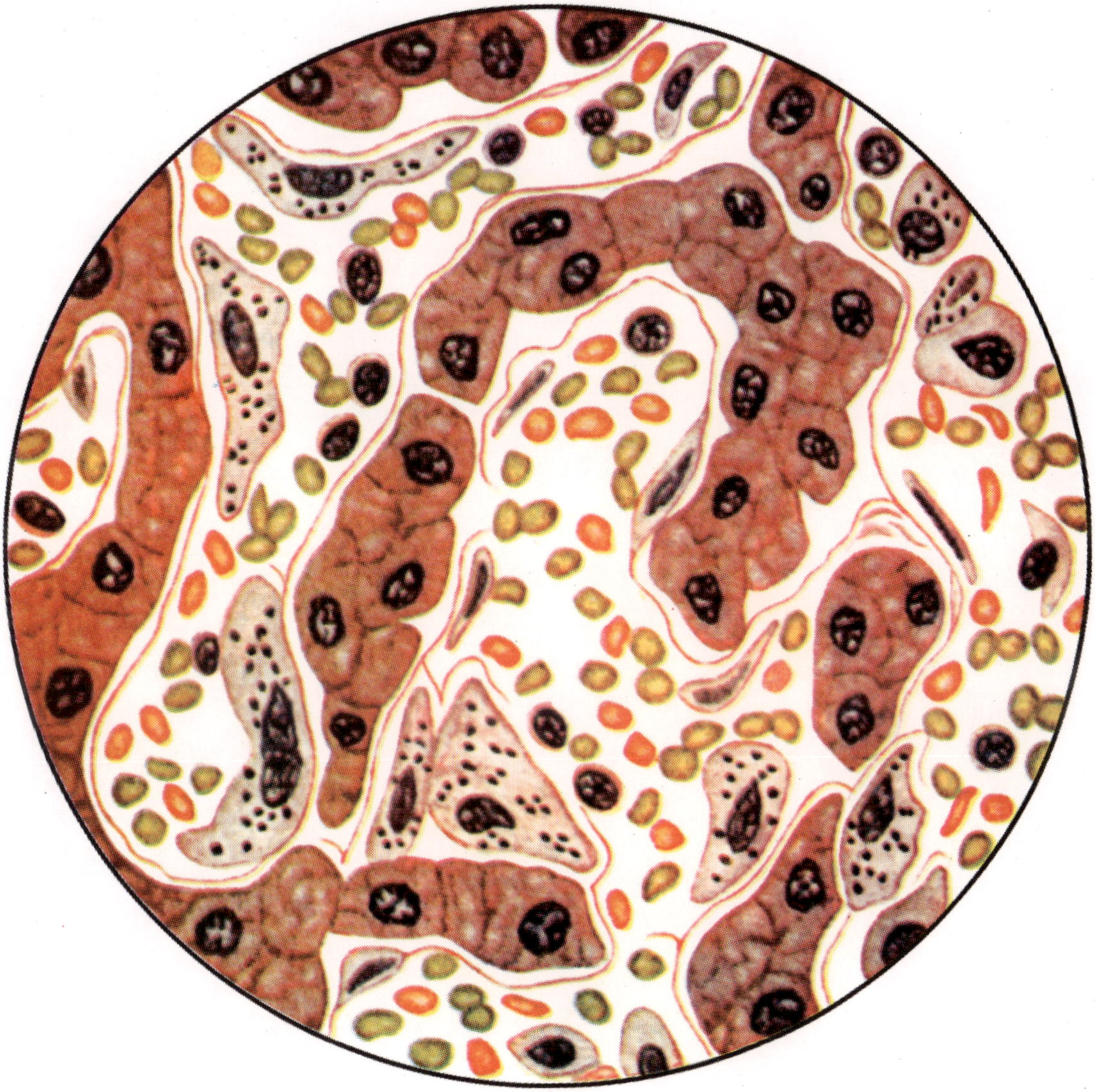

Microscopic appearance of the liver in kala-azar showing marked dilatation and congestion of liver sinusoids, parasitised Kupffer cells with L-D bodies. but healthy parenchymal or liver cells (Iron-haematoxylin and Eosin; × 1000)

PLATE 4.IV
BONE-MARROW FEATURES IN KALA-AZAR

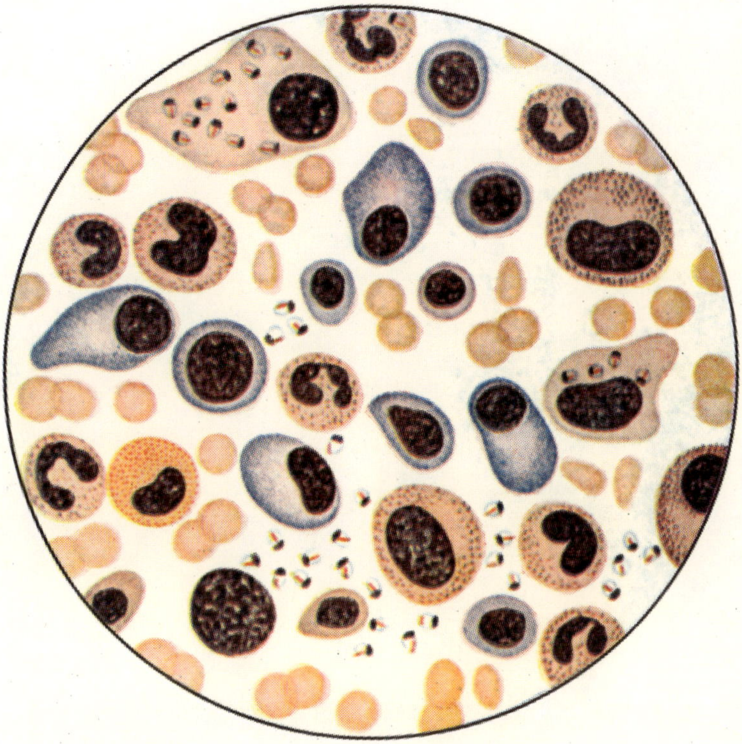

A
(× 1200)

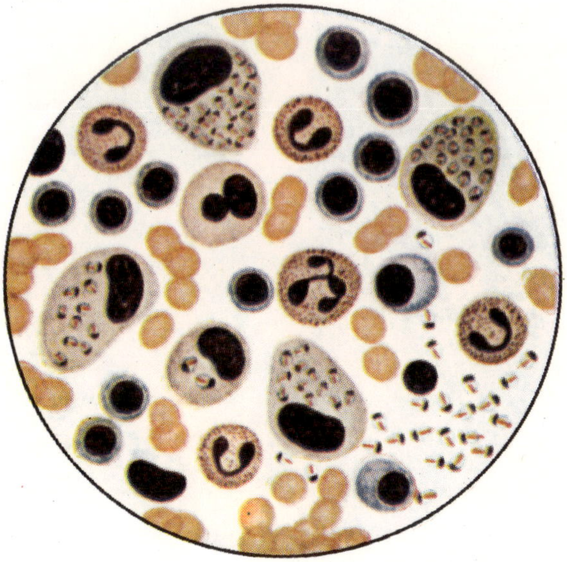

B

Bone-marrow smear from sternal puncture material showing free and phagocytosed L-D bodies in Littoral (endothelial) cells (Leishman; × 800)

ture (12%) is specific. In chronic cases *stage of apyrexia* occurs.

(b) Appetite: At times there may be *VORACIOUS* or PERVERTED APPETITE.

(c) Skin: Entire body is *DRY, ROUGH, with BLACK PIGMENTATION* (*disturbed melanin metabolism* by hepatic and adrenal cortex involvement). Hair is *BRITTLE* and falls out. In African Kala-azar warty eruptions appear.

(d) Constitutional symptoms: weakness. lethargy, fatiguability are less, euphoric.

(e) Haemorrhagic manifestations bleeding gums, menorrhagia, petechiae *HYPOPROTHROMBINAEMIA, Thrombocytopenia*).

(f) Emaciation in late stage.

SIGNS

(a) General–Anaemia (normocytic normochromic). Pulse is high in absence of fever.

(b) Pitting oedema.

(c) Pigmentation: perioral temple, forehead. Skin is shiny and scaly. Hair is brittle.

(d) Jaundice may be present (in severe liver infection causing gross enlargement; compression of bile canaliculi).

(e) Marked emaciation (Kala-azar CACHEXIA).

(f) Spleen–Invariably palpable, 2 to 3 cm after 1 month. It is soft in acute stage, firm and not tender in chronic cases. Tenderness indicates secondary infection (perisplenitis).

LABORATORY DIAGNOSIS OF KALA-AZAR

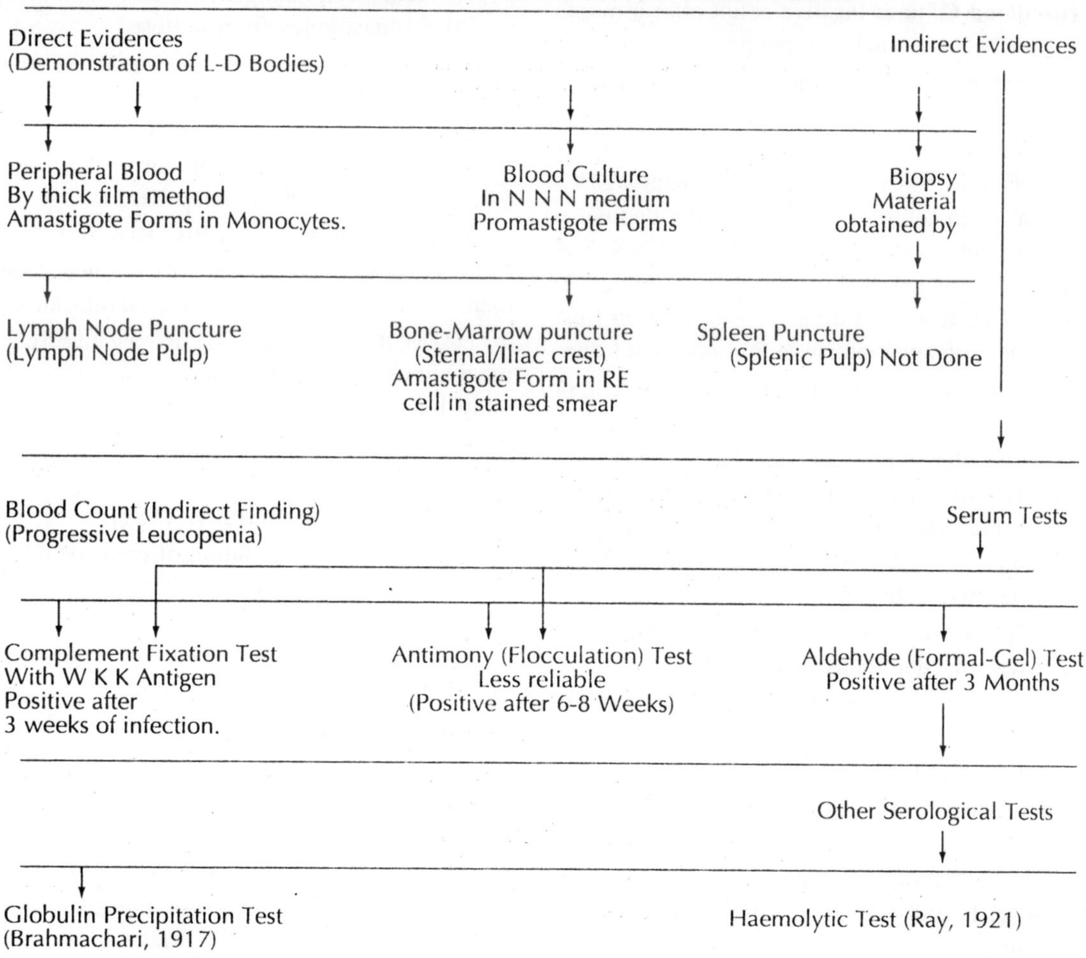

LIVER

Invariably enlarged. It is soft in acute cases but firm with share margins in chronic cases and is not tender.

(g) Lymphomatosis may be observed in African and Chinese forms.

(h) Heart shows tachycardia and haemic murmur. Blood pressure is usually low. Pulse remains high.

(i) Lungs show evidences of bronchitis.

I. DIRECT EVIDENCES

(i) **Peripheral Blood:** Microscopic examination of stained blood film. Thin blood film gives negative result

(i) By making a thick blood film.

(ii) By centrifuging citrated blood. (See Appendix I).

(ii) **Blood Culture:** Positive result after a month in N.N.N./Senekjie's medium.

Procedure: 1 to 2 ml venous blood taken aseptically and diluted with 10 ml. Citrated Saline solution (normal saline with 2% sodium citrate). Cells are allowed to settle in a cold incubator (22°C) overnight, then centrifuged. The cellular deposit is inoculated into water of condensation NNN Medium and incubated at 22°C for 1 to 4 weeks. At the end of each week a drop of condensation fluid is examined for development of Promastigote forms.

Bone Marrow Biopsy (From the Sternum or Anterior superior spine of Iliac Crest):

Anterior Iliac Crest puncture is the safest procedure; risk of haemorrhage is nil; whereas sternal puncture there is pain and shock. Amastigote forms (L-D bodies) are demonstrated in a stained film in Monocytes macrophages.

(iii) **Spleen Puncture:** It is abandoned due to high risk of continuous bleeding.

AMASTIGOTE FORMS are found in stained films within RE cells.

II. INDIRECT EVIDENCES

(i) **Blood changes (peripheral blood count)**

(a) Progressive Leucopenia (Pathognomonic feature). Diminution of Neutrophils and relative increase of Lymphocytes and Monocytes. (Cf. Enteric fever).

Average total W.B.C. count is 3,000 per cmm. in chronic cases. There is anaemia thrombocytopenia and leucopenia. So, PANCYTOPENIA occurs in Kala-azar. The proportion of WBCs to RBCs is 1 : 2000 or 1 : 1000 (normal 1 : 700).

Coagulability of blood is diminished; A : G ratio is altered.

(ii) **Serological tests**

(A) Complement Fixation Test (CFT) with WKK ANTIGEN: This is a nonspecific test but gives an early diagnosis within 3 weeks. Kastrowski's Antigen is also used instead of WKK antigen.

A. COMPLEMENT FIXATION TEST (CFT)

1. Antigen–Antibody System:
   Antibody–Patient's Serum.
   Antigen–Derived from either: (a) WKK antigen (from non-pathogenic strain of Human Myco. Tb. (**Whitebsky. Klingenstein and Kubn Antigen**).
   (b) Promastigotes from culture.
2. Complement: From Guinea pig's blood (From heart)–Linking and Reactionary agent
3. Haemolytic (Indicator) System:

(A) Anti-Sheep Cell Rabbit serum derived from rabbit after injection of sheep RBCs.

(B) 5% washed sheep cells (RBCs).

NO HAEMOLYSIS means CFT Positive (Complement used to bind Antigen with serum antibody).

HAEMOLYSIS means CFT is Negative (complement not used to bind non-specific antigen and antibody, but binds Sheep cell and Anti-sheep cell rabbit serum). So, complement becomes available to react with sheep cell.

B. ANTIMONY (CHOPRA) TEST:

Few drops of 4% solution of urea stibamine are added to (1 to 10) diluted patient's serum.

Result

Positive: A flocculant precipitate within 15 minutes indicates a positive reaction.

Negative: If there is no change two fluids mix without precipitation (NEGATIVE).

The test is positive after 2 months. Antimony test is less reliable than the aldehyde test.

C. ALDEHYDE (FORMAL GEL) TEST

The test depends upon an increase of serum gammaglobulin.

Procedure

1 ml SERUM taken from a case of Kala-azar in a small glass test tube. Add a drop or two FORMALIN. A positive results is indicated by Jellification—WHITE OPACITY like a hard-boiled egg. Gradation of test on Opacity and Solidification.

I. within 20 minutes, Reaction is Strongly positive (+ + +)

II. within 2 hours indicated by (+ +)

III. Occurrence within 24 hours (+).

In negative cases, serum remains liquid or forms a gel without any opacity. Opacity is the criterion for positivity.

The aldehyde test is not positive till three months. By then spleen is 4 fingers enlarged. This test is positive in infections with *S. japonicum* and *T. brucei*, Multiple myeloma and Cirrhosis liver. This test is Negative in *Cutaneous Leishmaniasis* (*Oriental sore*).

D. OTHER SEROLOGICAL TESTS

(i) **Immuno-Fluorescent Test** for diagnosis of Visceral leishmaniasis. Serum should be diluted 1 in 100. Antigen is prepared from promastigote forms in culture, and then it is smeared on slides (Sudan, 1968) tagging with Fluorescent dyes (Fluorescein isothiocyanate). Serum is applied. Immuno-fluorescence results.

(ii) **Indirect Haemagglutination** Test with tanned/untanned red cells.

(iii) A specific complement fixation test may also be carried out either with an antigen prepared from Promastigotes of *L. donovani* or from infected hamster spleen or liver.

(iv) **Globulin Precipitation Test** (Brahmachari, 1917). 10 serum is added to 5 ml distilled water. Turbidity by excess euglobulin precipitation indicates positive reaction (within 3 months).

(v) **Haemolytic Test** (Ray, 1921). If freshly drawn blood is added to distilled water, haemolysis is interfered. Test is negative with normal blood.

IMMUNOLOGICAL TESTS

(a) **Immuno-fluorescent test.** The immuno-fluorescent method is one of fluorescent antibody technique tests, where the patient's serum antibodies are tagged with **Fluorescein Isothiocyanate** (FI). The antigen is from promastigotes from culture. The antigen is smeared on a slide. One drop of processed serum (serum + FI) is kept on the antigen-smeared slide; incubated for 30 minutes at 37°C under a coverslip and examined under a fluorescent microscope showing bright apple green immuno-fluorescence of antigen-antibody conjugate with Lissamine-Rhodamine B (RB 200) dye, which is easier shows an orange fluorescence.

(b) **Leishmanin test** (Manson-Bahr, 1961); see before also under IMMUNOLOGICAL REACTIONS (Montenegro, 1926); There is a delayed type skin reaction with 0.1 ml suspension of killed promastigote culture from 6-10 million *L. donovani*/ml injected intradermally. Positive reaction occurs in 72 hours (induration and erythema). Test is positive in cured Kala-azar (8 weeks of recovery); but negative in untreated cases, of K-A and post-Kala-azar dermal leishmanoid.

(c) **Adler□s test.** In Locke's serum agar, the development of promastigote form of *L. donovani* is inhibited by adding specific immune serum of heterologous serum. It helps to differentiate 3-species of Leishmania, i.e., *L. donovani*, *L. tropica* and *L. brasillensis* Serologically: which are indistinguishable morphologically. culturally, by animal inoculation.

CULTURE

(PL. 4.VA)

For the details of culture of Leishmania and Trypanosomes see Appendix I.

PROPHYLAXIS

1. ATTACK ON THE PARASITES
   (a) In INDIA, treat human patients (reservoir host).
   (b) In China and Mediterranean areas, measures to be taken against dogs.
2. CONTROL OF VECTORS: D.D.T. spraying for sandflies control transmitter.
3. PERSONAL PROPHYLAXIS
   (i) Mosquito net (22 meshes/sq.inch).
   (ii) Cows are kept away from sleeping room.
4. ACTIVE IMMUNIZATION: Sub-cutaneous/intra-dermal inoculation of living promastigotes, which prevents K-A.

TREATMENT

CHEMOTHERAPEUTIC DRUGS

1. Antimony Compounds: Pentavalent antimony compounds: urea-stibamine, neostibosan. Sodium stibogluconate in visceral leishmaniasis.

   Dose: 600 mg. I.V. daily for 10 days in an adult. Repeated once or twice after 2 to 4 weeks interval. Initial dose is 0.5 mg/kg body weight daily.

   Contraindication: Pneumonia, tuberculosis.

   Disadvantages: Shock, collapse, breathlessness, cyanosis.

2. Synthetic non-metallic compounds are Aromatic diamidines–STILBAMIDINE and PENTAMIDINE ISETHIONATE.

   Dose: 5 mg/kg body weight, 7 injections (total dose 2 gms).

   Contraindication: Liver renal damage.

   Disadvantages: Produce trigeminal neuropathy.

DERMAL LEISHMANOID

(Post-Kala-azar Dermal Leishmaniasis)

An infective granuloma of skin caused by *Leishmania donovani* after cure of visceral affection.

1. Hypopigmented Macules:

(PL. 4.VII., Fig. 1 and 2)

This is earliest manifestation on trunk and extremities; face is least affected. Pin-point macules coalesce and form bigger patches.

2. Butterfly Erythema

Erythema on face is photosensitive, marked in middle of the day.

3. Nodules

They are on skin, rarely mucous membrane of tongue, and eyes, mostly on face on any other part, soft, painless and granulomatous.

Other clinical types are xanthomatous, verrucose, papillomatous and hypertrophic lesions of the skin.

DIAGNOSIS

Clinically history of Kala-azar (long continued fever) diagnosis is confirmed by finding of the parasite by microscope.

Procedure: From Nodular lesions → Biopsy fluid obtained → Smear is made : Stained by Leishman → examined under microscope → Amastigote forms in RE cells in the granuloma.

TREATMENT

It is same as in Kala-azar.

ORIENTAL SORE

Leishmania tropica

(Wright, 1903) Luhe, 1906

Parasite of cutaneous leishmaniasis

It is a granulomatous lesion of the skin caused by *L. tropica* which ulcerates but may heal spontaneously, leaving depressed scars. Organism is morphologically similar to *L. donovani.*

GEOGRAPHICAL DISTRIBUTION

Desert areas of India, West Pakistan. Afghanistan, Baluchistan, Middle East, Central Asia, Mediterranean region, and Central Africa.

Relationship to Kala-azar: *L. tropica* and *L. donovani* are not found in the same locality. (See Table 4.4).

DIFFERENTAL DIAGNOSIS

(a) Lepromatous Leprosy

- (i) *Mycobacterium leprae* is seen tion, when stained by Ziehl-Neelsen stain.
- (ii) Nodules involve ears less frequently.

(b) Oriental Sore and Espundia

Ulceration of nodules is a characteristic feature.

Habitat: *L. tropica* Promastigote form is in ulcers, and in granuloma RE Cells.

Cultivation: (1) NNN and (2) Chang's medium (same as *L. donovani*) Cultures live indefinitely by subcultures.

LIFE CYCLE

The sandfly having fed on the lesion of Oriental sore, develops the promastigote (Leptomonad) form in its gut similarly as in Kala-azar. The sandfly is found infected in nature and the disease spreads by the bite of infected sandflies (insect bite).

TABLE 4.4

L. donovani (Kala-azar)	*L. tropica* (Oriental sore)
(a) Rare in Iraq and Iran.	(a) Oriental sore is endemic in Iraq and Iran.
(b) Kala-azar is confined to moist Eastern parts of the country.	(b) Oriental sore is limited to dry Western parts.

TABLE 4.5

VARIOUS VECTORS OF *L. TROPICA*

India, Iraq and Persia	*Phlebotomus sergenti*
West Pakistan, North Africa and Eastern Mediterranean areas	*P. papatasii* and *P. sergenti*
Central Asia	*P. Papatasii* and *P. caucasiasus*
Latin America	*P. intermedius*

EPIDEMIOLOGY

(a) TRANSMISSION *Person* to person—transmitted by bite of sandfly.

(b) VECTORS (see Table 4.5).

(c) INFECTION IN ANIMALS

Dogs, wild rodents, cats, monkeys, hamsters and mice are susceptible,

(i) In monkeys, infection limits to skin.

(ii) In mice, infection may be cutaneous but sometimes involve the internal organs.

Supceptible Animals

(i) All laboratory animals.

(ii) In Syrian hamsters and sometimes in mice, intraperitoneal inoculations produce visceral infection.

(iii) Human Oriental Sore reproduced in Spermophile, *Citillus citillus.*

IMMUNOLOGY

In *L. tropica* infection cell-mediated immunity appears early, no serum antibodies. With delayed hypersensitivity reaction and elimination of parasites. Single attack gives lifelong immunity.

CLINICAL FEATURES

(i) *L. tropica* produces cutaneous Leishmaniasis (Oriental/tropical sore) or Delhi boil, Alpeppo button or other local names (PL. 4.VB).

(ii) Sores are on face or extremities, $^2/_3$ or single.

(iii) I.P. weeks to 6 months or more.

(iv) Found from endemic areas of Western India to Bengal, Assam.

(v) The lesion begins as a granulomatous nodule with a red margin. The nodule ulcerates in centre with a clean cut margin, indurated edge, and erythematous areola. Parasite is found along red margin. Sore heals spontaneously, slowly, in 6 months or more.

(vi) Ulcer is filled up by granulation tissue with depressed scar.

TYPES OF THE DISEASE (Fig. 4.8 & PL.4.VI)

Two types, based on clinical, immunology, and epidemiology:

(i) L. Tropica Minor: Dry type (Late-ulcerating type). Found in urban areas of Middle East, Mediterranean areas, N. Africa, N.W. India, Pakistan, runs a chronic course with parasites in lesion. skin is unbroken; after months ulcerates I.P. is 2 months to a year. Lesion is facial. Human and domestic dogs are reservoirs.

(ii) L. Tropica Major: Moist type (Ulcerating type). Found in rural areas of Central Asia and Iran. Runs an acute course, with scanty parasites, ulcerate in 1-2 weeks. Reservoir host is the desert gerbil *R. OPIMUS* and small rodents. Ulcers occurs on extremities with regional lymph-noditis 2-6 weeks after sandfly bite. Both types of cutaneous lesions are

L. tropica Major protects against L. tropica Minor (but not vice versa).

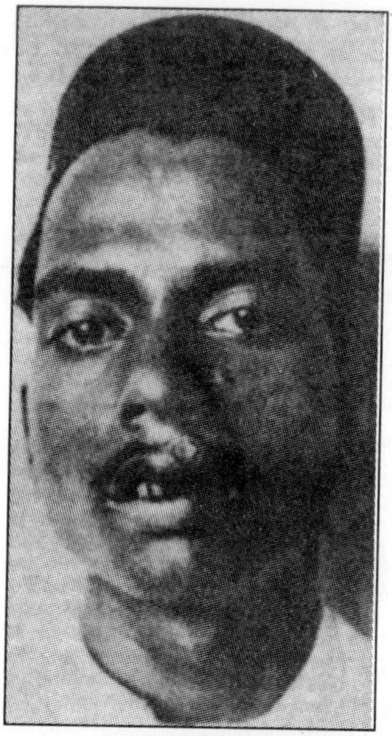

Fig. 4.8 Oriental sore on the upper lip of a man coming from Rajasthan

PATHOLOGY

(i) Oriental sore is a specific infective granuloma with fibrosis around it.

(ii) RE cells (skin), monocytes poliferate

(iii) Parasites are found in them.

(iv) Later, round cell infiltration, parasites reduced in number.

(v) Secondary organisms destroy parasites.

LABORATORY DIAGNOSIS

(a) Smear is made (puncture of indurated edge), stained by Leishman's; microscopic examination done.

(i) Amastigote form found in large number inside macrophages.

(ii) If the smear is negative, Cultures should be made on NNN medium.

(b) Skin test (Leishmanin Reaction): Intracutaneous injection of Leishmanin (suspension of promastigotes of *L. tropica*) gives a positive skin test in Oriental.

(c) Blood picture, serum gamma globulin are normal, Aldehyde test negative.

PROPHYLAXIS

(i) Elimination of the reservoir hosts.

(ii) Control of Sandflies.

(iii) Individual protection from sandfly bites by repellant dimethyl pthalate.

(iv) Prophylactic immunisation with *L. tropica* culture.

TREATMENT

(i) Pentavalent or trivalent antimony compounds intravenously.

(ii) Dehydro-emetine orally 100 mg. daily for 10-21 days.

(iii) Injection of Leishmania vaccine prepared from the dead culture.

ESPUNDIA

LEISHMANIA BRAZILIENSIS

Vianna, 1911

(Parasite causing espundia or muco-cutaneous Leishmaniasis)

Geographical Distribution: Central and South America.

Habitat: Intracellular parasite (amastigote) in macrophage cells (RE cells) of skin, and Oro-nasal mucosa.

Morphology: (i) Morphologically and culturally same as *L. DONOVANI.*

(ii) Differentiated on serological basis by agglutination.

Cultivation: (i) Cultivated in either NNN or CHANG□S medium.

(ii) Chorio-allantoin membrane of the chick embryo.

Susceptible Animal: Syrian hamster, inoculation of Cultures to skin causes local skin lesion.

NO VISCERAL LESIONS OCCUR BY INTRAPERITONEAL INOCULATION

The vector *PHLEBOTOMUS INTERMEDIUS*, a wild species, is found in endemic areas. Infection is transmitted to man by the bite of an infected sandfly. Auto-inoculation occurs by direct contact.

EPIDEMIOLOGY

Transmission (i) is caused by *Phlebotomus intermedius* a wild species of sandfly.

(ii) Auto-inoculable, and by direct contact (inoculated from man to man).

Vectors. These are *P. intermedius, P. verrucarum, P. peruensis* and others.

Animal Reservoir: Dogs in Brazil, and small forest rodents.

IMMUNOLOGY

L. brasiliensis infection causes metastasis in the skin and mucous membrane, cell-mediated immunity does not develop until they metastasise.

CLINICAL FEATURES

(i) I.P is few days to a few weeks.

(ii) Specific ulcerative granuloma of the skin.

(iii) Later, ulcer progresses, mucosa of buccal cavity, U R T, pharynx, nose are involved (20%).

(iv) Destroys the nasal cartilage and bone.

PATHOLOGY

MACROSCOPICALLY

(i) Produces local lesions, appear as a macule. followed by formation of a papule with a raised centre.

(ii) Papule breaks down in the centre.

(iii) Lesions develop more rapidly and ulceration occurs with secondary infections early in disease.

(iv) The lesion quickly reaches a large size; when the lesion reaches the mucosal surface, tissue destruction and scars occur.

MICROSCOPICALLY

(i) The skin and the mucous membrane show infiltration with lymphocytes, plasma cells and mononuclear cells.

(ii) The parasites are present in large number inside mononuclear cells, at the periphery of the lesion.

LABORATORY DIAGNOSIS

DIRECT METHOD

(i) **Finding of the parasite** (amastigote *L. brasiliensis*) in smear from infected tissue (skin and mucocutaneous lesions).

(ii) Culture shows promastigotes.

INDIRECT METHOD

Intradermal skin test by culture of *L. brasiliensis* shows delayed hypersensitivity.

PROPHYLAXIS

(i) Vaccination in endemic areas.

(ii) Personal Prophylaxis taken against bites of the sandflies.

(iii) Control depends on treatments.

TREATMENT

(i) Treated intravenously with antimony, e.g., neostibosan.

(ii) Antibiotics are used to combat secondary septic infection.

(iii) In resistant cases Pyrimethamine or Amphotericin B are tried.

TABLE 4.6

TRYPANOSOMES IN HUMAN AND ANIMALS

Species	Disease and Geographical Distribution
Pathogenic to human	
T. br. gambiense	**Gambian** Trypanosomiasis : Mid and West African sleeping sickness
T. br. rhodesiense	**Rhodesian** Trypanosomiasis : East-African sleeping sickness
T. br. Zambezi	**Zambezi** Trypanosomiasis : Acute form simulating Rhodesian Trypanosomiasis; chronic form resembles Gambian sleeping sickness
T. cruzi	**Chagas'** Disease : South American trypanosomiasis
Nonpathogenic to human	
T. rangeli	**Found** in the blood of human in Venezuela and Columbia
Pathogenic to animals	
T. brucei	**Causes** "Nagana" in domestic animals of tropical Africa. It is transmitted by *G. morsitans*
T. evansi	**Causes** "Surra" in horses and mules in India. It is transmitted mechanically by Tabanid horseflies
T. equinum	**Causes** "Mal de Caderas" in horses in South America. It is transmitted mechanically by Tabanid horseflies
T. epuiperdum	**Causes** "Dourine" disease in horses and donkeys of India, Europe, America and North Africa. It is transmitted by coitus
T. congolense	**Causes** a fatal disease in horses, mules, donkeys, cattle, sheep and goats
T. vivax	**Found** in horses, cattle, sheep and goats
Nonpathogenic to animals	
T. lewisi	A commensal of rats and transmitted by rat fleas from rat to rat

*T. vivax is larger and more active than *T. congolense* and has a free flagellum, whereas *T. congolense* is smaller, more active and has no free flagellum

TRYPANOSOMES

MORPHOLOGY

General Characters: See Figs. 4.2, 4.9 for general morphological structure of the trypomastigote form of a trypanosome.

Polymorphism of Trypomastigotes: These forms differ in: (a) size and shape, (b) presence or absence of a free flagellum, and (c) position of the nucleus. Trypomastigotes of *T. brucei* sub-groups are polymorphic.

METHOD OF REPRODUCTION

Reproduction occurs by binary longitudinal fission. Division of kinetoplast and basal body, followed by division of the nucleus. The flagellum with undulating membrane remains with one half of the basal body, while the other develops into a new one. The cytoplasmic body then splits longitudinally from the anterior end.

CLASSIFICATION

The PATHOGENIC TRYPANOSOMES are the following:

1. *T. brucei* subgroup (human strains)–Cause African trypanosomiasis (Gambian, Rhodesian and Zambezi forms of sleeping sickness), **PL.4.V.**
2. *T. cruzi*–Causes South American trypanosomiasis (Chagas' disease) **PL.4.VII.**

   T. rangeli–A non-pathogenic trypanosome found in the blood of man in Venezuela and Columbia.

Trypanosomes of Animals

A few of them are

NONPATHOGENIC: *T. lewisi* causes Trypanosomiasis in rats and transmitted by rat fleas.

PATHOGENIC: *T. brucei* (animal strain) found in wild games and domestic animals of tropical Africa; transmitted by sandfly *G. morsitans* causes "Nagana" in some domestic animals.

T. evansi causes "Surra" in horses and mules of India; mechanically transmitted by Tabanid.

T. equiperdum, causes "Stallion's disease" (venereal disease) in horses and asses of Europe, North Africa, America and India; transmitted by coitus.

T. equinum causes "Mal de Caderas" amongst horses in South America; transmitted mechanically by Tabanid; it has no kinetoplast and no insect cycle in its life history.

T. vivax and *T. congolense* cause disease in cattle; transmitted by Tsetse flies.

TRYPANOSOMA BRUCEI

(PLIMMER AND BRADFORD, 1899)

The parasite causing African Trypanosomiasis in man, and Nagana in domestic animals.

T. brucei produces a mild infection in cattle. Strain of Bruce had admixture of *T. congolense*.

TRYPANOSOMIASIS

(SLEEPING SICKNESS)

and *T. brucei* Subgroup

Based on clinico-epidemiological pattern, African trypanosomiasis is classified as "Gambian" and "Rhodesian" sleeping sickness caused by *T. gambiense* and *T. rhodesiense* respectively. Zoologists have amalgamated the species. *T. brucei* subgroups as follows:

1. The **animal strain** of *T. brucei* does not infect man.
2. The **human strains** *T. gambiense* and *T. rhodesiense* are recognised, e.g., *T. brucei*, rhodesiense.
   (a) "Rhodesian" is an acute disease.
   (b) "Gambian" is a chronic disease.
   (c) "Zambezi" is chronic but alike acute "Rhodesian" form.

Rickman and Robson (1970) introduced Blood incubation infectivity test, to identify *T. brucei* animal strain (*"T. brucei"*), and human infectivity strain (*"T. rhodesiense"*). The test runs as follows: The strain of *T. brucei* to be tested is at first inoculated into rats or mice and when *parasitaemia* is established a few ml of cardiac blood is withdrawn. About 0.25 ml each of same sample is taken in 2 Bijou bottles. To one bottle 2 ml of human blood and an anticoagulant (0.25 ml of 2% Pot. Oxalate with glucose added to a strength of 3 mg/ml of blood).

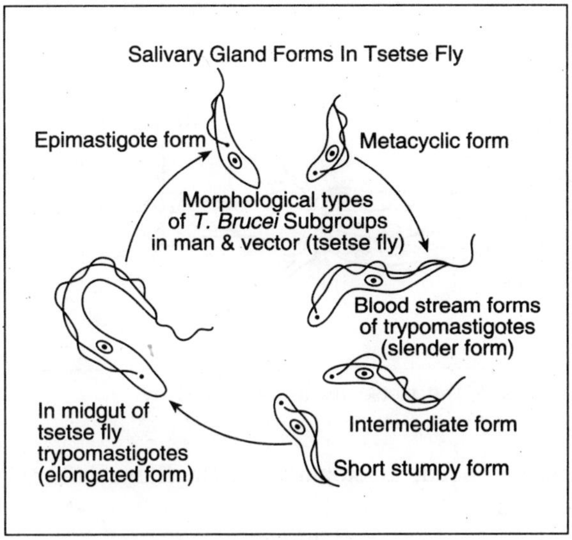

Fig. 4.9 Showing different forms of trypomastigotes of *T. brucei* subgroups which occur in the vector and man

To the other bottle 2 ml phosphate-buffered salaine (*p*H 7.4) is taken. This is the control sample.

Both the samples after gentle mixing are incubated in a water bath for 5 hours at 37°C. Each of the mixtures is then tested separately by inoculating a rat. If persistent parasitaemia occurs in both the rats, the result is positive, i.e., the strain is human infective form, and infectivity to rats persists. If the parasitaemia occurs only in the rat inoculated with the control sample, the test is *negative.* i.e., strain is of animal origin and inoculation with the human blood have rendered it non-infective to the rat.

HABITAT

T. brucei is essentially a parasite of connective tissues where it multiplies readily. It consumes enormous amount of glucose causing hypoglycaemic (drowsy/sleepy).

It invades regional *lymph nodes* and blood (parasitaemia) to localised in brain. African sleeping sickness is a disease of the central nervous system.

Prevalence of *T. brucei.* Human strains are not widespread.

The acute ''Rhodesiense'' strain is distributed only in East Africa (Tanganyika, Uganda, Zambia, Rhodesia and Malawi).

The chronic "Gambiense" strain is of West Africa (from Gambia to the Congo).

The chronic "Zambezi" strain (pathology similar to "Gambiense" disease) is found in Botswana, Protuguese East Africa, Rhodesia, Zambia. The acute "Zambezi" strain (resembling "Rhodesiense" disease) is found in Tanzania, Uganda and Kenya.

MORPHOLOGY (Fig. 4.9), PL. IV.VI

T. brucei exists in vertebrate hosts as *tropomastigote form.* It is an elongated, rather flattened, spindle—shaped organism with a blunted posterior end and a finely pointed anterior end. Nucleus is large, oval and central. Kinetoplast is small at the posterior end. The flagellum starts from the posterior extremity near kinetoplast. Curves around the body as undulating membrane and continues beyond the anterior end as free flagellum.

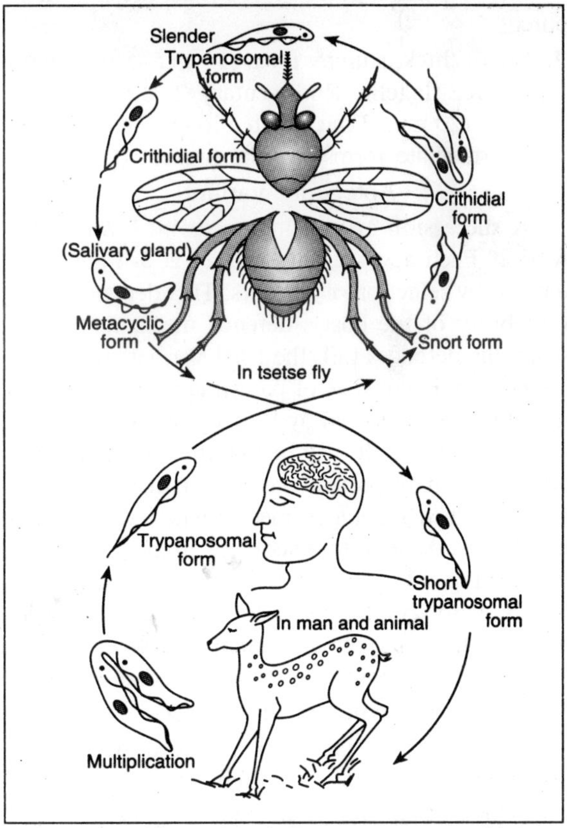

Fig. 4.10 Life cycle of *Trypanosoma gambiense* and *Trypanosoma rhodesiense.* Antelopes are hosts of *T. brucei* and reservoirs of *T. rhodesiense.* Domestic animals are subsidiary hosts of *T. gambiense*

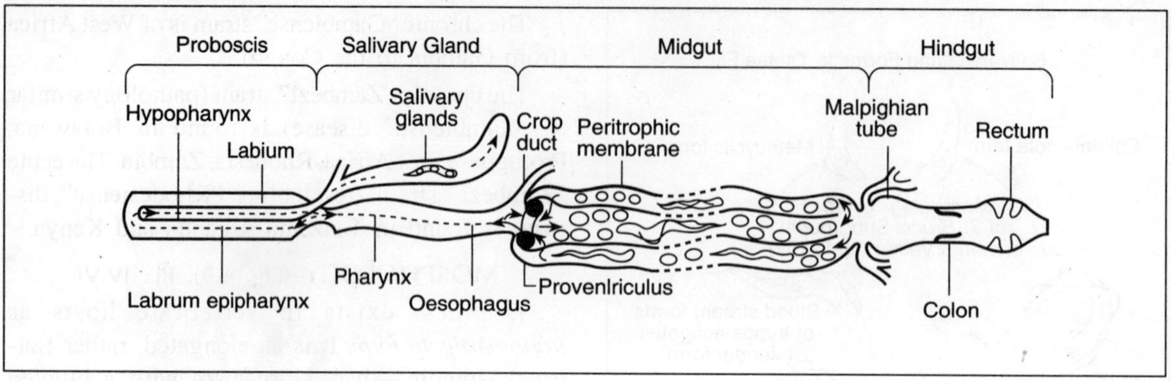

Fig. 4.11 Developmental stages of trypanosomes in the tsetse fly as indicated by arrows and their passage to different parts of the fly (After Hoare, 1949)

Undulating membrane is thrown into 3 to 4 folds. It is an *actively motile flagellate.*

POLYMORPHISM

The trypomastigotes of *T. brucei* are polymorphic.

I. Short; thick, stumpy form (10 mu.–5 mu.) with no free flagella. Rudimentary 2. Long slender form (20 mu.–3 mu.) with a long free flagellum intermediate forms may be present (Fig. 4.9).

Antegenic variant

A succession of variants occur in *T. brucei* infection. Each new variant emerges at 3-4 days' intervals, by selection of mutants. This depends upon (1) ability of the host's defence mechanism. And when the defences fail, the final variant multiplies unchecked. Each wave of parasitaemia is accompanied by fever followed by leucocytosis (monocytosis, neutrophilia). It may be that the outer proteinaceous coat may protect the organism in escaping from the host's defence mechanism result for (2) Antibodies develop to a series of immunologically distinct type of variant in the serum of hosts. Each rise in antibody titre coincides with the disappearance of the homologous variant and when this is eliminated, a new antigenic type immediately arises.

Occult Visceral Phase

Non-flagellate "latent forms" occur in capillaries of internal organs of vertebrate host. Choroid plexus and lungs are the sites of this phase (source of relapse).

Staining Reaction

With Leishman cytoplasm and undulating membrane appear pale blue; the nucleus reddish purple or red; kinetoplast and flagellum dark red (PL.4.II).

Cultivation

Medium of Ringer's solution with sodium chloride. Tyrode's solution and citrated human blood. Long slender forms of trypomastigote (mid-gut forms of Tsetse fly) develop in culture.

Animal Inoculation. Mice, rats and guineapigs are inoculated for demonstrating trypomastigotes when scanty in peripheral blood. They cause overwhelming parasitaemia and kills the animal in a few days. When inoculated in rats some 5-6% trypomastigotes develop posterior nuclear forms (nucleus situated posteriorly close to the kinetoplast) (see PL. 4.II; Top).

T. brucei a causes a chronic infection in rabbits and it dies after about 4 to 5 weeks.

IMMUNOLOGY

T. brucei infection stimulates formation of nonspecific IgM (19s) (no affinity for the organism). Host has no protective antibody (blocking effect of macrophage). African trypanosome has profound immuno-suppressive effects, so patients are unable to resist bacterial invasion.

Other serum antibodies found in trypanosomiasis are (1) *ablastin* which prevents multiplication of trypomastigotes. (2) heterophil antibody in *T. br. rhodesiense* infection, which agglutinates sheep RBCs.

LIFE CYCLE

Two different hosts are needed (Fig. 4.10). The vertebrate (definitive) host is human or animal. Insect

PLATE 4.V(A)

PROMASTIGOTE (LEPTOMONAD) FORM OF *LEISHMANIA DONOVANI*

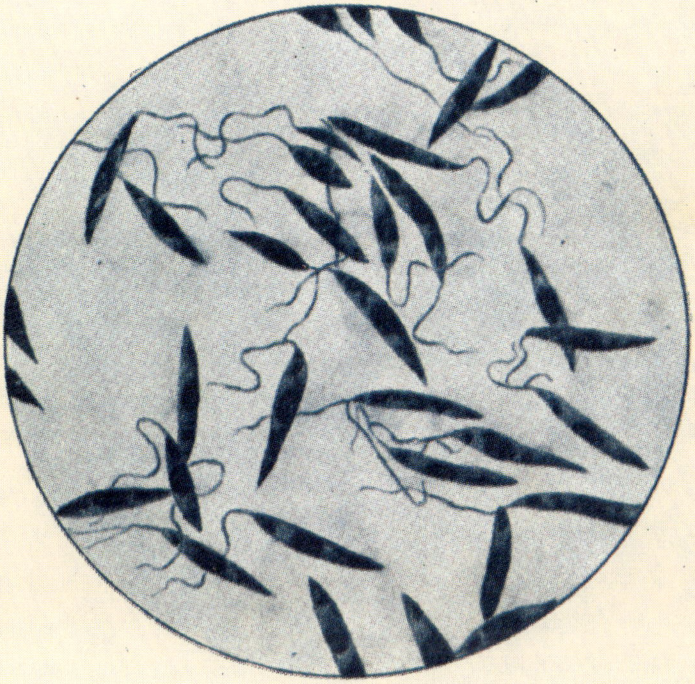

A smear from culture

PLATE 4.V(B)

ORIENTAL SORE

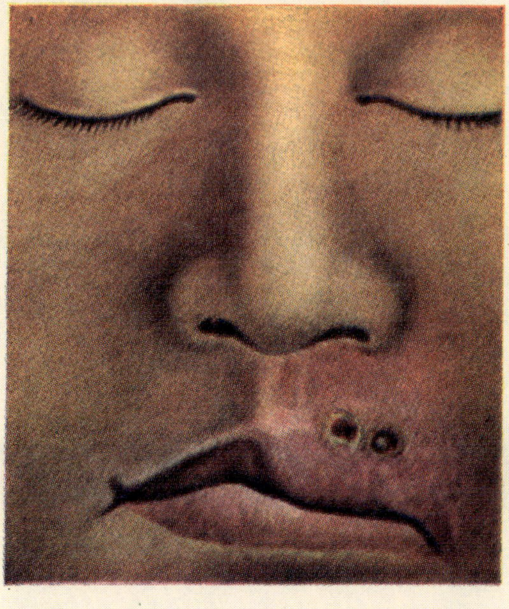

Oriental sore with granulomatous ulcers.
One of the ulcers is covered with a scab.
Note the erythema of the granulating area.

PLATE 4.VI
TSETSE FLY

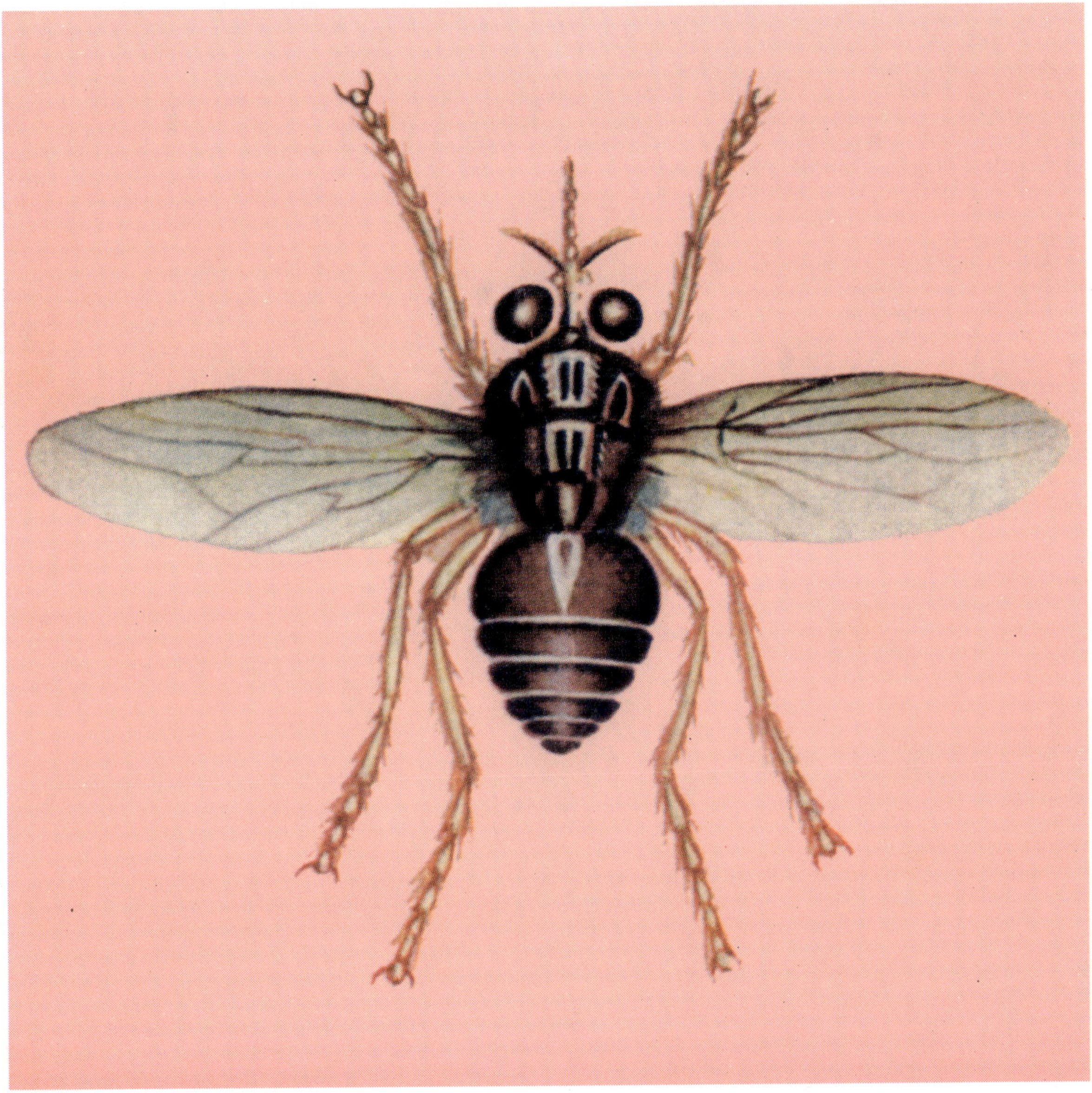

Glossina palpalis (Tsetse fly), the vector of Trypanosoma gambiense causing Gambian type of West African trypanosomiasis

PLATE 4.VII

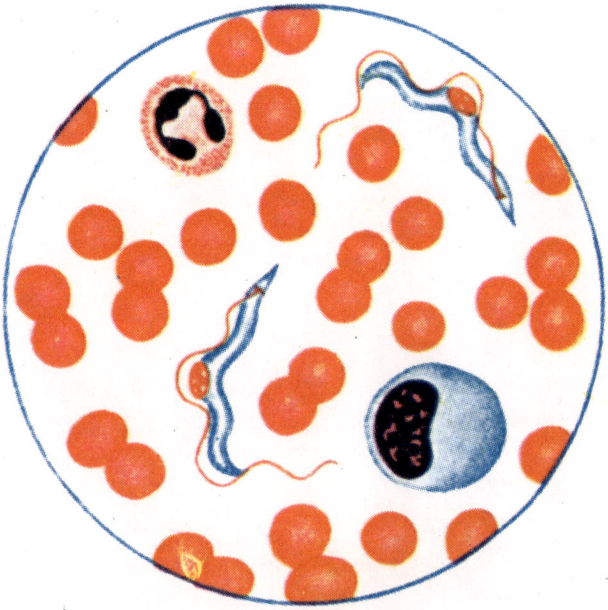

Peripheral blood showing the morphological appearance of Trypanosoma gambiense; Leishman × 1000

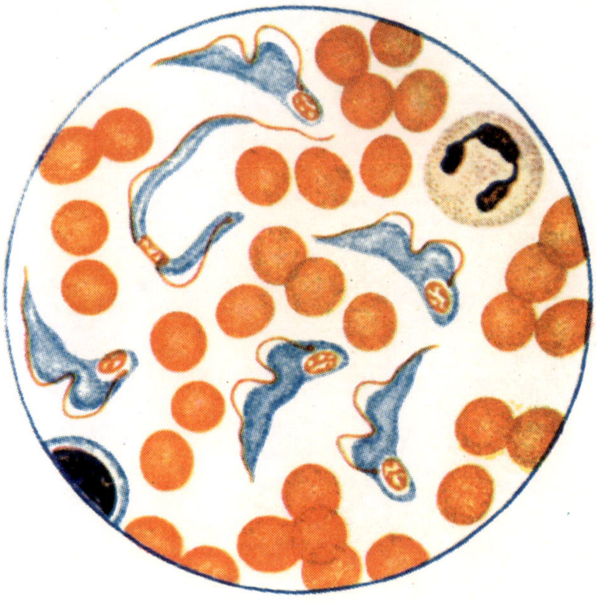

Morphological appearance of Trypanosoma rhodesiense in peripheral blood. Note the epimastigote and the slender trypomastigote forms; Leishman × 1000

PLATE XVII

PLATE 4.VIII

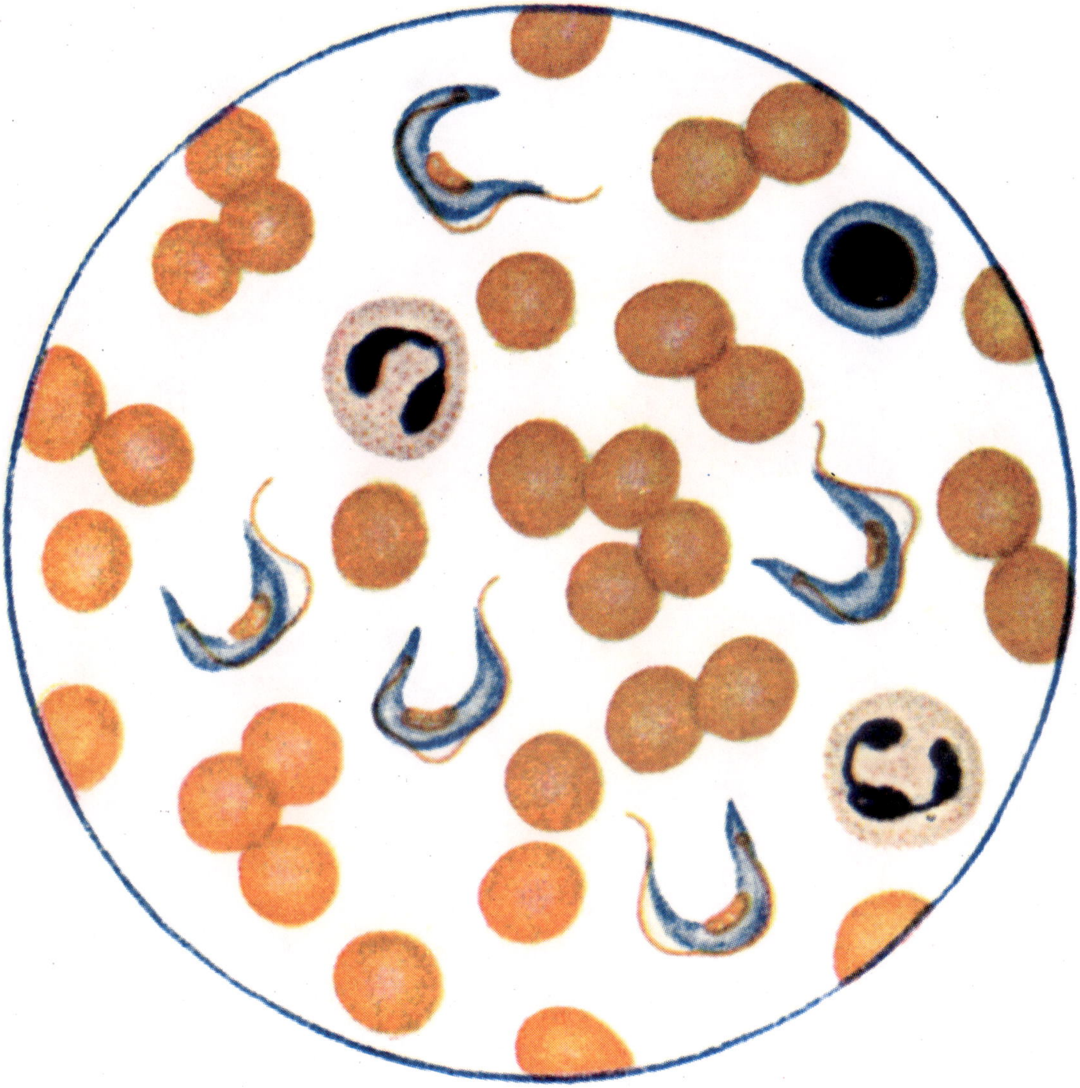

Peripheral blood showing 'C'-shaped forms of
Trypanosoma cruzi (American Trypanosome); Leishman × 1000

is Intermediate host: they are several species of Tsetse fly Glossina (**PL. 4.IV**). e.g., *G. palpalis*, *G. morsitans*. *G. tachinoides*, *G. pallidipes*, *G. swynnertoni*. Development in human and other vertebrate hosts: The metacyclic stage is infective form of trypomastigotes introduced by the bite of infected Glossina develop into long slender forms and multiply by binary longitudinal fission at the site of inoculation (bite). They become "intermediate" and "stumpy" form (**Fig. 4.9**). Parasites invade the blood (parasitaemia). The trypomastigote short stumpy forms are taken up by the Tsetse fly along with its blood meal and undergo a series of complex biological development inside the insect host (gut) before becoming infective to human.

Development in Tsetse Fly. Short stumpy forms of trypomastigote ingested by the Tsetse Fly (insect) first change the morphology in mid-gut. Long slender forms (the kinetoplast lying mid-way between the nucleus and the posterior end) appear which pass to the posterior end of the extraperitrophic space (a space between the peritrophic membrane and the epithelial cells—see **Fig. 4.11**), where they multiply for days. By 15th day they escape from the anterior end of this space and enter the lumen of proventriculus (proventricular form is same as that of midgut form).

They migrate forward to buccal catity, pass to hypopharynx to reach the salivary glands. There they multiply and change morphology, first into *epimastigote* and then into metacyclic stage (short stumpy forms of trypomastigote) which are infective to human.

Total period for evolution of the infective forms (metacyclic state) inside the Tsetse fly is 20 days. Once infected the Tsetse flies remain infective for the rest of its life (6 months). Offsprings are not infective. Tsetse flies produce a single larva at a time at 15 days interval and a total of 6 to 12 larvae during their life-span.

Transmitting Agents (*Vectors*) and *Reservoirs of Infection* (**Fig. 4.10**).

The *animal strain of T. bucei* is transmitted by *Glossina morsitans* to animals. The "Gambiense" (human) strain of *T. brucei* is transmitted by *Glossina palpalis*—**PL.4.V**. These are shade and moisture-loving flies found in shrubs and shady trees near water (Riverine species). They do not travel a distance.

"Rhodesiense" strain of *T. brucei*. The transmitting agents are *G. morsitans*. *G. swynnertoni* and *G. pallidipes*.

PATHOGENESIS & PATHOLOGY

Mode of infection (Inoculative method), by the bite of the infective Tsetse fly *Glossina* (both male and female) in daylight.

Trypomastigotes (Metacyclic stage) are introduced by bite with saliva into blood as it feeds.

TABLE 4.7

DIFFERENTIAL CHARACTERS BETWEEN GAMBIAN AND RHODESIAN SLEEPING SICKNESSES

	Gambian sleeping sickness	Rhodestian sleeping sickness
Causative organism	*T. gambiense*	*T. rhodesiense*
Reservoir	Human	Antelope
Vectors	*Glossina palpalis*	*G. morsitans*
Geographical distribution	West and Mid-Africa	East Africa
Course of disease in man	Chronic, prolonged, lasting for several years; involves the central nervous system (CNS) with pronouced nervous symptoms	Acute, shorter; duration—3-9 months, toxic symptoms predominate more than CNS involvement
Pathogenicity to laboratory animals	Low	High
Posterior nuclear from	Rare	Common
Reaction to tryparsamide	Sensitive	Resistant

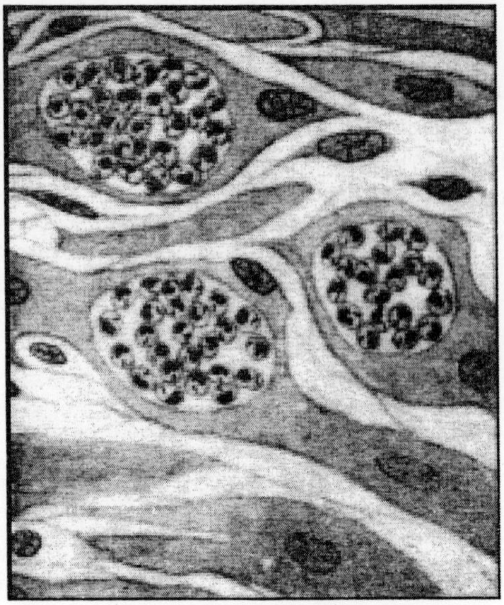

Fig. 4.12 Leishmania form of *T. cruzi* in heart muscle

Some enter blood stream directly, but majority entangle tissue spaces. Initial growth occurs in tissue spaces indus.

Trypomastigotes multiply in subcutaneous tissue spaces, cause damage; few organisms appear in peripheral blood.

Damage to connective tissue occurs by exaggerated immune (autoimmune) response (massive release of kinin) organism has low toxicity and excites response in host by two ways

1. Producing a large amount of non-specific in response to *exo-antigen*.
2. The infection triggers heavy macrophages; infiltration (no neutrophils).

Cellular defence plays an important role. Kinins (i) attract macrophage; (ii) increases capillary permeability and causes oedematous subcutaneous tissue at the site of bite. Severe damage of the perivascular connective tissues occurs. Collagen fibres and fibroblasts are disrupted (Collagenorrhexis). Pathology is found in the *lymph nodes* and the *central nervous system*, chiefly.

CSF is clear and pressure is raised. Cell count–50 to 100 lymphocytes/cu.mm. protein increased (100-150 mg%). Raised globulin content gives a ''tabetic'' *colloidal gold curve*. Parasites are demonstrated in CSF LYMPH NODE ENLARGEMENT. Generalised lymphomatosis occurs (posterior triangle in Gambian). Invasion of CNS is rapid in "Rhodesian". Symptoms of meningoencephalitis develop in classical sleeping sickness. Finally the patient becomes *thin* and *wasted* and suffers from *malnutrition*. Rhodesian disease is most dangerous and, if untreated, a patient dies rapidly. In Gambian and Zambezi disease, patients live for several years. Zambezi induces Healthy Carriers.

CLINICAL FEATURES

A history of the bite (uninfected fly causes severe reaction).

A hard painful trypanosomal chancre develops at inoculation site. It contains fluid containing actively dividing trypomastigotes. It subsides in a week.

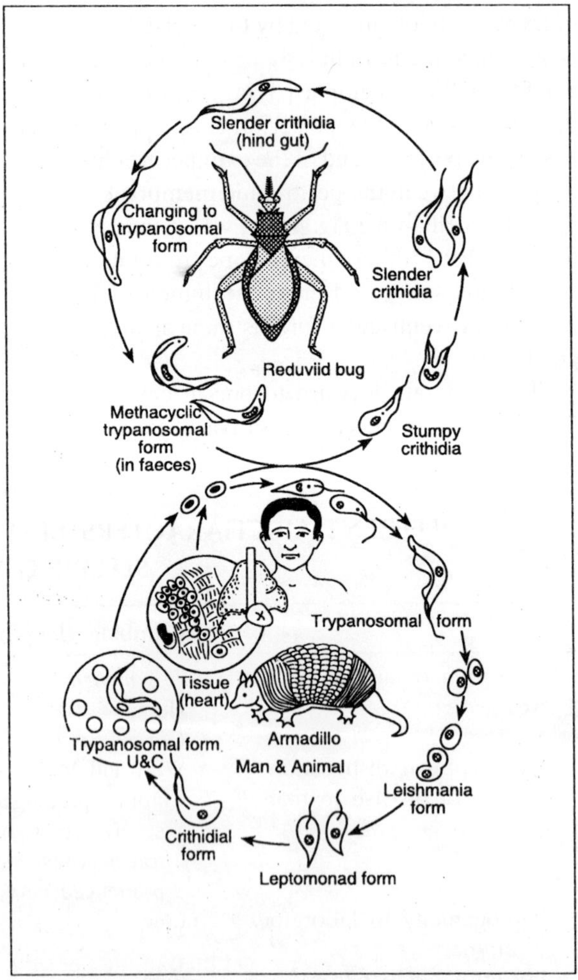

Fig. 4.13 Life cycle of *Trypanosoma cruzi* (American trypanosome)

TABLE 4.8

LABORATORY DIAGNOSIS OF TRYPANOSOMIASIS

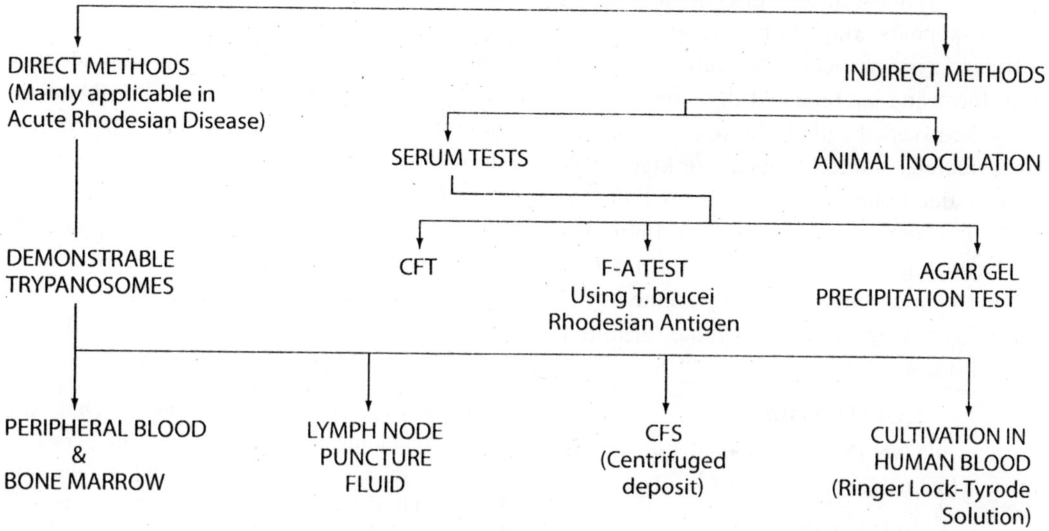

In "Rhodesian," symptoms appear after 2 weeks. In Gambian and Zambezi forms the symptoms may appear a year late. It is an infection of the blood which causes involvement and enlargement of regional and generalised lymph nodes. CNS invasion occurs. Early symptoms : fever (high and fluctuating in "Rhodesian"), severe headache, loss of nocturnal sleep and a feeling of oppression. A fleeting circinate erythematous rash on the chest and shoulders.

LABORATORY DIAGNOSIS (Table 4.5)

TREATMENT

Suramin and pentamidine in early acute infection, but cannot pass blood-brain barrier, are (useless in CNS involvement where Arsenical is used. Tryparsamide, Melarsen, Melarsoprol (Mel.B.) and *Trimelarsen* (water soluble). Tryparsamide is much better. Nitrofurazone (furacin) is used in resistant cases.

PROPHYLAXIS

This consists of:

1. Destruction of habitat of the vector.
2. Isolation of human population from areas harbouring infective games and treatment of all infected humans. This is effective in "Gambian".
3. Chemoprophylaxis. Pentamidine for "Gambian" disease. Single intramuscular injection of 4 mg/kg provide prophylaxis for 6 months.

TRYPANOSOMA CRUZI Chagas, 1909

(Organism of Chagas' disease or American Trypanosomiasis)

T. cruzi infection occurs in children; parasite is transmitted by Reduviid bugs in which the metacyclic infective form develops in hind gut. It is a "posterior station" parasite.

The disease is limited to South America (Peru, Ecuador, Columbia, Brazil), Panama and California.

T. cruzi amastigote form is seen in brain, muscles, thyroid, adrenals. Trypomastigote form "C" and "U"-shaped is found in blood.

T. cruzi is a plemorphic trypanosome having two phases of life cycle: (1) In man and other vertebrate hosts, (2) In insect vectors, invertebrate hosts. The morphology is best studied with Giemsa or Leishman.

IN HUMAN trypomastigotes are found in blood. Amastigote in RE cells, and tissues.

In blood. T. cruzi are spindle-shaped, 20 mu in length. Cytoplasm stains blue, nucleus and kinetoplast—violet, and flagellum red, (a) the long slender

'C' and 'U' forms, and (b) short, broad, *metacyclic* forms are seen **(Figs. 4.9 & 4.13, PL. 4.VII).**

In cells. As trypanosomes enter cells, undulating membrane disappears, flagellum is reduced to axoneme. Binary fission occurs in cell, producing amastigote form and by repeated division they fill and destroy the invaded cell. Their size is 1.5-4 mu, and a large nucleus stained ruby red, a kinetoplast with axoneme deep violet. Then parasites look like intracellular *L. donovani*, but in myocardium (**Fig. 4.12**) and Neuroglial cells amastigotes form collections, within a cystic cavity—showing all the forms: Amastigote, Promastigote, Epimastigote (crithidia) and Trypomastigote.

CULTIVATION

Cultivated in **NNN (Novy, MacNeal and Nicolla) medium**, in He La (cervical cancer) cells.

LIFE CYCLE

Life cycle of *T. cruzi* comprises two cycles of development. (**Fig. 4.13**):

(1) Human, Armadillo, Opossum. Bats, Monkeys act as reservoirs of infection. Disease spreads by bite of triatomid bugs. In man, no multiplication of trypomastigote occurs in blood. After entry in tissue cells, the Trypomastigotes take the Amastigote form intracellularly and divide by binary fission. As they escape from infected, destroyed cells, Promastigote, Epimastigote and then Trypomastigotes develop. Trypomastigotes appear in peripheral blood finally. The parasite multiplies in the human body in amastigote (leishmania) form, divides to invades tissue cells of spleen, liver, lymph nodes, bone-marrow, heart muscle and other tissues. The cycle is repeated. (2) Reduviid or Triatomid Bugs *Panstrongylus megistus* (*Triatoma megista*) or *Triatoma infestans* and *Rhodnius prolixus* are intermediate hosts and act as vectors. The trypomastigotes ('C' form) are ingested by the bugs *via* blood meal from an infected person. The development takes place in the bug intestine. *Trypomastigotes* become *stumpy epimastigote* (crithidia) *form* which multiplies to *slender epimastigote* (crithidia) *form* in the posterior part of the mid-gut. In 10 days, short *epimastigote* forms appear in bug rectum, and change to metacyclic trypomastigotes which are passed in the faeces (posterior station parasite). These are infective to man and animals, when rubbed into the punctured wound done by bug or in a abrased skin. The insect vector feeds on human skin at night and it deposits the liquid infective faeces on the skin while taking a blood meal, or after. Infection takes place when the metacyclic trypomastigote form is rubbed into the punctured wound by scratching. *Posterior Station Parasite* is called owing to faecal infection; African trypanosomes are *Anterior Station Parasites* as they infect through proboscis. The developmental cycle in the bug requires 2 weeks. Infection is carried through, during larval metamorphosis to growing adult bug which genetically transmits the disease.

EPIDEMIOLOGY

TRANSMISSION. Man becomes infected when the faeces containing the infective form of parasite enters into the skin as the organism is rubbed into the punctured wound caused by the bite of the transmitting insect; or through the abrasion caused by scratching.

VECTOR. The vector is a triatomid or cone-nosed bug *panstrongylus megistus* in Brazil, *Triatoma Infestans* in Northern Argentina and Uruguay, and *Rhodinus prolixus* in Northern South America, but numerous other triatomid bugs have been found naturally infected in endemic areas. In Panama *P. geniculatus* is the vector, and *Triatoma protracts* in California.

A VECTOR bites at mucocutaneous junction, outer canthus of eye, angle of lip and called *kissing bug*. Bite is painless and children sleep peacefully.

RESERVOIRS. In South America, dogs, cats, armadillos, opossums, ferrets, foxes, squirrels and monkeys are naturally infected. In Panama, bats are natural hosts in addition to armadillos and opossums.

SYMPTOMS

(See Fig. 4.14)

I.P. is within 1-2 weeks. Acute form occurs in children with parasitaemia, fever, severe toxaemia, followed by deposit of mucoid material in tissues causing tumefication of the entire body in 2 weeks. The face is swollen with oedema of the eyelids (dacryoadenitis) called Romana's sign (**Fig. 4.14**). Enlargement of regional lymph nodes (axillary and cervical) occurs. Trypanosomes are demonstrated in febrile stage), disappearing when temperature subsides.

More acute form is predominant in younger age groups with high mortality rate. Chronic disease

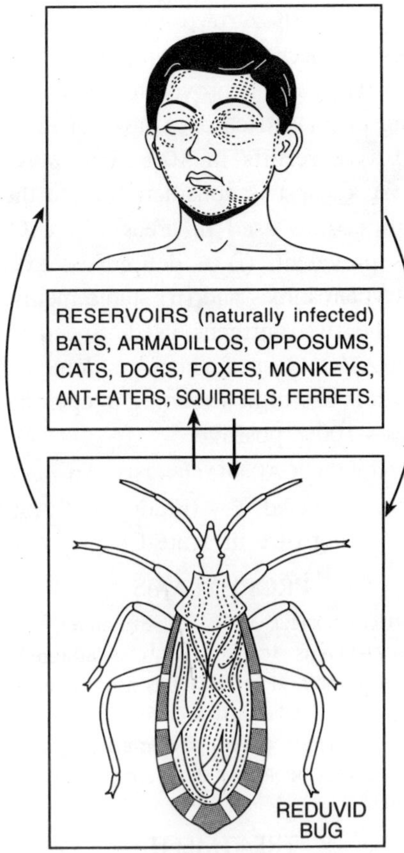

Fig. 4.14 *T. cruzi* infection in a child Reduviid bug acting as a vector

occurs in adult or children who survive acute infection, where amastigotes occur in visceral organs, and few/no trypanosomal form is seen in blood. In chronic infection symptoms are cardiac, meningoencephalitic, myxoedematous, pseudomyxomatous or Addison's type—according to involvement site (heart, brain, thyroid, ovary or suprarenals).

PATHOGENESIS

T. cruzi differs from African trypanosomes. Intracellular phase involves RE cells and also cells of myocardium, endocrine glands and glial cells of brain. After infection with the metacyclic trypomastigotes, parasites are engulfed by skin histiocytes forming a characteristic primary lesion "Chagoma" with cellular infiltration and fibrotic changes, encapsulating and blocking the lymphatics and capillaries, forming an oedematous area. They change to amastigote form after host cell destruction. When free they metastasise to satellite lymph nodes and soon enters blood stream (parasitaemia) assuming trypomastigote "C" and "U" forms. The parasite destroys cells of lymph nodes, lungs, liver, bone-marrow, where they multiply in fixed histiocytes, muscle fibres of the heart, neuroglia, and pyramidal cells of the cortex, adrenal glands, thyroid, gonads and intestinal mucosa, and where they produce destructive inflammatory reactions.

The parasites have a definite predilection for the cardiac and skeletal muscles, brain and endocrines. Therefore, chief pathological lesions are gross changes in the heart and brain and predominant symptoms are those of cardiac failure. The heart is greatly enlarged, pale, soft and haemorrhagic.

PATHOLOGY

T. cruzi is confined to body fluids. They absorb nutrient through body surface from the surrounding fluid at the expense of host blood sugar. The essential changes of trypanosomiasis are found in the lymph nodes and central nervous system. Inflammatory change after parasitaemia first occurs in lymph nodes with marked proliferation of sinus cells with infiltration of leucocytes round the blood vessels. In early stage lymphoid tissue proliferation, but in chronic stage there is enlargement of lymph nodes with histology like syphilis, productive endarteritis with endothelial proliferation of small arteries and by perivascular infiltration of plasma cells and lymphocytes. Lymph node puncture shows plenty of trypanosomes in early stage. Spleen is slightly enlarged.

Prior to CNS involvement, CSF is normal. With CNS involvement, CSF is under pressure, cell count increases to about 1,000 per cmm. *Globulin reaction*: Pandy's and Colloidal gold tests are positive, CSF reveals trypanosomes.

It produces meningo-encephalitis and meningo-myelitis, with perivascular infiltration of plasma cells and round cells in pia-arachnoid pons, medulla, and spinal cord. There is congestion with haemorrhages in areas and, at times, small cortical granulomatous lesions are seen.

There are large collections of organisms in the muscle fibres surrounded by interstitial infiltrate, of eosinophils, histiocytes and plasma cells. Brain is congested, oedematous containing scattered petechial haemorrhages. There are collections of organism associated with glial nodules. *Spleen* and *liver* are enlarged (cardiac failure). *Suprarenal cortex* involvement produces symptoms of Addison's disease, and *thyroid* produces myxoedema.

LABORATORY DIAGNOSIS

Direct Examination: (1) *T. cruzi* is found in *blood* (thick film) in febrile periods ('C' or 'U' trypomastigote).

(2) Amastigotes are present in tissue, demonstrated by *spleen, sternal* and *lymph node puncture.*

(3) Organism is cultivated at 22°C from blood in NNN. Chang's and He La cell culture media showing the epimastigotes and trypomastigotes.

(4) Laboratory animals: Guinea pigs/puppies show organism when 5 to 10 ml of infective blood is inoculated.

(5) *Xenodiagnostic test* is done for diagnosis. Laboratory-bred triatoma are allowed to suck blood from patient. The faeces or intestinal contents of the bug are examined after 10 days when epimastigote and/or metacyclic trypomastigotes are revealed in its faeces if organisms are present in patient's blood. Faeces is injected to mice or rats for confirmation of infection.

(6) Parasite is in CSF by direct methods (*centrifugation*), *culture, animal inoculation.*

(7) Amastigotes are demonstrated in *histopathology* of heart, brain or other tissues in operated or P.M. materials.

SERODIAGNOSIS. A (trypanosomal) *complement fixation test* has been devised with alcoholic extract of *T. cruzi* (antigen). It proved to be successful in diagnosing latent and chronic cases of the disease (false positive results in 10% with *Leishmania braziliensis*). CF test is considered to be the most reliable procedure used in areas where Chagas' disease is prevalent. (i) A delipidised extract of cultured trypanosomes and (ii) stable methylic extract are the two antigens used. Specific SLIDE AGGLUTINATION test of *T. cruzi* is done. An indirect HA test is useful in screening in epidemiological studies—100% positive.

IMMUNOLOGICAL DIAGNOSIS. An *intradermal test* has been devised. FA (Fluorescent Antibody) test shows rising titre in acute Chagas' disease.

PROPHYLAXIS

1. DRUG PROPHYLAXIS is not effective.
2. PROPHYLAXIS AGAINST VECTORS attained by residual spraying method of DDT has not proved successful in many cases. Residually sprayed Dieldrin markedly reduces the incidence (BHC or Gammexane).
3. PERSONAL PROPHYLAXIS is important by using mosquito nets.

TREATMENT

The drugs that are used in African trypomastigosis (trypanosomiasis) are not effective. No specific chemotherapy is known. Bayer 7602 (Ac) is regarded by some workers to be specific, and Bayer 9736 (As) is effective in cerebral symptoms. Primaquine and pentaquine are effective against experimental infections in puppies. Thyroid extract is disappointing in myxoedematous. □

CHAPTER 5

SUBPHYLUM : SPOROZOA

GENERAL CHARACTERS

The parasites belonging to this group of protozoa do not possess any special organ of *locomotion* (like flagella or cilia). They show slight amoeboid change of form. Reproduce asexually by fission (SCHIZOGONY) followed by sexual union or *syngamy* (SPOROGONY); alternation of generation. In plasmodia these two stages of life cycle take place in alternate hosts (HUMAN and MOSQUITO). So there is an alternation of generation and alternation of host. Human Pathogenic Sporozoa are divided into two main groups according to Site of affection:

I. INTESTINAL SPOROZOA

After sexual union, development of oocyst occurs in faeces and passed on soil. Infection is transmitted by contamination.

II. BLOOD-INHABITING SPOROZOA

HAEMOSPOROZOA

Sexual union (and SPOROGONY) takes place inside insect host (Mosquito). Infection is transmitted by *inoculation* (Mosquito bite).

TABLE 5.1

SIMPLE CLASSIFICATION OF MEDICALLY IMPORTANT SPOROZOA

SUBPHYLUM :	SPOROZOA		
CLASS :	TELOSPOREA		
SUBCLASS :	COCCIDIA		
ORDER :	EUCOCCIDA		
SUBORDER :	*EMIERIIDEA*		HAEMOSPORIDIIDEA
FAMILY :	*EIMERIIDAE*		PLASMODIIDAE
GENUS	ISOSPORA	TOXOPLASMA	PLAMODIUM
SPECIES :	*I. belli* *I. hominis*	*T. gondii*	*P. falciparum* *P. malariae* *P. ovale* *P. vivax*

SUBORDER: HAEMOSPORIDIDEA
Denilewsky, 1886
Family: Plasmodidae Mesnil, 1903
GENUS: PLASMODIA

This family contains one genus, Plasmodium, which includes the parasites causing malaria in man and other animals. The parasites are characterised by production of pigment during the asexual life cycle in RBCs with multiplication of parasite within these cells. Besides man, monkeys, birds, bats, rats, squirrels, flying foxes and lizards, are parasitised. The sporogony is completed in the invertebrate host, a mosquito.

The genus plasmodium contains more than 40 species and only 4 are pathogenic to man.

The plasmodia infecting monkeys and birds are extensively used in the laboratory in experimental studies of the developmental stages and screening new plasmodicidal drugs.

DEFINITION AND EXPLANATIONS OF TERMS

Sporozoite. It is the infective phase of the parasite which develops in the invertebrate hosts (anopheles mosquitoes) and infects the salivary glands of these vectors.

Pre-erythrocytic schizogony (PL. 5.I & 5.II). This is the stage of asexual reproduction which takes place before the infection of the erythrocytes. As sporozoites of the erythrocytes. As sporozoites are inoculated by a mosquito, by repeated division of the nucleus, they show development of schizonts in the parenchymal cells of the liver in 6-10 days (6 days in case of *P. falciparum* but 8-10 days in case of *P. vivax*). They do not show development of any pigment. By the rupture of the liver cell containing mature schizont, a large number of cells containing chromatin fragments and protoplasm, are liberated forming *cryptozoites* and the process is known as *cryptozoic schizogony*. These are likely to re-enter other liver cells for further multiplication, producing *metacryptozoites*. After the first or after 3 or 4 generations metacryptozoites enter the RBCs to start the erythrocytic schizogony. Thereafter, all developments in cells other than erythrocytes are known as *exo-erythrocytic schizogony* resulting in *phanerozoites* which infect RBCs. This stage is considered synonymous with pre-erythrocytic cycle and responsible for relapses. This stage is improbable and yet unknown in *P. falciparum*.

Erythrocytic schizogony. This is the stage of asexual reproduction in red blood corpuscles in which, division of chromatin takes place followed by the division of cytoplasm. In a fully grown schizont there are 8 to 32 newly formed merozoites. After rupture of the infected cell which is known as sporulation, liberation of merozoites takes place. These merozoites are small young parasites which attack new erythrocytes and the cycle repeats.

Trophozoite. It is the intracellular growing form of the parasite in red blood corpuscles of man and shows ring form in its young stage

Schizont (*schizo*—to split; *ont*—a being). This is the form of parasite in the process of asexual division. It is called immature when the division has just started or it is incomplete but it is mature or full grown when the division is complete forming a *rosette*.

Sporogony. This is a process of sexual reproduction, which occurs in the case of malarial parasites, in the mosquito giving rise to sporozoites.

Gametocyte. This is the sexual stage of parasite which occurs in man. There is cytoplasm, chromatin and pigment but the chromatin does not show any division whatsoever. The gametocytes are differentiated into males and females and are called *microgametocytes* and *macrogametocytes* respectively. This is based on the morphology, i.e., staining character and distribution of chromatin and pigment.

Gametes are derived from gametocytes and formed in the stomach of the mosquito. Male gamete corresponds to a spermatozoa and female gamete to an ovum.

Zygote. It is a fertilized macrogamete.

Ookinete (Travelling vermicule). It is an elongated zygote capable of moving in the wall of the stomach which is limited by tunica elastica muscularis investing the outer surface of the stomach wall.

Oocyst. An ookinete which settles down in the stomach wall of the infected mosquito, becomes rounded and covered by a membranous wall forming a cyst. *Sporoblasts* and *sporozoites* develop in the oocyst.

PLATE 5.I

FIG. 1 & 2: PRE-ERYTHROCYTIC SCHIZONTS OF *P. VIVAX* (HUMAN LIVER)

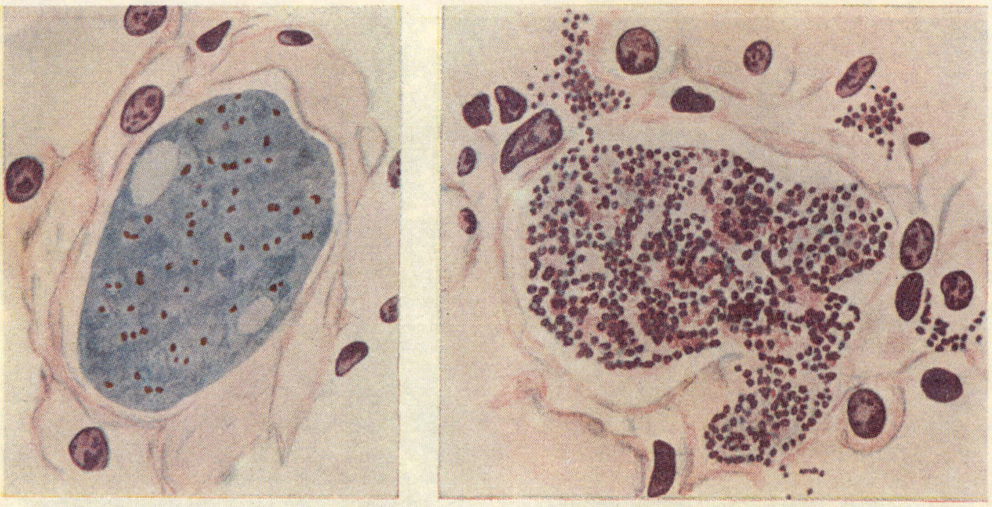

FIG. 3 TO 6: PRE-ERYTHROCYTIC SCHIZONTS OF *P. FALCIPARUM* (HUMAN LIVER)

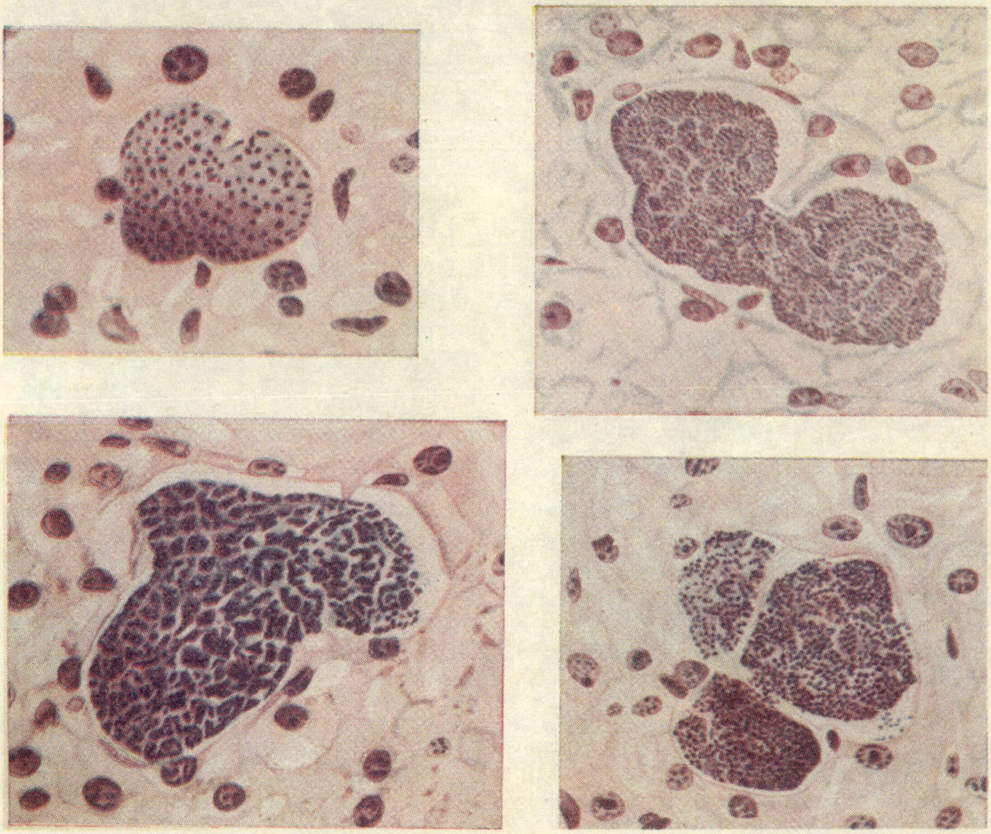

(1) 7th day form with vacuolation. (2) Advanced 7th day schizont (lobulated) with release of merozoites. Shortt and Garnham, 1948; courtesy of *Trans. Roy. Soc. Trop. Med & Hyg.* (3) 4 days. (4) 5 days. (5) 6 days after mosquito bite and (6) Mature schizont (lobed) ready to burst. Shott *et. al.,* 1951; courtesy of *Trans. Roy. Soc. Trop. Med. & Hyg.*

PLATE 5.II

PRE-ERYTHOROCYTIC SCHIZONTS OF *P. OVALE* (HUMAN LIVER)

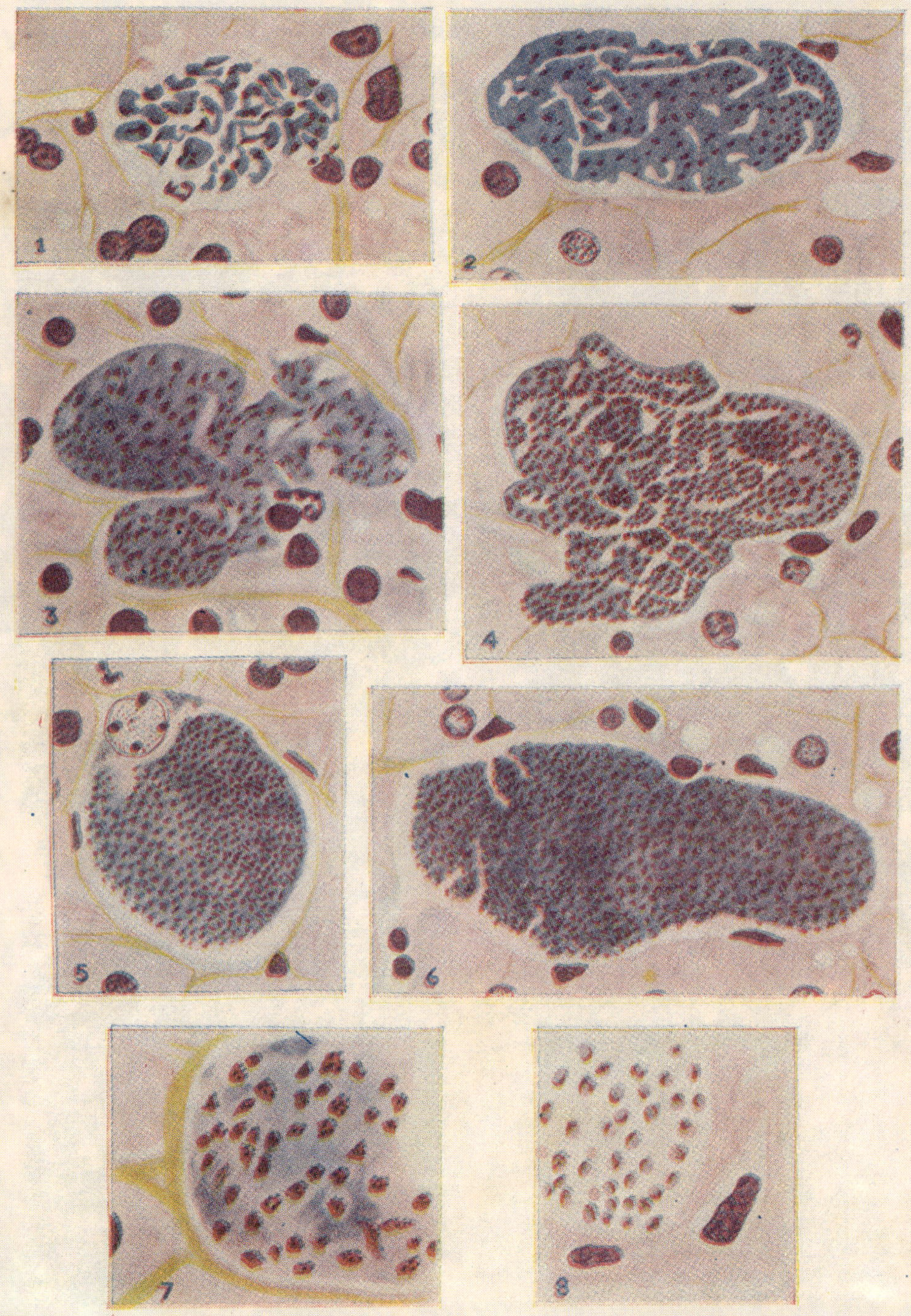

Immature: (1) 5th day form. (2) Form showing clefts. (3) Lobular form with larger nuclei. (4) Form with whorls and pallisade arrangements of nuclei. (5) Form with nucleus pushed to one side. (6) Mature 9th day form packed with merozoites. (7) Portion of Fig. 3 showing nuclear structure. (8) Portion of Fig. 6 showing arrangement of merozoites. Garnham *et al.,* 1955; courtesy of *Trans. Roy. Soc. Trop. Med. & Hyg.*

MALARIAL PARASITES AND MALARIA

History. A disease resembling malaria was mentioned in *Susruta Samhita*, where the spread of the disease was attributed to the bite of an insect. The disease was described in the 5th century BC by Hippocrates.

In 1638, the Countess of Cinchon, wife of a Spanish Viceroy of Peru, was cured with the bark of an indigenous tree of Peru. The plant was brought by her to Europe. It was subsequently named Cinechona in honor of the Countess. In 1820, quinine was isolated from CInchona bark. In 1753, the name malaria (*mal*—bad; *aria*—air) was given by an Italian writer. In 1847, Meckel discovered malarial pigment in the blood and viscera. In 1880, Laveran, a French military surgeon, discovered malarial parasites in the blood. In 1885, Golgi described stages of the quartan parasite in red blood corpuscles and exactly determined thye periodicity of fever to be 72 hours. In 1894, Manson suggested that the mosquitoes might be the vector of malaria. In 1898, Surgeon-Major Ross proved that infection of Proteosoma in sparrow was transmitted by Culex mosquitoes. This was supported by finding of sporozoites in the salivary gland of mosquitoes.

Italian workers, namely, Birnami, Grassi, and Bastianelli described the development of human and mosquito cycles of malaria parasites in a series of papers (1898-99). On 3rd November, 1898, Bignami succeeded in experimentally infecting man with malaria from Anopheles mosquito.

Since 1930 many workers on avian malaria demonstrated the tissue phase of avian malarial parasite in the RE cells and other mesodermal cells in *P. elongatum, P. relictum*, and *P. cynomolgi* and in human parasite—*P. cynomolgi* malaria.

In 1949, Shortt and his associates discovered the pre-erythrocytic schizogony of *P. falciparum* in a human volunteer in the liver after sixth day, and in 1952, Jeffrey and others demonstrated 3 days old pre-erythrocytic schizont of *P. falciparum* in human liver. In 1954, Garnham and his associates discovered the pre-erythrocytic schizogony of *P. ovale*.

In 1960 Bray demionstrated the pre-erythrocytic cycle of *P. malariae* in the parenchyma cells of the liver by inoculating sporozoites obtained from *A. gambiense* into a chimpanzee with the formation of mature schizont after twelve and half days.

GENUS: PLASMODIUM

Marchiafaya and Celli, 1885

General characteristics. Parasites of the genus plasmodium infect not only man but also apes, monkeys, birds and other vertebrate hosts. They complete their life cycles in two hosts. The asexual cycle (schizogony) occurs inside the red blood cells of the vertebrate host (the intermediate host); whereas the sexual cycle (sporogony) occurs in the invertebrate host (definitive or final host), a mosquito. Thus there is an *alternation of generations* associated with *alternation of host*; i.e., sporogony in mosquitoes and schizogony in man or other hosts. Sporogony → Schizogony → Sporogony, etc.

Staining reaction. When stained with Leishman, Giemsa or Romanowsky stain the red blood corpuscle is stained pink, cytoplasm of the parasite blue and chromatin superb ruby red. The pigment is stained brown or brownish black, cytoplasm of male gametocytes greenish blue and that of female gametocytes blue.

Species parasitic to human. Four species of parasites of the genus plasmodium are pathogenic to human causing malaria which manifests as an acute or chronic disease characterised by successive attacks either primary or relapses with paroxysm of fever, typically intermittent with periodicity and associated with anaemia and splenomegaly. The species are as follows: (1) *Plasmodium vivax* (Grassi and Feletti, 1890), causing benign tertian malaria. (2) *Plasmodium malariae* (Laveran, 1881) Grassi and Feletti 1890, producing quartan malaria. (3) *Plasmodium falciparum* (Welch, 1890) producing malignant tertian, subtertian, aestivo-autumnal or falciparum malaria. (4) *Plasmodium ovale* (Stephens, 1922) producing ovale tertian malaria.

Species parasitic to animals. A large number of species of vertebrate hosts are infected with plasmodia; namely, higher apes, monkeys, birds like sparrows, canaries, domestic fowls, ducks or bats, cold blooded animals like lizards, etc. In man (human malaria) or in monkey (simian malaria) the parasites are transmitted by ANopheline mosquitoes but in birds (avian malaria) it is done by Culicine mosquitoes. The species parasitic in monkeys and birds are tabulated (Table 5.2).

TABLE 5.2

In Monkey	In Birds
P. knowlesi	*P. gallinaceum, P. relictum*
P. cynomolgi	*P. cathemerium, P. elongatum*
P. inui etc.	*P. lophurae* etc.

Malaria Parasites in Human

Geographical distribution. Malaria is seen in all countries extending from 40°S to 60°N of the equator, covering a large portion of the tropical and subtropical regions. Highly endemic areas are often seen in the tropical regions, where humidity and temperatures are favourable for the breeding of the Anopheline mosquitoes and growth of the parasite in the insect vector. *P. vivax* is the specially prevalent species in the temperate zone, whereas *P. malariae* is a parasite of the subtropical zone in India specially in Assam. *P. ovale* has been specially reported from East Africa, West Africa (Nigeria) and Philippines.

Habitat. The parasite, after infection caused by the bite of a mosquito, enters the blood and carried to the parenchyma cells of the liver, where they multiply enormously. This is called the *pre-erythrocytic* or *tissue phase.* By rupture of the infected cells of the liver they enter the red blood corpuscles, the *erythrocytic phase* (*Schizogony*) and reach all the organs of the body *via* the circulating blood, producing parasitaemia.

Life cycle. The life cycle of malaria parasite occurs in *two hosts*; namely; (i) *the human or intermediate host* in which the schizogony or asexual cycle takes place — the human cycle and (ii) *mosquito, the definitive host*, in which sexual cycle or sporogony occurs — the mosquito cycle (PL. 5.III & 5.IV).

HUMAN CYCLE (SCHIZOGONY/ASEXUAL CYCLE)

(Table 5.4)

The malaria parasites undergo several developmental phases in the human host. The *infection* in man is produced by the bite of an infected female Anopheline mosquito which harbours in its salivary gland the sporozoites of the plasmodium of any of the species mentioned above. Shute (1945) found that in the salivary glands of mosquitoes the number of sporozoites may vary from 950 to 200,000 or more from the fourth to the eleventh day after infection. A mosquito can inject 3000 sporozoites into a person at each bite. The sporozoites are thread-like curved organisms, measuring about 12μ in length, with a central elongated nucleus but without any pigment. Available evidences indicate that the sporozoites enter into the circulation, where they remain for 30 to 60 minutes after which they disappear from blood.

PRE-ERYTHROCYTIC SCHIZOGONY. A developmental phase occurs in the tissues of the host before the sporozoite becomes infective for the erythrocyte to start the stage of erythrocytic schizogony. This is referred to as pre-erythrocytic schizogony. The complete course of phase lasts for about 8 days in case of *P. vivax*, 6 days in *P. falciparum*, 9 days in *P. ovale* and about 15 days in case of *P. malariae* (Table 5.3).

It was formerly believed that sporozoites directly infected the erythrocytes and developed in it. Observation of Yorks and Macfie (1929) clearly indicated that malaria induced by inoculation of blood from malaria induced by inoculation of blood from malaria patients in which merozoites are concerned, is much easier to cure than natural malaria following inoculation of sporozoites by mosquitoes. Boyd *et al.* (1934), Fairley (1947) and others observed that during a period of 6 days in case of *P. falciparum* and 7 to 9 days in case of *P. vivax* after infection with sporozoites, the blood of the inoculated person was not infectious to others. It was also observed that about 30 minutes after inoculation the sporozoites disappeared from blood. It was suggested by James (1931) and Ruge (1936) that these sporozoites must have been multiplying in the fixed RE cells before entering the red cells. Many workers demonstrated the pre-erythrocytic and exo-erythrocytic stages in avian parasites; namely, *P. elongatum, P. relictum, P. gallinaceum* and other species in the RE cells and other parts of the mesoderm.

Shortt and Garnham (1948) demonstrated the pre-erythrocytic stage of simian parasites *P. cynomolgi* in the liver parenchyma cells and this closely resembled *P. vivax* (Plate 5.I), and later in 1949 the pre-erythrocytic form of *P. falciparum* in the parenchyma cells of the human liver; (Plate 5.I). Jeffery and his colleagues confirmed the latter finding in 1952. A similar pre-erythrocytic form of *P. ovale* was found by Garnham *et al.* (1954) located in the parenchyma cells of the human liver (Plate 5.II). In *P. cynomolgi*, the pre-erythrocytic schizogony is observed from the second day onward, when the parasite is round or oval 2.5μ in length with an undivided nucleus. By the fourth day, it is compact, measures 11μ in diameter with 24 nuclei. With the growth of the parasite, the nucleus of the host cell is pushed to one corner and one or more vacuoles appear in the cytoplasm of the parasite. On measures 38μ and contains about 10,000 merozoites devrived from the schizonts but some of the schizonts may be 100μ or larger in size. Most of the merozoites derived from these schizonts enter erythrocytes, but some of them re-enter into parenchyma cells of the liver to continue to persist in the parenchyma cells of the liver for over 3 months and these forms are likely to be responsible for relapses. The pre-erythrocytic forms of *P. vivax* are similar to those of *P. cynomolgi*, and indirect evidences suggest that they also persist to live in the parenchyma cells of liver to produce relapses.

In case of *P. falciparum*, the youngest form observed is about 3 days old, measuring about 15μ in diameter. The schizont grows rapidly. According to Garnham (1954), the parasite pushes out in any direction, where the pressure of the tissue is least, resulting in lobes and protuberances on the surface of the schizont. *Vacuoles are absent* in the sixth day, measuring about 60μ and containing 40,000 merozoites. As there is no relapse in this case, exo-erythrocytic schizogony is considered to be absent.

The exo-erythrocytic form of *P. malariae* has not been studied in man, but similar parasite is known in simian quartan parasite — *P. inui*, which closely resembles *P. malariae* in (*a*) general morphology, (*b*) erythrocytic cycle (72 hours) and (*c*) duration of sporogony. Cytomeres form on the 11th day and mature schizont measures about 24μ in diameter, containing 2000 merozoites.

Bray (1960) demonstrated the pre-erythrocytic cycle in a chimpanzee, the duration of this cycle being about 15 days and the merozoites are about 1500.

In *P. ovale*, there is a prepatent period of 9 days. The mature pre-erythrocytic schizont is irregular and measures about 42μ with an unusually large nucleus and there is the suggestion of division into 'cytomeres'.

Various stages of pre-erythrocytic form of development have been postulated. The first stage consists of ***cryptozoic schizogony*** resulting in the formation of ***cryptozoites***. These perhaps enter other liver parenchyma cells, initiating further pre-erythrocytic schizogony and forming ***metacryptozoites***. After 3 or 4 generations or immediately after the first, the metacryptozoites attack RBCs in circulation to initiate the erythrocytic schizogony. After this all forms of development in cells other than those in erythrocytes are referred to as *exo-erythrocytic schizogony* producing *phanerozoites*.

GROWTH IN PARENCHYMA CELLS OF THE LIVER. *Garnham* (1954) suggested that, malaria plasmodium, a coccidian parasite of man, is likely

TABLE 5.3

DIFFERENTIAL CHARACTERS OF THE TISSUE PHASE OF MAMMALIAN MALARIA PARASITES (Modified from Garnham, 1954)

Species	Duration of pre-erythrocytic	Size of mature schizont cycle in days	No. of merozoites liberated in μ	Special features (approximate)	Existence of exo-erythrocytic cycle
P. cynomolgi	8	34	< 10,000	Vacuoles	Yes
P. vivax	8	42	> 10,000	Vacuoles	Probable
P. falciparum	6	60	40,000	Irregular contour	Improtable
P. ovale	9	45	? 10,000	Large nuclei	Protable
P. malariae (chimpanzee)	12	48	1294-1739	Vacuoles (5-8)	Protable
P. inui	11	24	2,000	'Cytomeres'	Protable

to develop in the parenchyma cells of the liver due to the following causes: (1) Phylogenetically, malaria parasites are probably derived from coccidia, developing in the intestinal epithelium which is the same as that of the liver; (2) the richness of the nucleoprotein and aminoacids in parenchyma cells makes it specially suitable for rapid nuclear multiplication of the parasite; (3) it may be recalled that parenchyma cells have well known allied parasites like Hepatozoon.

ERYTHROCYTIC SCHIZOGONY. In this phase the pre-erythrocytic merozoites free in the circulating blood, attack the RBCs and develop in these cells through stages of trophozoites, schizont and merozoites. The parasites in these stages of development can be demonstrated in the smears of peripheral blood, 3-4 days after the completion of the pre-erythrocytic schizogony. Each cycle of schizogony occurs regularly after 48 or 72 hours according to the species. The sporulation occurs after 48 hours in case of tertian fevers, but it is 72 hours in case of quartan fever caused by *P. malariae* (see charts 1 & 2). The cycle continues with precise regularly for considerable period, but there may be anticipation in case of malignant tertian, giving an asynchronous cycle with a continuous or remittent temperature (see chart 3). This is why it is called subtertian malaria. In course of time the infection wanes out due to the exhaustion of the asexual reproductive power or due to the spontaneous destruction of the parasite.

GAMETOGONY. After a variable period of erythrocytic schizogony, depending on the host developing into trophozoites develop into gametocytes in the RBCs of the capillaries of the internal organs like spleen and bone marrow but mature forms of gametocytes often appear in the peripheral blood. The lag periods after which gametocytes. The asexual parasites taken with the blood meal are destroyed in the stomach of the mosquito, where blood forms a clot. In the first phase of development, the crescents as other gametocytes become rounded. The pigment of microgametocyte shows violent movement and soon exflagellation occurs, characterised by the development of 4-8 filamentous structures. They become detached and form the microgametes. The exflagellation can also be observed outside the mosquito host in a moist chamber preparation of peripheral blood. The flagella are extremely motile and only one of them penetrates the ***macrogamete*** which develops by undergoing a process of nuclear division and extrusion of polar bodies. One macrogamete develops from one macrogametocyte. When the macrogamete is ready for fertilisation, the microgamete is attracted towards the macrogamete by a process of chemotaxis. The microgamete attaches itself to the macrogamete at the site of a protrusion and penetrates it. This is followed by fusion of the male and female pronucleus and within a short time the fertilised macrogamete is transformed into a zygote. The whole process of development is complete within 20 minutes to a hours after the blood meal of the mosquito, depending on the moisture and temperature of the atomosphere. The zygote now acquires the power of active movement and the body is now called ookinete or *travelling vermicule*

TABLE 5.4

ASEXUAL CYCLE (SCHIZOGONY)
(Sporozoite Inoculated by Mosquitoes)
1. TISSUE PHASE
↓

P. vivax, P. ovale, P. malariae		*P. falciparum*	
Pre-erythrocytic → schizogony	Exo-erythrocytic schizogony	Pre-erythrocytic schigony	Exo-erythrocytic schizogony is unknown
↓	↓	2. ERYTHROCYTIC PHASE	↓
Erythrocytic schizogony Malaria (primary infectior) with recrudescences	Erythrocytic schizogony Malaria (secondary infection) with relapses	Erythrocytic schizogony Malaria (primary infection) with recrudescences	No erythrocytic schizogony No relapse of malaria.

with a pointed end. It penetrates through the epithelial lining and the muscular wall and lies below the outer limiting membrane of the stomach wall, forming a rounded body called *oocyst*. It measures 6-12μ in diameter containing a single vesicular nucleus and pigment granules of the macrogamete. With the further development, the oocyst increases to a size of about 60μ in diameter by the successive nuclear division containing several hundreds or thousands of sickle shaped bodies called **Sporozoites**. The cyst is now called a **Sporocyst**. The number of oocysts varies from 20 to 30 in the stomach wall. The oocysts are matured in about 10-14 days after the infective blood feed. Sporocyst ruptures; sporozoites liberated in body cavity (haemocele) of the mosquito. The sporozoites are carried through the circulatory fluid to all parts of the body of the mosquito except the ovaries. The sporozoites which have special predilection for the salivary glands, pass through the gland and ultimately reach the lumen of the duct, where a maximum concentration of sporozoites is attained. The mosquito is now infective and is capable of transmitting the infection to man. It has been observed that certain species of Anopheline mosquitoes are capable of transmitting the disease even by a single bite. These species of mosquitoes contain oocysts in the stomach wall and sporozoites in the salivary gland, and hence a survey of the mosquitoes forms an important part for the epidemiological study and control of malaria in endemic areas. It should be noted that different species of the parasite can develop in the same mosquito and the bite of such an infected mosquito can transmit the infection and produce a "mixed infection" like that of *P. vivax* and *P. falciparum*.

Development of mosquito or sequal cycle (*sporogony*). Different species of parasites take different periods for their development of sexual cycle at a given temperature. The period taken for the development of different species of plasmodia in Anopheles is tabulated (Table 5.4).

INFECTION. When an infected mosquito bites, infection takes place by the escape of sporozoites contained in the salivary secretion into the blood of the human host. The cycle in mosquito is complete in 10-14 days or so. Though **sporozoite-induced malaria** is the natural mode of infection, erythrocytic stage of the malaria parasite is also infectious to man producing **trophozoite-induced** malaria. It differs from sporozoite-induced malaria in not occurring of the pre-erythrocytic stage. This type of tramsmission may occur through placenta or accidentally from blood transfusion from infected donors. It is used therapeutically in the treatment of general paresis. This is easily controlled and amenable to quinine therapy (Table 5.5).

TABLE 5.5

Species	Optimum temperature for development	Development of sexual cycle in the mosquitoes
P. vivax	25°C	8-10 days
P. ovale	25°C	14-18 days
P. falciparum	30°C	10-12 days
P. malariae	22°C	18-21 days

Summary. Two phases of development of malaria parasites are present in man:

I. TISSUE PHASE IN THE LIVER—(a) PRE-ERYTHROCYTIC (PRIMARY PRE-ERYTHROCYTIC) phase without any clinical symptoms or pathological destruction of liver. (b) EXO-ERYTHROCYTIC (SECONDARY PRE-ERYTHROCYTIC) phase responsible for relapses.

II. ERYTHROCYTIC PHASE, occurs inside the RBCs. (a) SCHIZOGONY—causing overt attacks of malaria. (b) GAMETOGONY—being the source of infection for mosquitoes.

The essential difference between the tissue phase and erythrocytic phase is that **haemozoin** pigment is absent in the former; whereas it is always present in the latter.

MOSQUITO CYCLE (PL. 5.III & 5.IV)

(SPOROGONY/SEXUAL CYCLE)

It has already been stated that gametogony with formation of gametocytes start about 10 days on an average after the malarial paroxysm has started in man. The male and female gametocytes are called *microgametocyte* and *macrogametocyte*, respectively. The insect vector in this case is a female Anopheline mosquito. The mosquito during her blood meal from an infected person or a carrier sucks blood containing sexual or both sexual and asexual malaria parasites. The presence of mature male and female sexual parasites (full grown *gametocytes*) is essential for the further development of the mosquito/sexual cycle (*sporogony*) in the mosquitoes. It has been estimated that at least 12 gametocytes must be present per cent of blood and the macrogametocyte must be in excess to the number of microgametocytes. The asexual parasites taken with the blood meal are destroyed in the stomach of the mosquito, where blood forms a clot. In the first phase of development, the crescents as other gametocytes become rounded. The pigment of microgametocyte shows violent movement and soon exflagellation occurs, characterised by the development of 4-8 filamentous structures. They become detached and form the microgametes. The exflagellation can also be observed outside the mosquito host in a moist chamber preparation of peripheral blood. The flagella are extremely motile and only one of them penetrates the ***macrogamete*** which develops by undergoing a process of nuclear division and extrusion of polar bodies. One macrogamete develops from one macrogametocyte.

When the macrogamete is ready for fertilisation, the microgamete is attracted towards the macrogamete by a process of chemotaxis. The microgamete attaches itself to the macrogamete at the site of a protrusion and penetrates it. This is followed by fusion of the male and female pronucleus and within a short time the fertilised macrogamete is transformed into a zygote. The whole process of development is complete within 20 minutes to 2 hours after the blood meal of the mosquito, depending on the moisture and temperature of the atmosphere. The zygote now acquires the power of active movement and the body is now called ookinete or ***travelling vermicule*** with a pointed end. It penetrates through the epithelial lining and the muscular wall and lies below the outer limiting membrane of the stomach wall, forming a rounded body called *oocyst*. It measures 6-12μ in diameter containing a single vesicular nucleus and pigment granules of the macrogamete. With the further development, the oocyst increases to a size of about 60μ in diameter by the successive nuclear division containing several hundreds or thousands of sickle shaped bodies called Sporozoites. The cyst is now called a sporocyst. The number of oocysts varies from 20 to 30 in the stomach wall. The oocysts are matured in about 10-14 days after the infective blood feed. Sporocyst ruptures; sporozoites are liberated in body cavity (haemocele) of the mosquito. The sporozoites are carried through the circulatory fluid to all parts of the body of the mosquito except the ovaries. The sporozoites which have special predilection for the salivary glands, pass through the gland and ultimately reach the lumen of the duct, where a maximum concentration of sporozoites is attained. The mosquito is now infective and is capable of transmitting the infection to man. It has been observed that certain species of Anopheline mosquitoes are capable of transmitting the disease even by a single bite. These species of mosquitoes contain oocysts in the stomach wall and sporozoites in the salivary gland, and hence a survey of the mosquitoes forms an important part for the epidemiological study and control of malaria in endemic areas. It should be noted that different species of the parasite can develop in the same mosquito and the bite of such an infected mosquito can transmit the infection and produce a "mixed infection" like that of *P. vivax* and *P. falciparum*.

Development of mosquito or sexual cycle (*sporogony*). Different species of parasites take different periods for their development of sexual cycle at a given temperature. The period taken for the development of different species of plasmodia in Anopheles is tabulated (Table 5.6).

INFECTION. When an infected mosquito bites, infection takes place by the escape of sporozoites contained in the salivary secretion into the blood of the human host. The cycle in mosquito is complete in 10-14 days or so. Though sporozoite-induced malaria is the natural mode of infection, erythrocytic stage of the malaria parasite is also infectious to man producing trophozoite-induced malaria. It differs from sporozoite-induced malaria in not occuring of the pre-erythrocytic stage. This type of transmission may occur through placenta or accidentally from blood transfusion from infected donors. It is used therapeutically in the treatment of general paresis. This is easily controlled and amenable to quinine therapy.

LIFE CYCLE OF MALARIAL PARASITE (*Plasmodium vivax. P. ovale, P. malariae, P. falciparum AND SITES OF ACTION OF ANTIMALARIAL DRUGS*)

MALARIAL PARASITE

HUMAN CYCLE
i.e., Asexual cycle
(SCHIZOGONY)

HUMAN IS INTERMEDIATE HOST

MOSQUITO CYCLE
i.e., Sexual cycle
(SPOROGONY)

MOSQUITO IS DEFINITIVE HOST

HUMAN CYCLE

ASEXUAL CYCLE: STARTS WITH INTRODUCTION OF SPOROZOITES BY THE BITE OF AN INFECTED FEMALE ANOPHELINE MOSQUITO

FOUR PHASES EXIST IN THE HUMAN CYCLE

NO LIVER DAMAGE NO CLINICAL MANIFESTATION

I. PRE-ERYTHROCYTIC PHASE (PRIMARY EXO-ERYTHROCYTIC PHASE, P-E PHASE, OR PRIMARY OR EARLY TISSUE PHASE IN LIVER

Sporozoites injected to host (By Mosquito bite)

Spreads To Surrounding Tissue

Peripheral Circulation (Remains for Half Hour)
Does not enter RBC

Liver Parenchyma (PRE-ERYTHROCYTIC or PRIMARY EXO-ERYTHROCYTIC before infecting RBC)

This phase occurs in all the FOUR SPECIES (PL. 5.III)
(Not yet proved in *P. malariae*)

This phase lasts for in case of :

P. falciparum—6 days

P. vivax—8 days

P. malariae—9 days

MEROZOITES liberated at the end of the phase called PHANEROZOITES (CRYPTOZOITES)

Animal inoculation. Human malaria parasites cannot be successfully inoculated into lower animals, and likewise malarial parasite of lower animals cannot infect the human host.

Mode of transmission. The VECTOR is the female Anopheline mosquito. The sporogony develops in 8-10 days after biting an infected person or a carrier, having mature gametocytes in the blood.

PORTAL OF ENTRY. The infected mosquito bites a person and the sporozoites enter the blood through the skin. The INFECTIVE FORM is the sporozoite escaping from the salivary gland of the mosquito during bite. The sporozoites disappear from the circulating blood in about 30 minutes and multiply in the liver cells (**pre-erythrocytic phase**). The merozoites from the liver escape into the circulating blood about 8-10 days after maturation and attack the RBCs (erythrocytic phase). The infection may be artificially induced by injection of sporozoites contained in the emulsion of the salivary gland, the so called **sporozoite-induced** malaria.

RESERVOIR. Human hosts, the gametocyte carriers, act as the reservoir of infection. The gametocytes harboured in their blood, may develop in the female Anopheline mosquitoes, when they bite the carriers.

SPOROZOITES- AND TROPHOZOITES-INDUCED MALARIA

The infection may be artificially induced by injection of sporozoites contained in the emulsion of the salivary gland, the so–called **sporozoite-induced** malaria.

Trophozoite-induced malaria may be seen: (i) after blood transfusion when persons with latent malaria infections become donors; (ii) in congenital malaria when the foetus is infected *in utero* through some leakage in the placenta, or (iii) as therapeutic malaria, when malaria is artificially induced in neurosyphilis (general paresis).

According to revised scheme SUBPHYLUM SPOROZOA is divided into 3 classes: I. TELOSPOREA, II. TOXOPLASMEA. III. Haplosporea (no human representative). Class Telosporea has 2 subclasses:

1. Gregarinia (*no human representative*). 2. COCCIDIA. Subclass Coccidia has 2 orders : 1. PROTOCOCCIDA (no human representative) 2. EUCOCCIDA. Order Eucoccida is divided into 3 suborders:

1. Adeleidea (no human representative)
2. Eimeriidea
3. HAEMOSPORIDIIDEA (Medically important)

Two types of Cryptozoites form in the Liver in Pre-erythrocytic phase : Larger ones occur in 3 species, smaller Cryptozoites occur in *P. falciparum* only.

Larger Cryptozoites called

I) MACROMEROZOITES

↓

Re-enter Liver (SECONDARY EXO-ERYTHROCYTIC PHASE. (see later *EXO-ERYTHROCYTIC CYCLE*). They occur in case of : *P. vivax, P. malariae, P. ovale.*

(Secondary) EXO-ERYTHROCYTIC PHASE (RE-ENTERING LIVER) DOES NOT OCCUR IN *P. falciparum* (PL. 5.IV).

ii) **Smaller Cryptozoites** called **MICROMEROZOITES (OCCURS IN *P. falciparum*)**. The MICROMEROZOITES enter circulation directly (Erythrocytic Phase) in *P. falciparum* only : it does not reenter liver; does not pass the liver twice.

TABLE 5.6
DIFFERENCE BETWEEN SPOROZOITE AND TROPHOZOITE-INDUCED MALARIA

	Sporozoite-induced Malaria	*Trophozoite-induced Malaria*
PRE-ERYTHROCYTIC SCHIZOGONY	Present	Absent
INCUBATION PERIOD	Long	Short
EXO-ERYTHROCYTIC SCHIZOGONY	May be present	Absent
RELAPSE	May occur	Does not occur
SCHIZONTICIDAL DRUGS	No radical cure, may be due to the presence of exo-erythrocytic forms	Can be radically cured, as there is no exo-erythrocytic form

In this stage. neither any clinical manifestation nor any pathological damage occurs in the liver. Parasites are not found in peripheral blood (till RBCs are affected in Erythrocytic Phase).

DRUGS EFFECTIVE AT THIS STAGE ARE : 8—AMINOQUINOLINES, PROGUANIL. PYRIMETHAMINE (DARAPRIM)

II. *ERYTHROCYTIC PHASE*

During this phase parasites reside inside the red blood corpuscles.

***ERYTHROCYTIC PHASE* (IN RBC)**

('*E*' *Phase*)

Macromerozoites

(*P. vivax, P. malariae, P. ovale*)

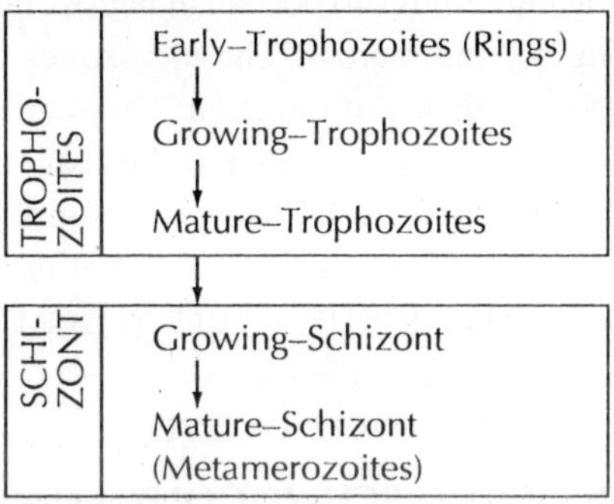

MEROZOITES (OLD RBCs Burst, Liberated MEROZOITES Attack Fresh RBC

A SINGLE 'E'-PHASE LASTS FOR

36-48 HOURS IN

P. vivax

P. falciparum

P. ovale.

AND

For 72 hours in *P. malariae.*

P. vivax. P. falciparum and *P. ovale* stay in RBCs for 48 hours (for completion of a single Erythrocytic Cycle); the temperature occurs after that time by (haemolysis) on every 3rd day (at 40 hours interval.

P. vivax is called BENIGN as it does not produce malignant (harmful) effect, and temperature occurs every third day (tertian). So, the infection is called BENIGN TERTIAN (B.T.) INFECTION. Similarly as *P. falciparum* causes malignant (harmful) effect and temperature occurs at every 40 hour interval. It is called MALIGNANT TERTIAN (M.T.) INFECTION.

So also *P. malariae* stays in a single Erythrocytic Cycle for 72 hours, hence temperature occurs every 4th day (Quartan) and the infection is called QUARTAN (Q.T.) FEVER or Q.T. infection.

These asexual forms of parasites can be demonstrated in peripheral blood by :

(a) Thin Smear

(b) Thick Smear

(c) Culture by Bass & John's method.

(For detail see **Appendix I**)

III. *EXO-ERYTHROCYTIC (E-E) PHASE,* OR *SECONDARY EXO-ERYTHROCYTIC CYCLE* OR LATE TISSUE PHASE IN LIVER

No. E-E Phase in *P. falciparum* so there is no relapse of M. T. infection

E-E cycle takes place in *P. vivax, P. malariae* and *P. ovale* by macromerozoites which do not enter circulation immediately after coming out of the liver. A part of Macromerozoite population may directly attach an RBC to start *Erythrocytic Schizogony*. But Rest of the Macromerozoites RE-ENTER OR RE-INVADE FRESH LIVER CELLS (PARENCHYMAL CELLS OF LIVER) TO MAINTAIN EXO-ERYTHROCYTIC CYCLE. So it is also known as SECONDARY EXO-ERYTHROCYTIC CYCLE. (while pre-erythrocytic cycle is known as PRIMARY EXO-ERYTHROCYTIC CYCLE).

In *P. falciparum*. There is no *Exo-erythrocytic phase*. So, there is NO RELAPSE (only Endogenous Recrudescence is there). In *Exo-erythrocytic schizogony* the parasites remain Dormant or potentially Infective to give rise to infection from time to time which is 1-3 years for *P. ovale*, 3-years for *P. vivax*, while 40 years for *P. malariae*.

EXO-ERYTHROCYTIC CYCLE ALWAYS PRECEDES ERYTHROCYTIC CYCLE. *EXO-ERYTHROCYTIC* CYCLE *NEVER OCCURS AFTER ERYTHROCYTIC PHASE*. So, LIVER is the potent reservoir of parasites for years in case of *P. vivax, P. ovale* and *P. malariae*, but **not in *P. falciparum*.**

A sexual division occurs in all four phases of Human Cycle (Pre-Erythrocytic, Exo-Erythrocytic, Erythrocytic and Gametocytic Schizogony). But in *PRE-ERYTHROCYTIC* and *EXO-ERYTHROCYTIC PHASES PARASITES ARE IN ASEXUAL FORM*. Only from Erythrocytic Schizogony phase, the Schizonts become sexually marked either MALE or FEMALE. Thus the MATURE Schizonts, which do not burst or spherulate, become either MALE or FEMALE GAMETOCYTES. Again, those bursting or spherulating schizonts which liberate MEROZOITES, are possibly also marked as MALE or FEMALE MEROZOITES, which when attack Fresh RBC and develop into SCHIZONTS are also accordingly sexually marked as MALE or FEMALE SCHIZONTS, respectively.

Hence, the sexual differentiation starts from 'E' Schizogony.

IV. GAMETOCYTIC SCHIZOGONY

(GAMETOGONY OR GAMETOCYTIC PHASE OR GAMETOCYTIC CYCLE).

Some of the ERYTHROCYTIC SCHZONTS are marked for SEXUAL FUNCTION, and Differentiated into having biological potentiality to liberate MEROZOITES. These RBCs do not burst, and contain MATURE Schizont (not sporulating schizont) passes to the Capillaries of Spleen and Bone-Marrow (Internal Organs) and settle there for about 3 days, where they change their form, and rearrange the merozoites within them to give rise to Gametocytes.

Individual Merozoites as such cannot give rise to Gametocytes as there is no RBC sheath around merozoites. They are liberated after bursting of RBCs. So, it is proper to say gametocytes arise from unburst RBC containing Schizont (of biological potentiality) containing merozoites. The Gametocytes are sexual forms arising from Asexual division after ERYTHROCYTIC SCHIZOGONY.

A particular Schizont gives rise to either a Male or a Female Gametocyte. To do this, some of the Erythrocytic Schizonts (which are biologically potential for performing sexual functions) are already sexually marked. Hence, Sexual Form is also found in Erythrocytic Cycle.

So, Sexual Forms are strictly found in all 2 Phases of Human Cycle, namely

(i) In ERYTHROCYTIC PHASE for those mature Schizonts destined for developing into Male or Female Gametocytes is SEXUALLY MARKED.

(ii) GAMETOCYTES—either Male or Female.

PLASMODIUM *FALCIPARUM* (Welch, 1897)

The parasite of Malignant Tertian (M.T.), or falciparum malaria. ''Falciparum'' (Latin 'falx = a sickle) is derived from its appearance of sickle-shaped gametocytes.

PRE-ERYTHOCYTIC SCHIZOGONY

(Early tissue phase)

(PL.5.I, Figs. 3-6)

This comprises a single cycle lasting for 6 days. The youngest Pre-Erythrocytic form (growing schizont) in the parenchymal cells of the liver (3 days' growth from sporozoite) measures 15 μm in diameter. The mature P-E schizont measures 60 × 30 mm containing numerous (40,000 small merozoites, each measuring 0.7 mm across. The merozoites are liberated on seventh day of infection. They enter RBCs (ERYTHROCYTIC CYCLE) after 6 days of the bite. P-E Schizonts completely disappear from the liver, and do not re-enter new liver cells. That is, there is no EXO-ERYTHROCYTIC CYCLE (LOCAL LIVER CYCLE or Late Tissue Phase).

P-E CYCLE IN LIVER

ERYTHROCYTIC SCHIZOGONY ('E'-CYCLE)

(E-PHASE—Plate 5.V)

P. falciparum invades both Reticulocytes and RBCs (young and old). 'E'-Schizogony occurs inside the capillaries of internal organs (Liver, Spleen and Bone Marrow). It is said that only ring forms appear in the peripheral blood, but this statement is not correct. The authors have found growing Trophozoites in peripheral blood and sometimes Schizonts as well, in a number of occasions. Erythrocytic cycle is completed in 36-48 hours. Multiple infections of the corpuscle, i.e., more than one parasite (2 to 6) invading a single RBC may occur.

'E' CYCLE occur in capillaries of Internal Organs and in Peripheral Blood.

TROPHOZOITE (*P. falciparum*) (Plate 5.V)

The early ring-form measures 1.5 μm in diameter and comprises a fine, uniform, Bluish Cytoplasmic Ring, with a Red Chromatin (nucleus) projecting beyond the ring, or lying outside it (Leishman

PLATE 5.III

LIFE CYCLE OF MALARIAL PARASITES (*PLASMODIUM VIVAX*)

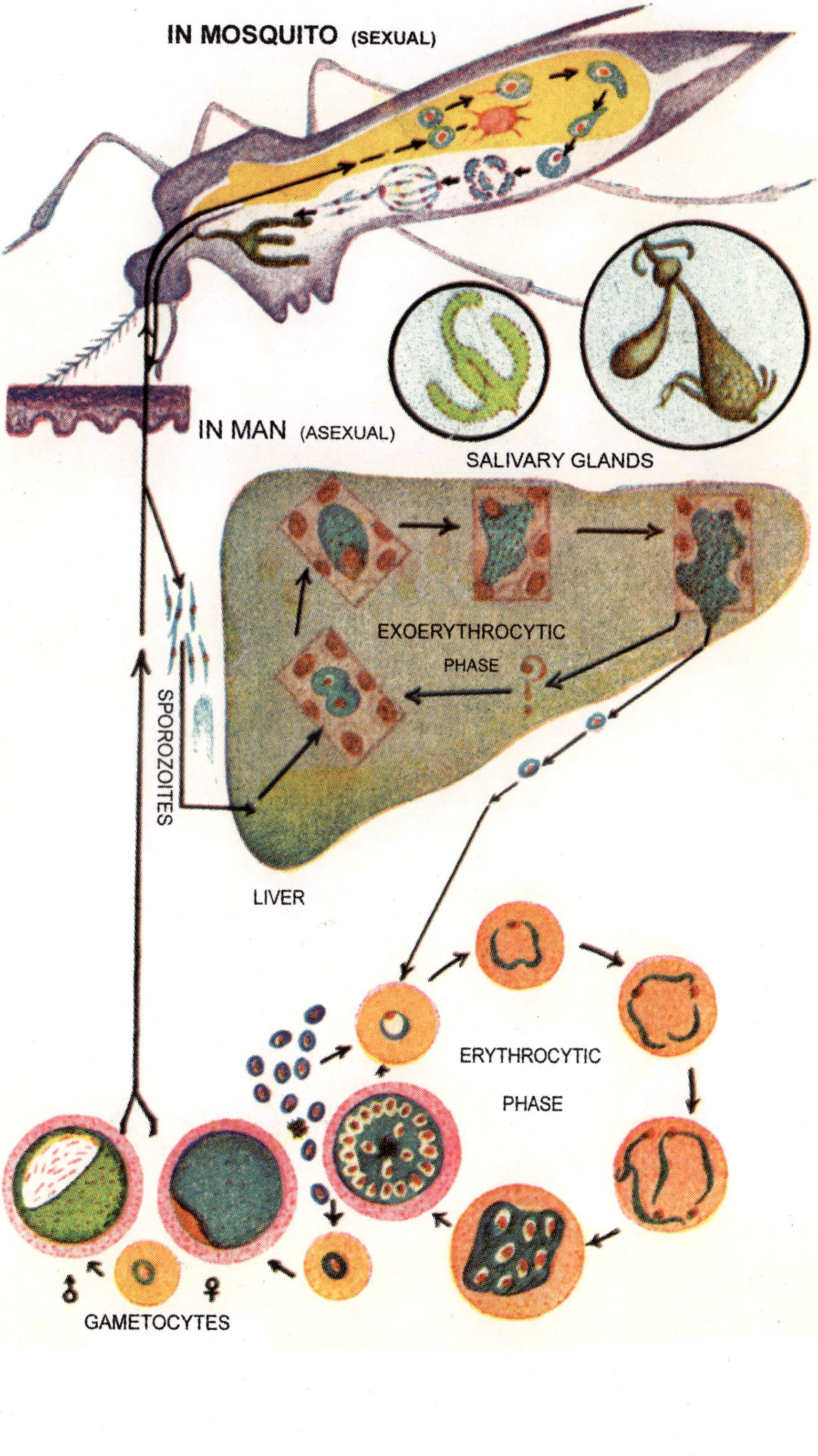

PLATE 5.IV

LIFE CYCLE OF MALARIAL PARASITE (*PLASMODIUM VIVAX*) IN HUMAN AND MOSQUITO

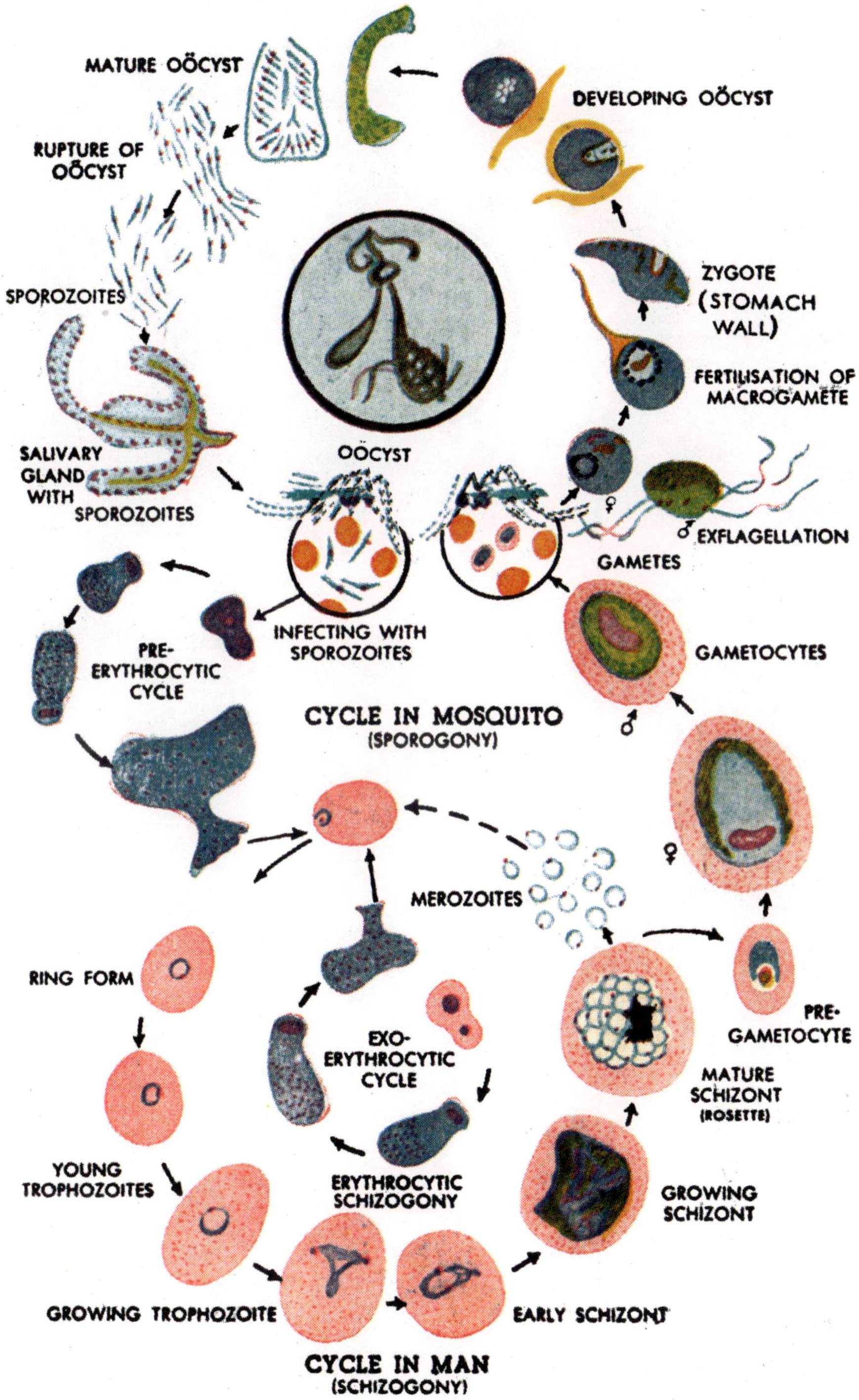

stain). The parasite adheres to the margin of RBC making a bluish curve in one arc of RBC, called Forme Applique or **Accole Form**. The nucleus is often divided into two parts which may either remain close together or situated at opposite poles (**Binucleate or Bichromatin Ring**).

The pigment granules (**Haemozoin**) are dark brown or black, collect into a single mass at early stage. Infected RBCs may sometimes show a crenated appearance. RBCs may show Maurer's dots (brick-red in Leishman's).

GROWING AND MATURE TROPHOZOITES

As soon as the pigment appears, the Ring enlarges to 4μm. The vacuole disappears and the parasite assumes a compact solid form with a single nucleus; the pigment granules form a single dark brown or black mass.

SCHIZONT (*P. falciparum*) (Plate 5.V)

As the growth continues, the nucleus divides into 8-32 masses. Cytoplasm dividies into the same number forming segments arranged around the central pigment mass. The mature schizont measures 4.5-5 μm across and occupies about two-thirds of the RBC.

MEROZOITE (*P. falciparum*)

(Metamerozoite or Erythrocytic merozoite)

It measures 0.6 μm across. About 20 merozoites are found in each affected RBC.

GAMETOGONY (*P. falciparum*)

(GAMETOCYTE FORMATION)

(Gamete = Sex Cell; Gony = formation)

Gametocytes of P. falciparum are sickle-shaped, called "Crescents". Gametogony occurs inside the capillaries of spleen and bone marrow. With the growth size of gametocyte, RBC is gradually used up and only its skin (or RBC) remains in the form of a sheath enclosing the parasite. The size of the mature gametocyte is 11 μm RBC is stretched beyond recognition, and the remains of RBC can i.e., recognised on the concave side of the parasite only, projecting outward in the form of an arched rim. Pigment granules in crescent assume "Rice grain" appearance.

In primary infection, gametocytes appear in 10 days after the appearance of Rings in peripheral blood, and in 21 days after sporozoite inoculation. "Crescents" not sucked by mosquito with her blood meal remain alive in peripheral blood for 30-60 days or longer (cf. *P. vivax*—7 days).

The differences between a microgametocyte (Male Gamete) and a macrogametocyte (Female Gamete) are shown in Table 5.7.

EXO-ERYTHROCYTIC SCHIZOGONY

(LATE TISSUE PHASE)

ABSENT IN *P. falciparum*.

PLASMODIUM MALARIAE

(Laveran. 1881)

Grassi and Feletti, 1890

The parasite of Quartan (Q.T.) malaria

Laveran (1880) named it malariae as it caused Malaria. MALARIA = MAL or bad; Aria comes from AIR : BAD AIR

PRE-ERYTHROCYTIC SCHIZOGONY (*P. malariae*)

(EARLY TISSUE PHASE)

Although Tissue phase has not been observed in man but identical organism P. inui causing Simian

TABLE 5.7

	MICROGAMETOCYTE (Male)	MACROGAMETOCYTE (Female)
SHAPE:	Broader, shorter; ends blunted	Longer, narrower; ends pointed.
SIZE:	10 × 3 μM	12 × 3 μM
CYTOPLASM:	Light blue	Deep blue
CHROMATIN:	Finely granular scattered over a wide area	Punctate, condensed into a small mass at the centre
HAEMOZOIN: PIGMENT	Scattered throughout cytoplasm	Aggregates form 'wreath-like' round the chromatin

(Monkey) Q.T. infection shows this phase. Hence, it may be inferred that a Pre-Erythrocytic Schizogony exists in this species. Duration of the cycle is 15 days. The Pre-Erythrocytic (P-E) Schizont was observed in the liver from the 7th to 12th day. The youngest form measure 5.5 μm across, with 5 nuclei; the mature P-E schizont is 22 μm containing over 2,000 merozoites.

ERYTHROCYTIC SCHIZOGONY (*P. malariae*)
('E'-PHASE) (**PLATE 5.V Figs. 22-28**)

P. malariae tends to invade Older Erythrocytes. The 'E'-cycle is completed in 72 hours (3 days) which occurs in peripheral circulation.

'E'-cycle occurs in Peripheral Circulation.

TROPHOZOITE (*P. malariae*)

The young Ring form has the appearance of P. vivax type. P. malariae often stretches right across the RBC giving a band-like appearance. In 6 to 8 hours, coarse pigment granules (dark brown or black) appear in cytoplasm. RBC is not enlarged; Schüffner's or Maurer's dots are absent.

SCHIZONT (*P. malariae*—**Plate 5.V**)

It is circular and measures 7 μm in diameter. Chromatin divides, and, after 50 hours, when segmentation is complete, about 10 merozoites arrange themselves around the central pigment mass giving the parasite a "daisy-head" appearance.

MEROZOITE (*P. malariae*)

It measures 2.5 μm in diameter.

GAMETOGONY (*P. malariae*)

It is similar to *P. vivax* gametocytes, are round, measuring 7.5 μm in diameter; macrogametocytes (females) are larger. Maturation of gametocytes is complete in 6 days. They appear in peripheral blood a few days after the first fever. Morphological differences between the male (Micro-) and female (Macro-) gametocytes are the same as P. vivax. RBCs containing gametocytes are not enlarged.

EXO-ERYTHROCYTIC SCHIZOGONY (*P. malariae*)

Occurrence of relapses suggests the existence of a late tissue phase. Garnham suggested the presence of dormant schizonts in the liver cells.

PLASMODIUM OVALE (STEPHENS, 1922)

Parasite of ovale tertian malaria. The name is derived from oval shape of both parasite and of the infected RBC.

PRE-ERYTHROCYTIC SCHIZOGONY (*P. ovale*)
(PLATE 5.II)

The cycle is for 9 days in the liver. A mature schizont measures 75 μm × 50 μm and contains 15,000 large merozoites each measuring 1.5 μm spherical bodies with chromatin on one side.

P-E Cycle occurs in the Liver.

ERYTHROCYTIC SCHIZOGONY (*P. ovale*)
(PLATE 5.V)

The schizogony cycle is completed in 48 hours and occurs mostly in the peripheral blood. It combines the features of P. malariae and P. vivax. Morphologically it resembles the P. malariae; whereas its effect on host-cell and duration of schizogony are similar to P. vivax.

TROPHOZOITE (*P. ovale*)

The ring-form measures 2 to 2.5 μm in diameter and resembles *P. malariae*. Band-form is not seen. Haemozoin pigment-granules are coarse and dark bown. Schüffner's dots appear in RBC at early ring stage. The infected RBC is little enlarged, oval, and fimbriated.

SCHIZONT (*P. ovale*)

It is round or oval measuring 6.2 μm across. Nuclear material is divided into 10 masses; in relapses, masses are more.

MEROZOITE (*P. ovale*)

It measures 2.5 μm across. Nucleus is crescentic.

GAMETOGONY (*P. ovale*)

Gametocytes develop from merozoites in the same manner as in other species. The gametocytes are distinguished from *P. malariae* by the oval shape of RBC, and the presence of Schüffner's dots; and from those of *P. vivax* by the smaller size of the infected RBC and its irregular outline.

EXO-ERYTHROCYTIC SCHIZOGONY (*P. ovale*)

Relapses occur in ovale tertian malaria and, hence, it may be inferred that a late tissue phase also exists

PLATE 5.V

MALARIA PARASITES OF HUMAN (*ERYTHROCYTIC PHASE*)

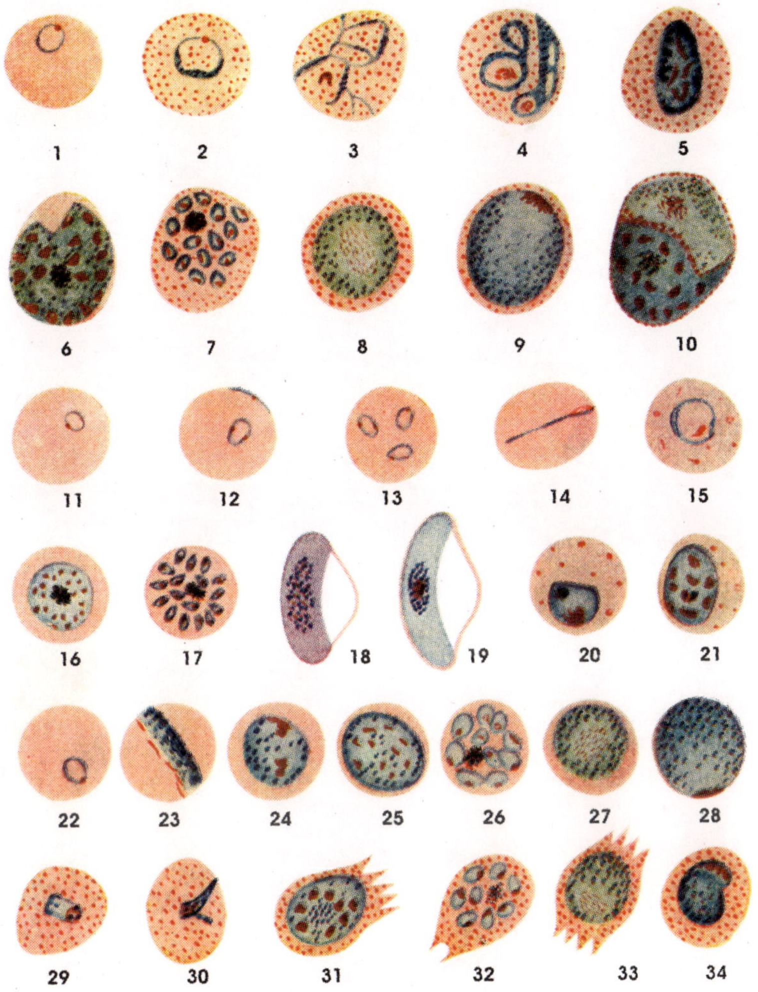

P. vivax (1-10). 1 and 2—Young trophozoites (ring form). 3—Amoeboid form 4—Growing trophozoite. 5 and 6—Developing schizonts. 7—Sporulating schizont. 1—Mature male and 9—Mature female gametocytes. 10—Mature schizont and microgametocyte in one cell. Note—Red cells are paler and larger than normal and show Schüffner's dots (2-10).

P. falciparum (11-21). 11—Young trophozoite (ring form). 12—Ring with double chromatin and marginal or accole form 13—Multiple infection of the cell. 14—Tenue form. 15—Larger ring form with Maurer's dots. 16—Growing and 17—Sporulating schizonts (in the capillaries of internal organs). 18—Male and 19—Female gametocytes (crescents). 20-21—Forms in Culture. 20—Growing trophozoite, and 21—Developing schizont. —Red cells show Maurer's dots, coarser than Schüffner's dots.

P. malariae (22-28). 22—Young trophozoite (ring form). 23—Growing trophozoite (band form). 24-25—Developing schizonts. 26—Sporulating schizont. 27—Male and 28—Female gametocytes.

P. ovale (29-34). 29—Young and 30-31—Growing trophozoites. 32—Sporulating schizont. 33—Male and 34—Female gametocytes. Note- Stipplings are coarser than Schüffner's dot's and cells are slightly enlarged and distorted.

PLATE 5.VI

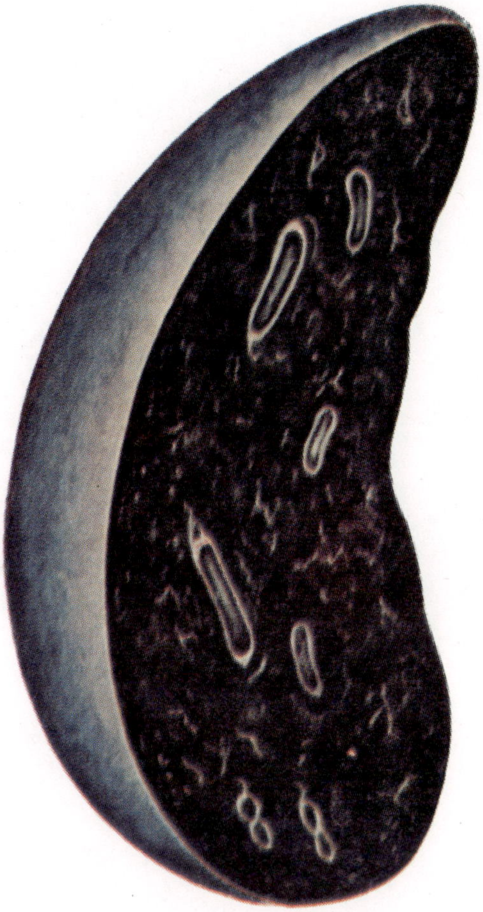

A
SPLEEN IN MALARIA

Gross appearance of the spleen in malaria. Note the characteristic slaty grey or bronze colouration. The cut surface assumes the bronze black or tarry appearance

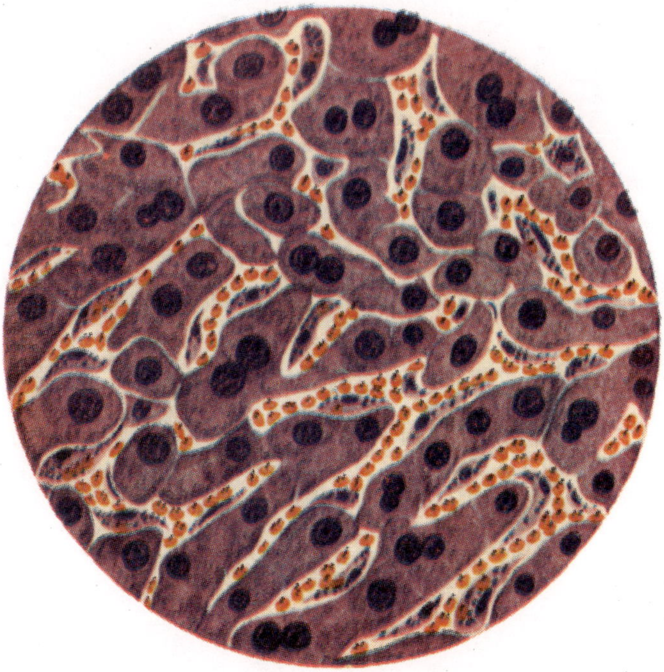

B
LIVER IN MALARIA

Micro-histological appearance of the liver in malaria. Note the sinusoidal spaces are filled with parasitised RBCs with malaria parasites within Stellate cells of van Kupffer are packed with phagocytosed haemozoin pigment, and infected and un-infected RBCs. *H & E*; × 900

in this species.

PLASMODIUM VIVAX (Grassi and Felatti, 1890)

The parasite of benign tertian (B.T.) or vivax malaria.

Vivax. Latin Vivere = to live; activity of movement.

PRE-ERYTHROCYTIC SCHIZOGONY (*P. vivax*)
(Plate 5.I.; Fig. 1 & 2)

After remaining in peripheral circulation for half hour, sporozoites settle in liver and development occurs inside the parenchymal cells of the liver (liver cells). Pre-Erythrocytic (P-E) Cycle is a single cycle in the liver, which lasts for 8 days. Mature 'P-E' schizont measures 42 μm in diameter. It contains a large number (12,000) of merozoites. Each merozoite has a fragment of chromatin with little cytoplasmic mass. Merozoites may either enter (attack) RBC (to start Erythrocytic Schizogony) or re-enter into fresh parenchymal cells of the liver (Liver Cells or Hepatocytes) to continue Exo-Erythrocytic ('E-E') Schizogony. The parasite multiplies by Asexual Method (Schizogony) during development in liver or RBC. But the merozoites are Sexual Forms.

P-E Cycle occurs in the LIVER ONLY

ERYTHROCYTIC SCHIZOGONY (*P. vivax*)
(After P-E Cycle)

P. vivax invades younger RBCs and Reticulocytes. During Erythrocytic ('E') Schizogony the parasite passes through the following stages: Young Trophozoites (Rings), Growing Trophozoites, Mature Trophozoites, Growing Schizont, Mature Schizont, Sporulating Schizont, and Merozoites. The cycle of Erythrocytic ('E') schizogony lasts for 48 hours (2 days) in blood circulation and when all the growth stages are over, usually each RBC is invaded by a single parasite.

'E' Cycle occurs within RBC in circulatory BLOOD

TROPHOZOITE (*P. vivax*—**PL.5.V**)

Early (young) trophozoites with Leishman's stain looks like a signet ring (Blue Cytoplasm) and Red Chromatin (nuclear mass), and unstained vacuole. The Ring diameter is 2.5 to 3 μm (about one-third of RBC). The ring is thicker on one side, and the nucleus is on the thinner part. The trophozoites have constant active amoeboid (pseudopodial) movement showing diverse forms. After 10 hours, yellowish brown pigment granules appear in the cytoplasm of the parasite called haemozoin pigment. While developing, the parasite induces certain changes in RBC as follows:

(i) It enlarges (double the original size)
(ii) It becomes rhomboidal or irregular
(iii) It becomes pale.
(iv) The RBC cytoplasm shows pink dots or stipples, called Schuffner's dots.

Early Trophozoites mature to Growing trophozoites and Late (Mature) Trophozoites.

SCHIZONT (*P. vivax*—**Plate 5.V**)

Schizonts appear after 36-40 hours. It is a Mature Trophozoite ready to divide. It loses its amoeboid movement. Vacuole disappears and haemozoin pigment still scattered throughout cytoplasm. Enlarged Nucleus lies at the periphery.

A schizont measures 9-10 μm across. Nuclear division is complete in 6-8 hours, and 16 daughter parasites form. The small parasites are called *merozoites*. They arrange themselves in the form of a

TABLE 5.6

P. vivax

	MICROGAMETOCYTE	MACROGAMETOCYTE
Size	9-10 μm	10-12 μm
Cytoplasm :	Stains light blue	Stains deep blue
Nucleus :	Large and Diffuse, situated laterally (little away from the RBC border)	Small and compact, lies and extend peripherally (near the margin of RBC)

TABLE 5.7

MALARIAL PARASITES OF HUMAN

Differential Characters of Erythrocytic Phases (PL.V)

	P. vivax	*P. falciparum*	*P. malariae*	*P. ovale*
SCHIZOGONY :	48 hours	48 hours or under	72 hours	48 hours
FORMS IN : PERIPHERAL BLOOD	1. Trophozoites 2. Schizonts 3. Gametocytes	Ring and crescents Only growing. Schizonts Trophozoites and Schizonts rarely seen	1. Trophozoites 2. Schizonts 3. Gametocytes	1. Trophozoites 2. Schizonts 3. Gametocytes
TROPHOZOITE : RING-FORM	Size 2.5 μm Cytoplasm opposite the nucleus is thicker	Size 1.25 to 1.5 μm Cytoplasm fine and regular in outline. Often with 2 nuclei. Form accole. Multiple infection.	Same as *P. vivax*	Same as *P. malariae*
GROWING : FORM	Irregular with a vacuole. Actively amoeboid	Assumes a compact form. Pigments collect into a single mass early.	Band-like. Slightly amoeboid. Vacuole disappears early.	No Ribbon Bands. Slightly amoeboid
SCHIZONT : (MATURED)	Size 9 to 10 μm. Regular, almost completely fills an enlarged red blood cell	Size 4.5 to 5 μm. Fills two third of a red blood cell which is not enlarged	Size, 6.5 to 7 μm. Regular, almost fills a normal sized red blood cell	Size, 6.2 μm. Fills about three quarters of a red blood cell which is slightly enlarged
MEROZOITES :	12 to 24. Arranged in an irregular grape-like cluster	18 to 24 or more. Arranged in a grape-like cluster	6 to 12; usually 8. Arranged around a central mass of pigment like a "daisy" or a "rosette"	6 to 12, usually 8. Irregularly arranged

(contd.)

(contd.)

TABLE 5.7

	P. vivax	*P. falciparum*	*P. malariae*	*P. ovale*
HAEMOZOIN :	Yellowish-brown; fine granules.	Dark brown or blackish; one solid black.	Dark brown coarse granules	Dark yellowish brown; coarser than *P. vivax*.
INFECTED :	Enlarged, Pale, Schüffner's dots present	Usually unaltered. Crenation, reddish violet colour and Maurer's dots	Neither enlarged nor decolourised. No Schüffner's dots	Slightly enlarged, oval shape, fimbriated. Schüffner's dots appear early
GAMETOCYTE :	Spherical or globular. Much larger than a red blood cell. Host-cell enlarged with Schüffner's dots	Crescentic. Larger than a red blood cell. Host-cell hardly recognisable	Round or oval. Size of a red blood cell. Host-cell not enlarged	Oval. Size of a red blood cell Host-cell slightly enlarged with Schüffner's dots

"*rosette*" in 2 rows with the haemozoin pigment at the centre, giving a *mulberry* appearance to the RBC. When maturation is complete, the RBC bursts. This gives rise to *Malarial Paroxysm* with the *end of Erythrocytic Schizogony*. A Schizont may be:

1. Immature Schizont (undivided nucleus)
2. Mature Schizont (nucleus divided), and
3. Sporulating Schizont (liberating merozoites).

Some of the mature Schizonts having biological potentiality of performing Sexual Functions settle at capillaries of Spleen and Bone Marrow to form *Gametocytes*.

Biologically Potential Mature Schizont → Gametocyte.

MEROZOITE (*P. vivax*)

It is an oval mass of cytoplasm with a central nucleus measuring 1.5 μm × 0.5 μm. Free (Asexual) merozoites attack Fresh RBC to continue Erythrocytic Schizogony repeating the cycle every 48 hours, in absence of treatment.

Merozoites within Schizonts are of two types :

1. Asexual Merozoites—attack fresh RBC to continue Erythrocytic Cycle.
2. Sexual Merozoites within a Schizont, and that Schizont gives rise to Gametocytes.

GAMETOGONY (*P. vivax*)

Certain *schizonts* are biologically potential for performing *sexual functions*. The respective merozoites of those schizonts are differentiated into sexual forms. All (Sexual) Merozoites of a particular Schizont become either *all males* (*microgametocytes*), or *all females* (*macrogametocytes*). Such an RBC containing this type of Schizont containing a single class of male or female merozoites increase in size, becomes pale, containing Schüffner's dots. These Schizonts are carried to the capillaries of Spleen and Bone marrow for Gametocytic development within 3-4 days.

Gametocytes *appear* in peripheral blood from the *first day of fever* or 12-13 *days after inoculation* of sporozoites, i.e., 4 to 5 days after the initial appearance of the asexual (Ring) forms of parasites in Blood smears of 2-3 days from the beginning of 'E' Cycle. Gametocytes which remain in Blood–and not taken up by Mosquito–die out in a week.

The differences between a Microgametocyte (Male Gamete) and a Macrogametocyte (Female Gamete) are shown in TABLE 5.5.

EXO-ERYTHROCYTIC SCHIZOGONY (*P vivax*)

Exo-Erythrocytic Schizonts have been observed in *monkey* (*Simian*) *malaria* only, but due to close resemblance of it to vivax Malaria, this phase has been accepted in man. Morphologically Exo-Erythrocytic ('E-E') forms are identical to Pre-erythrocytic ('P-E') forms. Exo-Erythrocytic Schizogony (E-E CYCLE) is maintained throughout the course of infection in *P. vivax*, which is independent of Erythrocytic Schizogony, lasting for 3 years. For this fact, a single infection with *P. vivax* may cause Relapse at any time within this period. As long as Exo-Erythrocytic Phase Persists, *Erythrocytic Schizogony* may occur at any time or from time to time. If there is no further specific mosquito bite, the infection dies down after three years with guarantee.

The forms in 'E-E' Phase are :

1. 'E-E' Schizonts in Liver
2. 'E-E' Merozoites in Liver (identical to P-E Merozoites or Macromerozoites).

E-E Cycle occurs in the LIVER only.

GENERALISED CHARACTERS OF TROPHOZOITES : *P. VIVAX* TAKEN AS AN EXAMPLE

Early (Young) Trophozoite consists of :

(i) *Bluish Cytoplasmic* Ring (Signet ring appearance)

(ii) *Red Chromatin* Mass (Nuclear material) and

(iii) *Vacuole* (unstained area).

Measures 2.5 to 3 micrometre (1/3 of RBC).

One side is thicker than the other.

Nucleus is on *thinner side*.

It has pseudopodial (Active Amoeboid Movement) and shows diverse forms (of amoeba).

Haemozoin pigments appear in the bluish *cytoplasmic ring* 10 hours after Ring formation.

Affected RBCs show following changes :

(a) RBC *enlarges* to *double*

(b) RBC *distorted*, out-line *crenated*

(c) *Pale* and colourless with progressive infection.

(d) Unoccupied portion shows Reddish stipplings (Schuffner's Dots)

PRE-ERYTHROCYTIC PHASE
Sporozoites injected to host

↓

Surrounding Tissue

↓

Peripheral Circulation

↓ (Remains for Half Hour)

Liver parenchyma
("Pre-erythrocytic" before infecting RBC)

Remains :
P. vivax–8 days
P. falciparum–6 days
P. malariae–9 days

↓

Merozoites liberated at the end of this phase called Cryptozoites

(i) Larger cryptozoites called *Macromerozoites*

↓

Re-enter Liver
(Exo-erythrocytic) in *P. vivax*
P. malariae
P. ovale

(ii) Smaller cryptozoites called *Micromerozoites*

↓

Enter Circulation
Directly (Erythrocytic)
in *P. falciparum* only

ERYTHROCYTIC PHASE (in RBC)
(E-PHASE)

Macromerozoites (*P. vivax, P. malariae, P. ovale*)
& Micromerozoites (*P. falciparum*)

↓

Early Trophozoite (Rings)

↓

Growing Trophozoite

↓

Mature Trophozoite
Growing Schizont
MATURE SCHIZONT → MATURE SCHIZONTS (Sexually Marked Ones)
Sporulating Schizont

↓

MEROZOITES (Attack Fresh RBC) GAMETOCYTE

'E'-PHASE LASTS AS FOLLOWS :

(i) For 48 hours { *P. vivax*, *P. falciparum*, *P. ovale*

(ii) For 72 hours : *P. malariae*

As *P. vivax, P. falciparum* and *P. ovale* stay in RBCs for 48 hours, the temperature occurs after that time by lysis of RBCs every 3rd day. *P. vivax* is called BENIGN as it does not produce malignant (harmful) effect and as temperature occurs every third day (tertian), the infection is called BENIGN TERTIAN (B.T.) INFECTION.

CULTIVATION

Culture methods have been evolved to observe the erythrocytic schizogony of malarial parasite as it occurs in man. Only the development of one generation can be studied. Hence it is not a "culture method" in the truest sense but in reality a "concentration method". Base and Johns technique with a slight modification is being used for the cultivation of malaria parasite in artificial culture media.

ANIMAL INOCULATION

Human species of malarial parasites can now be transferred to several species of malarial parasites of primates (monkeys). Similarly, certain species of monkeys, when inoculated into man, are able to establish themselves in the human host. Two questions now arise—whether an animal reservoir of human malaria exists and whether a natural monkey-to-man transmission can take place.

Accidental laboratory infections of human with the simian parasite, ***P. cynomolgi bastianelli*** (Bastianelli strain of *P. cynomolgi*) has been reported (Eyles *et.al*, 1960) although the naturally acquired infections of simian malaria in man appears to be rare.

MODERN TRENDS IN MALARIA

Malaria has appeared in the 8th decade of twentieth century in a new form with varied clinical symptoms and signs. This new form might be attributed to some kind of mutation which might have taken place in course of 2 or 3 decades in dormant state. The following peculiarities have been observed in a study of a few thousand cases of Clinical as well as asymptomatic malaria, confirmed by blood examination.

CLINICAL PECULIARITIES

1. There may not be any fever in spite of presence of Malaria parasites (Tophozoites) in peripheral blood.
2. The reverse may also happen (Parasites detected in blood later, but at the outset, no or occasional

parasites found in peripheral blood).

3. There may be low grade fever persisting for months, not responding to common Antibiotics or Chemotherapeutic agents other than Antimalarials.
4. There may be high rise or moderate rise of temperature which may be *Remittent*, *Intermittent*, or *Continued* (due to multiple species infection or single species infection with multiple bites at different time or in different days).
5. The onsets may be tubercular, enteric or influenzal type. The presenting features may be of *Bronchial Asthma* type even.
6. There may not be any chill or rigor.
7. No other symptom except general malaise may be the presenting feature.
8. Tongue is usually mildly or moderately coated with lips even moderately red, which is to be differentiated from ENTERIC FEVER.
9. In chronic cases, jaundice may develop with yellowish skin. Jaundice may also appear after cure by Metakelfin (Trimethoprim and Sulfa Methoxazole) Therapy as a side effect; more so with a repeated dose in short interval.

PATHOLOGICAL PECULIARITIES

1. Rings (Early Trophozoites) transiting to growing Trophozoites may look like **tiny triangular shape** particularly in *P. falciparum* morphology, which may disuade the pathologist.
2. The film, if not prepared exactly, may not differentially stain chromatin and cytoplasm of M. P. Rings for which a negative report is made, which is not correct. Pathologist has to investigate and comprehend with his Analytical Sight and Mind. Rings may look black and chromatin may not be differentiated. Rings of *P. falciparum* may assume the size of a pinhead or just bigger than that.
3. Schizonts mostly look like a blackish mass within RBC, which should be carefully examined (if not properly stained).
4. Merozoites (Metamerozoites or 'E'-Merozoites) are rarely found which appear as blackish granules.
5. Gametocytes do not stain green or blue as shown in the picture but appear somewhat greyish blue or greyish violet.
6. Rare presence of Gametocytes may occur in peripheral blood even in a relatively long-standing case.
7. Association of 2 or 3 species together, e.g., *P. vivax* and *P. ovale*, or *P. vivax* and *P. falciparum*, *P. falciparum* and *P. malariae* both together found on many occasions.
8. Thin film is enough. But *at least Two Good Smears* must be examined thoroughly before giving a Negative Report.

Above finding commonly help to negate a positive slide. Not using the *Standard Quality of Distilled water* and *Reagents*, are common causes for such faults. Last but not the least, through search to be done to find out a parasite.

DRUG PECULIARITIES

Sometimes it is seen that in a confirmed case of Malaria, usual drugs cannot bring about total remissions of fever. 4-Aminoquinoline, particularly the brand 'Resochin', is supposed to be the best drug in Malaria. It is a SCHIZONTICIDAL DRUG. About 3% cases are hypersensitive to Resochin (Dey, 1987).

In view of this, they have to take pyrimethamine (DARAPRIM). The second drug of choice is Metakelfin. Resochin–Hypersensitive, or Resochin–Resistant cases should be put to a single dose treatment of 2 tablets of Metakelfin. If unsuccessful after repeating the single dose 1 week later, the patient should take **Daraprim** or **Primaquine** which are the next drugs of choice.

In spite of these lines of treatment, when temperature still persists, and when a month or more has passed while other investigations negate presence of any other disease, the patient should withdraw all antimalarials and be put to **anti-histaminics, alkaliser, good food** and **rest**. The toxic fever should then come down automatically after some time, possibly due to some acquired immunity and disappearance of drug toxicity.

Many of the early and late infections of *P. falciparum* are not creating alarming clinical features, as were feared in the past. The explanation for such occurrence remains obscure, but may be possibly due to some mutational change in the organism itself, which is left out for the young scientists to probe in.

Last but not the least, total dose of any tablet (treatment) other than trimethoprim-sulpha, must be 15 tablets. For chloroquin (Resochin), it is 1 tablet (200 mg. Chloroquin base) 2 times daily for 7/8 days; or 3 tablets T.D.S. for 2 days, then 1 tablet B.D. for 5 days.

STEROID SHOULD NOT BE GIVEN AS IT SUPPRESSES IMMUNITY.

CLINICAL CONSIDERATIONS

CLINICAL FEATURES IN MALARIA

INCUBATION PERIOD. This connotes the period between the entrance of the sporozoite in the body and clinical manifestations of malaria characterised by actual onset of fever. During this period the parasite undergoes developmental (Preerythrocytic) cycle in the liver followed by the erythrocytic cycle in RBCs. During the erythrocytic schizogony the parasites multiply in geometrical progress. The febrile stage is indicated by a sufficient concentration of the parasite in the blood. Therefore, the incubation period will depend on various factors including the power of multiplication of the different species of parasite. It is usually taken to be about 10-15 days, but the period is definitely longer in *P. malariae*. When acurately observed, it is 12-17 days (average 14 days) in case of *P. vivax* and *P. ovale*; 8-14 days (avarage 12 days) in *P. falciparum* and 21 to 35 days (average 28 days) in case of *P. malariae*. Incubation period, the number of plasmodia in blood, duration of disease and relapse period in malaria are shown in Table 5.8.

COLD STAGE

COLD STAGE. The fever is ushered in with rigor or "cold stage" which lasts for 1 to 2 hours when the extremities are cold, followed by rise of temperature. Children may have convulsions.

HOT STAGE

HOT STAGE. It follows the cold stage and lasts for about 4 hours with a feeling of warmth, headache and vomiting. The pulse is full and bounding. The temperature may rise up to 105°F (40°C) or more.

SWEATING STAGE

SWEATING STAGE. This lasts for 1 to 2 hours, when the patient has profuse sweating with a feeling of relief; temperature comes down to normal or subnormal.

TYPES OF FEVER

TYPES OF FEVER. The febrile attack corresponds approximately to the sporulation of the parasites in the erythrocytic schizogony. Therefore, in tertian malaria, the cycle repeats with recurrence of fever after every 48 hours, i.e., every third day, giving a characteristic **tertian fever**. It recurs every 72 hours in case of quartan fever. On the other hand, the fever may recur at intervals of every 24 hours (the quotidian fever) in infection of *P. vivax* or *P. ovale*; when two broods of parasites undergo sporulation

TABLE 5.8

Species	Incubation period in days		Number of plasmodia per cmm of blood		Duration of first attack, if untreated	Relapse period
	Range	Average	Maximum	Average		
P. vivax	12-17	14	50,000	20,000	3 weeks	2-5 years
P. ovale	12-17	14	30,000	10,000		Relapse rare
P. falciparum	8-14	12	Innumerable		11 days	Recrudescence 1-6 months
P. malariae	21-35	28	20,000	6,000	6 months	10-40 years

on two successive days—it is **tertiana duplex**. In case of quartan malaria the quotidian temperature may be possible, when three generations of parasites undergo maturation on three successive days; it is **quartana triplex**. But the fever may occur on two successive days followed by an apyrexial day; it is **quartana duplex**—when two successive generations of the quartan parasites undergo sporulation on two successive days (Charts 1 and 2).

The falciparum malaria is often called *malignant tertian* as it is always dangerous and may be fatal, in contrast to other types which are free from dangerous complications and menace to life. Its capacity to invade both mature erythrocytes and reticulocytes is directly related to the intense, rapidly increasing parasitaemia in this infection. Moreover, the infected RBCs tend to agglutinate and adhere to capillary endothelium, forming thrombotic emboli; causing anoxia and ischaemia in the viscera. The fever often comes with regular periodicity in benign tertian or quartan malaria, but in *P. falciparum* infection this regularity of paroxysm is less definite and it is called **subtertian**, that is, less than tertian periodicity. It often lacks three definite successive stages; namely, the cold, hot and sweating stages. In these cases the fever is often insidious in onset which becomes continuous or remittent instead of being intermittent. This may be explained by anticipation and retardation of the schizogony which varies from 36-48 hours and also as a result of the sporulation of new generation of parasites, released into the circulation over a prolonged period. There is sensation of chilliness instead of a frank chill, a prolonged intensified hot stage and lack of marked terminal sweating. The fever curve shows prolongation of fastigium. The prostration is more marked and pernicious symptoms may develop in some cases with greater tendency for delirium (Chart 3).

PERNICIOUS MALARIA

(by *P. falciparum*)

The term refers to serious or fatal attacks produced by *P. falciparum*, when the schizogony occurs in the capillaries of important internal organs. This may also be called septicaemic type of malaria. This causes: (a) **Agglutination** of the infected red cells in the capillaries due to *adhesive properties of infected RBCs* showing the trophozoites, schizonts and sexual forms of the parasites. A very high concentration of parasites is necessary (50,000 per cmm) for this. The agglutinated RBCs thus act as emboli and block the capillaries. (b) **Endothelial**

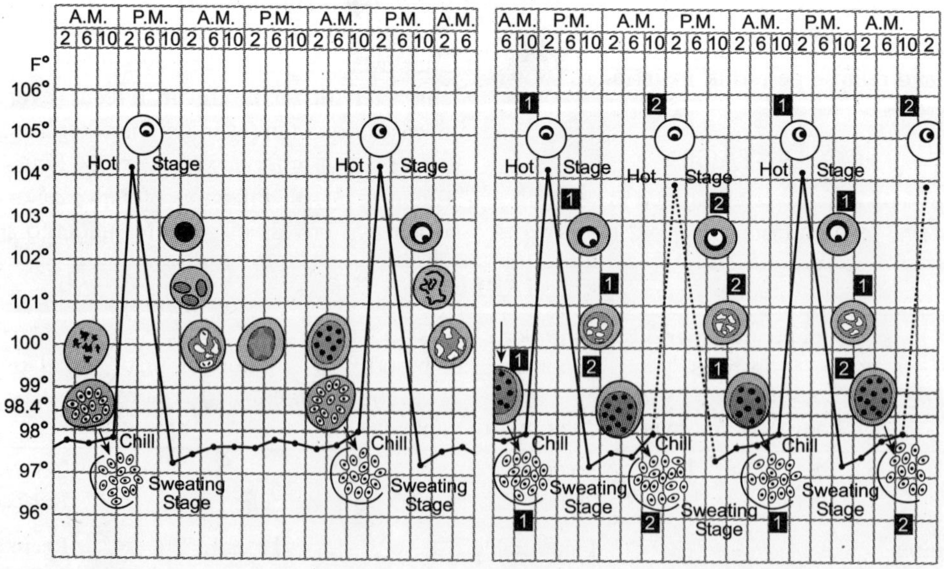

Chart 1—Left: Fever with simple tertian periodicity in *P. vivax* infection (Cycle after 48 hours). Right: Quotidian periodicity in double infection with *P. vivax* (two generations of parasites sporulating alternately)

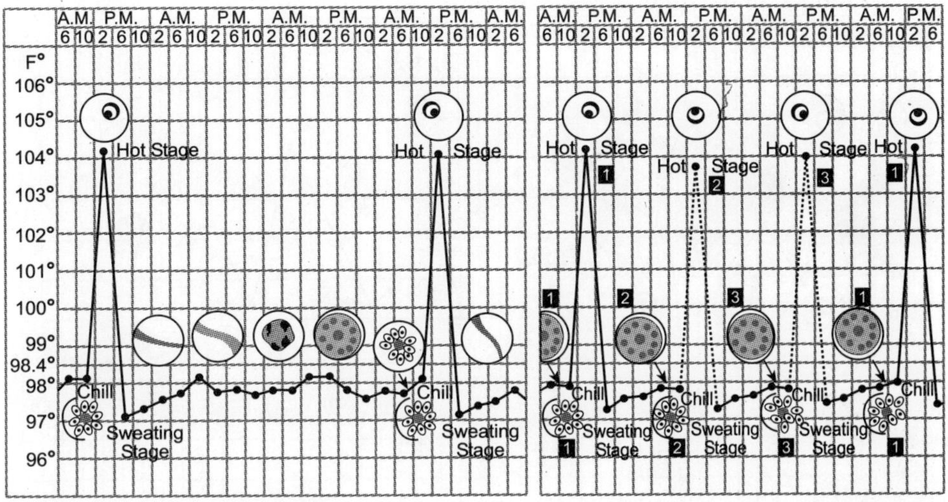

Chart 2—Left: Fever with simple quartan periodicity in *P. malariae* infection (Cycle after 72 hours). Right: Fever with quotidian periodicity in triple infection with *P. malariae* (three generations of parasites sporulating successively)

damage is done by the *haemozoin pigment* liberated by sporulation. The pigments are engulfed by the endothelial cells causing swelling and roughening of the intima and formation of thrombus. In this condition the parasites are present in large numbers in internal organs, but schizonts may sometimes escape in the peripheral circulation in moribund cases.

The different clinical forms are:

(A) **Cerebral forms.** There may be hyperpyrexia, delirium, convulsion, coma, hemiplegia, aphasia, bulbar paralysis, etc. **are all due to hypoxia/anoxia due to capillary blockage of cerebral vessels by adhesion and thrombus formation by erythrocytes (see later under pathology).**

(B) **Algid forms.** Symptoms of these forms depend on the organ where the blockage of capillaries occurs as follows:

Gastric form with epigastric pain, persistent vomiting and haematemesis.

Choleraic form with purging and vomiting followed by collapse as in cholera.

Dysenteric form. Blood and mucus appear in the stool resembling bacillary dysentery.

Haemorrhagic form. Sudden haemorrhage from the stomach (haematemesis), from bowels (melaena) or skin (petechiae) may take place.

Syncopal form. Sudden death may occur from cardiac failure due to blockage of coronary vessels by parasites.

The other associated types of malaria are:

Latent malaria. In endemic malarious areas individuals may show plasmodial parasites in the peripheral blood without evidence of symptoms of malaria and such infections are known as *latent malaria*. Most of these individuals have gametocytes in their blood and act as carriers.

Malaria in pregnancy. This may occur before the onset of the labour by any of the common malaria parasites, the relative incidence being related to relative prevalence of the species. The frequency estimated to be about 1 per cent of the cases, when the mother may have attacks of malaria.

Congenital malaria. Intrauterine transmission of malaria from mother occurs when the placental barrier has been disturbed, but there is no evidence that the infection may take place by passage of sporozoites, or exoerythrocytic forms of plasmodium through the *placental barrier*.

Relapses in malaria. These are common in untreated cases of malaria (90 per cent). In untreated cases of malaria, the exoerythrocytic and erythrocytic cycles continue for some days but *spontaneous termination* follows. The erythrocytic plasmodia

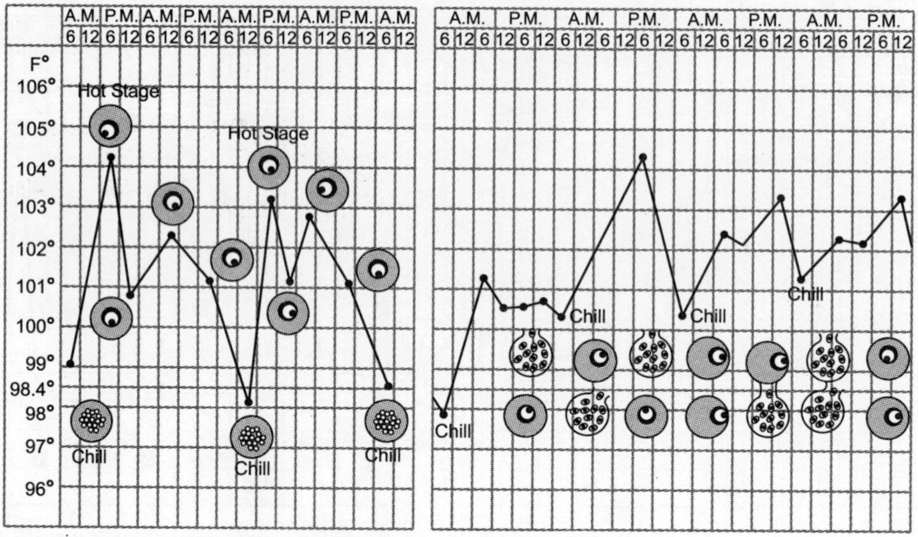

Chart 3—Left: Fever with subtertian periodicity with short fever-free period (sporulation occurs in the capillaries of internal organs). Right: Subtertian fever has become remittent due to irregular sporulation of *P. falciparum*

disappear probably due to development of **cellular immunity**. The exo-erythrocytic cycle, which may remain latent for the time being, may develop to start the erythrocytic cycle again. The frequency of relapses varies with the species or even the strains. Climatic conditions also greatly affect it. In a tropical climate, relapses of *P. vivax* are frequent within a few weeks after the primary attack but, with the strains of temperate zone, the primary attack may be delayed and relapses may follow after 10 months or during the next year.

Clinical attacks of malaria may be precipitated by supervening conditions which reduce the patient's resistance. These are amoebiasis, bacillary dysentery, typhoid fever, hookworm disease, respiratory or renal infections, surgical operations, shock, etc., which might precipitate an attack of malaria from reactivation of latent malaria.

TERMS USED IN EPIDEMIOLOGY

The term *endemic* connotes natural transmission confined to an area also called *autochthonous* or locally contracted malaria which is *indigenous*.

Imported malaria is acquired from an outside source and cases derived from it are called *introduced* malaria in contrast to autochthonous malaria. When there are only a few scattered cases, the disease is called *sporadic*. The prevailing frequency and intensity of endemic malaria is termed as *endemicity* of malaria; this is qualified by the Expert Committee on Malaria of World Health Organisation, according to spleen rate in age-group 2-9 years as follows:

Hypo-endemic malaria. Spleen rate not exceeding 10 per cent.

Meso-endemic malaria. Spleen rate between 11 and 50 per cent.

Hyper-endemic malaria. Spleen rate over 50 per cent and the adult spleen rate is also very high.

Holo-endemic malaria. Spleen rate over 75 per cent with adult tolerance high and adult spleen rate low.

Epidemic. When the morbidity rate of malaria rises sharply above average endemicity it is said to be *epidemic*. The epidemic may be seasonal, regional or localised.

Epidemiology. The spread of malaria in a locality depends on 3 factors: (1) mosquito vector, (2) gametocytes, and (3) immunity of the host.

MOSQUITO VECTOR. Female anopheles of about 50 out of 200 species can transmit the disease. The developmental cycle of plasmodia in mosquitoes depends on moisture, external temperature, rainfall, topography, soil, density of susceptible species, etc.

The plasmodia develop between 15.6°C (60°F) and and 37.8°C (100°F). On an average it requires *P. vivax* to develop in 10 days at 25°C or 16-17 days at 20°C; *P. falciparum* develops in 22 days at 20°C and *P. malariae* in 30-35 days at 20°C.

Malaria infection in mosquitoes is never congenital. The sporozoites may remain infective in mosquitoes as long as 90 days. They were found to be non-infective after 155 days. The plasmodia may remain dormant during the winter but renew their development in the mosquitoes in the spring. A particular species of mosquito *acts as a vector* due to: (1) its *susceptibility to infection* by the parasites; (2) its presence in *effective numbers* in the human habitation; (3) its capacity to take human blood repeatedly rather than the animal blood; (4) its life, long enough for the development of the gametocyte to sporozoites. **Sporozoite index** is also important. There may be endemicity of malaria even with low index depending on the blood-sucking habits of the mosquito. Thus *A. culicifacies* may show a lower sporozoite index (1 per thousand) than *A. fluviatilis* (10-20 times higher). The former may be a less important vector as the vector is much more easily deviated to cattle for its blood meals.

GAMETOCYTE. The development of gametocyte to sporozoites depends on the age, number, sex distribution and the species of gametocytes. All these influence the infectivity of blood for mosquitoes. According to Green (1929), to infect *A. maculatus*, the peripheral blood must contain 1 gametocyte of *P. falciparum* to 200 leucocytes, but 1 of *P. vivax* to 1000 leucocytes, or 1 of *P. malariae* to 300 leucocytes. He also observed that predominance of macrogametocytes over microgametocytes showed a reduction in the number of mosquitoes infected. Very young or overripe gametocytes cannot develop in mosquitoes. Boyd (1942) is of the opinion that some gametocyte carriers are "good infectors" while others are "poor infectors".

CARRIERS. The principal carriers are often children between the age of 1-4 years who may not show symptoms of attacks of malaria but contain gametocytes in their blood. Two factors, i.e., vectors and gametocytes, combined are important in the rise and fall of malaria incidence. There is a **critical density** of mosquito population for the disease. When the incidence of the vector falls below the critical level in a locality, the incidence of malaria falls. *Gametocytes have also a critical density* in a community. When the gametocytes carriers are few, malaria transmission will be less, and the reverse is also true when there are many carriers in human population. But there is a fluctuating minimum level below which transmission is unlikely; whereas, when these two factors rise concomitantly, an epidemic may take place.

IMMUNOLOGY

IMMUNITY OF THE HOST. Covel *et al* (1935) referred to immunity in malaria as the processes involved in preventing *infection*, *reinfection* and *superinfection*, or which assist in destroying the plasmodia, or in limiting their multiplication or modify the physical effects of their invasion or help specifically in the repair of tissues. **Acquired immunity** to malaria develops as a result of antigenic stimulation of the parasite or its products. It is active as a result of malaria infection but passive when it is transferred from the mother to the child. The active immunity may be concomitant when there is parasitaemia or it may be *residual* after eradication of the parasite. Premunition or **infection immunity** is the concomitant immunity.

Tolerance indicates a condition which lessens the effect of a given quantum of the parasite on the host. The terms immunity and tolerance are not synonymous, as tolerance does not prevent but makes endurable to increased quantum of parasitic infection. It is often seen in holo-endemic areas and such individuals may show parasitaemia without clinical symptoms, often seen in adolescents, but in adults parasites are scanty. The immunity in malaria is of the nature of infection immunity or premunition depending on the persistence of the infection. It is related to activity and quantum of the erythrocytic and not to the exo-erythrocytic form of the parasite. The mechanism of immunity lies in the destruction of plasmodia by RE cells acting as phagocytes (Craig *et. al.*). It involves not only **cellular** but also **humoral responses** as complement fixing antibodies develop in cases of malaria towards group specific antigen (*specific to the genus,* e.g., all plasmodia). But type (species) specific **agglutinin** also develops. Individual may become immune to a particular strain employed in inoculation but he may be reinfected by another strain of the same species. Again, infection with one species does not immunise against another species.

Immunity is acquired in childhood, when children get repeated attacks of the disease. Adult human subjects develop some immunity and resist infection to a certain extent due to previous attacks (see later under Malarial Antibodies). Therefore, the splenic index is of value only in children, who constitute the susceptible population.

PLASMODIAL (MALARIA) ANTIGENS. The plasmodial antigens, being soluble, are present in the sera of patients which can be detected by the **agar gel double diffusion precipitation** technique of Ouchterlony. The antigen has been extracted from the infected erythrocytes. Plasmodial antigens may be classified on the basis of thermostability:

(a) 'L' antigen–Heat labile at 56°C for 1/2 hour.

(b) 'R' antigen–Thermoresistant at 56°C for 1/2 hour.

(c) 'S' antigen–Thermostable at 100°C for 5 minutes.

The 'L' antigen has 2 subclasses: (i) $'L'_a$ (4 subclass antigens), and (ii) $'L'_b$ (3 subclass antigen).

MALARIAL ANTIBODIES IN RELATION TO IMMUNOGLOBULINS. The *protective* antibodies exist in the 7S IgG fraction of immune sera (who had previous attacks). But the *precipitating* antibodies (as in Ouchterlony's test) exist in both serum IgG and IgM fractions.

The anti $'L'_a$ antibody is found in the IgG fractions. This antibody crosses the placental barrier and is responsible for conferring immunity to the newborn babies. Very high percentage of newborn infants were seen to possess specific IgG antibodies in their sera (congenital immunity) in Gambia, which was a real *hyperendemic area* for *P. falciparum*. Even in absence of any specific infection, the serum antibodies persist for months or years. But later on, the protective antibody level falls to nil in absence of infection (lack of antigenic stimulation).

However, antibodies to 'S' antigen are of precipitating nature, and are found in the serum IgM fraction. Anti-'S' antibody does not cross the placental barrier, does not persist for a long time, and are present in the sera of adults only.

POSTMALARIAL IMMUNOLOGICAL REACTIONS. The effects of immunological responses are:

I. Immunopathological States

1. PROTECTIVE IMMUNITY. (a) There is a chance of **congenital immunity** against 'L' antigen (for 6 months postnatal). The antibody is serum **IgM**, which crosses the placental barrier and is also transferred *via* milk (breast feeding).

(b) The older age group may bear an antitoxic immunity (no protection from malaria; only toxic parasitic metabolites are neutralised).

II. Immunopathological States

They are: (i) **Nephrosis** in malaria caused particularly by *P. malariae* infection in children.

(ii) **Idiopathic splenomegaly** (*Banti's syndrome*) in adults associated with fibrous tissue proliferation.

(iii) **Auto-immune haemolytic anaemia** (AIHA) due to auto-antibody formation against erythrocytic antigen in pregnant women after *P. falciparum* infection.

(iv) **Immunosuppression** against antigenic stimuli. This has been demonstrated by failure of production of antitoxin against tetanus toxoid in Gambian children (McGregor & Burr, 1962).

(v) Association (*synergism*) of **Plasmodial immunosuppression** with **proliferation of Onchogenic virus.** The chief example is Burkitt's lymphoma caused by an onchogenic virus. It may be possible that the plasmodial antigen may be analogous to that of Burkitt's lymphoma virus. Immunosuppression freely allows the virus multiplication, or interferes with the immune reactions against neoplastic cells.

(vi) There is a definite *antagonism* between **kala-azar** and **malaria** in man. Patients of kala-azar show proliferation of immunologically competent (round) cells and they are not likely to contract malaria during the course of **kala-azar**.

Pathogenesis. In malaria the parasite grows inside the red blood corpuscle at the expense of the haemoglobin which is converted into haemozoin pigment. After the introduction of sporozoites of plasmodium, the organism promptly enters the liver and develops in the parenchyma cells of the liver, where **pre-erythrocytic** and **exo-erythrocytic schizogony** occurs. When sufficient merozoites are produced, the schizont bursts and merozoites escape into the circulating blood. Some of them invade erythrocytes and initiate destruction of the RBCs. This destruction is increased in multiples with **new asexual reproduction** till clinical manifestations of chill and fever start at the end of the incubation period.

Sporulation occurs in the peripheral circulation or in the internal organs and the pigment is engulfed by endothelial cells and deposited specially in the organs rich in reticulo-endothelial cells, i.e., the spleen, liver, bone marrow, lymph nodes, etc. In the case of *P. falciparum*, sporulation invariably occurs in the internal organs.

The red cells infected with *P. falciparum* have a tendency to adhere to the walls of the capillaries, and produce symptoms by blocking the capillaries, leading to ischaemia, oedema, necrosis and capillary haemorrhage, and these give rise to grave manifestations.

During sporulation of mature schizonts the infected red cells burst with liberation of numerous *merozoites*, *haemozoin pigment*, *oxyhaemoglobin*, *disintegrated* RBCs and parasites.

The foreign substances together with broken down products of destroyed RBCs are set free and might probably sensitise the host at the end of each erythrocytic cycle and primarily produce **allergic reaction**. This produces a "haemoclastic shock" of the nature of a protein shock followed by rigor, vomiting, fall of blood pressure, leucopenia, thrombocytopenia, and diminished coagulability of blood.

Clinical pathology. BLOOD. Malarial parasites are present in the blood in their various forms, namely *rings*, *trophozoites*, *schizonts* and *gametocytes* during or in between the attacks. These are demonstrated by a **thin blood film** method, but a **thick film** examination is more reliable and less time-consuming. In case of *P. falciparum*, only the **rings** and **gametocytes** (crescents) are seen in the peripheral blood. But in moribund cases, **schizonts** may appear in peripheral blood.

As a result of the infection, **monocytes** increase in greater number in circulating blood and may engulf free parasites (merozoites) and pigment in the plasma. After a few episodes the parasites become less and less in the circulating blood and the patient becomes free of symptoms. But the parasites tend to reappear in the circulating blood as a result of return of parasites from quiescent centres in the liver, in the **late tissue phase**, the **exo-erythrocytic cycle**.

As the disease becomes chronic, there is iron deficiency anaemia, marked enlargement and hardening of the spleen, enlargement of the liver, pigmentation of cortex of the *brain*, *spleen*, and *kidneys*. The spleen, liver and bone marrow may contain infected RBCs, pigmented leucocytes and free pigment. The anaemia produced is **microcytic hypochromic** in nature.

In **anaemic patients**, RBCs show abnormalities like anisocytosis, poikilocytosis, punctate basophilia and polychromasia. Cabbot's ring and Howell-Jolly bodies are also found. Blood shows presence of malarial parasites and monocytes with ingested haemozoin pigments. The latter by themselves are proof of malarial infection in the absence of malarial parasites in the blood. **Haemolytic** (retention) jaundice occurs.

There is **hyperbilirubinaemia**, with indirect van den Bergh reaction; a *delayed direct reaction* indicates liver damage.

URINE. The urine is usually normal in *P. vivax* and *P. malariae* infection except that it may be high coloured. In infections with *P. falciparum*, especially in pernicious malaria, the urine is dark brown in colour with increase of **urobilinogen** and **urobilin** due to haemolysis. Bile salts and bile pigments appear in urine and this is marked in malarial hepatitis. In the acute stage there may be albuminuria, chloride and urea may increase in chronic cases.

Pathology. The characteristic pathological changes in malaria in general are as follows: (1) **Pigmentation** occurs in various organs of the body including the brain, giving a slate-grey appearance. This is due to the ingestion of haemozoin particles by the macrophages of different organs. (2) Increased activity of the reticulo-endothelial cells is characterised by **proliferation of RE** cells to deal with the parasites, their effete products like haemozoin, toxins, etc. and formation of reticulin fibres. (3) **Vascular congestion**, *engorgement* and *dilatation* in organs is marked specially in sinusoidal vessels. (4) The **parasitised erythrocytes which adhere to the intima may block the capillaries. This occurs specially in P. falciparum infection, in which** the *sporulations* take place in the capillaries of internal organs and, as such, **thrombi** are produced in internal organs. (5) Damage and destruction of the capillary endothelial lining may result in **perivascular haemorrhage** in *P. falciparum* infection showing *petechial haemorrhage*. (6) *Anoxaemia* is responsible for **degenerative changes** in vital organs like liver, kidney, etc. This may cause fatty degeneration and **ischaemic fibrosis**. (7) **Marked haemolysis** may occur specially in *P. falciparum* infection. Due to the massive haemolysis, there may be **bilious vomiting**. Haemolysis is partly due to the **destruction of RBCs** by the parasites and partly due to **haemolysin** liberated by them.

In *chronic cases*, there is enlargement of the spleen and liver (hepatosplenomegaly). This is partly due to *congestion* and partly due to *proliferation* of RE cells as a result of ingestion of the pigment (**PL.5.VI**).

CAUSES OF ANAEMIA IN MALARIA. Anaemia in malaria is principally due to (i) *destruction of infected RBCs* by the sporulation of the parasite but haemolysis may also be due to (ii) *haemolysin production* in *P. falciparum* infection, causing intravascular haemolysis of the non-infected RBCs. Intensity of haemolysis may produce a condition of **haemoglobinuria** and **Blackwater fever**. In *chronic cases*, **anaemia is refractory**. In addition to continued destruction of erythrocytes, factors like (iii) failure of organs to *reconvert liberated iron into haemoglobin*, and (iv) *selective parasitisation* of reticulocytes in *P. falciparum* infection are contributory to anaemia. (v) *Phagocytosis of RBCs* by macrophages of the spleen (**hypersplenism**) might be another factor responsible for producing anaemia in chronic cases with enlarged spleen.

Morbid changes in organs depend on whether the infection is **acute** causing pernicious symptoms of cerebral or algid malaria, or **chronic**.

SPLEEN. The main pathological changes are: (a) In acute *cases* of *P. falciparum* infection, the organ is congested, soft and enlarged. The colour is slate-grey or chocolate. The capsule is stretched. CUT SURFACE shows a slate-grey or chocolate colouration (see **PL.5.VIA**). The pulp is tar-like and diffiuent. The Malpighian corpuscles are pale grey. HISTOPATHOLOGY. There is marked congestion; parasitised red cells are present in the sinuses and pulp; brownish **haemozoin pigments** are in the macrophage cells of the *Billroth cords* and less so in *littoral* cells.

(b) In ***chronic cases***, the spleen is moderately enlarged due to hyperplasia. It is firm or hard in consistency and had a typical *slaty colour*. The weight of the spleen may reach up to 1000g or more. The capsule is thick and stretched. There may be adhesions here and there, and even with the diaphragm. Old areas of infarcts are often seen. CUT SURFACE shows a typical slaty colour and the ogan cuts with a gritty sensation. HISTOPATHOLOGY. The capsule and the trabeculae show overgrowth of the connective tissue. There is great hypertrophy and hyperplasia of the RE cells, which contain malarial pigments; parasites are present in RBCs in sinuses. The Malpighian corpuscles are **atrophied, lymphoid tissue** is practically absent and the central artery is prominent. This area is usually free from pigment. The spleen shows marked **fibrosis**. In the splenic arteries half-grown or full-grown parasites may be seen. **Monocytes** containing the **haemozoin pigment** are present in the branches of the splenic artery.

LIVER. Gross (a) It is congested, soft and more friable than normal in acute cases. (b) It is enlarged due to congestion of hepatic capillaries and hyperplasia of the Kupffer's cells laden with pigment. (c) The colour is chocolate red in *acute cases* but in *chronic cases* slate-grey or black. The left lobe is specially pigmented as it received blood from the spleen. (d) It is firmer in chronic cases due to certain amount of fibroblastic reaction. (e) The CUT SURFACE may show fatty changes.

MICROSCOPY. (i) The *liver* (*parenchymal*) *cells* contain **haemosiderin**. (ii) There is **cloudy swelling** and **fatty degeneration** specially in *P. falciparum infection*. (iii) **Parenchyma cells** show different stages of degeneration and sometimes there may be necrosis **around central vein** and this is due to anoxia as a result of interference with hepatic venous blood supply. (iv) The sinusoids are congested, parasites are present in the red blood corpuscles in the sinusoids. (v) **Kupffer's cells** are distended with

haemozoin pigment, which persists for about four months after infection (**PL.5.VIB**).

GALL BLADDER. It is distended with *thick bile* which is *deep brown* in colour.

BONE MARROW. In acute cases, red bone marrow of the sternum, ribs and vertebrae is *dark red* or *chocolate* in colour due to congestion and deposition of pigment. In **chronic cases**, yellow marrow of large bones changes to chocolate brown, due to *erythropoietic response* and deposition of pigment. **HISTOPATHOLOGY**. The *hyperplastic bone marrow* shows many erythroblasts and normoblasts. There is also *hyperplasia of the RE cells* but *hypoplasia of myeloid tissue* with decrease of granulocytes. Parasites are present and the bone marrow is sometimes seen packed with crescents. The *pigment* is seen engulfed by the cells.

STOMACH AND INTESTINE. Features differ in acute and chronic cases. In **acute cases**, there is generalised congestion of the intestine. Peyer's patches show "shaven bread" appearance due to minute punctiform haemorrhages. Capillaries are blocked with RBCs containing parasites. In **chronic cases**, serous membranes and mucosa of the stomach and intestine are lead-coloured.

CHANGES IN ORGANS MARKEDLY INVOLVED IN ACUTE CASES OF *P. falciparum* INFECTION ONLY:

BRAIN. Meninges are hyperaemic, the cortex smoky, lead-coloured due to deposit of pigment. **Punctiform haemorrhages** are seen in the white matter of the subcortical zone specially in the corpus callosum and corpus striatum (**PL.5.VIIA**). There are *areas of focal degeneration* with formation of subcortical malarial granuloma of Durck. **HISTOPATHOLOGY**. Capillaries are filled with mature schizonts and sporulating forms of *P. falciparum* and blocked by swollen endothelial cells, parasites and haemozoin pigment (**PL.5.VIIB**).

Blockage of capillaries results in haemorrhage and necrosis, aggravated by anoxaemia. Granuloma of Durck is due to perivascular proliferation of glial cells which may show formation of giant cells.

KIDNEYS. The organ is enlarged and congested. CUT SECTIONS show relative increase in thickness of the cortex and pigmented greyish dots and lines in the pyramids. The dots represent Bowman's capsule full of parasitised RBCs. **MICROSCOPY**. *Bowman's capsule* may show parasites; convoluted tubules show degenerative changes or necrosis. *Blood casts* are seen in the tubules in acute cases.

SUPRARENALS. The organs is affected as a result of toxaemia or arteriolar occlusion which may be responsible for a hypertensive or a poorly functioning heart. The yellow colour of the cortex is lost. The organ shows areas of haemorrhage due to degeneration and necrosis as a result of thrombosis of capillaries. **HISTOPATHOLOGY**. Cortical cells show degeneration with reduced lipoid content. Parasites and ingested haemozoin pigment are present in the capillary endothelium.

PANCREAS. The organ shows **focal necrosis** due to **blocking of capillaries**. In rare cases **acute haemorrhagic pancreatitis** may occur.

HEART. Fatty infiltration of the myocardium is sometimes present. Ecchymosis of mycocardium and pericardium may be seen. Blood capillaries in *P. falciparum* infection contain parasitised RBCs and the endothelial cells contain haemozoin pigment. There is blocking of furthest capillaries, especially noticed in the apical region. This may result in myocardial infarction in some cases.

According to Merkel (1946), **coronary occlusion** by plugging or thrombosis results from the tendency of free and infected red cells to adhere to the capillary walls. In these cases, anoxaemia of the myocardium due to coronary occlusion by the parasites is *fatal* as in the case of cerebral capillaries. Heart may show flabbiness and fatty change.

LUNGS. Pleurae and lungs are pale and anaemic in chronic cases. There is congestion of alveolar capillaries which may be blocked with parasitised RBCs. Deposit of pigment may give bluish grey colour to the organs. Haemorrhage with occasional **infarcts** may occur.

PLACENTA. Maternal sinuses may be blocked resulting in **abortion**.

Laboratory diagnosis. This depends on the following:

MICROSCOPIC EXAMINATION OF A BLOOD FILM PERIPHERAL BLOOD SMEAR. **Thin film**. This is the most useful method for the diagnosis of malaria by finding the malaria parasite in a blood smear stained with Leishman or Giemsa stain. **Thick film**. This is a method of concentration and when the parasites are few in the peripheral blood, a thick film is useful (**PL. 5.VIII**). Therefore, as a routine, Sinton's thick and thin film method should be adopted specially in the field work (For details, see Appendix I). In a well-stained thin film, where the parasites are numerous, there is no difficulty in recognising them for the knowledge of morphology of the parasites, but possibility of a mixed infection should always be remembered. It is, however, difficult to differentiate the species of the parasite, particularly in the ring form, when thick film is used.

Difficulties in finding the parasite in blood films are due to scanty parasites in the peripheral blood. This is evident: (i) in case of *early primary infection*, (ii) blood film taken during the *apyrexial period*, specially in case of *P. falciparum* infection, (iii) after administration of *anti--malarials*, or (iv) any other suppressive drug.

STERNAL OR ILIAC CREST PUNCTURE. This may be used to supplement blood film method of diagnosis, when the parasite is not found in the peripheral blood. In general, this method of diagnosis has not been popular and useful, as it requires experience as far as technique is concerned **(See App. I)**.

CULTURAL EXAMINATION. This may be necessary only in special circumstances, when there is difficulty in identifying the ring form of *P. vivax* and *P. falciparum* or other ring forms. Further developmental stages of the parasite can be studied in **Bass and John's culture**, which is not true culture but an *enrichment process*, as it is questionable, whether any new generation occurs by this process **(See App. I)**.

SEROLOGICAL TESTS. The following tests are positive for malaria. They may be divided into *specific* and *nonspecific*.

(i) Specific. Precipitation and complement fixation tests may be carried out with antigen preferably from *P. knowlesi* or in the latter test from *P. gallinaceum* as well. At NCDC both FA (fluorescent antibody) and HA (haemagglutination) tests are employed for the diagnosis of malaria.

FA TEST. With the introduction of FA test, there has been a renewed interest in the serological diagnosis of malaria. Works of Tobic *et. al,* 1966; and Collins *et al,* 1966 have contributed much to the evaluation of this procedure. In the Parasitology Laboratory of NCDC (National Communicable Disease Centre), a thick smear antigen is adopted for use of FA test prepared from washed parasitised blood cells (Sulzer *et al* 1967). Evaluation of antigen indicates a false positive rate of 1 per cent at a titre of 1 : 16, and the sensitivity of the test is 95 per cent.

HA TEST. Stein and Desowitz (1964) described indirect haemagglutination (HA) test with formation and tannic acid-treated sheep red cells sensitised with antigen from *Plasmodium cynamolgi* and *P. coatneyi*. Mahoney *et al*, (1966) prepared antigen by disruption of parasite. Rogers *et al*, (1968), who used the antigen of *P. knowlesi* prepared by method of Mahoney *et al*., has shown that it is both sensitive and specific for malaria. The HA test revealed the antibody titres of 1 : 16 or greater in 98% of slide positive cases of malaria and in less than 1 per cent of sera from individuals without a history of malaria. But the major problem of this technique is the lability of the antigen.

Prophylaxis. Personal prophylaxis depends on protection against mosquito bites by the use of mosquito nets, repellants, mosquito–proof houses.

Chemoprophylaxis is useful by the systematic use of antimalarial drugs.

General prophylaxis is applicable to the community. It consists of prevention of carriers by the use of 8-*aminoquinoline* (pamaquine, plasmoquine or less toxic primaquine) and/or along with quinine. The drugs have destructive effects on gametocytes and exo-erythrocytic forms but they have not become popular for mass prophylaxis due to toxicity.

Antimosquito measures. This consists of destruction of adult mosquitoes by spraying insecticides like DDT or gammexane. The antilarval measures depend on the elimination of breeding places of Anopheline mosquitoes and also by use of larvicides, e.g., oil, parish green, solutions of DDT in kerosene oil, etc.

PLATE 5.VII
APPEARANCE OF THE BRAIN IN MALARIA

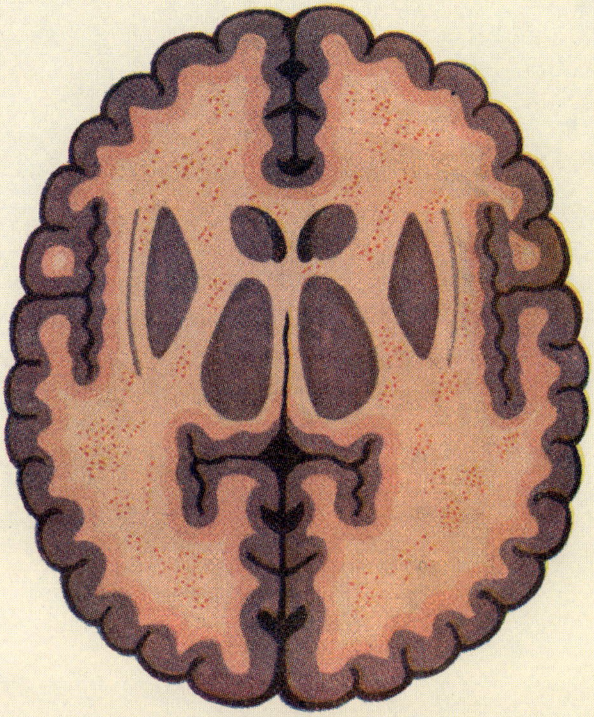

A

Showing punctiform haemorrhages in the brain

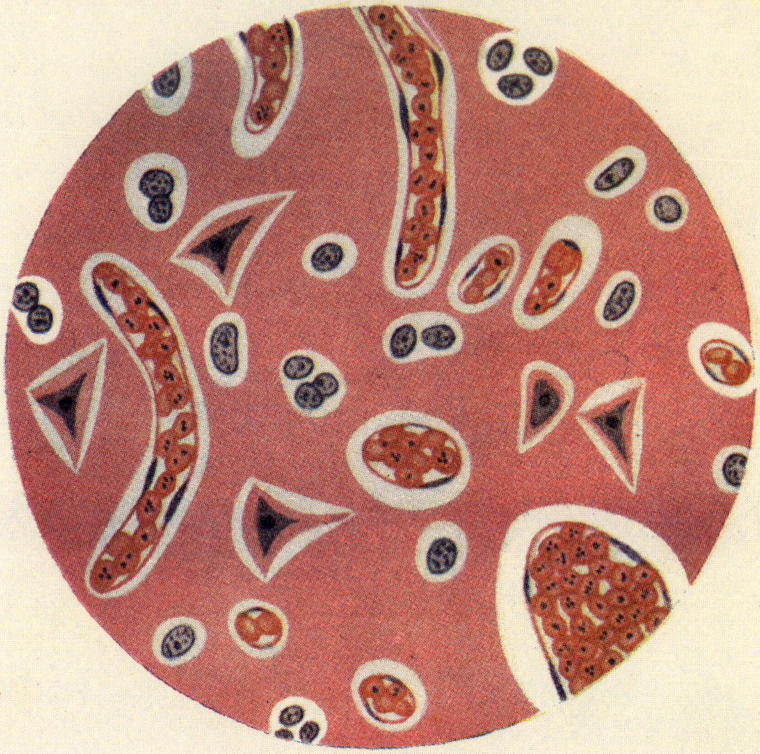

B

Showing marked congestion and dilatation of the capillaries in the brain.

PLATE 5.VIII

THICK FILM PREPARATION (*GIEMSA STAIN AFTER DEHAEMOGLOBINISATION*)

A

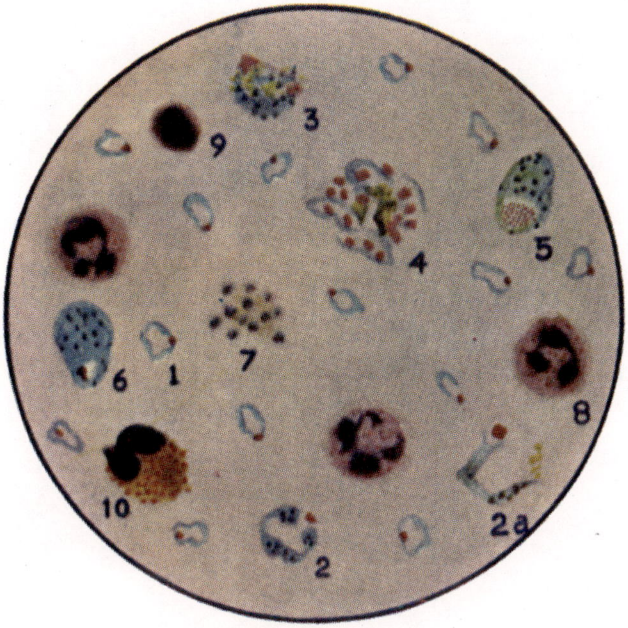

B

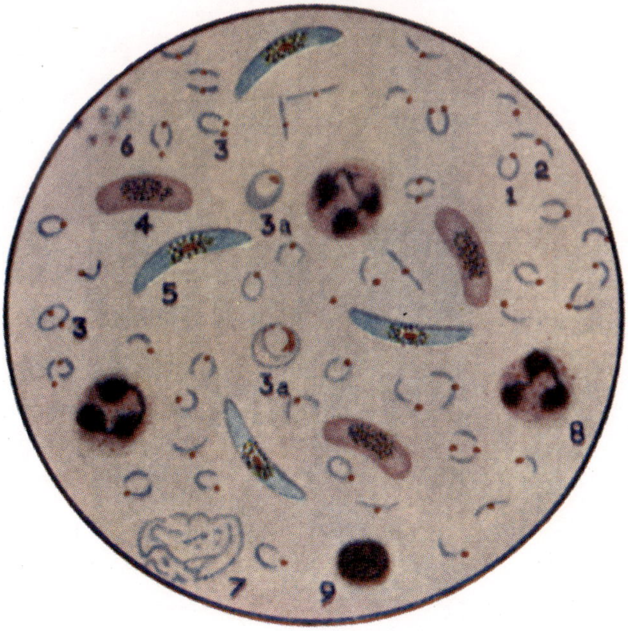

A. *P. vivax* infection. 1. Ring form. 2. and 2a. Growing trophozoities. 3. Developing schizont. 4. Full-grown, mature schizont. 5. Male and 6. Female gametocytes. 7. Platelets. 8. Neutrophil. 9. Lymphocyte. 10. Eosinophil.

B. *P. falciparum* infection. 1. Ring form. 2. Accole form. 3. Ring with double chromatin. 3a. Growing gametocyte. 4. Male and 5. Female gametocytes. 6. Platelets. 7. Cellular remains of young RBCs. 8. Neutrophil. 9. Lymphocyte.

TREATMENT OF MALARIA

The treatment may be divided into (i) *Supportive treatment*, and (ii) *Specific therapy*.

(I) *Supportive treatment*. Malaria patients do not require hospitalisation, except the cerebral or algid forms of pernicious malaria. Symptomatic treatment with antipyretic analgesics during the attack gives relief to the patient when administered along with specific therapy. In the convalescent state, the patient should have good food, vitamins and iron tonics or Rarical tablets (Ethnor).

(II) *Specific therapy*. Specific antimalarial drugs are:

(a) NATURAL ALKALOID: Quinine which is one of the important alkaloids of Cinchona. It is schizonticidal in its action.

(b) Synthetic drugs: (i) *Schizonticidal drugs*: They are (a) Mepacrine (9-aminoacridine) also known as atebrine or quinacrine; (b) Chloroquine (4-aminoquinoline derivative), also avilable in the market as "Resochin" or "Nivaquin", or (c) Camoquine (4-aminoquinolines) are active against overt attacks of malaria. Chloroquine has been proved to be one of the most effective drugs in malaria but it may not be used in three instances:

(1) *There are cases where malaria parasites gradually grows resistance to the drug.* (2) *Occasional untoward effects are noted by the authors which are giddiness and allergic or exfoliative dermatitis.* (3) In subjects with congenital G6PD deficiency. The adult dose of chloroquine is 1 tablet 3 times daily for 2 days, then 1 tablet B.D. for 4 days which should eradicate malaria. But more drastic dose has been recommended at present which is 4 tablets at a time initially, then a maintenance dose of 1 tablet B.D. for 1 day. The *prophylactic dose* is 1 tablet every week on a fixed day in endemic areas.

The dose of camoquine is two tablets stat and then 1 tablet B.D. for 1 week.

(ii) *Suppressive therapy*: Proguanil hydrochloride (a biguanide) or Paludrine is a suitable suppressive drug, but *cannot control an acute falciparum malaria*. It is a suitable suppressive drug specially after an acute attack, and is useful also against *early vivax relapses*; with this *falciparum cases* (if not acute) are also cured.

(iii) *Preventive* drugs: Pamaquine, Plasmoquine (8-aminoquinolines) and Daraprim (diamino pyrimidines or pyrimethamine) are gametocidals and act against *exo-erythrocytic forms*.

(iv) Other drugs: A broad spectrum antimalarial drug has come to the Indian market in or around 1977. This is a combination of *sulfamethopyrazine* 500 mg, and *pyrimethanine* 25 mg per tablet and the trade name is "Metakelfin". Sulfamethopyrazine acts by double sequential blockade in the metabolic pathways and eventually inhibits the formation of nucleotides. It inhibits the formation of dihydrofolic acid from PABA. Pyrimethamine acts by inhibiting the enzyme *di-hydro folic acid reductase* of the malaria parasite, which is responsible for conversion of dihydro-folic acid to tetrahydro-folic (folinic) acid. The latter is the basic factor for nucleic acid synthesis. The adult dose is two tablets stat, which is a single dose treatment. Two tablets may be repeated after about a week. The side effects are iatrogenic (drug-induced) jaundice and the other effects noted post sulfa-therapy. Indeed metakelfin resistant and chloroquine responsive malaria, or metakelfin responsive chloroquine resistant malaria have been noted which is cured by repeating metakelfin therapy within a week. The children dose of metakelfin is 25 mg/kg of body weight.

Along with specific therapy antipyretics and alkalies are absolutely indicated.

The treatment of malaria should always be completed by the drug therapy. Inadequate therapy may lead to serious complications like, acute relapses, Black-water fever, etc.

SUMMARY OF TREATMENTS

1. **Antipyretics**
2. **Alkaliser**
3. **Antimalarials**
4. **Robinaxol for myopathy**

SUMMARY OF IMMUNITY IN MALARIA

The essence of immunity in malaria is Tolerance to infection. Parasitaemia may persist, but there is remission of clinical disease. The immunity is Strain-specific (immunity to respective and specific strain which infect the host). Infection, if occurs by *P. falciparum*, immunity will develop against the particular strain of *P. falciparum* only and not to any other species. That is to say, there is no cross-immunity amongst the species.

The host tolerance to malaria develops by active immunity which is both humoral and cellular type. The phagocytic activity of R-E cells in the liver and spleen triggers the development of immunity to malaria. Some workers believe that Post-Infective Parasitaemia is essential for Immunity Development and the parasites are kept at subclinical condition. So many authors are of the opinion to label this immunity as Infection Immunity or Premunition. Immunity is short lasting.

Cellulo-humoral defence mechanism is effective against parasite in the Erythrocytic Phase only. Therefore, relapses are not protected (in persistence of Exo-Erythrocytic Forms). Hence, Exo-Erythrocytic Merozoites ('E-E'–Macromerozoites) attack RBCs and, ultimately, bring about the clinical attack of malaria. But, when immunity forms, the antibodies paralyse the Pre-Erythrocytic Merozoites (of the liver) as soon as they appear in circulation. So they cannot invade RBC any more. But, when Immunity is low or nil, then only the Macromerozoites escaping from the liver can bring up a clinical attack or Relapse (Shortt, 1950).

BLACKWATER FEVER

Blackwater fever is a manifestation of an attack of malaria caused by *P. falciparum* on a subject previously suffering from this infection. It is characterised by a sudden intravascular haemolysis of RBCs with a chill and fever followed by *haemoglobinaemia* and *haemoglobinuria* (haemoclastic crisis). The mechanism of haemolysis is not fully understood, but it is possible an allergic response to reinfection with *P. falciparum* resulting in sensitisation of self RBCs. Therefore, according to the modern concept, it is an auto-immune (auto-allergic or autosensitisation) disease. Many persons acquire a certain degree of immunity but a few become allergic.

Experimental immunological test tecomes positive in them when intradermal injection of the suspension of ground up parasities is given.

Geographical distribution. Blackwater fever occurs irregularly in hyperendemic malarial regions. In India, it is common in hyperendemic areas of Assam and the Dooars.

Aetiology. It is now universally agreed that malaria in some unexplained manner is the cause for haemolysis in blackwater fever. The patient usually gives a history of repeated attacks of malaria over a period of months with irregular administration of quinine. It *commonly occurs in susceptible individuals specially immigrants or visitors after their stay for some days or months in an endemic area and having had* repeated attacks *of malignant tertian malaria*. There is no racial immunity and Indians or Asian are as susceptible as Europeans. Blackwater fever may occur during the coarse of an overt falciparum attack. In some cases, it may develop after a single attack of malignant tertian infection. It may be seen amongst the local inhabitants but mainly in children or in those, who live under conditions of low immunity or incomplete protection.

Cold, exertion, alcohol and specially irregular administration of quinine may precipitate an attack. It has been noticed that Blackwater fever occurs in persons incompletely protected by drug against malaria. It is likely that there is development of some state of sensitivity resulting from partial loss of hard-earned immunity which lead to sharp haemolysis upon successful reinfection with *P. falciparum*, specially when the strain is homologous. Quinine when taken, irregularly probably increases the fragility of red cells.

MECHANISM OF INTRAVASCULAR HAEMOLYSIS. The exact mechanism of haemolysis in Blackwater fever is not fully understood. It appears that some haemolysin (lecithinolysin) develops. This causes sensitisation of RBCs followed by haemolysis, resulting in liberation of oxyhaemoglobin in the blood stream. The attractive hypothesis is that, the infection changes the composition of the red cells, rendering them AUTOANTIGENIC. The antibodies *sensitise* the erythrocytes and the antigen in presence of *complement* causes lysis of the RBCs.

The hypersensitised or the **pre-Blackwater fever state** is produced by previous infections of *P. falciparum*, and an allergic type of reaction is precipitated by the action of a heavy infection of a homologous or a slightly heterologous strain of the parasite. It is likely that there is development of some homologous or slightly heterologous or a slightly heterologous development of some homologous or slightly heterologous strains at the cost of **hard-earned immunity** which leads to sharp haemolysis upon successful reinfection with *P. falciparum*, when the strain is homologous or slightly heterologous. Quinine when taken irregularly probably increases the **fragility** of red cells, due to the liberation of antigen and thus precipitating an attack.

Parasites in the blood. In the majority of cases of blackwater fever, *P. falciparum* is not usually detected in the peripheral blood but occasionally the parasites may be found in the early stage of the attack. This is probably due to the fact that they are destroyed by the **haemolytic crisis**. In case the patient survives, the parasite may reappear in the peripheral blood in one or two weeks after the haemoclastic crisis.

Pathogenesis. The pathological manifestations are due to **intravascular haemolysis** with the onus (burden) on the kidney. Haemolysis is rapid and resembles that of incompatible transfusion. **Severe anaemia** occurs as a result of haemolysis and even half the total RBCs of the body may be lysed within a short time during a paroxysm.

RESULTS OF INTRAVASCULAR HAEMOLYSIS. As a result of excess of haemolysis, oxyhaemoglobin liberated into blood circulation is excreted through glomeruli, causing *haemoglobinuria* and *blockage of urinary tubules* by formation of **acid haematin**, insoluble in the acid urine, resulting in anuria. The *renal failure* tubular lesions. *Decreased urinary flow* is due to failure of glomerular filtration and obstruction and degeneration of tubules. So, alkali must be given.

The haemoglobin liberated by intravascular haemolysis is converted into: (a) **methaemalbumin**, (b) **haemobilirubin** by separation of **haemosiderin** ingested by the RE cells. This is far in excess of what the liver can dispose of and results in *hyperbilirubinaemia* and escape of excess of *urobilinogen* in urine. The van Den Bergh gives an *indirect positive* reaction.

The oxyhaemoglobin in blood is split up into glogin and haematin, a ferrous salt, which after oxidation is converted into ferric salt. (i) This combines with serum albumen forming methaemalbumen. This is unable to be excreted by the kidney tubules and retained in the plasma producing a condition of **methaemalbuminaemia. Haemoglobinuria** results from excess of haemoglobin in the circulating blood and as the amount exceeds the renal thresholds, it is excreted through the kidney tubules. (iii) Oxyhaemoglobin may be converted into methaemoglobin in the renal tubules and excreted in the urine or deposited in the tubules forming acid haematin casts.

To sum up, the pigments are: (a) **In blood** oxyhaemoglobin, methaemalbumen and bilirubin are formed; the last one is responsible for indirect van Den Bergh reaction. (b) **In urine** oxyhaemoglobin, giving a red colour and *methaemoglobin producing a black/dark brown colour of urine,* haematin forming a deposit, and excess of urobilinogen is present; the last one on oxidation gives *urobilin.*

Morbid anatomy. Main changes are seen in the liver, spleen and kidneys. The changes in these organs are like those in falciparum malaria. The *liver* is enlarged and soft. The *gall bladder* show thick and tarry bile. The *spleen* is enlarged and soft and the pulp is diffluent. The *kidneys* are swollen, dark and congested. Renal failure is the common of haemosiderin pigment in RE cells of different organs.

MICROSCOPICALLY: Haemosiderin and haemozoin abound in the liver and spleen. Necrosis of liver cells is often seen in the centre of the lobule. Kidneys show granular debris in the tubules and there may be toxic or anoxic degeneration of convoluted tubules.

CLINICAL PATHOLOGY. Blood. Malarial parasites are found in the early stage of the disease but they disappear from peripheral blood within 48 hours after an attack or after administration of quinine. Severe normocytic anaemia is produced as a result of haemolysis and abnormal red cells appear in circulation; van Den Bergh reaction gives a strongly positive indirect reaction. There is leucopenia with increase of monocytes which may show ingested haemozoin pigment. In severe cases, direct biphasic reaction is positive due to hepatocellular damage. Icterus index is very high. Plasma contains oxyhaemoglobin and later methaemalbumen; the latter is formed by combination of serum albumen with methaemoglobin. Blood urea and NPN are slightly raised but the rise is marked in cases of oliguria or anuria.

Urine. The urine is almost black in colour and when held in a conical glass shows granular debris at the bottom. It contains methaemoglobin, albumen oxyhaemoglobin, haematin and *uribilinogen* in excess. *Methaemalbumen* is *absent in urine*. Chloride and urea concentration are greatly reduced owing to insufficiency of renal tubules with corresponding retention of blood. Bile and ketone bodies may appear in urine in severe cases. *Microscopic examination* of urine shows haemoglobin casts and crystals of haematin but RBCs are absent. *Spectroscopic examination* of urine shows bands of oxyhaemoglobin absorption in the spectrum.

Complications. The patient may die of uraemia due to renal failure, acute liver dysfunction or circulatory failure. Anaemia is marked after the attack of Blackwater fever when the patient survives the attack. Pigment calculi may form due to overproduction of bilirubin and its excretion through the bile ducts.

Treatment. Big doses of alkali containing potassium salts are necessary for the excretion of haematin which blocks the tubules due to formation of acid haematin. Atebrine may be used as an antimalarial therapy but quinine is totally avoided. An infusion or extract of leaves of *Vitex pèduncularis* found in large quantities in Assam forests (local name *Ashui paata*) prevents haemolytic crisis and soon makes the urine clear.

A FEW CONFIRMED SPOROZOA

CLASS :	FAMILY :	EIMERIIDAE	
TELOSPOREA	GENUS :	1. ISOSPORA 2. EIMERIA	TOXOPLASMA

ORDER : EUCOCCIDA

(*Rare intestinal parasites of human*)

The coccidia parasitic to man belong to two genera, e.g., Isospora and Eimeria. The former includes rare parasites of human causing infection in the epithelial cells of the mucous membrane of the small intestine (ileum) but the pathogenicity of the latter is doubtful.

(1) The genus Isospora is characterised by formation of 2 sporocysts, each containing 4 sporozoites (Fig. 1). (2) The genus Eimeria is characterised by formation of 4 sporocysts each containing 2 sporozoites (Fig. 5.2).

Habitat. *Isospora belli* and ***hominis*** are the parasites of the small intestine of man and they are most probably present in the last portion of the ileum or in the caecum, like those of *I. canis* in the dog or *I. felis* in the cat, Schizogony occurs in the intestinal epithelium, where gametocytes also form. The gametes undergo fertilisation, and development of oocysts follows with the secretion of the cyst wall occurring in the intestinal lumen.

Cultivation. These parasites have not been cultivated *in vitro*.

Life cycle. (Fig. 5.3). The life cycle of human coccidia has not been fully observed in human but

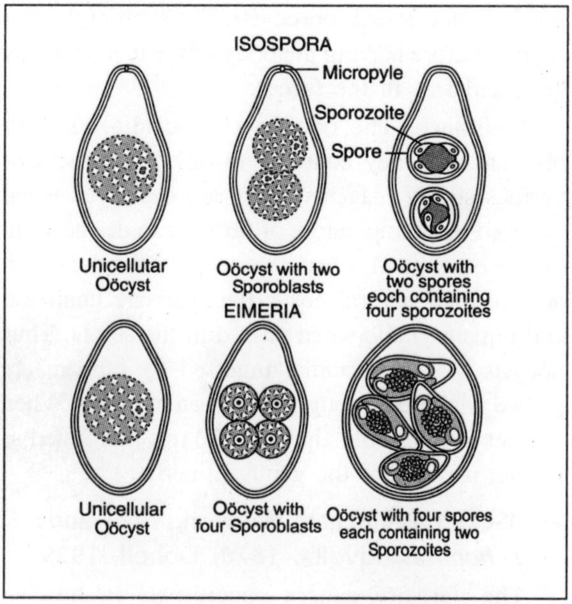

Fig. 5.2 Development of sporozoites in the oocysts of genera Isospora and Eimeria

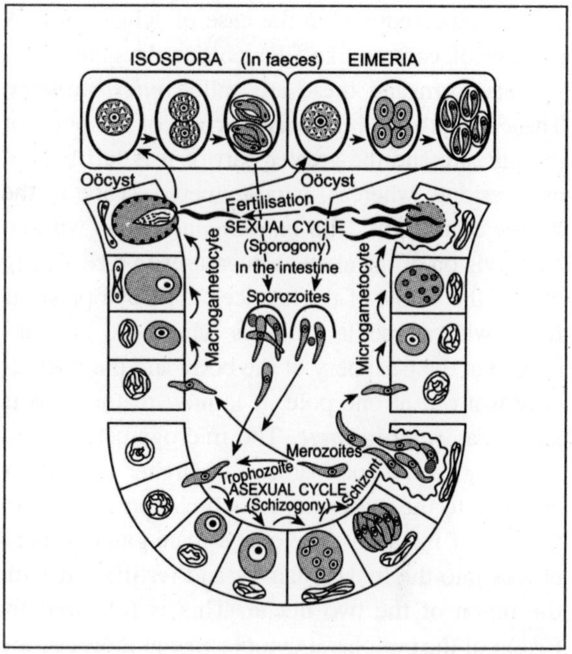

Fig. 5.3 Life cycle of Coccidia (Isospora and Eimeria), representing infection in two adjacent intestinal villi. *Asexual cycle*–The ingested ripe oocyst contains spores and sporozoites which are liberated in the intestine. The development occurs in the intestinal epithelium with the formation of trophozoites developing into a schizont and merozoites. *Sexual cycle*–Some of the merozoites form microgametocytes and macrogametocytes and respective gametes. After fertilisation, oocysts with a single sporoblast are passed in the faeces. In *Isospora*, 2 spores are seen with 4 sporozoites in each spore; whereas, in *Eimeria*, 4 spores are seen, each containing 2 sporozoites in the cyst

as the course and development of most coccidia are similar, the typical life cycle of Isospora is being described, starting from the alimentary tract. The coccidia shows ***alternation of generations***, e.g., asexual and sexual, both being passed in the same host. The parasite lives in the epithelial cells of the small intestine of the host. Here the life cycle consists of several asexual generations followed by a sexual generation, terminating into an encysted stage called *Oocyst*. The oocyst, when passed in the faeces, undergoes further development outside the body by formation of sporocyst containing sporozoites.

INFECTION IN HUMAN HOST. **Schizogony.** After ingestion of a sporocyst, the sporozoite, the youngest coccidium liberated from sporocyst, infects the epithelium of the small intestine, becomes rounded in form, with a single, vesicular nucleus remaining within an epithelial cell and this is called *trophozoite*. This gradually increases in size and undergoes multiplication by a process of schizogony forming a schizont. In this the nucleus of the parasite divides repeatedly in rapid succession by mitotic divisions into two with the formation of new spindles before the preceding division is complete. After the splitting of the requisite number of nuclei, the cytoplasm accumulates around each daughter nucleus and the schizont undergoes segmentation into vermiform merozoites, with many nuclei in the mature schizont. The motile merozoites escape from the infected cells into the lumen of the gut and infect new epithelial cells in which development takes place and the asexual cycle is repeated.

Sporogony. After some generations of the asexual cycle merozoites become sexually differentiated into male and female gametocytes known as microgametocytes and macrogametocytes, respectively, and the development of sexual cycle begins. The microgametocyte increases in size at first and the nucleus divides repeatedly as in the case of schizogony. A number of comma-like filamentous daughter individuals form and these are called *microgametes*. These are extruded from the surface of the body of the parasite and the greater part of it is left behind as a residue; whereas, microgametes escape in the lumen of the gut. The ***macrogametocyte***, without any division of the nucleus, increases in size, filling almost the whole of the host cell. The cytoplasm is filled with refractile globules which are later arranged at the periphery of the body and the nucleus is drawn out at one pole. It is now mature and is known as ***macrogamete***. The microgamete, corresponding to the spermatozoa of higher animals is attached to the macrogamete which corresponds to the ova of metazoa. One of the male gametes penetrates into the female gamete and fertilises it with the union of the two nuclei. This is followed by fusion of the peripheral cytoplasmic granules of the macrogamete, forming a tough membrane or cyst, surrounding the body. The fertilised body contracts to form a rounded body, the ***zygote***. The encysted zygote, now known as ***oocyst***, drops into the lumen of the gut and is discharged with the faeces.

OUTSIDE THE HUMAN HOST. The oocysts are colourless oval bodies having a cyst wall and a protoplasmic mass inside. They are 32μm by 16μm. Further development of the oocyst takes place outside the body by a process of sporogony within several days. In *Isospora* the nucleus of oocyst divides into two and the zygote develops into two uninucleate, ovoid *sporoblasts*, each being invested with a cyst wall of its own, called a *sporocyst*. Within each sporocyst 4 sausage-shaped vermiform uninucleate *sporozoites* arise by further subdivision. The sporozoites measure about 14μm by 7μm. In the course of development of the zygote and sporoblasts, the oocysts invested with thick, hard cyst walls, are discharged in the faeces in an immature state and further stages of the development of sporogony are completed outside the body of the host. It should, however, be noted that in some coccidia the entire development including sporogony is completed in the subepithelial tissue. The oocysts, when voided in faeces, are already mature, containing fully developed sporocysts. The sporocysts may rupture before leaving the body of the host and may be found free in the faeces.

Resistance. The oocysts of coccidia are very resistant and they continue to develop in acid or various strong reagents. They are destroyed when exposed to a temperature of 56°C or to desiccation. On the other hand, when ingested by animals, which are not their natural hosts, the cysts are unaltered and remain viable when passed in the stools. Thus oocysts of fish-coccidia, ingested by human, are passed unaltered through the human intestine. When present in the stools, they may be misinterpreted as human parasite of the genus Eimeria.

ISOSPORA BELLI* Wenyon, 1923 and *I. hominis* (Rivolta, 1878) Dobell, 1929

The parasite causes coccidiosis in human, characterised by enterocolitis. They are found in the stool and cause pathological lesions in the small intestine of human. Both asexual and sexual cycles develop in the epithelial cells. Closely related parasites are found in cats and dogs.

Morphology. The oocysts passed in the faeces are ovoid with a double layer of cyst wall with a micropyle, sometimes seen at the narrow end. Their sizes vary from 22-23μm by 10-19μm. The oocysts are passed in the zygote state but sometimes oocysts containing two sporoblasts which are seen in the freshly voided faeces. The sporogony is complete in 1-4 days outside the body. By the division of the nucleus of the zygote, two sporoblasts and finally two oval sporocysts form, 12-14μm by 7-9μm. Each mature sporocyst contains 4 sporozoites and a residual mass of cytoplasm. The life cycle is complete in human volunteers in 9-16 days.

Clinical symptoms. *I. hominis* has been reported in British soldiers, returning from Gallipoli, Salonika and the Balkans. Mukherjee (1947) reported 14 cases amongst British soldiers in Arakan and India and stated that this occurred as a mild outbreak in the monsoon season. The infection causes diarrhoea and enterocolitis in human but it causes debilitating di-

* According to Wenyon (1923-1926) *I. hominis* has smaller oocysts than those of *I. belli*

arrhoea in domestic animals. The disease is self-limited and **the subject is cured in 3 weeks without any treatment**.

Diagnosis. It depends upon recognition of oocysts in the faeces. These are coloured ovoid bodies measuring 18μm by 28μm on average with a clear-cut wall of two or more layers. The protoplasm is unsegmented, and when they are passed in stools and appears as a rounded granular mass the protoplasm does not fill the cyst. They may be mistaken for eggs of some unknown worm.

EIMERIA GUBLERI Guirat, 1922

This has been claimed to be responsible to cause **hepatic coccidiodosis** in human. It is a very rare condition and only a few cases have been reported until now. □

REFERENCES

Bamatter, F. (1952). Neuere gegichtsputspunkte in der toxoplasmoseforschung. *Wein. Klin. Wochenschr.* 64, 185-189.

Biocca, E. (1949). Observazoini sulla posizioni sistematica del *Toxoplasma. Riv. Parassitol.* 10, 73-81.

Collins. W. E. Jeffery. G. M., Guinn. E. and Skinner, J. C. (1966). Fluorescent antibody studies in human malaria. IV. Cross reactions between human and simian malaria. *Amer. J. trop. Med. & Hyg.* 115, 11-15.

Frenkel. J. K. (1949). Pathogenesis, diagnosis and treatment of human toxoplasmosis. *J. am. med. Assoc.* 140, 369-377.

Gustafson, P. V., Agar, H. D. and Cramer, D. L. (1954). An electron microscope study of toxoplasma. *Am. J. trop. Med. Hyg.* 3, 1008-1021.

MacDonald, A. M. (1963). *Personal communication.*

Mahoney, D. F., Redington, B. C. and Schoenbechler, M. J. (1966). Preparation and serologic activity of plasmodial fractions. *Mill. Med.* 131 (Suppl.), 1141-1151.

Nicolle, C. and Manceaux, L. (1908). Sur une infection a crops de Leishman (ou organismes voisins) du gondi. *Compt. rend. Acad. Sci.* 147, 763-765.

Nicolle. M. M. C. and Manceaux, L. (1909). Sur un protozoaire nouveau du gondi (Toxoplasma n. sp.). *Arch. Inst. Pasteur Tunis.* 2, 642.

Rogers, W. A. Jr., Fried, J. A. and Kagan, I. G. (1968). A modified indirect microhaemagglutination test for malaria. *Amer. J. trop. Med. & Hyg.* 17, 804-809.

Sabin, A. B. (1941). Toxoplasmic encephalitis in children. *J. am. med. Assoc.* 116, 801-807.

Sabin, A. B. (1943). Toxoplasma neutralizing antibody in human beings. *Proc. Soc. exptl. Biol. & Med.* 51. 6-10.

Sabin, A. B. (1949). Complement fixation tests in toxoplasmosis and persistence of the antibody in human beings. *Pediatrics* 4, 443-453.

Sabin, A. B. and Feldman, H. A. (1949). Dyes as microchemical indicators of new immunity phenomenon affecting a protozoon parasite (Toxoplasma). *Science* 108, 660-663.

Sabin, A. B. and Ruchman, I. (1943). Characteristics of the toxoplasma neutralizing antibody *Proc. Soc. exptl. Biol. & Med.* 51, 1-6.

Stein, B. and Desowitz, R. S. (1964). The measurement of antibody in human malaria by a formalized shep cell hemagglutination test. *Bull. W.H.O.* 30, 45-49.

Sulzer, A. J., and Wilson, M. (1967). The use of thick-smear antigen slides in the malaria indirect fluorescent antibody test. *J. Parasitol.* 53, 1110-1111.

Tobie, J. E., Abele, D. C., Hill, G. J., Contacos, P. G. and Evnts, C. B. (1966). Fluorescent antibody studies on the immune response in sporozoite-induced and blood-induced vivax malaria and the relationship of antibody production to parasitemia. *Amer. J. trop. Med. & Hyg.* 15, 676-683.

Warren, J. and Sabin, A. B. (1943). The complement fixation reaction in toxoplasmosis. *Proc. Soc. exptl. Biol. & Med.* 51, 11-14.

CHAPTER 6

MISCELLANEOUS SPOROZOA AND MICROSPORA

Sporozoa are the Protozoa that produce spore-like occysts containing sporozoites. They live partly intracellularly during their life cycle. At some stage in their life cycle, they possess a structure called the apical complex, by means of which they attach to and penetrate the host cells. They are absent in the malaria parasites, Sarcystic species, (Cryptosporidium) Coccidia, and Babesia. The unclassified organisms of uncertain origin (Pneumocystis carinii) were also grouped with sporozoa at present. But it has been dealt with in different chapters in this book at the end of Protozoa.

The life cycle of sporozoa show alternation of generations consisting of a sexual sporogonic phase and an asexual schizogonic phase. Some of them, in addition, show alternation of hosts, i.e., a vertebrate host and an insect vector, or a definitive and an intermediate host. There is no organ of locomotion. Motility is by flexion or gliding movements. Flagella are present in the microgametes.

Many minute intracellular protozoa have been classified under microspora. They infect a large number of hosts including vertebrates and invertebrates. Invasion of subjects remain asymptomatic or it may cause clinical illness in immunodeficient persons. Many of the infections are associated with AIDS.

The trophozoite and tissue cyst represent stages of schizogony (asexual multiplication). Oocyst is formed by gametogony or sexual reproduction i.e., sporogony. All the 3 forms occur in domestic cat and other felines which are the definitive hosts. Only the asexual forms—i.e., the trophozoites and the tissue cysts stages—are present in humans, other animals and birds, which behave as the intermediate hosts. Both oocysts and tissue cysts are infective. Infection occurs by ingestion of infected cysts.

TOXOPLASMOSIS AND *T. GONDII*

It occurs in 3 morphological forms: See Fig 6.1, Fig. 6.2.

T. gondii occurs in three forms—trophozoite, tissue cyst and oocyst (Fig. 6.1).

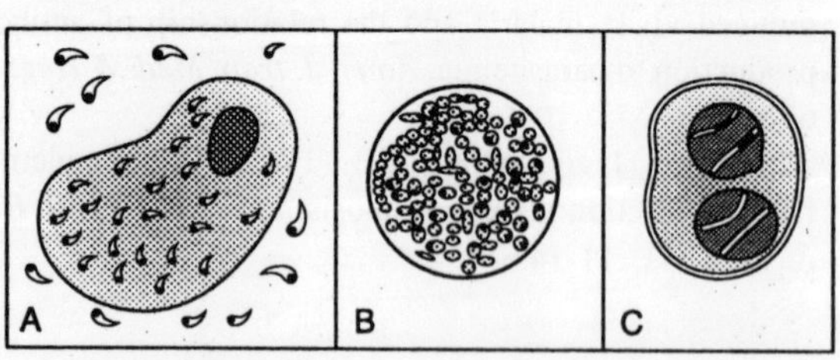

Fig. 6.1 Toxoplasma gondii: (A) Smear from peritoneal fluid of infected mouse, showing crescentic tachyzoites—extracellular trophozoites and intracellular form within macrophage. (B) Thick-walled tissue cyst containing rounded forms—**bradyzoites**. (C) Oocyst containing two sporocysts with sporozoites inside.

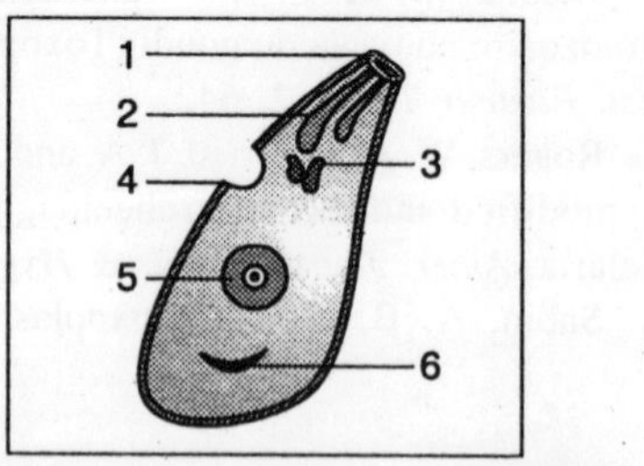

Fig. 6.2 Electron microscopy of **Toxoplasma gondii**. Trophozoite (tachyzoite), fine structure seen by electron microscopy. 1. Conoid; 2. Rhoptery (Toxonemes); 3. Golgi body; 4. Cytostome; 5. Nucleus; 6. Mitochondrion

TROPHOZOITE: The trophozoite is crescent-shaped with one end pointed (containing an apical complex) and the other end rounded. That is why the name of the subphylum is apicomplexa. It measures approximately 3 μ by 7 μ. The ovoid nucleus is situated near the blunt end. Electron microscopy reveals the pointed end of the apical complex.

STAINING REACTION: The trophozoite stains with Giemsa stain, the cytoplasm is azure blue and the nucleus red. It is intracellular in various tissues and organs of the host during the early acute phase of infection. Extracellular trophozoites are seen in impression smears. These invade any nucleated cell and replicate within the cytoplasmic vacuoles by the process of endodyogeny (internal budding). As a result, daughter trophozoites are formed that are surrounded by its own membrane itself within the parent cell. When the host cells are distended with the multiplying parasites, they disintegrate and release the trophozoites that infect other host cells.

ACUTE INFECTION: In acute infection, the proliferating trophozoites within the host cells appear spherical and are enclosed by the host cell membrane. This is called the pseudocyst' or 'colony'. That is differentiated from true tissue cysts by staining reactions. The rapidly proliferating trophozoites (in acute infection) are called tachyzoites. Trophozoites are propagated in the laboratory in the eggs in tissue culture, and in the peritoneum of mice by incubation for the maintenance of stains, and antigens preparation for the serological tests. The trophozoites are susceptible to gastric digestion, drying and thawing.

CHRONIC INFECTION

The Tissue Cyst (in Chronic Infection): Tissue cysts occur in the muscles and other tissues and organs, e.g., the brain. The parasite multiplies slowly within the host cell and produces a cyst wall within the host cell membrane. The cyst wall is eosinophilic. It stains with silver (in contrast to the 'pseudocyst'). With PAS stain, the cyst wall stains light magenta and the parasites stain deep magenta inside the cyst wall. Slowly multiplying parasites within the cyst are called bradyzoites. The cyst is spherical to oval. It measures 10 μ to 200 μ in size and contains numerous bradyzoites. Cysts remain viable in tissue for several years. In normal hosts, the cysts are silent; in the immuno-compromised hosts cysts are reactivated, and cause clinical toxoplasmosis. The cysts are relatively resistant. When meat (containing the cysts) is eaten raw or under-cooked, toxoplasmosis infection occurs. The cyst wall is disrupted by peptic and trypic digestion, when parasites are released. The released parasites invade the intestinal epithelial cells and cause infection. They reach various tissue and organs via circulation and lymphatic spread. Cysts are susceptible to desiccation and thawing. They are thermostable at 60°C.

THE OOCYST: Oocysts develop in a definitive host, i.e., the intestine of cats (and other felines). Cats get infected by ingestion of tissue cysts and oocysts. The parasites develop in the intestinal (brush border) epithelial cells of cats where schizogony and gametogony take place. Male and female gametocytes develop there. After fertilization the zygote gets surrounded by a thin, resistant wall. Oocyst is spherical to ovoid; 10 μ in diameter and contains a sporoblast. Cats shed millions of oocysts daily in the faeces for two weeks during the primary infection. Freshly passed oocysts are noninfective. They become infective after development in the soil or water for a few days. During this state of sporulation, sporoblasts divide into sporocysts; 4 sporozoites develop inside each sporocyst. A mature oocyst contains sporozoites. Oocyst is resistant to many environmental conditions and remain infective in soil for one year. When the infective oocyst is ingested, it releases sporozoites in the intestine and initiate infection.

Life Cycle of *T. gonodii* (Fig. 6.3)

Three stages are there: (a) Tachyzoites—which are rapidly multiplying trophozoites—invade host cells and multiply there.

(b) Bradyzoites—which are slowly multiplying cysts form inside the tissue cysts. This occurs in latent and in chronic infection.

(c) Sporozoites inside oocysts are shed in cat faeces that remain in the environment.

THE ENTERIC CYCLE: Cats are the definitive hosts where schizogony and gametogony take place in the intestinal epithelial cells. This is the enteric cycle. The oocysts produced by gametogony are shed in faeces. They develop into the infective forms in soil and water. They are ingested by cats (felines) to repeat the enteric cycle.

When oocysts are ingested by animals and birds they become the intermediate host.

THE EXOENTERIC CYCLE: The oocysts release sporozoites that infect the intestinal epithelial cells. They multiply by endodygeny and form tachyzoites. The host cell ruptures releasing numerous trophozoites that spread through blood and lymph, infecting the nucleated cells in various tissues and organs. This is known as exoenteric cycle.

ASEXUAL CYCLE: Primary infection with the parasite may be either asymptomatic or acute and chronic. In chronic infection tissue cysts are produced within the muscles and other tissues. At this stage, other intermediate hosts ingest the tissue cysts when the asexual cycle is repeated. When cats ingest the tissue cysts they become infected and, in them, Schizogony and gametogony cycles are repeated (Fig. 6.3).

The life cycle of parasites and the human infection occurs as follows:

1. Eating uncooked and undercooked infected meat containing tissue cysts.
2. Ingestion of mature oocysts through food, water, fingers and flies contaminated with cat faeces—directly and indirectly.
3. Vertical intrauterine infection from infected mothers to babies.
4. Infection is possible by blood transfusion or tissue transplantation from infected donors.

Transmission. The infection of *T. gondii* may occur in two ways; namely, congenital or acquired.

Pathogenesis. The PORTAL OF ENTRY is not definitely known in man or in the reservoir host. Once the infection takes place, toxoplasma may localise in the **brain, lungs** or other organs. It is characteristically associated with the RE cells, or the endothelial cells of the circulatory system. It tends to produce serous exudation in body cavities, minute areas of consolidation, necrosis and granulomatous tissue with calcification of cerebral lesions. *Protean clinical manifestations* are due to its power of invasion of different types of tissue cells. The **toxotonin** formed in days before the death of

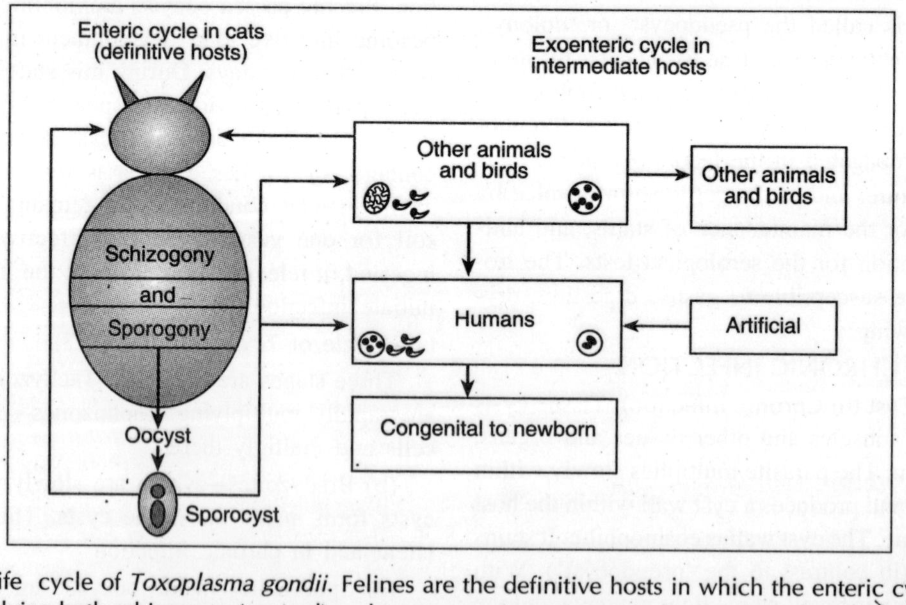

Fig. 6.3 Life cycle of *Toxoplasma gondii*. Felines are the definitive hosts in which the enteric cycle takes place involving both schizogony (asexual) and sporogony (gametogony). Cat is infected either by ingestion of oocyst shed in its faeces or by eating flesh of other animals and birds containing tissue cysts. Oocysts in cat faeces sporulate and develop into sporocysts containing sporozoites. When ingested they infect animals, humans and birds. Human infection also occurs from flesh of animals and birds containing tissue cysts. Artificial methods of human infection are laboratory contamination, blood transfusion and organ transplantation. Congenital infection occurs as well.

the animal is highly toxic for mice. According to Sabin (1950), toxoplasma-infected pregnant women exhibit no characteristic signs; whereas the developing nervous system of the foetus is specially vulnerable, if the foetus is exposed during the *third trimester*.

Symptoms. *Clinically*, the condition may be **congenital** due to infection of the mother in the early or later months of pregnancy. The infection in these cases is due to transmission of the organism from the mother to the foetus through the placenta. Younger the foetus is, the greater is the damage.

In later *embryonic months* it may produce encephalitis, chorioretinitis, hydrocephalus, microcephalus or intracerebral calcification and the issue dies soon. In *acquired conditions* it may produce fever with *lymphnoditis, pneumonitis* or *hepatitis* with *jaundice, myocarditis, skin rash, hepato-splenomegaly*, but in about 50 per cent cases the infection is inapparent and detected only serologically.

CLINICAL FEATURES

Clinical toxoplasmosis may be congenital or acquired. Most human infections remain asymptomatic.

CONGENITAL TOXOPLASMOSIS

Congenital toxoplasmosis occurs when infection is transplacentally transmitted from mother to the foetus. When the mother gets asymptomatic or symptomatic primary toxoplasma infection during pregnancy, the foetus gets infected from the mother.

Most infected newborns are asymptomatic during child birth. Some children develop clinical toxoplasmosis in months and years after birth. The clinical manifestations are chorioretinitis, strabismus, blindness, deafness, epilepsy, mental retardation. A few babies are born with manifestations of acute toxoplasmosis at birth like fever, jaundice, diarrhoea, petechial rashes, hydrocephalus, microcephaly, cerebral calcifications, microphthalmis, cataract, acute congestive glaucoma, chorioretinitis, optic atrophy, lymphadenitis, pneumonitis, myocarditis, hepatosplenomegaly, etc. 35% babies are infected in the first trimester which is dangerous than those 65% which get infected during the 3rd trimester.

ACQUIRED TOXOPLASMOSIS

The most common manifestations of acute acquired toxoplasmosis is lymphadenopathy. Cervical lymph nodes are most frequently affected. Fever, headache, myalgia and splenomegaly are other manifestations. The illness is self-limited and may resemble 'flu' and infectious mononucleosis which is self-limited. Lymphadenopathy may persist in some cases typhus-like exanthem is present with pneumonitis, myocarditis and meningoencephalitis, which is indeed fatal. Another type is ocular toxoplasmosis. About 35% cases of all chorioretinitis is due to toxoplasmosis. Some cases may be so severe as to require eye enucleation. Toxoplasmosis primarily involve the CNS which is usually fatal and the rest is associated with AIDS where brain involvement is common.

IMMUNITY AND TOXOPLASMOSIS

Host defence is by way of both humoral and cellular immunity, like TB. Specific IgG antibody lyse extracellular trophozoites. Activated T cells and NK (natural killer) cells are important and are the potential reservoirs or sources of infection, and, at the same time preventing the clinical disease.

However, ELISA is the simplest test and is the test of choice for IgM and the IgG antibodies.

The presence of IgM antibody in absence of IgG indicates a current infection while the presence of IgM antibody with high titre of IgG indicates the recent past infection. But the negative IgM titre with positive IgG indicates a remote past infection. It is also true that, in some cases, IgM antibody titre persists more than 1½ years. For such a confusion, Serial ELISA test should be done for a decisive opinion.

EPIDEMIOLOGY (and brief cycle)

The infection is worldwide in cats. The natural cycle is maintained by the cats and the mice.

The mice eat the excreted materials containing oocysts (shed by the cats). Mice get infected and develop toxoplasma cysts in their tissues. When these mice are eaten by cats, they get infected. Infected cats shed oocysts in faeces.

Toxoplasmosis is a zoonosis. Humans are infected through:

(i) Food and
(ii) Water contaminated with mature oocysts,
(iii) By ingestion of raw and undercooked meat, pork and beef containing the tissue cysts,
(iv) Flies and cockroaches act as mechanical vectors by contaminating food with oocysts from soil,

(v) Water-borne infection oocurs when the source of water is contaminated with the faeces of the cat,

(vi) Infection can also be transmitted through blood and leucocyte transfusion as well as organ transplantation,

(vii) Toxoplasmosis is acquired by laboratory infection also.

Symptoms. *Clinically*, the condition may be **congenital** due to infection of the mother in the early or later months of pregnancy. The infection in these cases is due to transmission of the organism from the mother to the foetus through the placenta. Younger the foetus is, the greater is the damage.

In later *embryonic months* it may produce encephalitis, chorioretinitis, hydrocephalus, microcephalus or intracerebral calcification and the issue dies soon. In *acquired conditions* it may produce fever with *lymphnoditis, pneumonitis* or *hepatitis* with *jaundice, myocarditis, skin rash, hepato-splenomegaly*, but in about 50 per cent cases the infection is inapparent and detected only serologically.

Clinical diagnosis. Toxoplasmosis can be presumably diagnosed by: (*a*) *cerebral calcification* found by ventriculography; (*b*) *chorioretinitis*, specially in the macular region or (*c*) evidences of *hydrocephalus, microcephalus, microphthalmos*, changes in the CSF, and (*d*) other conditions like pheumonitis, myocarditis, splenomegaly, hepatomegaly etc.

Laboratory diagnosis. DIRECT METHODS: (1) *Microscopic demonstration* of the parasite. *T. gondii* in Giemsa stained smears of the material from blood, splenic or bone marrow puncture, centrifuged deposit of CSF, ventricular aspirate or smears from brain or other tissues removed by biopsy, or at autopsy is the direct method of diagnosing the disease. (2) As an alternative method, the *animal inoculation* of the suspected material in mice, hamsters or guinea pigs is done intraperitoneally, for the demonstration of the parasite in the peritoneal exudate. Mice die in about three weeks, but guinea pigs die in about one week. The organisms may by recovered from the brain of these animals.

Isolation

Isolation is done by intraperitoneal injection of body fluids or ground tissues into cell cultures (Fig. 6.4), or immunosuppressed mice (Fig. 6.5). Peritoneal fluid and spleen smears show the trophozoites after 7 to 10 days. Serial blind passages are necessary for isolation: Sera of inoculated animals are tested for antibodies.

INDIRECT METHODS. The disease can be diagnosed indirectly by **immunological and serological** methods or by skin sensitivity test.

Many serological tests are prevalent. **(a) Sabin-Feldman dye test, (b) Indirect immunofluorescence, (c) Indirect Haemagglutination, (d) Complement fixation text, and (e) ELISA tests.**

(Macdonalt, 1949) is done by using the chorio-allantoic membrane of the chick embryo and it has been found to be satisfactory.

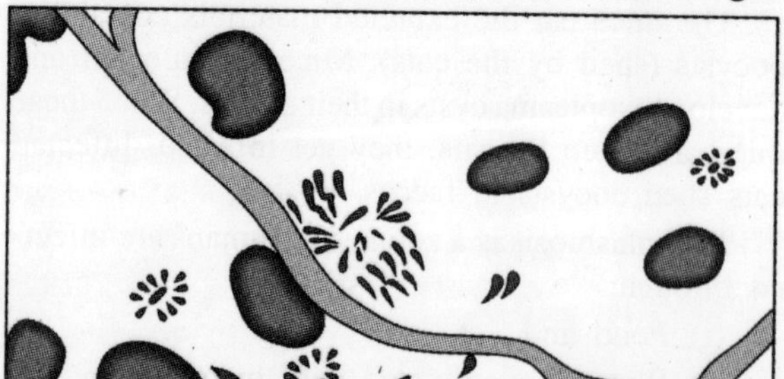

Fig. 6.4 *T. gondii.* Trophozoite grows in tissue culture. Smear shows trophozoites arranged in different patterns—singly, in cluster or as rosette (Giemsa stain)

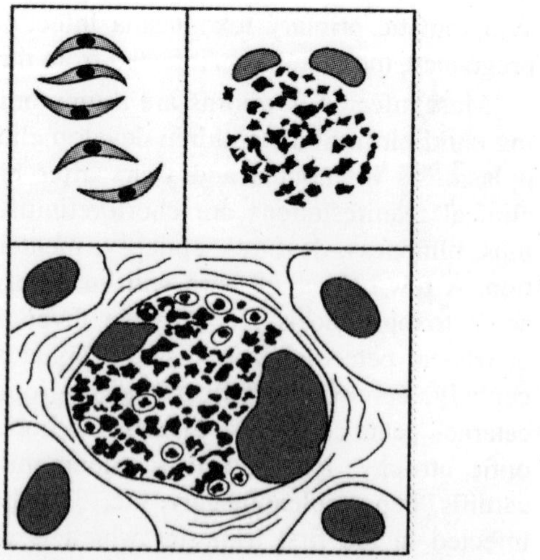

Fig. 6.5 *Toxoplasma gondii*—Upper left—free in the peritoneal exudate; upper right—pseudocyst in the film from brain. Lower—intracellular. × 1000 (After Dr. A. B. Sabin in J. A. M. A., Vol. 116)

NEUTRALISING ANTIBODY TEST (Sabin and Ruchman). This consists of the intracutaneous injection of patient's serum mixed with living toxoplasma into a rabbit. Failure of toxoplasma to produce any skin reaction characterised by erythema and oedema in 3 to 4 days indicate a positive reaction.

TOXOPLASMIN SKIN TEST (Frenkel). Suitable dilutions of toxoplasmin is injected intradermally. A delayed reaction with induration and erythema over 10 mm after 8 hours indicate a positive reaction. The test is not conclusive. Some observers (Bamatter, 1952 and others) consider Sabin's neutralisation and Frenkel's toxoplasmin tests of doubtful value.

IMMUNODIAGNOSIS NEUTRALISATION TEST

Sabin-Feldman dye test is based on the specific inhibition by antibody of the staining of the trophozoite by alkaline methylene blue. The Toxoplasma trophozoites propagated in mice peritoneal cavity are used in the test. An accessory factor present in fresh normal serum is needed for the test. The highest dilution of the test serum that inhibits the staining is the antibody titres of 1,000 or more in 4 to 8 weeks that remain positive at lower titres for years. Fluorescent antibody titre. The test becomes positive within 1 to 2 weeks after infection, reaching test results are of similar nature.

CYTOPLASM-MODIFYING ANTIBODY REACTION (Sabin and Feldman, 1948). It is also known as methylene blue dye test of Sabin and Feldman. The test is based on the fact that the organism, acted on *in vitro* by specific antibodies, fails to take up and stain with methylene blue.

The test modified by **Jacob** and **Cook**, 1954, is carried out as follows:

1. Peritoneal exudate of mice, inoculated 3 days earlier by the intraperitoneal route, is obtained by paracentesis. The fluid containing the maximum number of *T. gondii* is used.

2. Stock buffer solution of soda borax is made at a *p*H 10.8; 1.5 ml of the stock buffer is added to 0.1 ml of saturated alcoholic solution of methylene blue.

3. A volume of 0.1 ml of the dye solution is added directly to tubes of exudate containing the Toxoplasma, incubated for 1 hour with different dilutions of the serum to be tested.

Neutralising antibodies present in positive serum refrain *free parasites* from taking the stain, but parasites intact in cells or with negative serum stain well. Choice of the strain of toxoplasma is essential to give a clear cut reaction. The test when positive indicates acute, chronic or previous infection.

The test may, however, be positive in other protozoal infections like *Trichomonos hominis*, *Trypanosoma cruzi*, etc.

COMPLEMENT FIXATION TEST (Sabin and Warren). The antibody can be demonstrated by this test. The antigen utilised in the test is the toxoplasma material derived from chick-embryo culture. The test becomes positive about a month after the infection, when the serum should be positive in a dilution of 1:8. It remains positive after an acute phase of infection.

The CF test becomes positive only 3 to 8 weeks after infection when titre rises over the next 2 to 8 months and declines to low or undetectable levels within a year. The dye test required live toxoplasma and can be done only in reference laboratories.

ELISA tests give better results. The standard test used at present is ELISA which is separately done for IgM and IgG antibodies under the range of tests called "TORCH".

INTERPRETATION

The presence of IgM antibody in the absence of IgG denotes current infection; IgM with positive IgG indicates past infection. This is subject to individual variation. In some cases IgM antibody may persist upto 18 months. Serial ELISA provides better information than a single test.

EPIDEMIOLOGY

The infection is worldwide, being found whereever there are cats. Numerous species of mammals, reptiles and birds are naturally infected. The full natural cycle is maintained predominantly by cats and mice. The mice eat materials contaminated with oocysts shed by cats. Mice get infected and develop cysts in their tissues. When such mice are eaten by cats they get infected. Infected cats shed oocysts in faeces. Besides this cycle, several other cycles have been documented.

Human toxoplasmosis is a zoonosis. It is acquired through food or water contaminated with mature oocysts or by ingestion of raw or undercooked meat containing tissue cysts. Pork and beef frequently have tissue cysts. Flies and cockroaches may act as mechanical vectors by contaminating food with oocysts from soil. Infection may be water- borne when the source of water is contaminated with cat faeces. Rarely, infection may be transmitted through blood and leucocyte transfusion, and organ transplantation. Toxoplasmosis may also be acquired by laboratory infection. The incubation period is usually 1 to 3 weeks.

The outcome of infection depends on the immune status of the infected person. Active progression of infection occurs in immunocompromised individuals. Toxoplasmosis has acquired great importance as one of the major fatal complications in AIDS.

The incidence of congenital toxoplasmosis is estimated as 1 in 1,000 live births.

Prevention

Eradication of toxoplasmosis appears unlikely because it is so widely disseminated in nature. But some simple measures may reduce the risk of infection. These include proper cooking of meat and washing of hands before eating as a measure against soil contamination.

Prophylaxis depends on measures directed against the transmission of the disease specially during pregnancy.

Treatment

Daraprim (Pyrimethamine) in combination with sulphadiazine has been found to be effective in human toxoplasmosis.

Combined treatment with Pyrimethamine and Sulphonamides or Pyrimethamine and Cotrimoxasole can cause clinical cure, though the parasites may not be eliminated. Spiromycin and Clindamycin have also been used. Treatment is effective only against trophozoites (and not against cysts).

SARCOSPORIDEA Butschlii, 1882

The parasites of this group belong to the genus "Sarcocystis" of the subphylum sporozoa, occurring in the muscle fibres of domestic animals, e.g., sheep, cattle, horses, pigs, rabbits and ducks. The toxin **sarcocystin** secreted by the parasite is toxic to rabbits. The infection is often fatal to the infected animal.

SARCOCYSTIS LINDEMANNI, Ribolta, 1878

The parasite is found in the muscle fibres as a tubular, fusiform, elongated body, called **"Miescher's tube"**, hyaline in appearance, containing a large number of crescentic spores, called **Rainey's corpuscles**. Each spore measures 10μ in length and 1-2μ in breadth, containing a single nucleus.

Man is rarely infected by ingestion of uncooked meat, food or drink, contaminated by excreta of animals harbouring the parasite. The parasite usually does not produce any symptom; it is accidentally detected at autopsy in the skeletal muscles, or larynx.

SARCOCYSTIS

Sarcocystis belongs to sporozoa that show alternation of generations, as well as alternation of hosts. There are three human pathogenic species. They are: S. hominis (Fig. 6.6), *S. suihominis*, *S. lindemanni*,. Human is the definitive host for hominis and suihominis species; and intermediate host of lindemani species. The genus sarcocystis produce cysts in the muscles of intermediate hosts. These cysts are the sarcocysts that contain numerous merozoites (bradyzoites). When the definitive host eats the flesh, the merozoites are liberated in the intestine. There they develop into male and female gametes. After fertilisation the zygote develops into an oocyst containing two sporocysts; each sporocyst has four sporozoites. The oocysts are shed in faeces and are ingested by the intermediate host. In these intermediate hosts the sporozoites invade the bowel wall and reach the vascular endothelial cells, where they undergo schizogony production producing merozoites (tachyzoites). Tachyzoites spread into the muscle fibres and develop into sarcocysts.

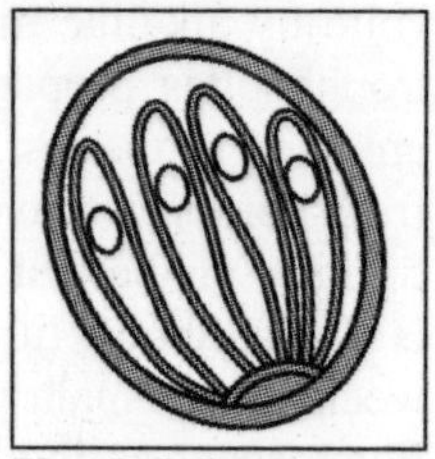

Fig. 6.6 *Sarcocystis hominis* oocyst

Cow is the intermediate host for S. hominis. Human infection is acquired by eating raw and undercooked beef. Oocysts are shed in human faeces that contaminate grass—the fodder eaten by the cows. In case of S. suihominis, pig is the intermediate host and human infection is obtained through pork meat. Human infection with S. hominis and S. suihominis is related to the food habits, though the clinical symptoms are negligible.

Humans are the intermediate host for *S. lindemanni*, the definitive host of *S. lindemani* is unknown. S. lindemani is not a single species; a group of unidentified species constitutes together *S. lindemani*.

CRYPTOSPORIDIUM PARVUM

Tyzzer, in 1907 first observed cryptosporidia in the crypts of the gastric mucosa of laboratory mice. Cryptosporidium frequently causes intractable diarrhoea in immunocompromised subjects and in AIDS patients. It causes a wide range of intensity of diarrhoea starting from mild diarrhoea in healthy subjects to chronic life-threatening diarrhoea in immunocompromised subjects.

Cryptosporidium is a worldwide distribution. It is a minute cocoidian parasite. Natural human infection occurs with cryptosporidium parvum (C. parvum) apart from infections in birds including cats, turkeys, and cattle, sheep, goats, etc. The infection can spread from one host species to some other animal species. The parasite has its both sexual and asexual phases of life cycle in a single host which is called monoxenous parasite (Fig. 6.7).

Crystosporidium infection is contracted by ingesting the oocyst in contaminated foods or drinks. After ingestion of the oocyst, four sporozoites are liberated in the intestine. Sporozoites infect the intestinal brush border epithelial cells, remaining restricted within the brush border cells.

There they develop into trophozoites that undergo schizogony asexual multiplication and release the merozoites. Some of the trophozoites develop into mature oocysts which are shed in faeces. They are infective or oocyst is 5 μ in diameter which remain viable for long period. Oocysts are resistant to most disinfectants.

EPIDEMIOLOGY

C. parvum contamination causes outbreaks of food poisoning. It survives in chlorinated water. Sequential application of ozone and chlorine and water is effective. There are asymptomatic carriers.

They may show febrile illness with watery diarrhoea. It can cause childhood and traveller's diarrhoea, and water-borne outbreaks as well. In immunodeficient persons and AIDS patients, infection leads to persistent and severe diarrhoea, fever and emaciation. The parasites invades the bronchial and biliary tracts which are demonstrated in sputum of AIDS patients.

DIAGNOSIS

(i) Direct demonstration of oocysts in the faeces. With Jenner-Giemsa stain, oocysts infected smears appear as blue spherical bodies containing a few eosinophilic granules. By cold Ziehl-Neelsen technique, the internal structures acid fast staining cysts (Fig. 6.8).

(ii) Fluorescent staining with auramine phenol is a useful staining technique.

(iii) Indirect immunofluorescence using specific antibody is also a useful technique.

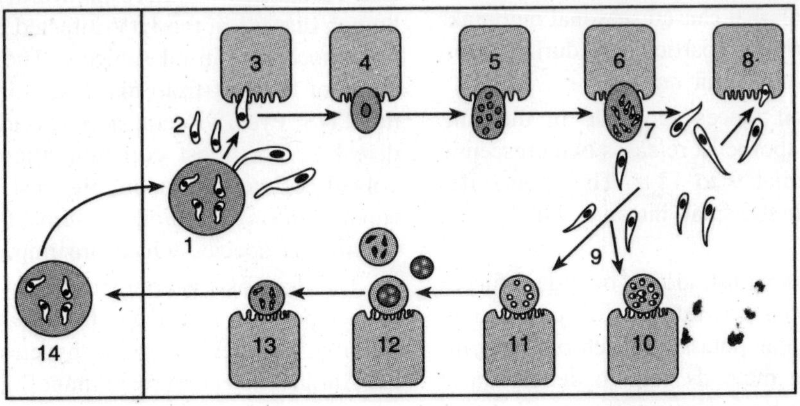

Fig. 6.7 Life cycle of *Cryptosporidium parvum*. 1. Infection occur by ingestion of oocyst containing four sporozoites. 2. In the small intestine, excystation releases the sporozoites. 3. The motile sporozoites penetrate enterocytes, remaining intracellular but extracytoplasmic. 4. to 6. Trophozoite, early schizont and mature schizont respectively, comprising of the asexual cycle (merogony). 7. Release of merozoites from schizont. 8. Merozoites infect neighbouring enterocytes to continue merogony. 9. Initiation of sexual cycle (sporogony). 10. Macrogametocyte. 11. Microgametocyte. 12. Zygote. 13. Oocyst. 14. Thick-walled oocyst the infective form, shed to exterior

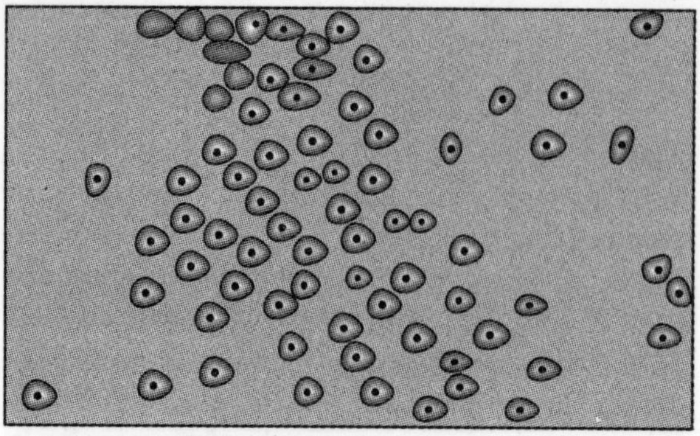

Fig. 6.8 Cryptosporidium sp. Oocyst of stained by Ziehl-Neelsen technique.

(iv) In acute diarrhoea, the oocysts are abundant, but when they are scanty, concentration by the formol-ether technique is useful.

Seroconversion occurs within 2 months of acute infection.

(v) Antibodies persist for one year—this is demonstrated by ELISA and immunofluorescence.

(vi) ELISA technique for detection of cryptosporidium in stools using monoclonal antibody is a highly sensitive and specific technique.

In persons with normal immune response, the disease undergoes spontaneous cure. There is no specific therapy.

C. parvum is an intestinal pathogen that has an association with HIV-related diarrhoea. It was first reported from Nepal, that caused seasonal outbreaks of prolonged diarrhoea—particularly during monsoon season in warm Terai regions.

Oocysts shed in faeces sporulate in the soil. Excystation of the sporocyst releases two crescentic sporozoites measuring 9 to 12 μ. The sporozoites infect enterocytes in the small intestine which causes diarrhoea.

Diagnosis is by demonstration of oocysts in faeces (Fig. 6.8). They can be induced to sporulate in presence of 5 percent potassium dichromate solution. Concentration methods help to demonstrates the cysts. The parasite is also seen in small bowel biopsy material examined by electron microscopy.

Infection is through faecal-oral route. The incubation period is 1 to 7 days. Drinking water is the important source of transmission. No specific therapy is known.

PROPHYLAXIS

Therapy: Specific potable water should be boiled.

MICROSPORIDIA

Microsporidia are minute intracellular parasites. They reproduce by spores. Spores are 2 to 4 mm in size, which have polar filaments (tubules). The spore is the infective form. Infection is contracted by ingestion of the spores. Spores transmit the sporoplasm through the tubules into enterocytes (intestinal brush border epithelia). Merogony (schizogony) and sporogony occur and the spores are shed in the faeces. Infection also occurs outside the intestine, in any viscera, muscle, and in the CNS.

In 19th century Europe, the silkworm disease pebrine caused great damage to the silk industry. Louis Pasteur was assigned to solve the problem in 1863. By 1870, Pasteur could control pebrine and could secure safe the silk industry in France. The causative agent of pebrine is Nosema bombycis, a microsporidian parasite.

Microsporidia are classified under the Phylum Microspora. It was recognised as a human pathogen in the 1980s with the spread of AIDS. Nine genera and 13 species of microspora are associated with human disease in the HIV-infected as well as other immunocompromised subjects. They cause a wide range of illness—from diarrhoea to involvement of the CNS, eyes, viscera, muscles and disseminated diseases. The most common microsporidium involved is Enterocytozoom biuneusi. Others are Encephalitozoon, Brachiola, Nosema, Pleistophora and Vittaforma species which are important.

The diagnosis is confirmed is by demonstration of the spores in faeces and tissues after appropriate staining, and demonstration by electron microscopy. Antigen detection by immunofluorescence is the best method. Regarding therapy—metronidazole, primaquine and albendazole from the line of treatment.

CERTAIN SPECIES OF PROTOZOA, PARASITIC TO HUMAN, ARE OF UNDETERMINED RELATIONSHIP. THEY BELONG TO SPECIES PNEUMOCYSTIS

AT PRESENT PNEUMOCYSTIS IS CONSIDERED TO BE A FUNGUS. THIS ORGANISM IS SO MUCH DEBATABLE AS REGARDS TO ITS TAXONOMICAL POSITION THAT THE ORGANISM HAS BEEN TEMPORARILY KEPT AS SUCH IN THE CHAPTER ON PROTOZOA

CHAPTER 7

PROTOZOA OF UNDETERMINED RELATIONSHIP

PNEUMOCYSTIS CARINII

Delanoe and Delanoe, 1912

Pneumomycosis carinii is considered to be a protozoa of **undetermined relationship infecting** animals, and rarely man—especially the newborn and young children. It produces **interstitial plasma cell pneumonia** with massive lobar involvement and this is often fatal (Figs. 7.1 & 7.2).

Incidence. It affects almost exclusively the newborn, premature infants or debilitated children with **hypogammaglobulinaemia**.

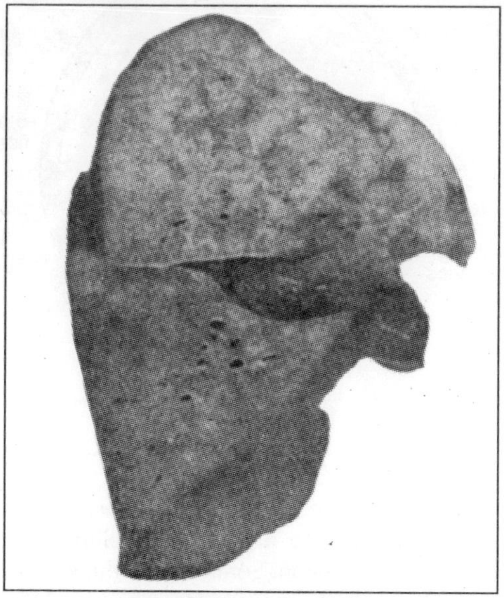

Fig. 7.1 Massive pneumonia caused by *Pneumocystic carinii* infection

Parasite. The nature of the parasite is believed to be a protozoa, but others believe it to be of *vegetable nature*, a fungus e.g., **Blastomyces** or **Candida**.

According to the English summary of Vanek and Jirovec (1952), *P. carinii* forms *foam-like masses* in the lung alveoli and bronchioles.

Morphology. The parasites having **foam-like wrapping** substance are small, unicellular, roundish or elongated bodies; they reproduce by binary fission and ultimately form eight **germinal sporozoites**, 5-7μ in size. These are best seen after staining with

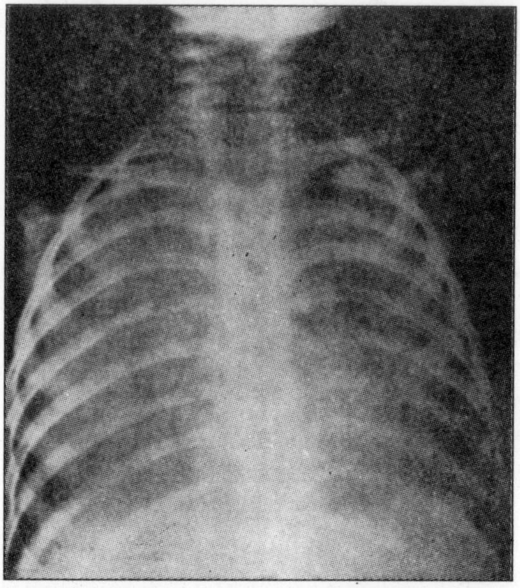

Fig. 7.2 Skiagram of the chest in pneumonia caused by *Pneumocystis carinii*

Giemsa stain. According to Herzberg *et al* (1952), these foam-like agglomerations are rounded uninucleate forms of the parasite and cysts having 8 nuclei, formed in the macrophages. According to **Westphal** (1953), octonucleate cysts represent the most important stage for differential diagnosis. He also found foam-like coagulation zones round the parasites which produce it. He found *P. carinii* to be Gram-negative. *Dab smears* of lung tissue should be stained with Giemsa stain.

Postmortem. Autopsy shows **interstitial pneumonia** in which *P. carinii* is present.

GROSS. The lungs are distended and pleurae thickened.

The CUT SURFACE is grey, consolidated and airless with thickened interlobular septa. Both the lungs are equally affected (Figs. 7.1 and 7.2).

MICROSCOPICALLY, the thickened septa are infiltrated with mononuclear cells, mainly the **plasma cells (Fig. 7.5 & 7.6)**. The alveolar epithelium is thickened and desquamated in places. The alveoli are filled with foam-like agglomerations, exudate and numerous irregular bodies identified as *P. carinii*. **Microcysts** may be present containing epithelial cells of the alveoli, macrophages, connective tissue cells and blood corpuscles. Honeycombed masses of parasites are present within alveoli of the lungs. **Cytomegalic inclusion** bodies were found by Baar in the cells of parotid ducts.

Epidemiology. The mode of transmission is not definitely known. Rats and mice are the probable carriers of the organism.

Pneumocystis carinii. P. carinii lives within the alveoli of the lungs. It occurs in two forms, namely trophozoite (Fig. 7.3) and cyst (Fig. 7.4). Trophozoite is 1 to 5 μm in size, amoeboid in shape and has a central nucleus. Its cytoplasm contains mitochondria, ribosomes, endoplasmic reticulum and various granules.

It divides by binary fission. Some trophozoites become encysted and produce granules.

Within the cyst, eight daughter trophozoites, also known as intracystic bodies or sporozoites—are found (Fig. 7.8). The mature cyst is thick-walled and measures up to 10 μ in diameter. The cyst collapses, releasing trophozoites that initiate another cycle of multiplication, either in the same host, or in others. The collapsed cysts can be seen as irregular crescentic bodies (Figs. 7.3 and 7.4).

P. carinii is normally a commensal in the lung, spread by respiratory droplets and many healthy persons carry the organisms in the lungs. It is an opportunistic infection—the clinical disease is found only in the subject with poor resistance as in premature and malnourished infants, immunocompromised hosts, AIDS and other immunodeficiency patients. The multiplication of the parasite in the lungs induces a hyaline or foamy alveolar exudate containing numerous lymphocytes, macrophages and abundant plasma cells.

Neutrophils are absent. Hence, it is called plasma cell pneumonia.

In stained sections, the exudate in the alveoli forms a honey-combed pattern.

Clinically, there is non-productive cough, breathlessness and cyanosis. *P. carinii* pneumonia (PAP) is a life-threatening opportunistic infection in AIDS patients.

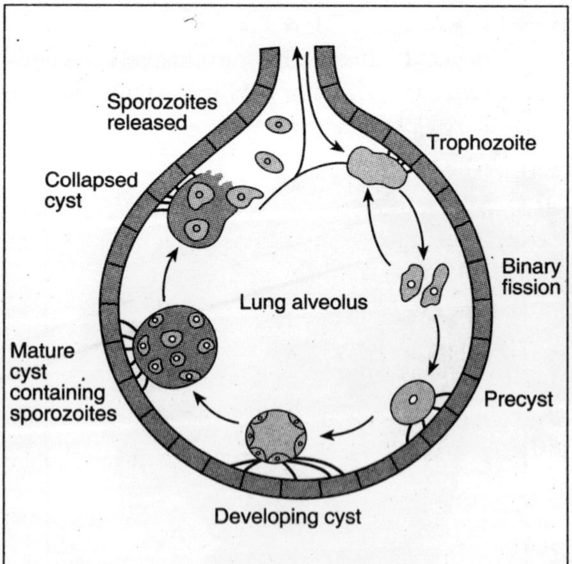

Fig. 7.3 Life cycle of *Pneumocystis carinii.* The parasite enters the lung in respiratory droplets and gets affected to alveolar epithelium. It divides by binary fission. Some form a thick-walled cyst within which sporozoites develop. When mature cysts rupture, sporozoites are released that initiate fresh cycles of infection

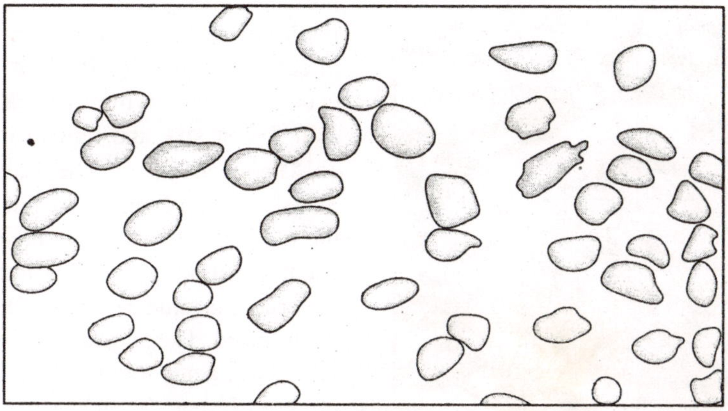

Fig. 7.4 *P. carinii* cyst (Gomori's methanamine silver stain)

Diagnosis. Diagnosis can be made by demonstration of the intraerythrocytic parasites in Giemsa-stained blood films. Blood from suspected cases may be inoculated into hamsters and, after a month, blood films from the inoculated animals show the parasites.

Regarding therapy, pentamidine with cotrimoxazole, clindamycin and oral quinine are the line of treatment.

Diagnosis is made by demonstrating the parasite in sputum, tracheobronchial lavage or transbronchial biopsy specimens. Sputum examination shows cyst as cyst as stained by Gamri's silver methenamine stain. Open lung biopsy may be necessary to establish the diagnosis.

Diagnosis is often made in autopsy specimens. The cysts can be stained by Giemsa and methanamine-silver staining technique.

Immunofluorescence has been used for demonstrating cysts. *P. carinii* antigen can be demonstrated by ELISA Test.

X-ray shows **diffuse mottling** of the lung fields (Fig. 7.2). **Acute serum reactants** like C-reactive protein, and erythrocyte sedimentation rate (**ESR**) may be elevated (Robbins *et al* 1965; Robbins (1967).

HISTOPATHOLOGY. The pathological diagnosis is based on characteristic microscopic picture (Fig.7.3 and 7.4). The alveoli are filled with granular, foamy honeycomb-like material, fuchsinophilic to **PAS stain**, but negative to fibrin, mucin and glycogen stains. The material is acellular. The alveolar walls are infiltrated with mononuclear cells amongst which plasma cells are numerous.

SEROLOGICAL REACTIONS. Complement fixation test (CFT) is a sensitive and reliable method for diagnosis—when done accurately—and a significant titre is obtained in–between 20 and 30 days of illness (Vivell, 1960). There had been 82 per cent positive correlation of CFT with clinical cases.

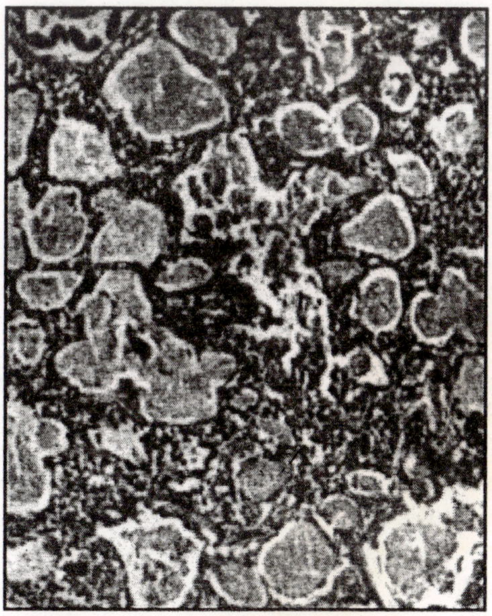

Fig. 7.5 The alveoli are filled with granular, foamy honeycomb-like material and alveolar septa are showing infiltration with mononuclear cells and plasma cells; × 100

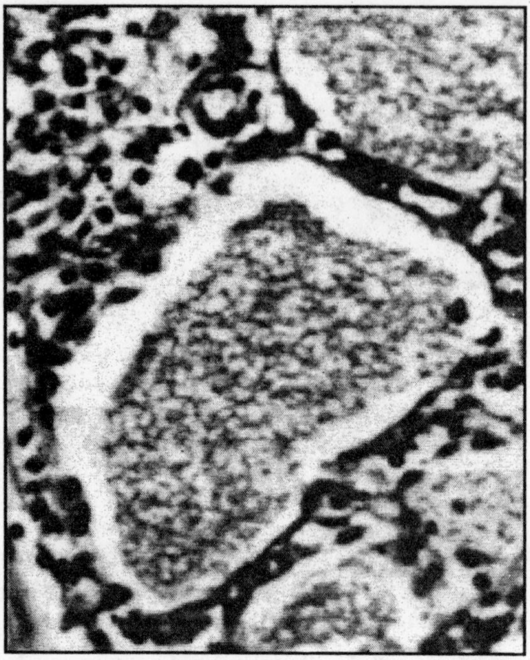

Fig. 7.6 The alveolar walls are showing infiltration with mononuclear cells and plasma cells to high power.

IMMUNOLOGICAL REACTION (Immunofluorescence). Gaedeke (1960) and Goetz (1995) have employed *fluorescein-labelled antibodies* (direct and indirect methods) for the specific demonstration of Pneumocystis in lung sections with excellent results.

Prophylaxis. The mode of infection is not definitely known and, therefore, little care can be taken about its prevention. In each of the 16 cases of **Vanek** (1951), the infants and children were housed in old buildings infested with rats and mice, which are presumed to be the **carriers**. So proper care should be taken.

BABESIA

Babesia is named after Babes who, in 1888 described the intraerythrocytic parasite in the blood of cattle and sheep in Romania. In 1893, the parasite was shown to cause the 'tick-borne Texas fever' which is an acute haemolytic disease of cattle. This was the first arthropod-borne disease found in the USA.

Infection in vertebrates is caused by the bite of ixodide ticks in which the parasite undergoes its sexual cycle. The sporozoites present in the tick-salivary glands are inoculated into the vertebrate host, when they enter the blood stream and invade erythrocytes in which they undergo asexual multiplication by budding..Release of daughter parasites occur. The intraerythrocytic parasite is pear-shaped; 2 to 5 μ in size and remain in pair.

The appearance in Giemsa-stained films may be mistaken for Plasmodium falciparum rings within the red cells. The parasite digests haemoglobin, no haemozoin-like pigment is formed—as opposed to malaria (plasmodia). Ticks feeding on vertebrates get infected. The parasite can be maintained through successive generations in ticks by transovarial transmission. Hence the ticks can behave as a reservoir host as well as a bilogical vector.

The name Piroplasm (from its pear-shape) was given to Babesia because of its pear-shape (from *pyrum*, i.e., pear) and the disease caused by the parasite is known as piroplasmosis.

Human infections caused by *bovis*, *Babesia*, *B. divergans* and *B. microti* are in record—they occurred in Europe and in the USA. After an incubation period of 2 to 3 weeks, the clinical illness starts with fever, chills, headache and myalgia. Anaemia and jaundice may follow.

PROTOTHECA

Prototheca are algae. They cause opportunistic infections in immunocompromised hosts, like many other parasites.

Prototheca infections occur in the skin and subcutaneous papules, plaques and erythematous lesions. The infection may become disseminated in the immunodeficient subjects involving the liver, the gall bladder and peritoneum. Biopsy of the lesion shows sporangia with multiple septa, containing spores, 5-15 μ in diameter. Cultures are obtained in Saboraud's medium showing creamy yeast-like colonies.

Treatment is not effective with tetracycline and amphotericin *B. Surgical* excion of the lesions are needed for full cure.

TREATMENT

Cotrimoxazole and pentamidine have been used in treatment. Prognosis is poor in the immunocompromised subjects. □

REFERENCES

Delance, P. (M. and Mme.) (1912). Sur les rapports des kystes de Carini du poumon des rats avec. *Trypanosoma lewisi. Compt. rend. Acad. Sci.* (Paris) 155, 658.

Gaedeke, R. (1960). Morphologische antigen-antikorper-lokalisation mittles fluoreszierender antikorper im lungenkewebe bei interstitieller pneumonie. *Mschr. Kinderheilk.* 108, 152.

Goetz, O. (1965). Fluorescenmikroskopische untersuchungen bei interstitieller plasmacellularer pneumonie. *Mschr. Kinderheilk.* 113, 194.

Herzberg, K., Herzberg-Kremmer, H. and May, G. (1952). Uber *Pneumocystis carinii* bei interstitiellen pneumonien. *Klin Woch.* 30, 822-824.

Robbins, J. B. (1967). Immunologic and clinicopathologic aspects of *Pneumocystis carinii* pneumonitis. *Pediat. Res.* 6, 131.

Robbins, J. B. Miller, R. H., Arean, V. M. and Pearson, H. A. (1965). Successful treatment of *Pneumocystis carinii* pneumonitis in a patient with congenital hypogammaglobulinemia. *New Eng. J. Med.* 272, 708.

Vanek. J. (1951). Atypika intersticialni pneumonie deti, vyvolana *Pneumocystis carinii, C. L. C., Prague* 90, 1121-1124. (English summary).

Venek. J. and Jirovec, O. (1952). Parasitare pneumonie. Interstitielle plasmazellenpneumonie der fruhgeborenen, verursacht durch *Pneumocystic carini. Zentr. F. Bakt. 1. Abt. Orig.* 158. 120-127.

Vivell, O. (1955). Ein neues stabiles antigen fur die serodiagnoses der interstitielle plasmacellulare pneumonie junger Sauglingen und Fruhgeburten. *Deutsch. med. Wschr.* 80, 1357.

Westphal, A. (1953). Zur diagnose der *Pneumocystis carinii*—Infektion des Menschen. *Zeitscher. f. tropen Med. U. Parasitol.* 4, 549-554.

CHAPTER

8 SUBPHYLUM : CILIOPHORA

CLASS: CILIATEA; ORDER: HETEROTRICHIDA

General characteristics. The members of this group belong to the subphylum Ciliophora. Ciliates are one-celled organisms, provided with short thread-like prolongations of the *ectoplasmic membrane* called cilia, the organelles of *locomotion*. In the species of ciliates, there is a distinct cytostome (cell mouth) and a cytopyge (anal pore) at the posterior end. The cilia cover the entire body and are arranged in longitudinal or obliquely spiral parallel rows. The cytoplasm contains two kinds of nuclei; (a) macronucleus of massive type, slightly curved and vegetative in function; and (b) micronucleus of vesicular type, the *generative nucleus*. Many of the species are free-living; whereas, others live in a wide range of vertebrate and invertebrate hosts. The only species of medical interest is *Balantidium coli* belonging to the order: Heterotrichida; suborder: Heterotrichina; falimy: Balantidiidae. The parasite is capable of encystment.

GENUS: BALANTIDIUM

Claparede and Lachmann, 1858

The members of this genus are parasites in the digestive tract of vertebrate or invertebrate hosts. They have a conspicuous *cytostome*, *cilia* covering the entire body, contractile vacuoles, a large and conspicuous *macronucleus* and a small, vacuolated *micronucleus.*

Reproduction. The asexual multiplication takes by binary fission; encystment is characteristic. Conjugation of two individuals takes place by a process of interchange of nuclear material. After conjugation, individuals separate, each being rejuvenated by the process.

Pathogenicity. Species of Balantidium are natural parasites of hog, monkey, guinea-pig, frog and cockroach. The species pathogenic to man is *Balantidium coli.*

BALANTIDIUM COLI (Malmsten, 1857) Stein, 1862

(*Organism causing balantidiasis or ciliate dysentery in human*)

Distribution. *Balantidium coli* is the only ciliate pathogenic to human. It is prevalent in Philippines. In India, it is found in Assam.

Habitat. The trophozoite form is found in the large intestine of human and the pig. The cysts are also formed there.

Morphology (Fig. 8.1). The organism is the *largest protozoal parasite* of human. It has a *trophozoite* and a *cystic stage*. When observed in dysenteric stools the Trophozoite is large, ovoid and covered with short cilia relatively of uniform length, maintaining a constant synchronised motion, vigorously propelling the organism. The anterior end is somewhat pointed and on one side has a deep, slightly curved, inverted, conical, prominent depression, the cytostome. The posterior end is rounded with a small, less prominent opening in the cell membrane, the ***cytopyge***. The cytoplasm contains numerous food vacuoles and one or two contractile vacuoles, which empty periodically.

The trophozoites are 50 to 120μm in length and 40 to 70μ in breadth. The *cilia*, in a fixed iron-haematoxylin preparation, are found to arise from a basal granule, immediately under the cell membrane. Nucleus. The large trophic nucleus, the MA-

CRONUCLEUS is bean-shaped, containing densely packed chromatin granules forming a single mass. The MICRONUCLEUS lies in the centre of the inner curvature of the macronucleus. It is vesicular in character and is believed to function as a **kinetic nucleus** for organelles of locomotion.

REPRODUCTION (Fig. 8.1). The trophozoites of *Balantidium coli* feed on starch, the cells of the intestinal wall, bacteria and mucus as *lumen parasites*. Here they divide by **transverse binary fission**, where the *micronucleus* divides followed by division of the *macronucleus* and *cytoplasm*, reproducing two daughter organisms.

ENCYSTMENT. Encystation of the trophozoite occurs in the faeces, when it is dehydrated in the lower part of the gut, or it may occur in the evacuated semisolid stools. Cysts are 50-60μ in diameter containing a macronucleus, a micronucleus and a refractile body. In the cyst, the organism rounds up without completely retracting the cilia and it secretes a tough **cyst wall**. Unlike the encystation in amoebae, there is no multiplication of the nucleus or discharge of undigested food, and during excystation, only one organism emerges from the cyst.

Cultivation. The organism may be cultivated in various nutrient media or in the medium used for *E. histolytica*.

Life cycle. Pig is the natural host in which it develops in two stages; man is a rare and *incidental host*. The infective stage is the cyst of the parasite. The *portal of entry* is the oral route and infection takes place by ingestion of the cyst. The infection is carried from pig to pig and also from pig to man, man to man, or from man to pig.

Cysts when ingested, dissolution of the cyst walls occur; the trophozoites are liberated in the small intestine and pass into the large intestine (one trophozoite from one cyst), where it may remain in the lumen or in the epithelial cells. The trophozoites multiply in the epithelial cells by a process of transverse binary fission, producing two daughter ciliates (Fig. 8.1). This reproduction takes place successively, producing a large number of trophozoites. In this process, at first the micronucleus divides into two, followed by the division of the macronucleus and the cytoplasm, at the line of a transverse constriction in the middle of the body. The individual formed from the **anterior half** retains the

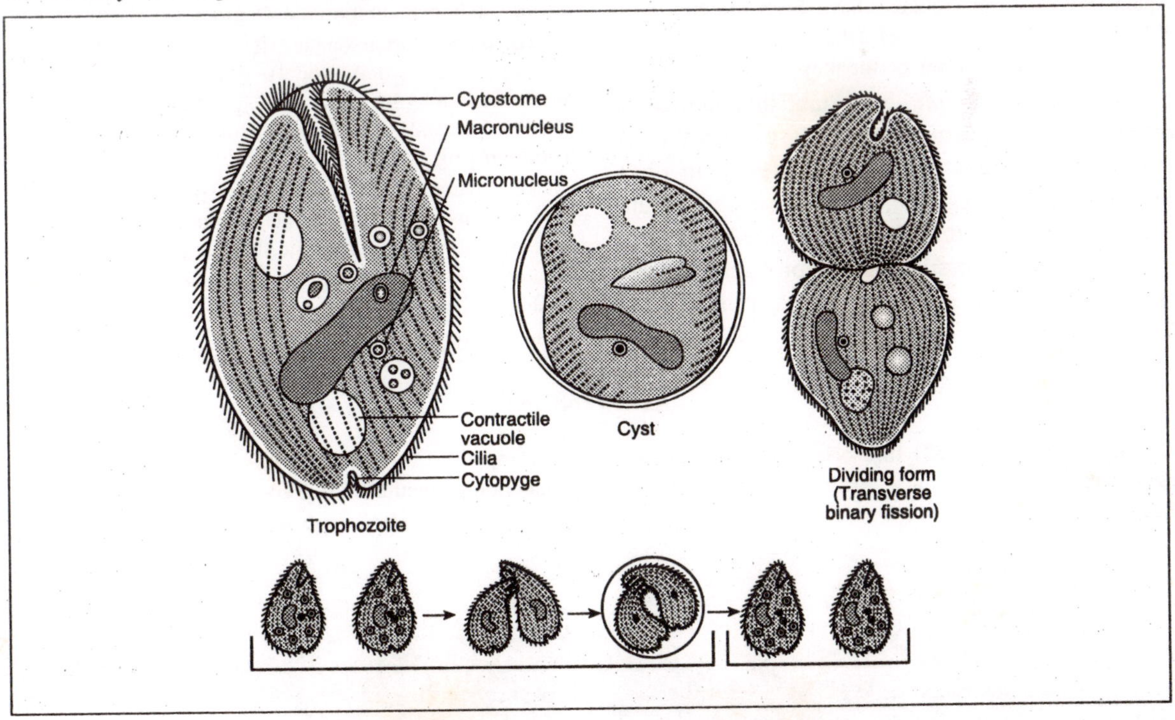

Fig. 8.1 Balantidium coli (Upper left × 700)

cytostome; whereas, reconstitution of the **posterior half** occurs with the formation of a *cytostome* and other structures. After a period of growth and multiplication, cysts develop in the lower part of the intestine, where the faeces undergo dehydration or they find conditions unsuitable for vegetative growth. Encystation may take place outside the body as well.

CONJUGATION. This takes place by a process, when the two trophozoites are found to be in a state of union and enclosed in a cyst, with the exchange of nuclear material. This is followed by separation of two **rejuvenated** individuals (**Fig. 8.1**).

Epidemiology. *Balantidium coli* that infects man is morphologically indistinguishable from *simian* or *porcine* strains. The high incidence of this organism in domestic hogs should have produced a greater incidence of balantidial dysentery in human hosts exposed to infection, especially among farmers and abattoirs through accidental ingestion of viable *B. coli* cysts. Therefore, it is regarded that *B. coli* of porcine origin is due to another species, namely, *B. suiss*, as *B. coli* infection has been found only incidentally in people exposed to pig excreta. In contrast, once the disease is established in human, the infection may develop as an epidemic under poor environmental sanitation and low grade personal hygiene. Again, the cats and monkeys have been infected with *B. coli* from human; whereas it has been impossible to transmit *B. coli* from pig or monkey to man.

Pathogenesis. *B. coli* once established in man, is often found to be a tissue invader. The parasite thrives mainly in abundant starchy food present in pig's intestine. Hoare suggested, in the presence of abundant starchy food, *B. coli* does not invade the epithelial cells of the intestine, and this probably explains the harmless behaviour of the parasite. Tempelis and Lysenko (1957) demonstrated that *B. coli* produces **hyaluronidase**. The enzyme depolymerises the substrate, hyalurate of connective tissue, thus helping mechanically and physiologically to play a complementary role for *B. coli* to invade the tissue. The organism may remain in the lumen of the human intestine without producing symptoms for a long time. It may produce diarrhoea and, in several cases, symptoms of dysentery may be produced accompanied by ulceration of the intestine. Within the tissue, *B. coli* multiplies and produces necrosis resulting in subsurface **abscesses** in the mucous or the submucous coat. The *ulcers* are like those of amoebic ulcers—round, ovoid or irregular in shape with undermined edges and the floor is covered with pus and necrotic material. Unlike one produced by *E. histolytica*, the parasite does not invade the liver.

Diagnosis. Diagnosis depends on the demonstration of *B. coli* in the faeces of the patient. The motile trophozoites are present in diarrhoeic or dysenteric stools, while cysts are found in semisolid of formed stools. For examination of stools, the technique is the same as that of intestinal amoebiasis.

Prophylaxis. It consists of measures against contamination of food and drink with faeces containing cysts of *B. coli* of human or porcine origin.

Treatment. Carbarsone is effective in the usual dosage of 0.25 g, thrice daily for 10 days, giving temporary relief. Di-iodohydroxyquinoline (diiodoquine) in doses of 10 tablets (0.21 g each) per day for 20 days is efficient in eliminating the parasite.

Tetracyclines and other broad spectrum antibiotics have been used successfully in **balantidiasis**. Oxytetracycline acts almost as a specific therapy in doses of 0.5 g, 6 hourly for 10 days, and the infection clears up within a week. Ciprofloxacin and ofloxcin may be tried and could be worthwhile. □

REFERENCES

Malmsten, P. H. (1957). Infusorien als intestinalthiere beim menschen. *Virchow's Arch. f. path. Anat.* 12 302-309.

Tempelis, C. H. and Lysenko, M. G. (1957). The production of hyaluronidase by *Balantidium coli. Exptl. Parasitol.* 6, 31-36.

CHAPTER

9

SECTION II

HELMINTHOLOGY

General consideration. Helminths or worms are animals belonging to the Sub-kingdom Metazoa, consisting of many cells, arising from more than one embryonic layers. The tissues are differentiated into (i) alimentary, (ii) excretory, (iii) reproductive and (iv) nervous systems, which developed partially or completely. They are mostly free-living, but some are endoparasites of human and animals. In man, they may produce disease by their presence in the tissues, depriving the host of its food, or by liberation of toxic substances. They are divided into 2 phyla:

PHYLUM: Platyhelminthes (Flat worms).

PHYLUM: Nemathelminthes (Round worms).

PHYLUM: PLATYHELMINTHES

(Flat worms)

This phylum includes worms, flattened dorsoventrally (leaf or tape-like), often bilaterally symmetrical. They are provided with a nervous system and an elaborate excretory apparatus. *Digestive* system may be absent, or—when present it is rudimentary and without an anus. The *excretory system* is formed by **flame cells*** (leash of cilia resembling flame of a candle), capillaries and tubules leading to the excretory vesicle. *Respiratory* and *circulatory system* and body cavity are absent. They are mostly **hermaphrodites**. Platyhelminthes parasitic to human belong to 2 classes—**Cestoidea** (Cestoda) and **Trematodea** (Trematoda).

PHYLUM: NEMATHELMINTHES

(Round worms)

The helminths of this phylum are round. They are unsegmented, bilaterally symmetrical, elongated,

* A *flame cell* (solenocyte) is a nucleated cell having in its protoplasm a space into which one of the capillaries leads; and in this space lie a bunch of vibratile cilia, rendering an appearance of a flickering candle flame with its movement (see Fig. 10.2, Ch. 10).

TABLE 9.1

CLASSIFICATION OF HELMINTHS

METAZOA

PHYLUM:	Platyhelminthes		Nemathelminthes
CLASS:	Cestoidea (Tapeworms tape-like)	Trematodea (Flukes—leaf-like)	Nematodea (round worms)
CHARACTERS:	Body—flattened dorsoventrally Body cavity—absent Alimentary canal—absent or rudimentary Suckers—present Sex—mostly hermaphrodite		Body—cylindrical Body cavity—present Alimentary canal—complete Suckers—absent Sexually differentiated

TABLE 9.2

DIFFERENCES AMONGST CESTOIDEA, TREMATODEA AND NEMATODEA (Fig. 9.1)

Body	Tape-like, segmented	Leaf-like, unsegmented	Cylindrical, unsegmented
Sex	Hermaphrodite	Usually hermaphrodite	Differentiated (male and female)
Head	Often with hooks and suckers	Without hooks but with suckers	Hooks and suckers absent; often with well-developed buccal capsule
Alimentary canal	Absent	Incomplete, without anus	Complete, with anus
Body cavity	Absent	Absent	Present

cylindroid worms having longitudinal axis of body. Their alimentary tract is complete. The body cavity is not lined by mesothelium. Flame cells are absent. The sexes are separate. They belong to the class *Nematoda.*

DIAGNOSIS AND TREATMENT OF HELMINTHIC DISEASES IN GENERAL

Diagnosis. In helminthic infections, the diagnosis is based on: (a) ***direct finding*** of (i) the parasite and/or (ii) their ova or larva, or (iii) encysted larvae in the body by X-ray examination; (b) ***indirectly*** by the finding of (i) ***precipitin*** and/or complement fixing antibodies, or allergic skin test like Casoni's or other skin tests, etc., (ii) ***anaemia*** as in hookworm disease, or (iii) ***eosinophilia*** in most of the helminthic infections, as they are likely to produce allergic states. Many parasitic worms contain, or secrete, mucoprotein containing a polysaccharide radical, which produces eosinophilic infiltration of the infected tissue. This response to parasitic infection occurs both as a direct chemotactic effect on blood and also as an allergic response. In trichinosis eosinophilic response may be inhibited by a simultaneous bacterial infection.

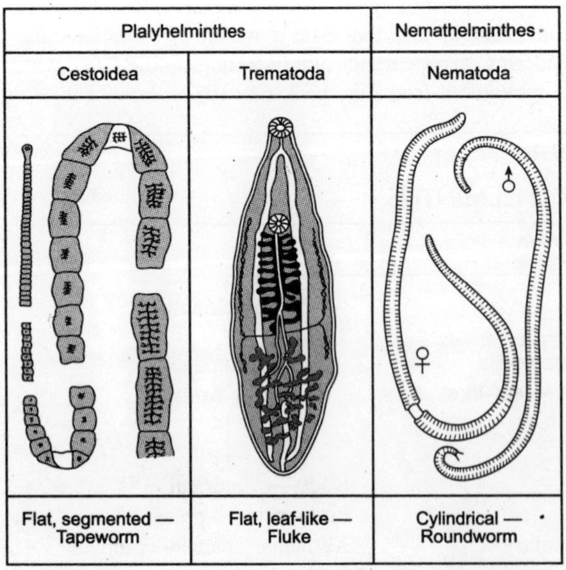

Fig. 9.1 Helminths of classes Cestoidea, Trematodea and Nematodea

Treatment. Anthelmintic drugs are either vermicides which may kill the worms, or vermifuge, helping to expel the worm, without killing them. A cathartic may, however, act as a vermifuge as it may expel the worms which are not anchored in the intestine and may remain free in the lumen.

GENERAL MEASURES. (1) Before the administration of anthelmintics, a specific diagnosis is made by examination of stools for ova of helminths. More than one parasite may be present and the appropriate drug should be selected for administration. One drug may be effective for more than one helminths. (2) The general condition of the patient should always be considered, e.g., anaemia, cirrhosis of the liver, nephritis, pregnancy, etc. Taking of alcohol should be forbidden during the treatment period. (3) A light liquid diet in the evening is always preferred, but with modern chemotherapeutic anthelmintics, a prepurgative is not often necessary (4) The drug is administered in an empty stomach and a postpurgative 1-2 hours after the specific therapy is administered. For this a saline purgative like magnesium or sodium sulphate is preferable to castor oil. *The effects of the purgative* are: (a) to eliminate the injured parasite and to remove the dead parasite which might otherwise be absorbed giving rise to toxic manifestations, and (b) to remove drugs which might show toxic manifestations after absorption. (5) The patient should remain in bed and no food is advised till the bowels have opened after purgative. (6) It is imperative that stools should be collected and examined for the worms expelled. (7) It is always necessary to make a follow-up examination of stools after about 10 days, when the treatment may be repeated if necessary (*vide* Plate 10.I). □

CHAPTER 10

CLASS: CESTOIDEA

PHYLUM: PLATYHELMINTHES

General characteristics of Cestoidea

1. Worms are tape or ribbon-like.
2. They are segmented; the segments vary from three or four to several thousands in number.
3. They have attachment apparatus.

   MODE OF ATTACHMENT. The scolex is attached to the mucosa either by cup-shaped *suckers* as in cyclophyllidea or by means of suctorial grooves called *bothria*, as in the case of pseudophyllidea.
4. Body cavity is absent.
5. Alimentary canal is absent.
6. Excretory and nervous systems are present.
7. They are hermaphrodites. The reproductive system is well-developed.
8. Eggs are hexacanth embryos and develop into a larval stage in an intermediate host.

TERMS USED IN DESCRIPTION OF TAPEWORMS AND DIFFERENT STAGES OF DEVELOPMENT (PLATE 10.II)

BROOD CAPSULE and HYDATID (Fig. 10.2C). The germinal layer producing multiple scolices developing into daughter bladders (bladder worm; brood capsules), each of which, in turn, produces many scolices internally (the *hydatid* type or *echinococcus*).

COENURIS (Fig. 10.2D). Multiple scolices develop from the inner germinal layer in a cysticercus type, called *coenurus*.

CORRACIDIUM is ciliated larva of Diphyllobothrium.

CYSTICERCOID (Fig. 10.2B) is a small cysticercus, which develops from the oncosphere with an invaginated scolex and a solid tail, e.g., *H. nana*.

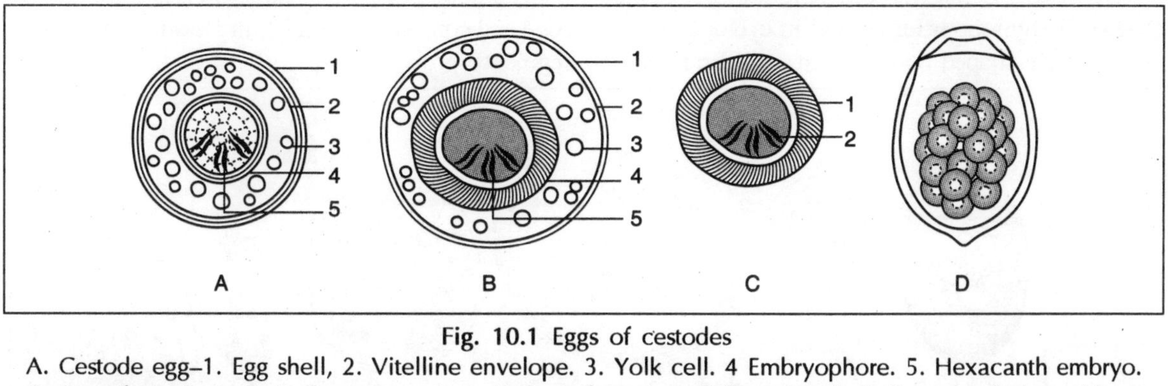

Fig. 10.1 Eggs of cestodes
A. Cestode egg–1. Egg shell, 2. Vitelline envelope. 3. Yolk cell. 4 Embryophore. 5. Hexacanth embryo. B. Egg of taenia–1, 2, 3, 5 same as A, 4. Embryophore is radially striated. C. Same as B, but without the egg shell. 1. Striated embryophore. 2. Hooklets in hexacanth embryo. D. Operculated egg of *Diphyllobothrium latum*

CYSTICERCUS (Fig. 10.1A) is the growing larval stage in the intermediate host, where it develops into a "bladder worm". A "bladder worm" consists of a vesicle containing fluid with a single invaginated scolex.

DEFINITIVE HOST is the host in which the adult worm lives. Man and other vertebrate animals may be *definitive hosts*.

EGG-SHELL (Fig. 10.1). The outer covering of the egg is the egg-shell. It is not often retained. The layer internal to the egg-shell is the vitelline membrane.

EMBRYOPHORE (Fig. 10.1) is the enveloping membrane round the onchosphere. It is often radially striated for the protection of the embryo within it.

INTERMEDIATE HOST is the host which harbours the larval stage of the parasite. When there are two intermediate hosts, the first one is called the *primary* and the other or the second one is called the *secondary intermediate host*. The larval stage in the intermediate host is the infective stage.

NECK is the narrow region between the body and the head.

ONCOSPHERE (Fig. 10.1) is an embryo with six hooklets (hexacanth embryo).

PLEROCERCOID (Fig. 10.2F) or *Sparganum larva* is the second larval stage of Diphyllobothrium which develops from procercoid. It loses larval hooks and develops into a worm-like body with anterior invagination of the head into the neck. It is found in fish, the secondary intermediate host.

PROCERCOID (Fig. 10.2E). It is the first larval stage of Diphyllobothrium found in cyclops. It is a solid, spindle-shaped body with a cephalic invagination and a caudal spherical protuberance which bears six larval hooks.

PROGLOTTIDES are segments or representative units which constitute the body. They are immature, mature and gravid. Anterior segments are immature and male and female reproductive organs cannot be differentiated; middle segments are mature, i.e., male and female reproductive organs can be differentiated. The posterior segments are gravid, and the uteri of these segments show branching and contain eggs.

ROSTELLUM is a beak-like projection on the head which carries hooklets in armed species.

SCOLEX denotes the head of the worm which carries suckers or organs of attachment. The term is applied to both adult and larval forms.

SPARGANUM is a *plercocercoid* larva infecting man.

STROBILA. It is either the entire body or the trunk of the adult worm and includes head, neck and segments (proglottides).

YOLK CELLS (Fig. 10.1) are present between the egg-shell and the embryophore.

Morphology.

INTEGUMENT. The body is covered with a homogeneous elastic cuticle and the cuticle is continuous from segment to segment.

MUSCULAR SYSTEM. This consists of an outer layer of circular and an inner layer of longitudinal muscles and also dorsiventral fibres.

The *scolex* or the head is small (size of a pinhead).

The posterior part of the scolex is the budding zone and consists of germinating tissue, from which segments grow. This merges with the neck. The

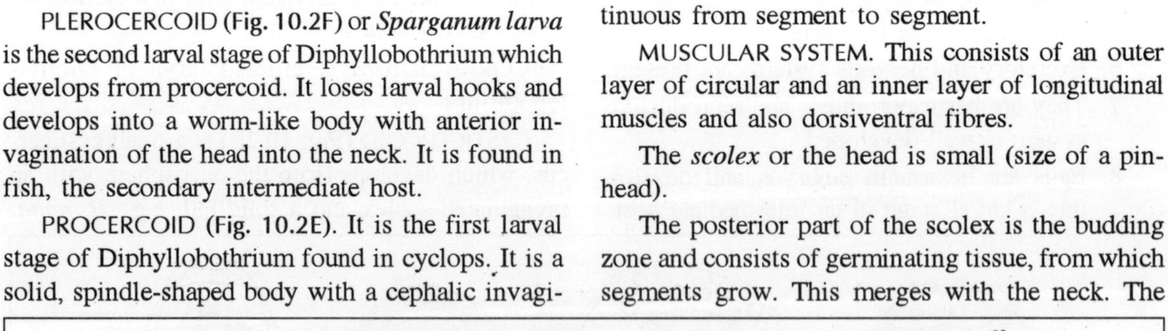

Fig. 10.2 (A) Cysticercus with invaginated scolex. (B) Cysticercoid with a solid caudal appendage. (C) Echinococcus (Hydatid stage). (D) Coenurus. (E) Procercoid. (F) Plerocercoid

PLATE 10.1

COMMON OVA OF THE PARASITIC WORMS OF MAN
(NEMATODA, CESTOIDEA AND TREMATODA)

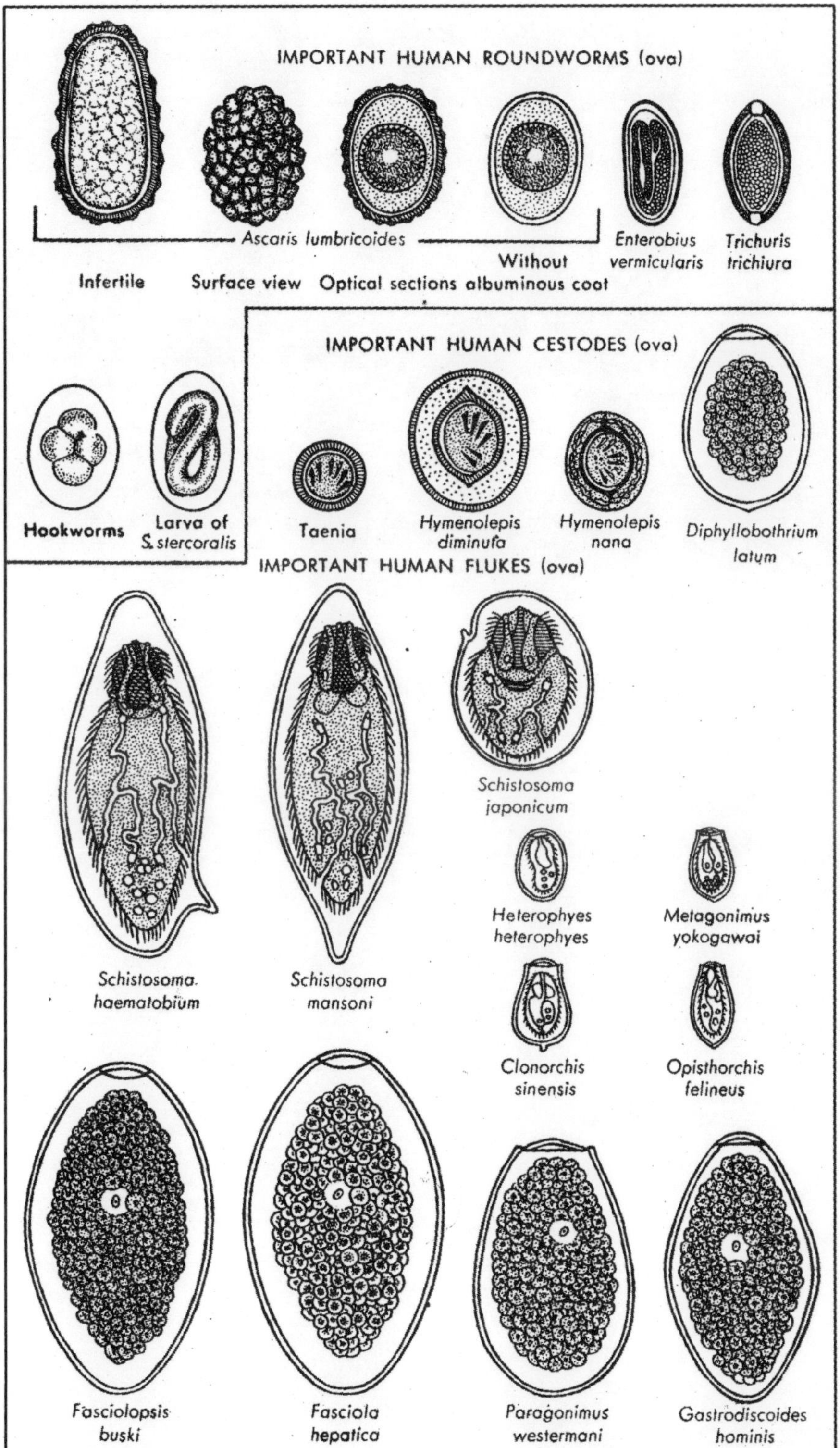

PLATE 10.II

DIFFERENTIATION OF CESTODES IN DIFFERENT STAGES OF DEVELOPMENT

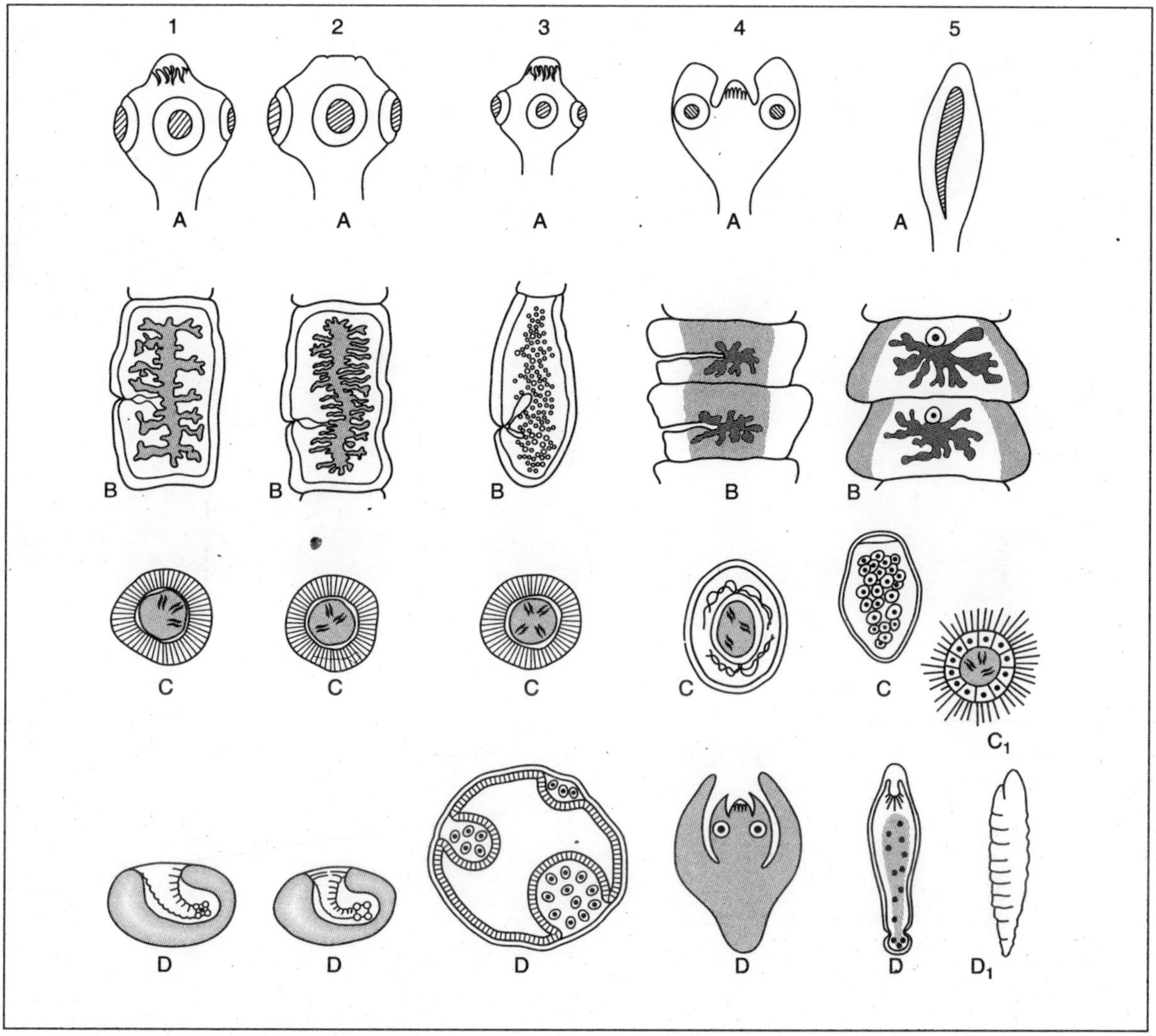

1. *Taenia solium*—A. Scolex armed with hooklets and has suckers. B. Gravid segment with branching uterus. The genital pore is marginal. C. Oncosphere (hexacanth embryo) in radially striated embryophore. D. *Cysticercus cellulosae* (larval stage).
2. *Taenia saginata*—A. Scolex, no hooklets; has suckers. B. Gravid segment shows branching of the uterus; branches are more in number than in the case of *T. solium*. The genital pore is marginal. C. Egg is like that of *T. solium* and cannot be distinguished. D. *Cysticercus bovis* (larval stage).
3. *Echinococcus granulosus*. A. The scolex is armed, hooklets and suckers present. B. The terminal segment is gravid. C. Egg is like that of other cestodes. D. Hydatid cyst (larval stage).
4. *Hymenolepis nana*. A. Scolex is armed, hookets and suckers present. B. The gravid segment shows uterus as an irregular sac. Genital pores are marginal and on the same side. C. The inner membrane (embryophore) has little knobs at either ends from which arise long, delicate wavy filaments which are characteristic. D. Cysticercoid of *H. nana* is with a tail.
5. *Diphyllobothrium latum*. A. Scolex is spoon-shaped with bothria. Not armed. B. Gravid segment shows rosette-shaped branching of the uterus. Genital pores open ventrally in the middle line. C. Egg operculated. C_1. The ciliated coracidium contains a hexacanth embryo, infective to a crustacean host. D. Procercoid larva (in crustacean host), D_1. Plerocercoid larva develops in fish, the secondary intermediate host.

PLATE 10

DIFFERENTIATION OF CESTODES IN DIFFERENT STAGES OF DEVELOPMENT

[illegible]

suckers are discoidal in shape and serve to fix the worm to the intestinal mucosa of the host.

STROBILA or body consists of a number of segments. According to maturity of the reproductive organs, *segments* are called **immature, mature** and **gravid**. The anterior segments are small, short and *sexually immature*. They are often longer transversely than lengthwise. The segments in the middle are *sexually mature* and adult, while the posterior ones are *gravid*. The ventral surface is determined by the position of ovary, which lies more ventrally than dorsally. In *T. solium* and *T. saginata*, the mature segments are longer than broad.

GENITAL PORES. In *Cyclophyllidea*, genital pores are at the margin of the segment, irregularly and alternately distributed in successive segments. In Hymenolepis they open unilaterally. In *Pseudophyllidea* they open on the ventral surface.

Nervous system. The nervous system (commissured plexus) is in the scolex and accessory nerves pass parallel to the length of the body.

Nutrition. The parasite derives its nutrition by *imbibation* of fluid material from the host through the entire surface of the body (**endosmosis**).

Excretory system. It consists of **flame cells** from which the collecting tubules drain into lateral, longitudinal excretory canals, ultimately opening into the terminal proglottid. A transverse canal joins them at the posterior part of each proglottid.

Organs of reproduction. Each proglottid is a hermaphrodite unit and consists of male and female reproductive organs (**Fig. 10.3**).

THE MALE GENITAL SYSTEM consists of a number of testes scattered throughout the proglottid. From each testis arises the *vasa efferentia* which collectively form a common duct called, the *vas deferens*. The proximal dilated part of the vas deferens is the *seminal vesicle* for storing spermatozoa. Passage of spermatozoa is facilitated by the *cirrus* (equivalent to penis) from the *cirrus pouch* to the vagina.

THE FEMALE GENITAL system consists of (1) a bilobed *ovary* situated on the ventral aspect of the proglottid in the posterior part of the segment; (2) the *oviduct* is the canal where eggs are discharged; (3) the *vagina* opens into the common genital atrium for male and female sex orifices. Medial to this is a dilated portion called the *seminal receptacle* which is followed by a constricted portion called, the *spermatic duct* ending in *ootype*; (4) the *uterus* is the tube arising from the ootype stores fertilised eggs; (5) the *ootype* is the chamber, where **fertilisation** occurs and the common vitelline duct opens in the ootype; (6) the *vitelline gland* is a bilobed mass in cyclophyllidea; but it is distributed all over the segment in pseudophyllidea. (7) *Mehlis' (shell) glands* consist of many unicellular glands, which open separately in the ootype.

Spermatozoa, after being transferred to the vagina by the protrusile cirrus, fertilises the ovum. Spermatozoa may be derived from the same segment or from different segments of the same worm or from another worm.

Birth pore. In Cyclophyllidea, the uterus does not communicate with the exterior (**Fig. 10.3A**) and,

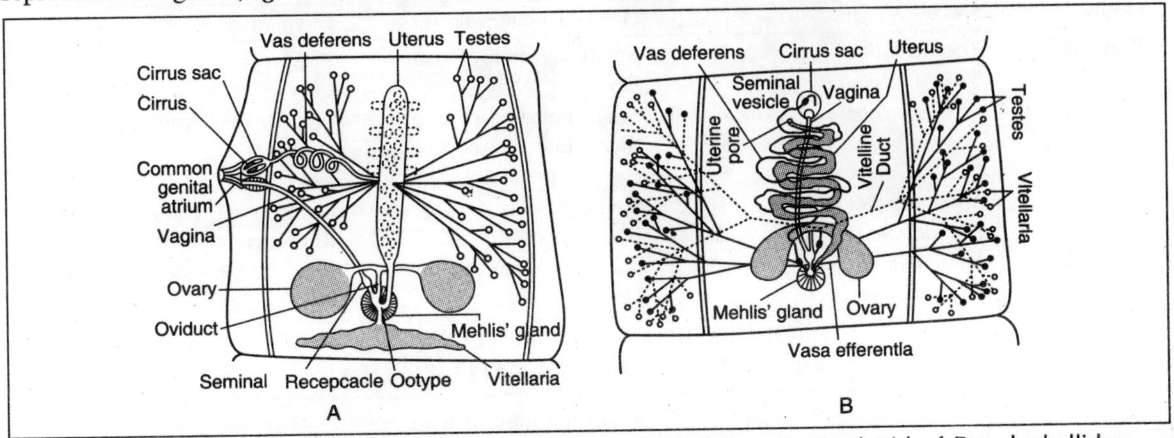

Fig. 10.3 Organs of reproduction. A. Proglottid of Cyclophyllidea. B. Proglottid of Pseudophyllidea

therefore, the eggs come out from the uterus by disintegration of segments which may occur in the intestinal tract of the definitive host or outside, when the segments are passed in the faeces. In Pseudophyllidea, the uterus opens to the exterior (Fig. 10.3B) by an opening called *uterine pore*, through which the eggs escape.

Eggs. In Cyclophyllidea, the eggs (Fig. 10.1) found in the faeces of the infected host contain a ball of cells, the morula with six minute hooklets called an *oncosphere*. It is usually enclosed in one or more envelopes. The one immediately surrounding the embryo formed by its own secretion is called the *embryophore*. The outer covering is the *egg-shell*. Internal to egg-shell is the *vitelline membrane*. Embryophore is the *vitelline membrane*. Embryophore is radially striated in cases of *T. solium* and *T. saginata*.

Eggs are ***colourless*** in the case of Hymenolepis, but ***brown*** (**bile-stained**) in case of Taenia.

In Pseudophyllidea, the eggs are oval, operculated and contain unsegmented ova surrounded by yolk cells. The egg develops into an embryo, within the egg-shell.

Larval stage. Two types of larvae are chiefly distinguished:

(A) CYSTIC LARVAL FORM (Fig. 10.2A, B, C, D)

Cysticercus is a bladder-like structure filled with fluid containing a scolex fixed to its wall, e.g., *Cysticercus bovis* and *C. cellulosae*.

Cysticercoid. In this, the larva has a tail and the bladder is rudimentary.

Coenurus is a bladder-worm with many scolices, e.g., in the genus Multiceps.

Echinococcus. It is a cyst containing daughter and granddaughter cysts and a number of scolices, e.g., *E. granulosus* (Taenia echinococcus).

(B) SOLID LARVAL FORM (Fig. 10.2E, F)

Procercoid. In this case, the hexacanth embryo of a coracidium (free-swimming ciliated embryo) develops without any central liquefaction, and forms a solid larva in the primary intermediate host, cyslops.

Plerocercoid. It is a solid tape-like and worm-like larva in the development of a tapeworm, following the procercoid stage with an invaginated scolex in the neck.

Life cycle. Full development of the worm from the oncosphere to the adult stage occurs usually in two or more different hosts. *D. latum* requires three hosts to complete the life cycle; whereas, *H. nana* requires only one. The definitive host is a vertebrate animal, which harbours the adult worm in its alimentary canal. The intermediate host harbours the larval stage of the parasite in its tissues.

When the eggs or segments are swallowed by an intermediate host with its food, gastric digestion liberates the embryo in the duodenum or jejunum. The naked oncosphere is amazingly active. With the

TABLE 10.1

ORDER I : CYCLOPHYLLIDEA
SUPERFAMILY : TAENIOIDEA

Family	Species	Habit of adult worms	Larval stage in
Taeniidae	*Taenia solium*	Small intestine of man	Pig or man
	Taenia saginata	Do	Cow or man
	Echinococcus granulosus	Small intestine of dog	Cyst in man, cattle, sheep, pig
	Echinococcus multilocularis	Small intestine of fox, dog, wolf	Do
	Multiceps multiceps	Dogs, jackals	Sheep, goat, cattle, man
Dilepididae	*Dipylidium caninum*	Dog and cat	Rat fleas
Hymenolepididae	*Hymenolepis nana*	Intestine of rat and man	Man, rat flea, beetles
	H. diminuta	Do	Rat flea, mealworm beetles

ORDER II : PSEUDOPHYLLIDEA
SUPERFAMILY : BOTHRIOCEPHALOIDEA

Family	Species	Habit of adult worms	Larval stage in
Diphyllobothriidae	*Diphyllobothrium latum*	Small intestine of man	Cyclops and fish
	D. mansoni	Intestine of dog or cat	Frog, snake or man

help of hooklets, it burrows into the wall of the investine and enters the portal circulation. The embryo is carried by blood stream into the liver, other organs, or muscle tissues of the intermediate host. The hooks are then lost and larvae grow in size, become encysted to form "bladder-worms", i.e., cysts containing fluid. The scolex with suckers and hooklets develop from the wall of the cyst, which is now called Cysticercus. This occurs in 2 to 6 months.

When meat infected with cysticercus is eaten by a suitable definitive host (in most cases man), the scolex, comes out of the cysticercus by absorption of the wall, evaginates, and attaches itself to the mucous membrane of the small intestine with the help of suckers. The bladder is dissolved and the scolex thus liberated, throws out a chain of proglottides forming a typical tapeworm.

Laboratory diagnosis (in general). The direct method of diagnosis depends on:

1. Finding of proglottides in the faeces. 2. Finding of ova in the faeces. 3. Finding of scolex of the adult worm, occasionally recovered after administration of anthelmintics. Expulsion of the scolex suggests cure; if only the head is removed, *proglottides develop again from the scolex.* So the scolex is always potentially infective.

The indirect method of diagnosis depends on eosinophilia, anaemia, and serological and immunological test.

CLASSIFICATION OF TAPEWORMS ACCORDING TO THE HABITAT OF THE PARASITE (Table 10.1)

(A) INTESTINAL TAPEWORMS OF HUMAN belong to the following groups:

(1) CYCLOPHYLLIDEA—*T. solium*, the pork tapeworm; *T. saginata*, the beef tapeworm, *H. nana*, the dwarf tapeworm of human; *H. diminuta*; the rat tapeworm.

(2) PSEUDOPHYLLIDEA—*D. latum*, the fish tapeworm.

(B) SOMATIC TAPEWORMS. The larval stage of tapeworm is found in the tissues and internal viscera of human and animals. The somatic tapeworms belong to the following groups.

(1) CYCLOPHYLLIDEA—(*a*) Genus : Echinococcus. (i) Hydatid cyst is the larval form of *Echinococcus granulosus* (the dog tapeworm); human is the intermediate host, definitive host being **dogs harbouring adult worms in their intestine**, and (ii) *E. multilocularis*–the larval stage causes alveolar or multilocular hydatid disease.

(*b*) Genus : Taenia. *Cysticercus*. It is the larval stage of *Taenia solium* or *T. saginata*, occasionally

TABLE 10.2

DIFFERENCES BETWEEN CYCLOPHYLLIDEA AND PSEUDOPHYLLIDEA (PL. 10.III)

	Cyclophyllidea	Pseudophyllidea
Mature proglottides	Longer than broad (A_1), PL. 10.III.	Broader than long (B_1), PL. 10.III
Scolex or head	Shape—Quadrate or globular. Sucking apparatus. Four cup-like round suckers (A_2)	Spoon-shaped Two bothria act as suckers (B_2)
Rostellum and hooks	Hooks are arranged in the rostellum in armed species (A_2)	Absent (B_2)
Genital pore	Opens at the lateral margin of the segment (A_3)	Very minute—opens at the flat ventral surface of the segment (B_3)
Uterus	It is a closed branched sac. Eggs escape by disintegration of the segment	Opens at the exterior at the uterine pore and forms a rosette. Eggs escape by the uterine pore
Ova	Contain hexacanth embryos (A_4)	Operculated (B_4), hatch out in water as a coracidium
Oncosphere	Non-ciliated (A_4)	Ciliated (B_5)
Larval form	A cysticercus develops in one intermediate host (A_5)	Develops in two intermediate hosts : procercoid in cyclops (B_6); plerocercoid in fish (B_7)

found in man. Man is usually the definitive host but, sometimes, may be an intermediate host.

(*c*) Genus : Multiceps (*synonym*: *Coenurus*). ***Coenurus***. It is the larval (bladder-worm) stage of *M. multiceps*, *M. glomeratus* and *M. serialis*; very rarely human may be the intermediate host.

(2) PSEUDOPHYLLIDEA—(*a*) Genus : Diphyllobothrium. It requires two intermediate hosts to complete its life cycle. The first larval form is the *plerocercoid form*; human or cat is the definitive host. (*b*) Genus : Sparganum. (i) *Sparganum mansoni*, may occur in man. Adults are found in cats and dogs.

(ii) *Sparganum proliferum—For both the species, man is the secondary intermediate host when accidentally infected.*

TAENIA SOLIUM Linnaeus, 1758

ORDER : *Cyclophyllidea*

SUPERFAMILY : *Taenioidea*

GENUS : *Taenia*

T. solium is commonly known as pig tapeworm, measly pork tapeworm or armed tapeworm. It is common amongst pork-eaters.

Geographical distribution. It is cosmopolitan but less common in India.

Habitat. The parasite inhabits the small intestine of human and the bladder worm (*C. cellulosae*) which is a somatic cestode, is seen in different organs of the body.

Morphology.

Adult worm. *Length* is 1.5–6 metres (5-20 feet). Strobila consists of 800-900 proglottides. *Head* is globular, about the size of a pin-head with a rostellum crowned with a double row of 26 to 28 hooklets, and 4 *suckers* at different angles. *Genital pore* is irregularly alternate.

Eggs. The egg has a thick embryophore with radially striated border, measuring 31 to 43µm in diameter. The embryophore encloses the six-hooked hexacanth embryo, which is called an oncosphere. Eggs escape from the uterus through a ventral longitudinal slit, either before or after ripe proglottides become free.

Larval stage. Lavae (*Cysticercus cellulosae*) are usually seen in pigs and are found in human. The pork containing *Cysticercus cellulosae* is known as "measly pork". They are 8 to 10 mm in length, and commonly found in the tongue, skeletal muscles and sometimes in other organs.

Human may occasionally become a larval host in the same way as the pig, by ingestion of eggs, and cysticercus develops in about 3 to 4 months. Man usually becomes infected by ingesting the eggs passed in his own stool by dirty habits, or by regurgitation of a gravid segment into the stomach during vomiting or by a reversal of peristaltic movement of the intestine. The *cysticerci* in human are usually multiple and may occur in skeletal muscles, skin and subcutaneous tissues, eye, heart muscle, bone marrow, brain, meninges or spinal cord. They commonly occur in striated muscles and brain and usually more than one organ is involved. In the skeletal *muscles*, the cysts are larger and about 5 mm in diameter, but in the *brain* they are smaller (1-5 mm). They are spherical, but a racemose form has been described, which may show symptoms of localised brain disease, like ***Jacksonian epilepsy***. When the larva dies, probably it absorbs fluid and rapidly increases in size. This together with toxic substance from the cyst that accounts for the symptoms of irritation. The cyst often undergoes calcification in 5 or 6 years. Localised fibrosis of the meninges may occur in superficial cerebral cysts.

LIFE SPAN of an adult *T. solium* is as long as 10-25 years.

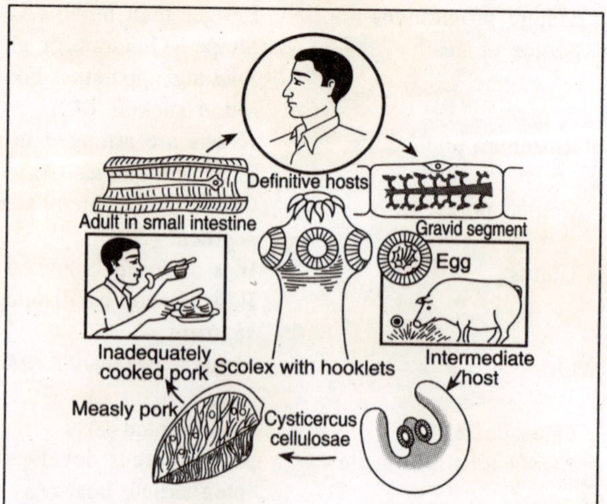

Fig. 10.4 Life cycle of *Taenia solium*

Source of infection. When a man eats insufficiently cooked measly pork containing the "bladder-worm" with immature scolex, the wall of the bladder is digested by the gastric secretion, liberating the larva. This now grows and fixes itself to the mucous membrane of the small intestine.

Life cycle. *T. solium* requires two hosts to complete the life cycle (Fig. 10.4): (1) Human is the Definitive host, while (2) Intermediate host is pig.

IN HUMAN. The infection takes place by ingestion of *C. cellulosae* in measly pork, which is undercooked. The wall of the bladder-worm is digested and the scolex is liberated. Coming in contact with bile, the scolex evaginates and anchors itself to the wall of the small intestine by means of its suckers. It now develops into an adult worm, and strobilisation takes place with astounding rapidity. The segments become sexually mature in about 10 weeks. The adult worm lives in the small intestine of man and gravid segments are passed in the faeces.

Man may act as an **intermediate host** due to auto-infection and, in such a case, *C. cellulosae* may develop in different organs and the cycle terminates.

IN PIG. The segments containing eggs are passed in the faeces by man and they contaminate the pasture. The pigs are also coprophagous. As the eggs or segments are taken by pigs, the radially striated embryophore rupture in the small intestine of the pig and hexacanth embryos containing six hooklets are liberated. They penetrate the wall of the gut with the aid of their hooklets and gain entrance to the portal tributaries or mesenteric lymphatics. Usually they pass through the portal vein and escape through the liver, lung capillaries and left side of the heart, and reach the systemic circulation. The hexacanth embryos are filtered out from the circulating blood by the muscular tissues. They now lose their hooks in the muscle, the cells in the centre are liquefied, and in about 8 days form small vesicles. The vesicles gradually increase in size and, in about 2 months, form a mature bladder-worm (*C. cellulosae*), containing the larva in which the scolex is *invaginated*. The cysticercus is commonly seen in the tongue, neck and shoulder muscles of the pig. Thus the cycle repeats.

Epidemiology. TRANSMISSION occurs by eating inadequately cooked pork containing *Cysticercus cellulosae*. Defective disposal of human faeces, or the use of faeces as fertilisers result in infection of animal vectors.

VECTOR. Pig is the important vector of the bladder-worm. In well-developed countries, incidence in pig is about 0.2 per cent, but it may vary from 10-25 per cent in many countries.

RESERVOIR. The only reservoir host is man.

Pathogenicity. The adult *T. solium* may not produce any symptom except vague abdominal pain of *colicky* nature or minor digestive disturbances. ***Gastrointestinal irritation*** or ***neurasthenia*** may develop later.

Human may become infected with *C. cellulosae* by auto-infection, *C. cellulosae* may develop in any organ, and ill effects are produced, depending on their location in the body. They tend to undergo calcification, which starts in the scolex and extends to the cyst capsule.

Laboratory diagnosis. (1) Presence of **gravid proglottides** of *T. solium* in the stool with 7-12 branchings of the gravid uterus (PLATE 10.IV). (2) Presence of **eggs (bile-stained)** in the faeces as found by microscopic examination, but the eggs of *T. solium* and *T. saginata* are morphologically similar. (3) Identification of the worm by inspection of stool for the **armed head** after a dose of anthelmintic. The cure of *T. solium* infection is not certain, unless the armed scolex i.e., scolex with rostellum is passed. (4) Calcified cysticercus can be detected by **roentgenogram**. (5) **Eosinophilia** is not a constant feature.

Prophylaxis. It consists of the following measures:

(*a*) Inspection of pork for cysticerci. (*b*) Refrigeration of pork at a temperature of 5°C for not less than 21 days. (*c*) Thorough cooking of meat (66°C is lethal for cysticerci). (*d*) Sanitary disposal of human faeces is very important as hogfeed should not be polluted with human faeces containing eggs of *T. solium*. (*e*) Rigid personal cleanliness is essential and contaminated food should be avoided. (*f*) Internal auto-infection is prevented by purgatives, (which do not cause nausea). (*g*) Above all, proper treatment is essential to terminate the infection, which reduces the risk of cysticercosis.

Treatment. Specific drugs are **filix mas, atebrine** and **dichlorophen.** Cestoidicide called *Yomesan*, a chlorsalicylamide derivative is useful. Filix (fern) mas (male) was the drug of choice in the past, but it is toxic and should not be repeated within one month. It is used in doses of 6 gm for an adult in an emulsion form.

Atebrine is quite effective and simple to administer. On the previous day, light diet is given in the evening after a saline purgative in the afternoon. Next morning, in an empty stomach 8 tablets (0.1 g each) of atebrine is administered, one every five minutes with a glass of water containing 6 gm of sodium bicarbonate. Two or three hours after the last dose, a saline purgative is administered. Results are satisfactory but nausea, vomiting or mental disorientation may follow the use of atebrine. The tapeworm is passed in 2-4 hours, but it may be delayed up to 7 days after this treatment. The worm is stained yellow. This treatment should not be given to children under 8 years of age. Cure by this method is 78 per cent. The highest success (90 per cent) is obtained with transduodenal intubation in an empty stomach, when atebrine solution acts directly on the worm. Expulsion of the armed head is the sign of eradication of the worm.

Transduodenal intubation. An hour before the operation the patient is sedated with 125 mg of phenobarbitone or 200 mg of sodium amytal. A Ryle's tube is passed, allowing sufficient time to enter the duodenum. The dose (1 gm of mepacrine hydrochloride) is suspended in 100 ml of water and introduced with the help of a syringe. Half an hour after, a saline purgative is introduced in the same way and the tube is withdrawn later on.

A dose of phenobarbitone 125 mg may be given at 6 A.M. to nervous patients, half an hour before administration of atebrine tablets. Hexylfesorcinol crystalloids, intubation transduodenally, are very effective. For cerebral cysticercosis, hetrazan may be administered.

Mebendazole (Mebex) is effective (see **Appendix III**).

Praziquantel and **niclosamide** are the drugs of choice for adult worm eradication. Also praziquantel and **metrifonate** are also useful. Surgical excision is the method of choice wherever possible.

TAENIA SAGINATA Goeze, 1782

SYNONYM. Beef tapeworm; **unarmed tapeworm** (without rostellum) of human.

Incidence. Infection in human with the adult *T. saginata* is commoner than that of *T. solium* in India, and the incidence of *Cysticercus bovis* is about 5 per cent in ox. The incidence of *C. cellulosae* in the pig is 10-25 per cent in many countries and it is higher in pig than the incidence of *C. bovis* in cattle.

Geographical distribution. Cosmopolitan, wherever beef is eaten.

Habitat. Small intestine of human.

Morphology. ADULT WORM. *Length* is 3.6–12 metres (12-40 feet) containing about 2000 segments. There may be 1,200 to 1,500 gravid proglottides, which are longer than broad. *Suckers*: These are four in number, pigmented and elliptical in shape, *Scolex*: Head has neither hooks nor rostellum and this is why it is called unarmed. *Genital pores* project markedly on the lateral margin of segments.

Larva (*Cysticercus bovis*). The larval stage occurs in the ox and cow, called *Cysticercus bovis*. The larvae are elliptical, 7.5 to 9 mm in length and 5.5 mm in breadth. The cysticerci are not numerous and are usually found **in the muscles of mastication.**

Eggs. They are oval in shape. Size is 30μm by 20μm. They are almost indistinguishable from those of *T. solium*. Embryophore is thick and radially striated.

LIFE SPAN is as long as 25 years.

Life cycle. *T. saginata* requires two hosts to complete the life cycle (Fig. 10.5).

DEFINITIVE HOST. Human is the only definitive host.

INTERMEDIATE HOST. The most important intermediate host is the cow or ox; but other herbivorous animals may be infected and act as intermediate hosts. In Egypt and Morocco, the camel is the most important intermediate host.

Eggs and gravid proglottides are passed in the faeces of man which contaminate grass and other vegetations. The eggs are swallowed by cattle while grazing, and eggs develop into *Cysticercus bovis* in the muscles of mastication and heart (For details see *T. solium*). If underdone meat of such animals is eaten by man, the wall of each cysticercus containing a scolex is digested by the gastric juice and the

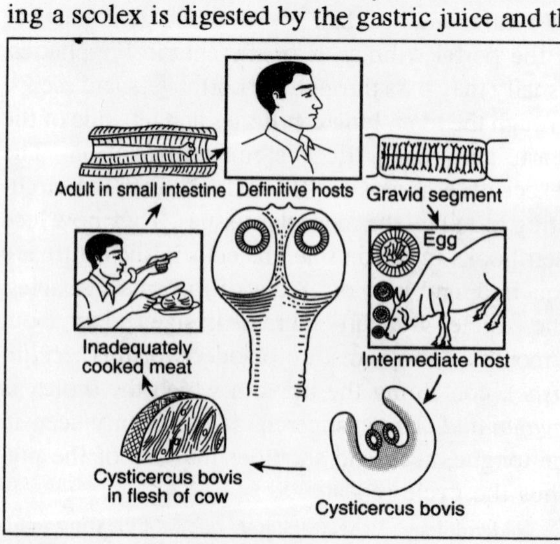

Fig. 10.5 Life cycle of *Taenia saginata*

free larva then attaches itself by means of suckers to the intestinal wall; proglottides grow from the scolex with great rapidity. The adult worm is found in the upper part of the small intestine of man.

The eggs or oncospheres are not infective to human.

Epidemiology. TRANSMISSION occurs by the ingestion of inadequately cooked infected beef.

INTERMEDIATE HOST (carrier) is ox. The common source of bovine infection is the flooded pasture along the rivers, where ova may survive for 6 weeks or more.

RESERVOIR HOST is human.

Symptoms and pathology. Usually a single worm is present without any symptom, but epigastric discomfort and vague abdominal disturbances may occur. The infection is detected by the passage of gravid segments in the stools. Anaemia and eosinophilia may be present.

Occurrence of adult *Cysticercus bovis* in human is practically unknown.

Laboratory diagnosis. This is same as that in the case of *T. salium*, but marked eosinophilia (6 to 34%) is an additional feature in case of *T. saginata*.

Treatment. Some as that of *T. solium*.

Dichlorophen. Anthiphen (M & B) is available as tablets of 0.5 gm. The adult dose is 6 gm given in a single dose; for children the dose is not less than 4 gm. No preparation of the patient or post-purgative is required as the drug is a mild laxative and may induce 2 or 3 motions. The drug is a **taeniacide** and destroys the head (scolex); immature and gravid segments are passed in the stool in a state of disintegration. Therefore, the head cannot be found in the stool. The cure is judged after 3 months by the absence of segments in the stool. The drug is more effective for *T. saginata* than other taenias.

HYMENOLEPIS NANA (Siebold, 1852) Blanchard, 1891

(The "dwarf" tapeworm producing Hymenolepiasis nana)

ORDER: *Cyclophyllidea*

FAMILY: *Hymenolepididae*

GENUS: *Hymenolepis*

SYNONYMS: Dwarf Tapeworm of human, *H. nana* var. *fraterna.*

H. nana dose not require any intermediate host for the development of larvae (cysticercoid). Human and murine strains are identical.

Geographical distribution. India, America, Egypt and Europe, i.e., worldwide distribution.

Habitat. Adult are found in the small intestine (upper three-quarters of the ileum) of human, rats and mice. Larvae develop in the intestinal villi of man, rats and mice. Eggs are found in the faeces.

Morphology. *H. nana* is one of the smallest human tapeworms.

ADULT WORM is small and thread-like, measuring 2 to 4 cm in length with a maximum breadth of 1 mm in its posterior portion.

TABLE 10.3
DIFFERENCES BETWEEN *T. SOLIUM* AND *T. SAGINATA*

	T. solium	T. saginata
Length	2-8 metres	5-10 metres
Scolex:		
Shape	Globular	Quadrate or pear-shaped
Size	Pin head	Larger than pin head, 1 to 2 mm
Sucker	Not pigmented	Pigmented
Rostellum	Present	Absent
Hooklets	Double row of hooklets	None
Proglottides	800 to 900	1,000 to 2,000
Segments:	In chain of 5 to 6	Disposed singly
Testes	300-400 follicles	150-200 follicles
Ovary	Trilobed (one accessory lobe)	Bilobed
Uterus in gravid proglottides	5 to 13 lateral branches (average 9)	15 to 30 lateral branches (average 20)
Vaginal sphincter	Absent	Present

HEAD. It is globular and is endowed with a short retractile **rostellum**, armed with a single row of 20 to 30 retractile hooklets, capable of invagination. There are four globular suckers. *Segments* (Fig. 10.6). The worm consists of about 200 segments. Each mature segment is broader than long and measures about 0.22 mm in length and 0.85 to 0.90 mm in breadth. *Genital pores* are marginal and they are situated on the same side. Each mature segment contains three *testes* and a pair of *ovary*. *Cirrus pouch* (Penis) is very prominent. The *uterus* is a transverse sac with lobulated wall.

Eggs are 30 to 45μm in diameter and colourless, as they are not stained with bile. Each has an inner and an outer membrane. *Embryo* is 16μ in diameter. *Embryophore* (inner membrane) is 20 to 30μm in diameter. The inner membrane exhibits little knobs at either end, from which four to eight delicate filaments arise. There is a wide space between the inner and the outer membrane, which contains yolk granules.

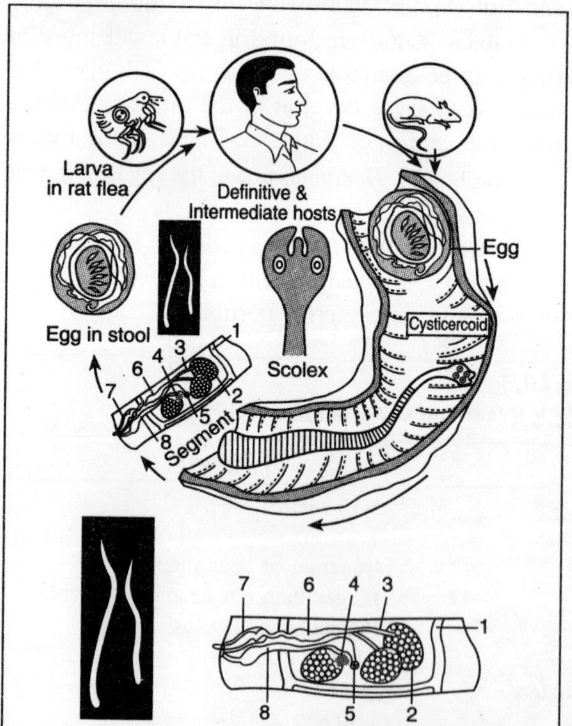

Fig. 10.6 Life cycle of *Hymenolepis nana*. Mature segment—1. Excretory vessel. 2. Testis. 3. Vas efferens. 4. Ovary. 5. Vitelline gland. 6. Seminal vesicle. 7. Cirrus pouch. 8. Vagina

Life cycle (Fig. 10.6). DIRECT CYCLE. Definitive host is human, in whom the life cycle is direct. No intermediate host is required. The larval development proceeds in the intestine of the same individual, where it later develops into an adult worm. *H. nana* is the solitary example of the egg developing into the adult form inside the body of the definitive host. Segments often rupture in the intestine and liberate the eggs.

When a fully developed hexacanth embryo in the egg passed in the faeces is swallowed, the hexacanth embryo is liberated. The embryo enters into an **intestinal villus**, where a small cysticercoid is formed in about 4 days' time. The villus ruptures when the cysticercoid is mature and the larva (scolex) re-enters the lumen of the small intestine. Later it attaches to another villus further down. Here the *strobilisation* is rapid and in course of one fortnight the cysticercoid develops into an adult worm. Eggs are passed in the faeces within 30 days after the infection. The **eggs which remain in the bowels can start a new cycle again.**

INDIRECT CYCLE. Besides the direct cycle mentioned above, rat fleas and beetles may act as intermediate hosts and help in the transmission of murine infection, indirectly to human. Development of the worm is rapid after ingestion of fleas often by children, and in about 30 days after infection, eggs begin to appear in the faeces. When the infection is established, autoinfection increases the number of parasites.

Natural mammalian hosts other than human are rats and mice, though the latter two hosts are not important.

H. nana var. *fraterna* in rats and mice being morphologically identical with *H. nana* has intermediate hosts, namely, fleas like ***Xenopsylla cheopis***, *Ctenocephalides canis*, beetles like *Tenebrio molitor*, or *T. obscurus*, which cause infection when ingested by rodents.

Epidemiology. TRANSMISSION occurs through ingestion of eggs, by faecal contamination of hands and foods. Eggs do not survive outside the body long after their passage in the stools. Occasional infection may occur from rodent sources.

VECTOR. None is responsible in human type infection.

RESERVOIR. Man is the important reservoir, but rodents are less important in this respect.

Pathogenicity. When the worms are present in large numbers in the small intestine, they may cause pain in the abdomen, diarrhoea, asthma and nervous symptoms, like convulsion and vertigo by reflex irritation.

Laboratory diagnosis. It is based on the finding of: (1) *Eggs* in the faeces; (2) Adult worms, which are very small and, as such, may be overlooked when passed in faeces. Eggs are **nonbile-stained.**

Prophylaxis. It depends on: (1) improvement of personal habits; (2) treatment of infected persons; (3) protection of food from rats and mice, which should be exterminated for worms.

Treatment. It is same as in the case of *T. saginata* in hyperinfection. In light infection, **cashewnut shell extract** or **cardol** is useful. The dose for both of them is 6 gm in capsules for adults; it is 4.5 g for children between 10 and 14 years and 2.5-3.5 g for children between 5 and 9 years of age. **Hexylresorcinol** may also be used in light infections.

HYMENOLEPIS DIMINUTA (Rudolphi, 1819) Blanchard, 1891

(*The rat tapeworm, producing hymenolepiasis diminuta*)

Habitat. It is a parasite found in the intestine of rats and mice and rarely in man. Eggs are infective to insects, and larvae are found in the haemocele of insects, e.g., fleas and cockroaches.

Morphology. ADULTS are 20 to 60 cm in length and have about one thousand segments. The *scolex* has 4 suckers and no hooklet. *Segments* are broader than long (0.75 mm by 2.5 mm). **Eggs** are like those of *H. nana*, but longer. They are subspherical and 60 to 80μ in diameter. They have a thicker transparent outer shell, yellowish in colour; the inner membrane around the oncosphere is the embryophore which has two knob-like thickenings, but without any polar filaments.

Life cycle. It occurs in two hosts: (1) the *larval* or *cysticercoid stage* occurs in fleas and (2) the *adult stage* in the rats, mice and occasionally in man. The *intermediate hosts* are various species of insects (fleas), which ingest the eggs. The more important intermediate hosts are larvae of rat fleas, like *Nosopsyllus fasciatus* and *Xenopsylla cheopis*; the mouse flea, like *Leptopsyllus segnis*; and the mealworm beetle, like *Temebrio molitor*. **Man acquires infection by accidentally swallowing infected insects.** The parasites are easily expelled by anthelmintics used for *H. nana*.

DIPYLIDIUM CANINUM (Linnaeus, 1758) Railliet, 1892

(*The double-pored dog tapeworm, producing Dipylidiasis*)

It is a double-pored short tapeworm of dogs and cats and rarely found in man.

Morphology. The ADULTS are about 15 to 60 cm in length and possess about 60-170 segments. The *gravid segments* are 12 mm by 2.7 mm. The *scolex* is rhomboid with 4 prominent oval or round *suckers* and a *rostellum* with 3 to 4 rows of hooklets. The *rostellum* can be retracted into the scolex. The **Eggs** are like those of *H. nana* measuring 35 to 60μ in diameter and they are grouped in masses of 5 to 25. Infection is acquired by ingesting rat fleas like *Ctenocephalides canis* which are the intermediate hosts. Most of the human infections have been reported in children (Manson-Bahr, 1961). If the infected flea is nipped by a dog and subsequently the dog licks a child or an adult, cysticercus may possibly be transmitted (Chandler, 1949). Accidentally, children may swallow and get infected (Dabidsohn, 1962). *Reproduction* takes place by **cross** or **self fertilisation.**

ECHINOCOCCUS GRANULOSUS (Batsch, 1786) Rudolphi 1895

(*The hydatid worm, producing Hydatid disease or Echinococcosis*)

Geographical distribution. It is found in all parts of the world; common in Australia, Iceland, Arabia, Africa, Egypt and Abyssinia; it is rare in India except in certain foci, like the Punjab, and Madurai in Southern India.

Habitat. The adult worm known as *E. granulosus* is found in the intestine of the dog, fox, jackal and

TABLE 10.4

DIFFERENCES BETWEEN *H. NANA* AND *H. DIMINUTA*

H. nana	*H. diminuta*
Adult:	
Measurement—2-4 cm	20-60 cm
Segments—200	800-1,000
Rostellum: with-hooklets	Without hooklets
Eggs: 30 to 60μ	60 to 80μ
The inner membrane has two distinct knobs with thread-like polar filaments	The inner membrane has two knobs without polar filaments

other carnivorous animals. Hydatid stage occurs in man and also in herbivorous animals, like cattle, sheep and pig.

Morphology (Fig. 10.7). ADULT WORM. *Length*: 4 to 5 mm. *Segments*: 4 segments only, but may be 3 or 5 including the head. The terminal one is mature and gravid. *Suckers*: Four. *Head*: Globular, smaller than that of *T. solium*. *Rostellum*: Prominent and armed with a double row of hooklets, 30 to 40 in number.

LIFE SPAN of the adult worm in the canine host is 5 to 6 months but the larval worm may continue to develop for many years.

Source of infection. Infection is acquired by dogs and other animals by ingesting infected viscera of animals containing innumerable scolices inside the hydatid cyst. The period between the ingestion of the scolices and passage of mature ova is about 40 days. Eggs are infective to human.

Life cycle (Fig. 10.7). *E. granulosus* requires two hosts to complete the life cycle.

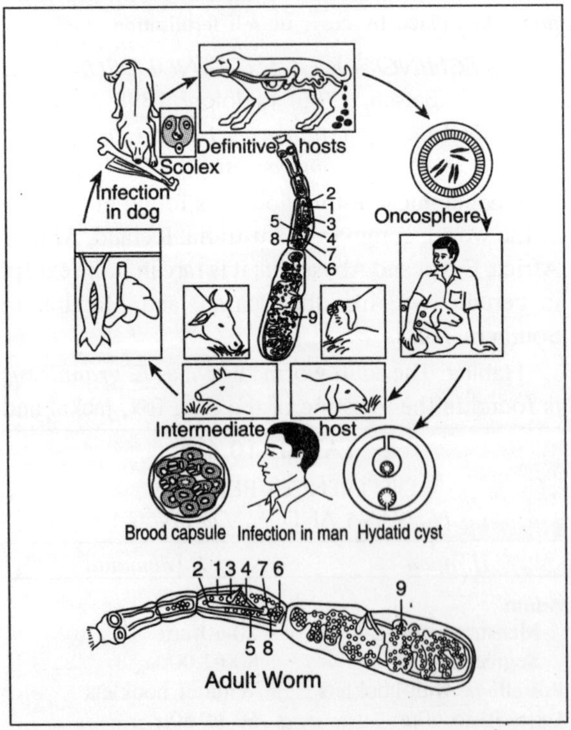

Fig. 10.7 Life cycle of *Echinococcus granulosus*. 1. Excretory vessel. 2. Uterus. 3. Cirrus pouch. 4. Vagina. 5. Ovary. 6. Testes. 7. Shell gland. 8. Vitelline gland. 9. Uterus (gravid)

1. Definitive hosts—dog, fox, jackal and other carnivorous animals.

2. Intermediate hosts—human, cattle, sheep and pig.

The adult worm is found in the dog, fox and other carnivorous animals after ingestion of infected viscera of cattle, sheep, or pig containing **hydatid cysts** full of ***scolices***. Eggs resembling those of ***T. saginata*** are passed by the definitive host (dog, etc.) in the stool.

Human is accidentally infected by handling infected dog or by ingesting water or green vegetables polluted by faeces of infected dogs. When the egg is ingested by man, the ***hexacanth embryo*** with ***six hooklets*** is set free in the duodenum after digestion of the wall of the embryophore in the stomach. The embryo is then active and in about 8 hours penetrates through the wall of the small intestine and escapes into the liver through portal circulation. In the liver, they are arrested by the liver filter in the sinusoidal capillaries. Escaping the liver filter, some embryos may reach the pulmonary capillaries to produce lesions in the lungs, while others may reach organs, like pleura, brain muscles and bones through general circulation. In the liver and other organs, the embryo changes into a **cystic larva** called **hydatid cyst** (Fig. 10.8).

DEVELOPMENT OF HYDATID CYST. After the embryo is arrested in the liver or other viscera, it settles down and the embryo develops into a spheroidal bud, and gradually forms a cyst with accumulation of fluid in it. The wall of the cyst is dif-

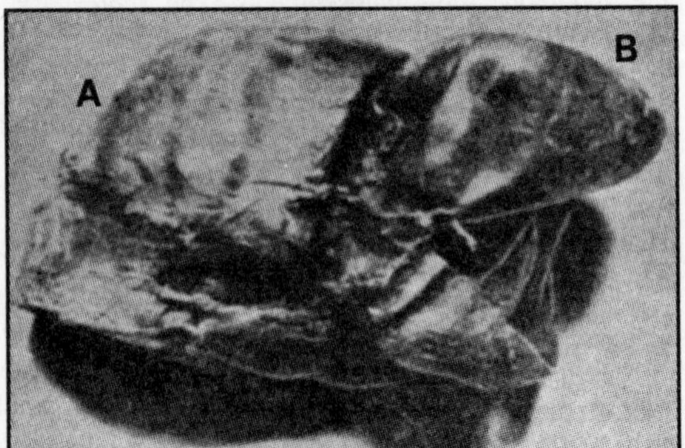

Fig. 10.8 Hydatid cyst in the liver. A. Normal liver tissue with compressed margin. B. Hydatid cyst cut open to demonstrate the size of the cyst

ferentiated into an ectocyst and an endocyst. A *pericyst* also forms as a result of formation of a fibrous layer around the growing embryo, but the parasite may derive its nutrition through it. It may be sclerosed and calcified; the parasite inside may die and degenerate for lack of nutrition.

Ectocyst consists of an outer laminated, chitinous layer about 1 mm thick. It is elastic and everted when cut, and has the appearance of the white of a hard-boiled egg.

Endocyst is the inner proliferating layer. The inner layer of the endocyst is a germinal layer containing a number of nuclei in a protoplasmic mass, and budding processes arise from them. This is the vital layer responsible for production of (1) scolices and brood capsule, (2) secretion of the hydatid fluid, and (3) the outer layer of daughter and granddaughter cysts, which contain scolices or immature heads of *E. granulosus*, characterised by hooklets and four suckers. The cysts contain brood capsules. **The secretion of the cyst is the hydatid fluid.**

DEVELOPMENT OF BROOD CAPSULE. The brood capsule is formed by proliferation of cells of the germinal layer. It differs from a daughter or granddaughter cyst in that it has only the germinal layer and not the outer laminated layer of the ectocyst. At first, from the germinal layer, a papule develops; it ultimately forms a vesicle held by a stalk inside the cyst. Within the wall of the brood capsule, tiny, stalked, invaginated scolices are formed containing hooks and four suckers. The number of the scolices in each brood capsule varies from 5-20 (**Fig. 10.9A**). The invagination acts as a protective covering to the growing scolex. The stalk of the brood capsule often breaks, detaching it from the wall of the cyst. The detached brood capsules disintegrated and the scolices lie free in the cyst. These scolices, free hooklets and disintegrated brood capsules in the cyst may form **hydatid sand**. When held in a conical glass, they form a sediment consisting of brood capsule, scolices and hooklets (**Fig. 10.9B**).

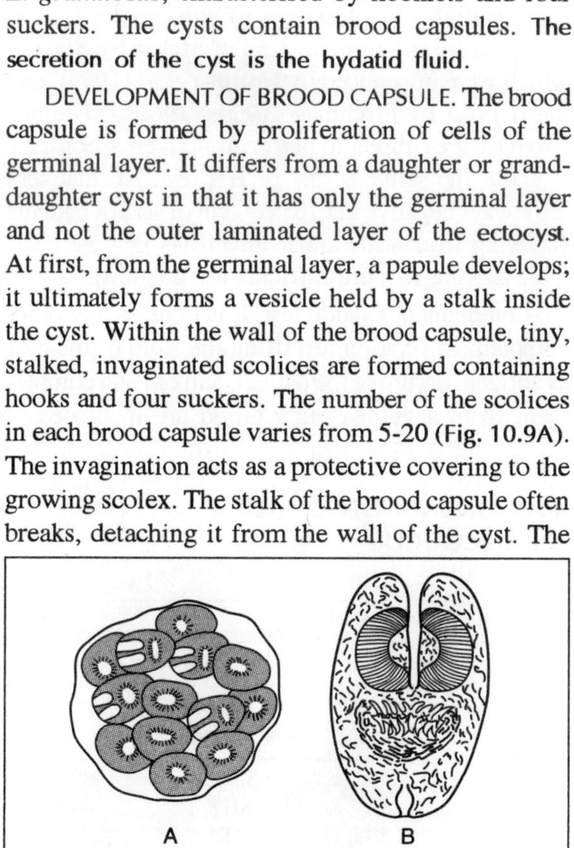

Fig. 10.9 A. Brood capsule showing scolices. B. Invaginated scolex (magnified)

RATE OF GROWTH OF HYDATID CYST. Hydatid in man develops slowly and it takes a long time before the cyst grows appreciably. At the end of 5 months it is just visible to the naked eye, at the end of one year it is about 1 inch in diameter, when brood capsules and scolices begin to appear. After 2 to 8 years it may assume the size of a foetal head or bigger. Endogenous daughter cysts formation occurs after a growth for many years.

VARIATIONS. (*a*) **Acephalocyst**. This is due to nondevelopment of brood capsules and is without any scolex. Such a cyst is also called a **sterile cyst**.

(*b*) **Exogenous cyst**. When the wall evaginates and comes out through the fibrous capsule, a daughter cyst is produced outside and it is known as **exogenous cyst**. This, in its turn, may be detached from the wall of the mother cyst and often it occurs in *hydatid cysts of bones*.

(*c*) **Multilocular** or **alveolar cyst**. They may be without any free fluid and filled with a jelly-like substance instead. These cysts are often sterile and have a great tendency to form irregular *multilocular infiltrating cysts*. They are regarded by some to be caused by *E. multilocularis*, a different species of Echinococcus.

(*d*) **Metastatic** or **secondary echinococcus**. This occurs when the cyst ruptures. The material of the cyst disseminates through the venous or arterial system; these are approximately of the same size as the primary ones.

INCIDENCE of hydatid cysts in **various organs** is as follows:

Liver–70%; **Lungs**–10 to 20%; **brain**–5% (primary and single in children, secondary and multiple in adults); **kidneys**–2%; **spleen**–2%; **bone**–1% (ribs, vertebrae, and upper end of long bones having the "blown up" appearance riddled with cavities); **pelvic organs** like the *urinary bladder, uterus, ovary* and *Fallopian tubes*–2%; *head, muscles and other organs*–1% to 3%.

FATE AND SECONDARY CHANGES. (1) Spontaneous cure may occur in some cases.

(2) The hydatid may die off and the fluid is gradually absorbed.

(3) Hydatid cyst may shrink with the contents degenerating, followed by calcification. In these cases, the hooklets may be persisting and they may be recognised microscopically for a long period. Such change may occur either by the entrance of bile in the cyst or by injury to the cyst wall.

(4) Inflammatory changes may be due to infection resulting in spontaneous evacuation of the cyst.

(5) If the cyst is in the liver, such evacuation may take place in the pleural cavity through the diaphragm or into the lung with expectoration of hooklets in the sputum.

(6) The cyst may rupture into the cavity with widespread growth of hydatid cyst.

DIAGNOSIS OF HYDATID DISEASE

1. CLINICAL: History of contact, local swelling, urticarial eruption with fever, hydatid thrill on percussion of the liver region are characteristic.

2. LABORATORY DIAGNOSIS: Examination of stool does not help, as there is no adult worm in the intestine. Hooklets or parts of the laminated cyst may be coughed out when the cyst bursts into the lungs. So *sputum examination* may be of help.

Blood. There is increased eosinophils (20 to 25%).

Immunological Test

ALLERGIC TEST (*Casoni's intradermal immunological test*). 0.2 ml of sterile hydatid fluid is injected intradermally. In positive cases, a wheal is formed in 15 to 20 minutes with blanching at the centre. The test is reliable and is the test of choice, except in old complicated cases, instead of ***complement fixation test***.

SEROLOGICAL TESTS

The tests of choice in the serodiagnosis of hydatid disease are (i) **indirect haemagglutination (HA) test**, (ii) benetonic flocculation **(BF) test** and (iii) **latex (L) fixation test** (Table 10.5). High titres of sera usually indicate hydatid disease, but low titres are equivocal, as they are positive with collagen diseases or cirrhosis of the liver (Kagan *et al*, 1960). Hydatid disease of the lung rarely gives positive results with these serological tests. Cysticercus antisera cross-react with echinococcus antigen.

HA test is more sensitive than others. The sensitivity varies from 82 to 88 percent in hydatid disease of the liver but 33 to 50 percent from patients with lung cysts (Kagar and Osimani, 1966). The specificity is high when the titres of antisera are 1 : 400 or higher by HA test and 1 : 5 or higher by BF test, which were introduced by Norman *et al* (1959). and the (L) test by Fischman (1960a, 1960b). The last two tests are simpler to perform and their specificity is about the same as that of HA test. Normal sera are always negative but 10 per- cent of sera of patients suffering from some other infections may be positive, making it more difficult for diagnosis.

Complement fixation test. It is done as any other complement fixation test using the fluid of the cyst as antigen. Serum of the patient, antigen and complement from a guinea pig's blood are incubated at

TABLE 10.5

SEROLOGICAL TESTS WITH SERA FROM INDIVIDUALS INFECTED WITH ECHINOCOCCUS

(After Kagan *et al,* 1960)

	SEROLOGICAL TESTS					
Infection	Haemagglutination		Flocculation		Latex Fixation	
Organs	No. Positive / No. tested	Percent Positive	No. Positive / No. tested	Percent Positive	No. Positive / No. tested	Percent Positive
Hydatid disease : Liver	52/59	88	50/58	86	55/62	89
Lung	6/18	33	9/18	50	8/18	44
Control (*Cysticercus cellulosae*)	9/9	100	4/8	50	NT*	NT*

*Not tested

37°C and sensitised sheep cells are then added. If there is no haemolysis, the reaction is positive; whereas, **haemolysis indicates a negative reaction.** The test is positive in 83 percent cases, and is valuable in old complicated ones.

Precipitin reaction. Patient's serum is layered with an equal volume of hydatid fluid (phenolised, unheated) and incubated at 37°C for one hour. A flocculation at the interface of the fluids suggests infection. A negative finding, however, does not exclude infection.

Haemagglutination test. As in any other bacterial haemagglutination test, fresh sheep red cells are treated with 1 in 20,000 tannic acid solution and then coated with echinococcus antigen as mentioned by Boyden (1951), and Kagan *et al* (1961). The cells so treated show agglutination with specific serum.

Flocculation tests. In this, bentonite particles or *polystyrene latex particles* are coated with antigen from hydatid cyst fluid (*cf.* rheumatoid arthritis; bentonite flocculation test of Norman *et al* (1959). The antigen is adsorbed on standard bentonite particles of 1 to 2µm size. To 0.1 ml of bentonite suspension, 0.1 ml of serial dilutions of serum with normal saline (1 : 5, 1 : 10, 1 : 20, etc.) is added on a large slide with concavities (as in VDRL test). The slide is then rotated for 15 minutes in a VDRL shaker and then the reading is taken. A positive result is indicated by aggregated floccules. The dilution at which at least more than half of the particles are aggregated into floccules indicates the positive reaction. The end point may be worked out in a positive case.

Latex fixation test (Fischman, 1960). The antigen is a standard suspension of polystyrene latex with a pooled hydatid fluid. The serum is used in double dilutions and mixed with the antigen. The mixtures are incubated in a water bath at 37°C for 90 minutes in a test tube rack, which is kept overnight at 4°C and the reading is taken next day. A heavy precipitate indicates a positive result.

RADIOLOGICAL: Circular shadows with a sharp outline and mottled appearance in the diaphysis or metaphysis of long bones are often suggestive. Walls are thin and poorly developed; cyst may spread along the canaliculi. The osseous cysts have blown-up appearance riddled with cavities.

EXPLORATORY PUNCTURE OF THE CYST is dangerous, as any leakage of fluid containing scolices might give rise to fresh hydatid cysts in other parts. Moreover, if the fluid escapes into cellular tissue, there may be **fatal anaphylactic shock**. The fluid contains an allergen which produces urticaria and also a toxin, which is depressant to the heart.

Composition and characters of hydatid fluid. The hydatid fluid is generally colourless, or pale yellow in colour. It is clear but may be opalescent of a specific gravity of 1004 to 1010 and pH of 6.7.

Albumin may be absent or present in trace. Little sugar is present. Sodium chloride content is 0.5 to 1%. Other sodium salts, like sodium and calcium succinate are present. The fluid contains scolices and hooklets demonstrable under the microscope; this is diagnostic. The fluid is antigenic and may be used for immunological tests. When absorbed, it produces anaphylactic reactions.

Prophylaxis. It consists of: (1) Prevention of infection in dogs in endemic areas, (2) deworming dogs by anthelmintics, (3) personal prophylaxis by washing hands after handling dogs.

Treatment. Surgical removal of the cyst as a whole may be successful when care is taken to prevent the escape of hydatid fluid into the peritoneal cavity or other tissues.

ECHINOCOCCUS MULTILOCULARIS

(Leuckart, 1863) Vogel, 1955

(The larval worm, producing alveolar hydatid disease in man)

DEFINITIVE HOSTS are dogs, foxes and wolves, and INTERMEDIATE HOSTS are field mice (Germany) and *tundra* voles (Alaska); men are accidentally infected from dogs. *E. multilocularis* is appreciably similar to *E. granulosus*. The size of the adult worm is 1.2 to 3.7 mm. In the sexually mature proglottid, the *genital pore* is anterior to the equatorial plane. The number of *testes* is 16 to 26 rather than 45-65 as in *E. granulosus*. They are situated posterior to the *cirrus pouch*. The *uterus* lacks lateral outpockets, often present in *E. granulosus*.

EPIDEMIOLOGY. According to Vogel (1955), in Europe, men get the infection sporadically from eggs of *E.*

multilocularis present in infected fox's excreta by direct contact with polluted ground, while picking berries and fruits.

Pathogenicity. The *multilocular* form of the cyst in fox and the *alveolar* form in human are not fundamentally different but transitional forms may also occur. Although the alveolar cyst is found in the lungs and other organs, its commonest site of development and occurrence is the liver. The hepatic disease may clinically resemble a slowly developing **mucoid carcinoma.**

Diagnosis. Immunological and allergic tests are positive with the antigenic fluid derived from hydatid cyst fluid.

MULTICEPS (COENURUS) MULTICEPS

(Leske, 1870), Hall, 1910

(The "gid" worm)

It is an armed tapeworm with 22-32 hooklets in double rows, and 40-50 cm in length, DEFINITIVE HOSTS are dog and wolf. The LARVAL STAGE is found in herbivorous animals (sheep, goats, cattle, horses, etc.) resulting from ingestion of eggs passed in dog's faeces. The egg appearing like that of other taenia species, with an average measurement of 31 to 36μm in diameter (Craig and Faust, 1964). The occurrence of *Coenurus glomeratus* in human in West Africa was reported by Turner and Leiper (1919). Usually the base of the brain, or the eye is affected in coenurosis, which essentially causes a condition of leptomeningitis (arachnoiditis) or **plastic meningeal fibrosis with foreign-body giant cell reaction** in the vicinity of the cyst-wall. Definite cases of intracerebral cyst formation have been recorded by Wainwright (1957). Frequently the cysts involving the central nervous system are sterile, having no scolices. Coenurus ophthalmitis have been recorded in Africa by Raper and Dockeray (1956), Wainwright (1957) and Epstein *et al.* (1959). The cysts are variable in size and look racemose, lobulated, or spherical. Different species of Multiceps may be determined on the basis of hooklet morphology and size (Clapham, 1942). *M. glomeratus*, *M. serialis* and *M. brauni* are responsible for subcutaneous and soft tissue cysts. However, Clapham (1941, 1942) regards *M. multiceps*, *M. glomeratus* and *M. serialis* as strains of the same species. Human is rarely infected. The oncospheres hatch out in the intestine of the intermediate host and lodge in various organs but usually in the brain and spinal cord. The larva metamorphoses into a *coenurus* (*C. cerebralis*), a bladder-worm with multiple scolices with the same hooklet pattern. They are capable of developing into adult worms, when a dog devours the brain of a sheep dying of the infection.

Other multiceps forming coenurus are: *Multiceps glomeratus* Ralliet and Henry, 1915. *Multiceps serialis* (Gervais, 1845) Stiles and Stevenson, 1905.

DIPHYLLOBOTHRIUM LATUM

(Linnaeus, 1758), Luhe, 1910

(Broad tapeworm, producing fish tapeworm infection)

ORDER: PSEUDOPHYLLIDEA **Carus, 1863.**

SUPERFAMILY: BOTHRIOCEPHALOIDEA **Braun, 1903.**

GENUS: DIPHYLLOBOTHRIUM **Cobbold, 1858.**

Geographical distribution. It is not seen in India, but found in Baltic countries and other parts of Europe, America, Central Asia and Japan.

Habitat. The adult worm inhabits the jejunum of man, where the worm attacks itself by the suctorial grooves (bothria).

Morphology. ADULT WORM is known as broad tapeworm; its ***length*** is 3 to 4 metres and ***breadth*** is 1 to 2 cm. It is greyish yellow in colour. ***Segments*** are broader than long, 3,000 to 4,000 in number. A mature segment is 2 to 4 mm in length by 10 to 20 mm in breadth. ***Head*** is minute, elongated, spoon-shaped, and flattened with two longitudinal suctorial grooves, called **bothria**, present one on each side. Hooklets are absent. Mature and gravid segments cannot be distinguished. **Genital pores** lie on the ventral flat surface. They are three in number and lie in the middle line. Antero-posteriorly, there are openings of **vas deferens, vagina** and **uterus.** ***Uterus***, when developed, is seen as a brownish area in the segment. It forms a coiled up mass in the centre of the segment in the form of a rossette, and opens into the **uterine pore. Ovary** is on the posterior third of a proglottid, ventral in position, symmetrical and bilobed. ***Testes*** are numerous and scattered throughout the superficial layer (dorsal plane of each segment).

LIFE SPAN of the adult worm in human is up to 20 years.

Eggs. Their size is 70μm by 34μm. They are oval and operculated, golden yellow in colour and contain immature embryos, which are unsegmented and surrounded by yolk. Under favourable conditions they hatch out in 9-12 days. The hexacanth embryo is surrounded by its ciliated **embryophore**, and this stage is called a **coracidium.** They swim about in water until ingested by a crustacean host, *Cyclops* or **Diaptome.** The eggs or coracidia are not infective to man. **The eggs do not float on saturated solution of common salt.**

PLATE 10.III

DIFFERENCES BETWEEN *A. PSEUDOPHYLLIDEA* & *B. CYCLOPHYLLIDEA*

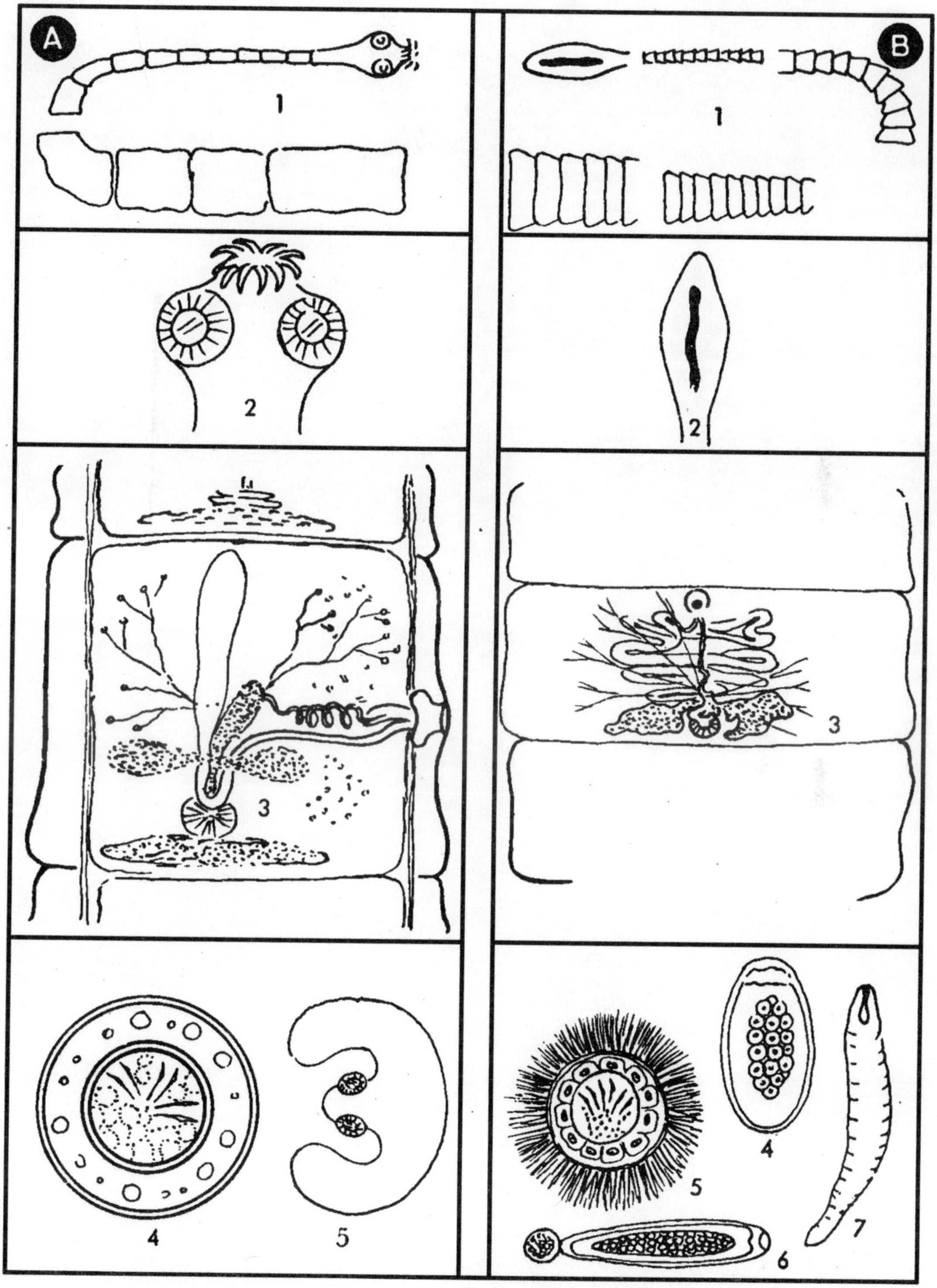

1. Mature proglottides. 2. Scolex. 3. Genital pore. 4. Ova. A5. Bladder worm. B5. Coracidium. B6. Procercoid. B7. Plerocercoid.

PLATE 10.IV

PASSAGE OF PROGLOTTIDES IN FAECES

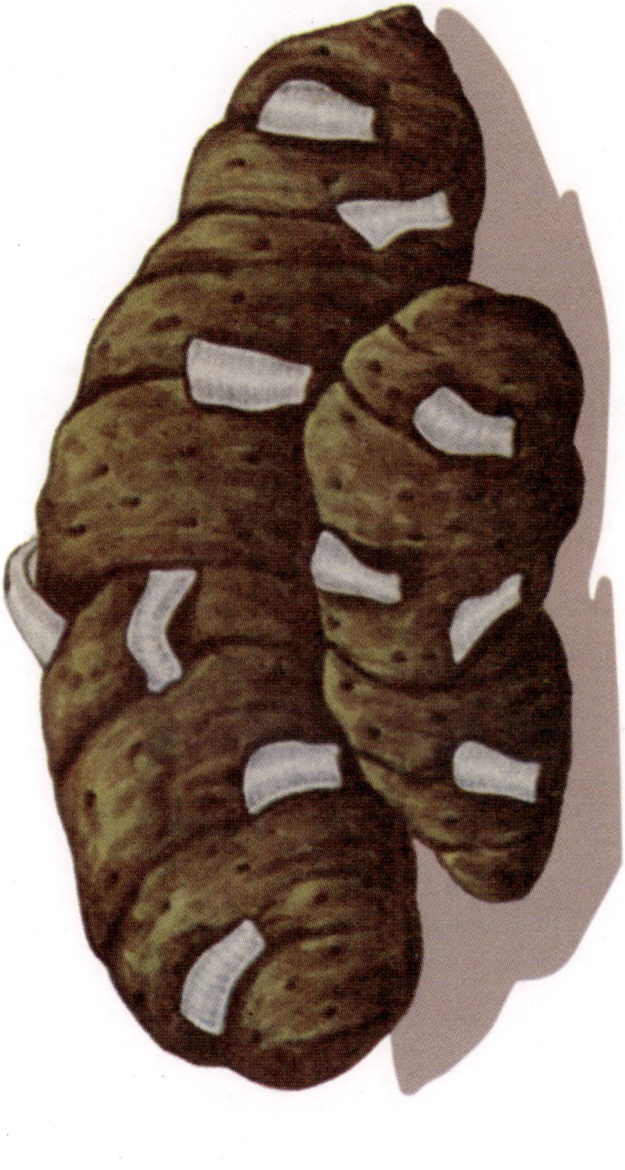

Whitish proglottides (segments) are seen in freshly passed stool. This is one of the most important criterion for diagnosis. After giving an effective anthelmintic, proglottides are passed. Stool examination is done repeatedly even upto 3 months following the course of the anthelmintic. Stool should be clear of proglottides. But the presence of proglottides in stool indicates either (a) failure of the drug, or (b) a fresh or repeated infection. In the latter instance, the source of infection should be traces; prophylactic measures should be taken.

Life cycle. *D. latum* requires 3 hosts to complete the life cycle (Fig. 10.10).

1. DEFINITIVE HOST is human or cat. 2. There are two INTERMEDIATE HOSTS, the primary being cyclops, and the secondary a **fresh-water fish**.

INFECTION IN HUMAN. A fully grown **plerocercoid** in fish flesh is 1.5 mm by 2 mm. It is infective to man when the fish is eaten insufficiently cooked. After ingestion of the fish, the plerocercoid containing the head of the future worm is liberated, and attaches itself to the intestinal wall. This then develops into an adult worm, which when discharges eggs in 6 weeks.

DEVELOPMENT OF EGGS. The egg develops in water within each egg-shell for 1 to 2 weeks and a spherical ciliated embryo with 3 pairs of hooklets, now called a ***coracidium***, comes out of the **operculated egg shell**, and swims about in water by means of cilia.

PRIMARY INTERMEDIATE HOST. The coracidium of *D. latum* is ingested by a small crustacean host, Cyclops or Diaptomus, and development takes place within these hosts. The free-swimming larva dies unless it finds its first intermediate host within 12 hours. Within the intestine of the crustacean host, the cilia are lost and the embryo finds its way into the body cavity of the host. After further development, it becomes a worm-like, **procercoid**, about 500μm in length and infective to the second host within three weeks. The primary intermediate hosts are *Cyclops strenuus* and *Diaptomus gracilis* in Europe, but in North America they are *Cyclops brevispinosus, C. prasinus* and *Diaptomus oregonensis*.

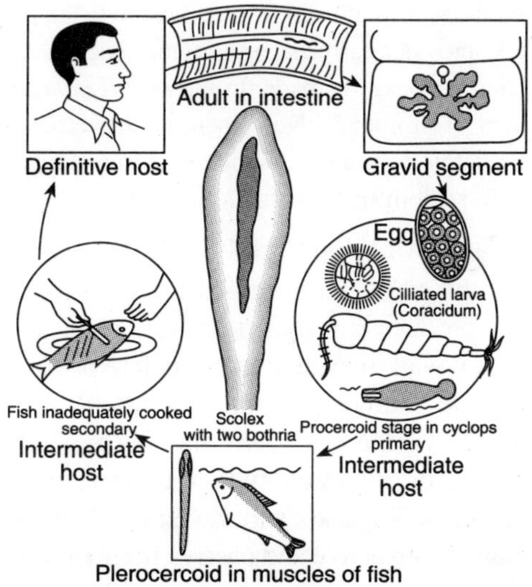

Fig. 10.10 Life cycle of *Diphyllobothrium latum*

SECONDARY INTERMEDIATE HOST. Various species of fresh-water fish act as the intermediate hosts. If an infected crustacean host is ingested by any of these fishes, the host is digested, and the larvae thus liberated, escape and bore their way through the intestinal wall of the fish, form plerocercoids, especially in the liver, muscles and mesentery of the fish. The plerocercoid larva is infective to the definitive host. It is to be noted that ***a single egg produces a single larva***, and ***plerocercoid represents the head of a future adult worm.***

Symptoms. Body weight may be lost to some extent in infection with *D. latum*. Indefinite nervous and digestive disorders, abdominal discomfort and pain resembling peptic ulcers may be present in *D. latum* infection within the first 6 months of infection. Macrocytic anaemia may develop later, and achlorhydria is often present.

Pathology. Usually a single worm is present but the attachment of the scolex to the mucous membrane causes irritation of the intestine. When the worm is high up in the jejunum, it absorbs vitamin B_{12} from the intestine and thus prevents its combination with the intrinsic factor. This results in **macrocytic anaemia.**

Epidemiology. TRANSMISSION of *D. latum* occurs by eating inadequately-cooked infected fresh-water fish.

VECTORS. Cyclops and fresh-water fish (see life cycle).

RESERVOIRS. Cats and dogs may be naturally infected, but man is the most important reservoir host. Incidence is high in Baltic countries and Russia, where the incidence may reach up to 50 per cent due to the practice of eating raw fish.

Laboratory diagnosis. 1. **Operculated eggs** are found in the faeces.

2. **Segments** passed are **broader than long** and can be identified by the presence of a brownish patch in the **middle of the segment**, where the **genital pores** are seen.

They are distinguished from *T. solium* and *T. saginata* by the absence of marginal genital pore.

Prophylaxis. This consists of: (1) proper disposal of faeces, (2) adequate cooling of fish, (3) survey and treatment of infected people in heavily infected areas, (4) fish inspection before sale, (5) freezing at 10°C for 24 hours, or thorough cooking, or proper drying and pickling which should kill the plerocercoid. A temperature of 50°C for a few minutes is lethal to the plerocercoid.

Treatment is same as that of *T. solium.*

SPARGANUM

Sparganum is the plerocercoid larval stage of unknown parentage of Diphyllobothrium, which has not been assigned to any particular genus.

SPARGANUM MANSONI Cobbold, 1882

(*Larval stage of Diphyllobothrium mansoni*)

THE DEFINITIVE HOSTS OF *D. mansoni* are the dogs and cats and the adult worm is found in their intestines.

PRIMARY INTERMEDIATE HOST. Cyclops in which the procercoid stage develops.

SECONDARY INTERMEDIATE HOST. Frogs, snakes, birds, etc., in which the plerocercoid stage (*Sparganum mansoni*) occurs.

Human is accidentally infected by:

(*a*) Drinking water contaminated by procercoid larvae in cyclops.

(*b*) The use of plerocercoid-infected frog tissue as a poultice for wounds or sore eyes, when plerocercoids are transferred to the human tissue.

(*c*) Ingesting the plerocercoids accidentally while handling infected frog fish.

SPARGANUM PROLIFERUM

(Ijima, 1905) Stiles, 1908

This is the plerocercoid stage of pseudophyllidean tapeworm producing encysted forms in large number in the subcutaneous tissues, intermuscular fasciae and internal organs, including the brain. So, the prognosis is grave in this infection.

Geographical distribution. China, Japan, Vietnam, Australia, Puerto Rico, etc.

Sparganum proliferum is flattened with anteroposterior polarity and near about 3 mm in length by 300μ in breadth. It is irregular in shape and shows branching of the body. The branching projections often get detached from the parent organism and develop into new larvae. Later they migrate into different tissues and form cysts. The procercoid stage occurs in cyclops, and plerocercoid (Sparganum) develops in man, when the infected cyclops are swallowed.

Diagnosis depends on finding of sparganum larvae from the subcutaneous cysts. Running of untreated sewage into fresh-water tanks may be a source of infection.

Preventive measures. In endemic areas all drinking water should be boiled or adequately filtered. The ingestion of raw tadpoles, frog, snake, fowl or mammalian flesh to be avoided. Poulticing of sparganum-affected ulcerated or inflamed areas of the skin, conjunctiva or vagina should be abstemiously avoided. According to Houdemer *et al* (1933), the unbranched sparganum may live more than nine years in the human host.

Treatment and Prognosis. In Vietnam, for ocular sparganosis Cornet (1933) recommended injection of 2 to 4 ml of 40 per cent *ethyl alcohol* with epinephrine-free *procaine* into the lesion to kill the worms *in situ.* This causes spontaneous absorption of the sparganum. Keller (1937) reported marked success from intravenous use of *novarsenobenzol* (300 to 450 mg per dose for adults, and 70 to 150 mg for children) every four or five days for 2 to 6 injections. *Tarsorrhaphy* has also been employed to preserve the cornea until the worms had been absorbed or discharged on the dressing. In *subcutaneous sparganosis*, which is the more frequent type of infection, commonly occurring on the anterior abdominal wall, and in which the worms are single or at most few, the prognosis is good, provided early diagnosis of the nodule and surgical excision *en masse* is made. In the *proliferating type*, on account of profound involvement of the tissues, except for palliative measures therapeusis is impracticable. The parasite seldom migrates and penetrates vital organs.

IMMUNITY IN TAENIASIS

As the adult taeniae are not tissue invaders and do not produce any significant lesion locally in the intestinal wall, they seldom stimulate production of detectable, humoral antibodies (Belding, 1942). Crude *T. saginata antigen* has been used in the treatment of infection with the respective worm (Machnicka-Roguska and Zweirx, 1966). Experimentally, both active and passive immunity has been produced in rats, cats, sheep and dogs (Belding, 1942). □

CHAPTER

11

CLASS: TREMATODA (Trematodea)

PHYLUM: PLATYHELMINTHES

Trematodea (Gr. *trematodes*—full of holes : Fr. *trema*—a hole; *eidos*—appearance) are commonly known as flukes. Species parasitic to man belong to the Subclass: Digenea.

Subclass: Monogenea. Species of the group inhibit only one host; they are ectoparasites of cold-blooded vertebrates, e.g., fishes, amphibians or reptiles and may inhibit the mouth cavities or urinary bladder of such hosts. They have a well developed adhesive organ at the posterior end with one or more suckers and chitinous hooks (anchors) as well. Only one or a few eggs are produced at a time, either laid in water, or attached to the host. A ciliated larva usually hatches out from the egg, and swims about to infect a host, or dies. The development is direct to adult form, and each egg, if successful, yields one fluke. There is *no alternation of generations* in their development, and no representative for human infection is known.

Subclass: Digenea. These flukes are internal parasites of man and animals. Each species has successive stages of development, which must live in certain organs of two or more hosts, in order to complete the life cycle. The larvae develop in certain snails as **intermediate host** and the adult stage is seen in some vertebrate hosts, the **definitive host**. Various species are peculiar to parts of the digestive tracts, lungs and urinary bladder. Some of them have two intermediate hosts to complete the life cycle before infecting human. Therefore, development takes place with **alternation of generations**. We are concerned with this subclass of medical importance.

ORDER: PROSOSTOMATA
Odhner, 1905

These are Digenea in which the mouth is surrounded by the anterior or oral sucker. All human trematodes belong to this order. They are divided into 3 sub-orders, namely *Strigeata, Distomata and Amphistomata*.

General characteristics. (1) Trematodes are unsegmented, **leaf-like** flatworms, but they may be cylindrical in exceptional cases, e.g., the female schistosoma.

(2) Their **size** vary from 1 cm to several centimeters in length.

(3) They have two **suckers** or muscular cup-shaped depressions; (a) one around the mouth called the *oral sucker*, and (b) another on the ventral surface of the body, the *ventral sucker* or the *acetabulum*.

(4) They are **hermaphrodites** or **monecious**, but schistosomes are **unisexual** (**diecious** or sexually distinct). The reproductive system is highly developed and the genital organs lie between the branching intestine.

(5) The **body cavity** is absent in them.

(6) The **alimentary canal** is present but incomplete; anus is absent.

(7) The **excretory system** consists of *flame cells* forming collecting tubules opening posteriorly into the excretory pore (Fig. 11.1, 11.2).

(8) **Eggs** are *operculated* except those of schistosomes which are *spined*. They are immature at the time of oviposition.

Morphology (Fig. 11.1). SUCKERS. Distomata have two suckers, an *oral* and a *ventral sucker*. In *amphistomata* the ventral sucker is placed at the posterior extremity of the worm, e.g., *Gastrodiscoides hominis* and *Watsonius watsoni*. In Heterophyes, a *third sucker* is present, which is called a *genital sucker*.

ALIMENTARY CANAL. The alimentary canal is incomplete and blind posteriorly; the anus is absent. Mouth begins from the centre of the oral sucker, which is anteriorly placed. The alimentary canal bifurcates behind the muscular pharynx into two blind tubes, each being called the *caecum*. They may be simple as in *C. sinensis*, branched as in *Fasciola hepatica*, or they may reunite to form a single caecum as in Schistosoma species.

THE NERVOUS SYSTEM. It consists of an oesophageal commissure, the brain of the organism. It is disposed like a saddle on the dorsum of the pharynx, or oesophagus. A main pair of nerve trunks from each of the saddle run anteriorly and posteriorly and are disposed in the dorsal, ventral and lateral aspects. In addition, there are special **ganglia** in the region of genital organs and special sensory nerve endings sensitive to light in the anterior part of the body, often referred to as **eye spots**.

EXCRETORY SYSTEM. It consists of bilaterally symmetrical excretory system with collecting tubules and capillaries terminating in minute vibratile ciliate structures called **flame cells**, as their cilia have a flickering movement like that of a candle flame. *Flame cells* are distributed all over the body. Form each flame cell a capillary arises. All the capillaries join to form a duct and terminate in the excretory bladder or *excretory vesicles*, at the posterior extremity of the body. The pattern of flame cells often provides the basis for species identification (Fig. 11.2).

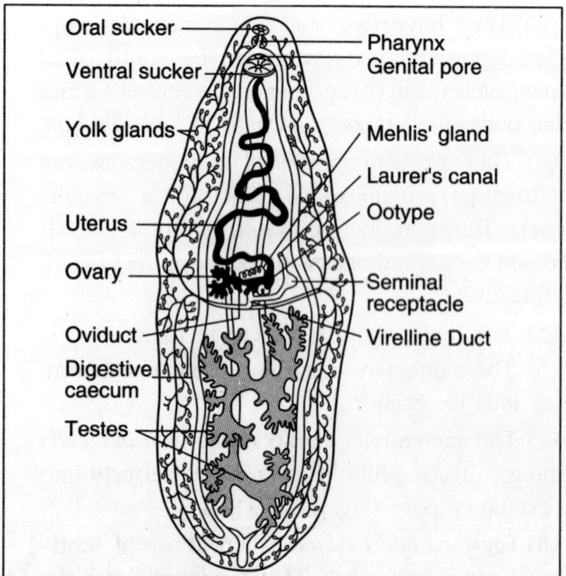

Fig. 11.1 Morphology of a Trematode

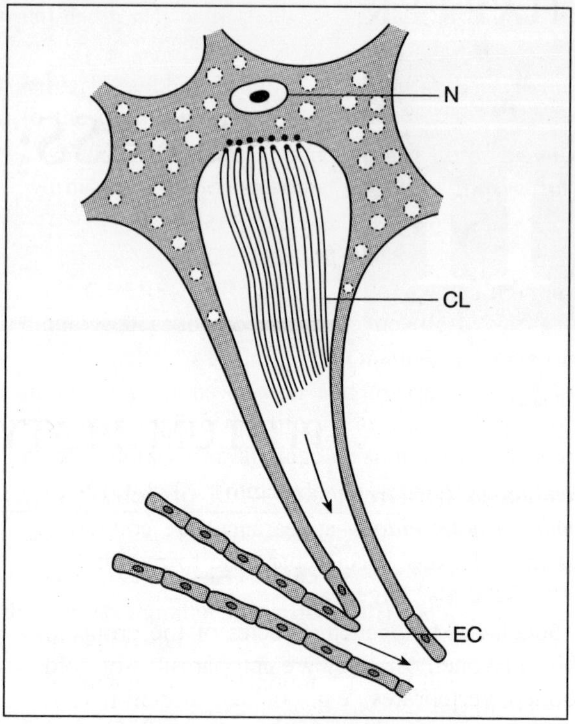

Fig. 11.2 Structure of a flame cell. N—Nucleus; CL—Leash of cilia; EC—Excretory capillaries draining into an excretory bladder

REPRODUCTIVE SYSTEM. Trematoda are hermaphrodites and contain male and female genital organs (Fig. 11.3).

Male genital system. These organs usually consist of two *testes*, but in Schistosoma they vary from four to eight. From each testis one *vas efferens* arises and join to form *vas deferens*, which passes forward to enter the *cirrus sac*, before opening into the common genital atrium adjacent to the ventral sucker. In the cirrus sac, *vas* leads to a *seminal vesicle*. A *cirrus*, the *copulatory organ*, is enclosed in a muscular *cirrus pouch*.

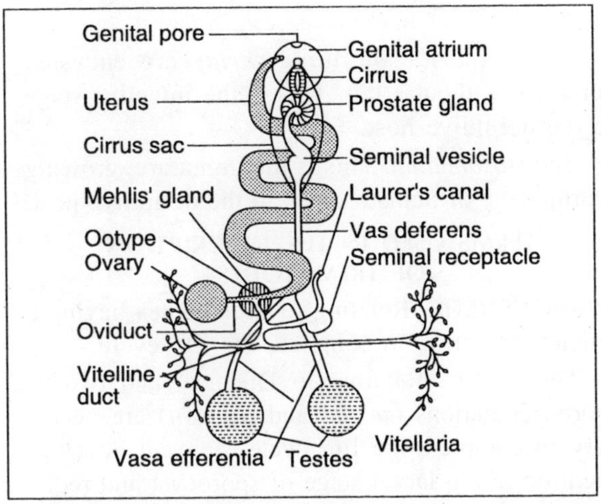

Fig. 11.3 Reproductive system of a Trematode

Female genital system. This consists of a single round or lobed *ovary* antetior to and smaller than testes, and its tube leads to the *oviduct*. The functionless **Laurer's canal** or the *vestigeal vagina* opens into the *seminal receptacle*, whose duct joins the oviduct. The Laurer's canal may open on the dorsal surface, when sperm may enter through it for a cross-fertilisation. The oviduct leads to the *ootype*, where ova are fertilised. Ootype is a muscular expansion continuous with the uterus and oviduct and surrounded by **Mehlis' gland** (shell gland). The *vitelline ducts* form a common duct, which opens into the oviduct. The *uterus* arises from the ootype and passes forward in a tortuous way and terminates by the side of the cirrus sac in the common genital atrium near the acetabulum.

Genital pore. Genital pore is very small. Vas deferens and uterus which are close to one another, open into the genital pore. Genital pore opens either anterior or posterior to the ventral sucker. It opens posterior to the ventral sucker in Paragonimus, Schistosoma, and Heterophyes. In Heterophyes, the genital pore is on one side of the midline.

Eggs. All the eggs are **operculated** except those of the genus Schistosoma (blood fluke), which are **spined.** In Fasciola and Paragonimus, eggs are fertilised and unsegmented, when passed. In Schistosoma and Clonorchis, the eggs, when passed contain miracidium. **They do not float in saturated solution of common salt.**

Developmental forms of eggs (Fig. 11.4).

Miracidium (Gr.—little boy). The ciliated larval stage of a trematode egg, which swims freely in water is infective to molluscan host.

Sporocyst. It is the intermediate (asexual) or second larval stage of the trematode occurring in the molluscan host, containing masses of germ cells. A second generation of asexual multiplication occurs only in Schistosomes at this stage, instead of the stage of redia, which is the usual next stage of development.

Redia. It is named after the Italian naturalist, Francesco Redi (1626-1698). It is the third larval stage occurring in the mollusc. These are produced

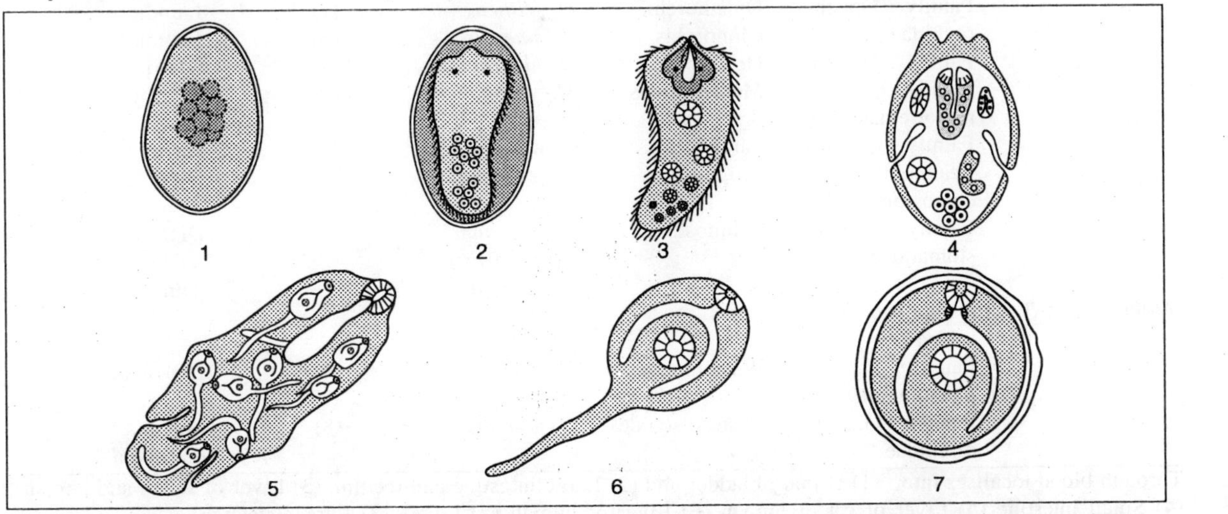

Fig. 11.4 DEVELOPMENT OF TREMATODE EGG 1. Operculated egg. 2. Embryonated egg. 3. Miracidium. 4. Sporocyst. 5. Redia containing cercariae. 6. Cercaria. 7. Metacercaria

parthenogenetically from cells in the sporocyst and come out by the rupture of a sporocyst.

Asexual multiplication occurs at this stage in all trematodes except the schistosomes, where the redia formation is absent. It is a vermiform structure with a blind gut and a genital pore.

Cercaria (Gr. *Keros*—tail). It is the fourth and the final larval stage, possessing a body and a tail. According to the nature of the tail, they are named as follows:

Furcocercus or fork-tailed *cercaria* as in Schistosomes.

Microcercus cercariae have short, stumpy rudimentary tails as in *Paragonimus westermani.*

Lophocercus cercariae have large fluted tail as in Clonorchis, Heterophyes and Metagonimus.

Pleurolophocercus cercariae have a long powerful tail and a pair of fin-folds as seen in Opisthorcis.

Metacercariae or *Adolescariae* are encysted cercariae without a tail. This is the infective stage to the definitive host.

Schistosomulum. This is the immature, growing worm-stage of Schistosomes in the definitive host.

TERMS USED IN THE DESCRIPTION OF TREMATODES

MONOGENETIC. Relating to Monogenea having a single generation to complete the life cycle.

DIGENETIC. Relating to Digenea, and two or more generations (*sexual* and *asexual*) are necessary to complete the life cycle. *Asexual* development occurs in larval stage of sporocyst and redia.

DISTOMATA. Trematodes possessing two suckers.

TABLE 11.1

CLASSIFICATION OF PATHOGENIC TREMATODES

Class: Trematoda; Subclass: Digenea; Order: Prosostomata: Sub-orders: Strigeata, Distomata, and Amphistomata

Sub-order	Superfamily and family	Genus	Species	Habitat	Clinical manifestations
STRIGEATA	Schistosomatoidea	Schistosoma	*S. haematobium*	(1)	Haematuria
	Family: Schistosomatidae		*S. mansoni*	(2)	Dysentery,
			S. japonicum	(2)	splenomegaly and cirrhosis of liver
DISTOMATA	Fascioloidea				
	Family : Fascioolidae	Fasciola	*F. hepatica*	(3)	Biliary colic
		Fasciolopsis	*F. buski*	(4)	Diarrhoea
	Opisthorchioidea				
	Family : Opisthorchidae	Opisthorchis	*O. felineus*	(5)	Jaundice
		Clonorchis	*C. sinensis*	(6)	Jaundice
	Family : Heterophyidae	Heterophyes	*H. heterophyes*	(4)	Diarrhoea
		Metagonimus	*M. yokogawai*	(4)	Diarrhoea
	Troglotrematoidea				
	Family : Troglotreamatidae	Paragonimus	*P. westermani*	(7)	Haemoptysis
		Troglotrema	*T. salmincola**	(4. 8)	Dysentery
	Echinostomatoidea				
	Family : Echinostomatidae	Echinostoma*	*E. ilocanum*	(4)	Diarrhoea, Abdominal pain
			E. lindoensis		
			E. revolutum		
AMPHISTOMATA	Paramphistomatoidea				
	Family : Paramphistomatidae	Watsonius*	*W. watsoni*	(4)	Diarrhoea
	Family : Gastrodiscoidae	Gastrodiscoides	*G. hominis*	(8)	Mucous diarrhoea

Through blood localises into : (1) Urinary bladder and (2) Large intestine and rectum. (3) Liver of sheep and human (4) Small intestine (5) Liver of cat or human (6) Liver of human (7) Lungs (8) Large intestine

* Rarely infects human

ACETABULUM (Lat. *acetum*—a venigar cruet). It is a cup-shaped, muscular organ of attachment and also called a ventral sucker.

GYNAECOPHORIC CANAL. A channel formed during copulation by infolding of the lateral margins of the body of the male to encircle the female.

The important order under Digenea is prosostomata, in which the ventral sucker is *subterminal*. The important species of Digenea parasitic to man are shown in Table 11.1.

MODES OF INFECTION. (a) Ingestion of encysted cercariae in:

(i) Vegetable; e.g., *F. hepatica*, *F. buski*, *W. watsoni*.

(ii) Fish; e.g., *C. sinensis*, *H. heterophyes*, *M. yokogawai*.

(iii) Carb or cary fish, e.g., *P. westermani*.

(b) Free cercariae with bifid tail penetrate through the skin, or the mucous membrane, e.g., *S. haematobium*, *S. mansoni*, *S. japonicum*.

On entering the definitive host, the young worms proceed to their site of localisation, where they grow into adult worms.

INTESTINAL FLUKES. On entering the digestive tract, they directly develop into adult worms, e.g., *E. ilocanum*, *F. buski*, *H. heterophyes*, *W. watsoni*, *G. hominis* and *M. yokogawai*.

LUNG AND LIVER FLUKES. Cercariae penetrate the intestinal wall and finally settle in their respective sites, e.g., *P. westermani* in the lung and *F. hepatica* in the liver. Some may enter directly through the bile duct into the liver, e.g., *C. sinensis*, *O. felineus*.

BLOOD FLUKES. Schistosoma cercariae pierce through the skin or mucous membrane and enter the blood stream and finally reach the vesical or haemorrhoidal plexus of blood vessels through the circulation.

CLASSIFICATION OF TREMATODA ACCORDING TO THE HABITAT

Blood flukes: *S. haematobium*, *S. mansoni*, *S. japonicum*.

Liver flukes: *F. hepatica*, *C. sinensis*, *C. endemicus*, *O. felineus*, *O. noverca*.

Intestinal flukes: *Fasciolopsis buksi*, *H. heterophyes*, *M. yokogawai*, *G. hominis*, *W. watsoni*, *E. ilocanum*.

Lung fluke: *P. westermani*.

SUBCLASS : *DIGENEA* Carus, 1863
(nec van Beneden, 1858)
ORDER : PROSOSTOMATA Odhner, 1905
SUBORDER : STRIGEATA La Rue, 1926
SUPERFAMILY : SCHISTOSOMATOIDEA
Stiles and Hassal, 1926

Schistosomes are unisexual; the females live in the gynaecophoric canal of male. Pharynx is absent. Intestinal caeca united posteriorly to form a single caecum. Eggs are spined or knobbed (*nonoperculated*) and parasitic while in circulation. *Redia stage is absent.*

GENUS : SCHISTOSOMA
Weinland, 1858
(*BLOOD FLUKES*)

ADULT WORMS are parasitic and are found especially in the lumen of small veins (venous plexus of the urinary bladder and rectum). Males are broader; lateral margins are folded ventrally to form gynaecophoric canal. Females are filiform, and longer than males (Table 11.2).

EGGS are spined and not operculated (Fig. 11.4).

THREE SPECIES ARE PATHOGENIC TO HUMAN

(1) *S. haematobium* (vesical schistosomiasis).

TABLE 11.2
DIFFERENCES BETWEEN MALE AND FEMALE SCHISTOSOMA

Male	Female
1. Cuticle—tubercular	Cuticle—not tubercular
2. Length—12.5 mm	Length—about 25 mm
3. Broad, leaf-like but ventrally folded like a tube (gynaecophoric canal)	Filiform in shape, often in the gynaecophoric canal

(2) *S. mansoni* (intestinal and visceral schistosomiasis).

(3) *S. japonicum* (intestinal and hepatic schistosomiasis).

Incidence. In highly endemic areas of Egypt, some parts of Africa and China, the incidence of schistosomiasis varies from 50 to 90 per cent in population; but in other parts, the incidence is low and infections relatively mild. It is commoner in males than in **females** and mostly found in the rural than in the **urban** areas. Workers in irrigated areas, like rice-fields, fishermen, or boatmen are

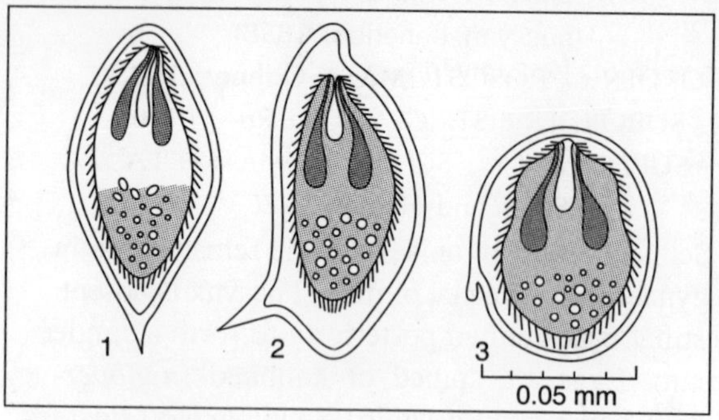

Fig. 11.5 Eggs of: 1. *S. haematobium* 2. *S. mansoni* 3. *S. japonicum*

infected. **Warm weather** and **sluggish streams** of water favour multiplication of snails, the **intermediate host**, with high infections rate. Sporadic cases are seen in Mumbai (Gadgil, 1968), India.

FAMILY : SCHISTOSOMATIDAE

SCHISTOSOMA HAEMATOBIUM

(Bilharz, 1852) Weinland, 1858

(*Vesical blood fluke producing bilharziasis*)

Geographical distribution. It is endemic in Egypt and some other parts of Africa, but sporadic in Arabia, Madagascar, Palestine and Iraq.

Habitat. Adult females usually live in the rectal and vesical venous plexuses, causing haemorrhage due to rupture of the venules in those parts.

Morphology. ADULTS. *Male.* It is 10 to 18 mm long by 1 mm broad. Sides are flattened and curved to form gynaecophoric canal, in which the long *filiform female* lies. The head of the male has 2 suckers. The body is rough and tubercular.

Female. It is filiform with pointed ends, about 20 mm long and 0.25 mm broad. It is smooth, except minute spines present at the sucker. It enters the gynaecophoric canal of the male during copulation. It then migrates to the smaller veins of the bladder and less commonly rectum, where eggs are laid.

Eggs. They are 112-170μm long and 40 to 70μm wide, oval or spindle-shaped with a terminal spine (Fig. 11.5). They are usually passed in urine and rarely in stool. Eggs are not operculated but **spined**.

Life cycle (Fig. 11.6). *S. haematobium* requires two hosts to complete the life cycle : 1. DEFINITIVE HOST, human. 2. INTERMEDIATE HOST, the snail.

For details of snails see molluscan hosts (Section III; PLATE 16.I; Table 15.1). These are *Bulinus truncatus* (*B. contortus*) in North Africa, *B.* (*Physopsis*) *africana* in Central Africa and *Planorbis dufourii* (*Planorbarius metidjensis*) in Morocco, Algiers, Portugal and Spain.

In the definitive host, the paired adult male and female pass *against the current of blood*, live in the vesical and rectal venous plexuses, and less commonly in the tributaries of portal veins, where the females lay eggs. Eggs are passed in the urine and less commonly in the stool. Eggs contain ciliated larvae called *miracidium*. They do not hatch out in urine unless diluted with water. When urine is diluted, there is imbibation of water and probably due to difference of osmotic pressure, the ciliated miracidium hatches out by rupture of the egg-shell. The miracidium swims about in water in search of intermediate host, a snail, which varies in different countries, such as ***Bulinus truncatus*** in Egypt. It is suspected to be ***Paludomus obsei*** var. ***philippi*** in Mumbai, where the disease is sporadic. In the absence of an intermediate host, they die in 24 hours. Embryos enter the intermediate host by penetrating its air sac or tentacle and lose their cilia. They migrate to the visceral mass and become a **sporocyst**. They multiply quickly, so that, within a month or so, visceral mass is filled with elongated tube-like **daughter sporocysts**, 25 to 50 in number. Unlike

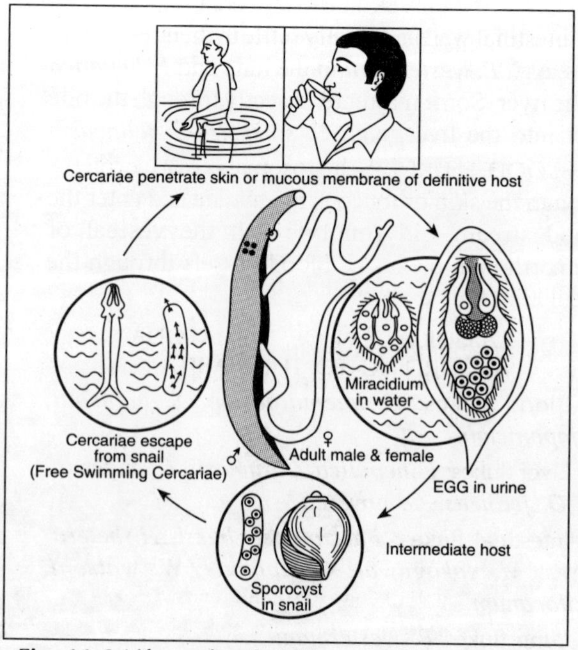

Fig. 11.6 Life cycle of *Schistosoma haematobium*

other trematodes, *rediae* are not produced and apharyngeal, *bifid-tailed cercariae* come out from the daughter sporocyst in the process of asexual reproduction, in 4-8 weeks. A single miracidium produces 100,000 to 250,000 cercariae (175 to 250μ by 35 to 50μm). They are phototactic and 50 to 100 emerge from the snail between 9 a.m. and 2 p.m., at an optimum temperature of 32°C to 33°C. No emergence occurs during a dark day. Their SPAN OF LIFE is 48 hours. The *cercariae* freely swim in water, as they require oxygen.

INFECTION IN HUMAN. Human is infected by wading, bathing and washing in infected water. The cercariae of *S. haematobium* penetrates the buccal mucosa, when man drinks infected water. As the water evaporates on the surface of the skin, cercariae penetrate the skin within 15 to 30 minutes. On entering the skin, they cast off their tail. By the action of the lytic ferment secreted by the penetration glands and their wriggling movement, the cercariae move till they enter venous circulation, or carried *via* lymph channels and reach the right heart. Through the lung they pass to the systemic circulation and then enter the portal vein through mesenteric artery and intestinal capillary bed. Those which do not reach the portal vein, die. By the 5th day after skin-penetration, young worms reach the portal vein. Once they reach the liver, they grow quickly and mature in 6 weeks. They pair and during copulation travel through the portal veins against the blood stream. The worms migrate *via* the inferior mesenteric vein, and haemorrhoidal and pudendal veins into the **vesical plexus**, where the female leaves the male and penetrates as far as possible into the venule. She lays eggs in 10 to 12 weeks. The venule contracts and thus holds the eggs in position, while the **spines of the eggs stick** *to the wall of the venule.*

Epidemiology. TRANSMISSION occurs by contact with water containing cercariae, which hatch out from the eggs. Water containing suitable vegetations and snails are polluted by faecal or urinary contaminations. Such water used for drinking, bathing, wading or agricultural purpose, etc. is the **source of infection**. The cercariae can penetrate the skin or mucous membrane with the help of the **lytic ferment**.

VECTORS. A large number of molluscan intermediate hosts are responsible vectors of schistosoma. These molluscan hosts belong to family BULINIDAE, e.g., *Bulinus trancatus*, *B. africana*, and *B. forskali* serve as reservoirs.

RESERVOIRS AND CARRIERS. Human is the most important reservoir host, but dogs, rats, cattle, cats and pigs may be naturally infected and serve as reservoirs.

Pathogenicity. The infection produces a condition of *bilharziasis* or *endemic haematuria* of Egypt.

Pathogenic effects. DUE TO ENTRANCE OF CERCARIAE. **Cercarial dermatitis** is produced with **pruritus** and **erythematous rash**.

DUE TO INVASION. Toxin liberated by the worm produces vague symptoms like anorexia, headache, generalised pain in the back and extremities, **rise of temperature** accompanied by rigor and **night sweat**.

ALLERGIC REACTION. Urticarial rash with localised oedema of the subcutaneous tissue is due to the passage of cercariae back to the skin when **eosinophilia** is **marked.**

DUE TO DEPOSITION OF EGGS. Eggs which are laid in vesical plexus pass to the mucous membrane of the bladder wherefrom they are voided in the urine. There is slight haematuria without pain at the end of micturition. The wall of the bladder shows papules with a red base, especially on the posterior wall. The mucous membrane is thickened and granular with congestion, catarrh and fibrous thickening of the wall. Many of these areas become calcified and give a **sandy patch** appearance.

Abscess formation and fibrosis, or **pseudotubercle**, formation around eggs, lodged in the perivascular tissue, are associated with inflammatory changes.

The inflammatory condition continues for months without subjective symptoms and is followed by **burning sensation** and **frequency** of micturition, with dull pain in the loin, suprapubic region, and colicky pain in the urinary bladder.

CHANGES IN THE URINARY BLADDER. **Papilloma** formation is usual and may be followed by **malignancy**. *Cystoscopy*. There is infiltration and hyperplasia of mucous membrane of urethra and base of the bladder. Papillomatous growth with **concretions** of **uric acid** and **oxalate** may be seen. Phosphatic stones may form with eggs which serve as nuclei.

ECTOPIC LESIONS. The **ectopic lesions** away from the site of primary infection are seen in case of heavy infection, when eggs and worms may escape into the pelvic veins and rectum, or carried to the lung *via* inferior vena cava, or to the liver *via* the portal system. By the *portal* or the *caval system* the eggs and adult worms may be carried to the distal parts of the body and cause lesions in the distal organs, like brain, skin and conjunctivae.

RECTUM. When rectum is involved, there is passage of blood and mucus simulating **dysentery**. The condition is, however, rare.

TABLE 11.3
SHOWING RESULTS OF CERCARIENHULLEN REACTION

Reaction	Symbolized		Findings
Negative *reaction*	(–)	:	If no envelope in 4-24 hours
(Doubtful) *reaction*	(±)	:	If a thin smooth membrane forms
Mild *reaction*	(+)	:	If a thin wrinkled membrane forms
Moderate *reaction*	(+) (+) to (+++)	:	If a discrete thick membrane forms
Strong *reaction*	(++++)	:	If a heavy loose membrane forms

CERCARIAL DERMATITIS. It is also known as **Swimmer's itch**. It occurs after a bath in infected water or due to the penetration of mammalian species of nonhuman cercariae of blood-flukes in the paddy field or avian cercariae after bath in salt water beaches, and a number of cercarial species are concerned with causing **dermatitis**. It is seen in Europe, the U.K., North America, Indonesia, India, New Zealand and elsewhere. The cercariae penetrate through the skin and when the skin dries, a pricking sensation is felt with erythematous macular, or **urticarial rash** persisting for several hours. After a lapse of 10-15 hours, **macules** are replaced by **papules** and the itching becomes intense for a few days. The papules persist for a week or so. In some cases, **vesicles** may occur after two or three days. In heavy infections in susceptible patients, there may be a generalised reaction with prostration.

Laboratory diagnosis. The DIRECT METHOD of diagnosis is established by finding of eggs: (i) in the **centrifuged deposit** of urine, or (ii) after removing vesical mucosa by a **cystoscopic biopsy** method. The excised, unfixed tissue is digested in a few ml of 4 per cent potassium hydroxide solution and the centrifuged deposit is examined for the presence of eggs. (iii) after hatching of **eggs** in warm water is a useful method. The water is previously heated to 60°C, to kill free-living potozoa and miracidia moving in water are sought for, through a beam of light (**miracidiascope**). Hatching confirms the presence of living eggs.

INDIRECT METHODS: **Serological** and **Immunological tests.**

They often show *group reaction* (common antigen for all species of schistosoma), and even nonhuman species of cercarial antigen may be used satisfactorily. These tests are applicable to all types of schistosomiasis.

The **Complement fixation** (CF) **test** is most widely used. **Fluorescent antibody** (FA) **test** is too sensitive. For routine use, two tests are desirable, namely, **Fairley's CF test**, and either the **Cholesterol-lecithin** (CL) **test** with undiluted serum, or the **Bentonite flocculation** (BF) **test** with a starting dilution of 1:5. The antigen used is a delipidised cercarial antigen. The CL test was adapted by Anderson (1960), and sensitivity and specificity were evaluated by Jackowski and Anderson (1961). Pellagrino (1964) tested 3,688 sera and found 90 percent sensitivity in parasitologically confirmed cases, but in the hand of Kagan *et al* (1962), only 77 percent cases showed sensitivity of the test. CL test cannot be performed with chylous or contaminated sera and to overcome this, (BF) test was improvised to give 70 per cent specificity. But it reacts with 15 per cent nonschistosomiasis sera as evaluated by Kagan (1968).

Trichina-positive antisera are positive with most schistosome tests.

SEROLOGICAL TEST

(i) **Fairley's complement fixation test** is group-specific. It is positive in early cases. For this, antigen is prepared by using an alcoholic extract of a snail liver infected with mammalian schistosome cercariae. It is helpful in the later part of incubation period and also in cases where eggs cannot be recovered.

IMMUNOLOGICAL TEST

(ii) **Miracidial immobilisation test** of Senterfit (1953), with development of pericercarial membrane around miracidia, and likewise around Schistosoma cercariae in (iii) **"Cercarienhullen reaktion** or **CHR"** of Vogel and Minning (1949) are useful and can be demonstrated using patient's serum. The CHR, as originally employed in *mansoni* infection, is equally applicable in case of *S. haematobium*. The test is specially applicable when eggs are not found in the stool, particularly in case of *S. mansoni* infection.

(iii) *Cercarienhullen reaktion* (CHR): Take a drop of cercarial suspension containing 30-50 organisms and 1 drop of antiserum (inactivated). Add a small drop of penicillin G sodium (400 units per ml) to prevent bacterial contamination in the chamber. Incubate for 4-24 hours at 22□C (cold incubator). The cercaria will be immobilised and surrounded by a membrane of precipitate, it antibodies are present in the serum.

(iv) Circumoval precipitin test of Oliver Gonzalez (1965) is quite specific. It was specially studied in *S. mansoni* cases, who were treated with fouadin (Table 11.4).

Circumoval precipitin test: It is more specific than the "CHR" for the species of schistosomes.

Take 1 drop of suspension of eggs (100 eggs) in 1.75 percent of saline; add 1 drop of 0.05 ml of serum which has been inactivated at 56°C for 30 minutes. Incubate at 37°C for 24 hours for recording percentage of ova showing *finger-like* shape of the precipitate with variable length.

TABLE 11.4
SHOWING RESULTS OF CIRCUMOVAL PRECIPITIN REACTION

Reaction	Findings
Weak	Precipitate length is 12.5μm or less
Moderate	Precipitate length is 25μm
Strong	Precipitate length is 37.5μm

(v) Globulin precipitation test of Sia-Wu becomes positive specially in *S. mansoni*, but it may be positive in other types of schistosomiasis (see Appendix I).

(vi) Intradermal test of Fairly and Williams (1927) is positive with cercarial antigen (see Appendix I).

(vii) Blood eosinophilia. Eosinophil count in peripheral blood may rise up to 50 per cent. Bilharziasis must be differentiated from renal calculus, anuria, oxaluria, filarial elephantiasis of colon and rectum.

Histopathologically, the nodules show eosinophils, monocytes and round cells with formation of giant cells. The nodules gradually disappear and are replaced by fibrous tissue. The centre may show degeneration and calcification with some eggs in it. The terminal spined eggs often erode or stick to the vessels of the urinary bladder producing haematuria.

Prophylaxis. ANTI-ORGANISM MEASURES. (1) Safe disposal of urine and faeces or their treatment to destroy the eggs.

(2) Chemoprophylaxis by mass treatment combined with control or elimination of snail vectors.

(3) Avoidance of cercarial contact.

ANTIVECTOR MEASURES. Eradication of snail vectors in endemic areas by removal of vegetations and by use of molluscocides.

PERSONAL PROPHYLAXIS. Avoidance of contact with infected water in endemic areas is rather impossible, but as far as possible, swimming, bathing, washing and wading in infected water should be avoided.

ANTIRESERVOIR MEASURES. Man is the only reservoir in case of *S. haematobium* and *S. mansoni*. Eradication of the disease in man by treatment is essential. The infected cases may be detected by intradermal tests, and treated. In case of *S. japonicum*, domestic animals and field mice are important reservoirs, so mass treatment is less effective in this case.

Treatment. CHEMOTHERAPY by trivalent antimony compounds (not pentavalent) are effective.

SODIUM ANTIMONY TARTRATE (tartar emetic) is administered intravenously in a freshly prepared 1 percent solution in distilled water or in 5 percent glucose solution on alternate days in graduated doses. *For adults*, start from 2 ml to a maximum dose of 8 or 10 ml and up to a total of 200 ml or 2 gm. A second course may be repeated if necessary. *Potassium antimony tartrate* is toxic, so, better not to use this.

FOUADIN (Stibophen B.P.; neoantimosan, Bayer) is indicated in all the three varieties of schistosomiasis. It is obtainable in 6.3 per cent solution and 1 ml of this solution contains 8.5 mg of trivalent antimony. This initial *adult dose* is 1.5 ml intramuscularly, which is gradually increased to 5 ml on alternate days to a total of 75 ml in 15 injections. *For children* 0.35 ml, per 10 kg body weight, gradually increased to 1 ml, is administered on alternate days. The drug is better tolerated, but less efficacious than sodium antimony tartrate in usual doses.

ANTHIOMALINE (*Lithium antimony thiomalate*). It is administered in daily doses of 2 ml containing 10 mg of stibophen up to a total of 66 ml. A maximum individual dose of 4 ml may be administered. The drug is entirely inadequate in doses usually administered.

T. W. Sb. (*Antimony dimercaptosuccinate*). The dose is 2 gm (containing 500 mg of Sb.) which is divided into equal daily doses for 4 or 5 days, preferably intramuscularly. It is effective in both urinary and intestinal schistosomiasis (*S. mansoni*).

MIRACIL D (Nilodon). It is a *thioxinate* derivative and proved to be of appreciable therapeutic effect in mice and rats experimentally infected with *S. mansoni*. It is obtained in 0.5 gm tablets. When administered orally in patients, in doses of 10-20 mg per kg body weight per day for one week, or a total dose of 60 mg per kg body weight in 3 to 6 days, it is effective against *S. haematobium* and *S. mansoni*, as found in Egypt. The daily dose may be administered in two doses, morning and evening. The drug is toxic, but effective specially in urinary schistosomiasis. The toxic effects are giddiness, nausea, abdominal pain, prostration, yellow colouration of the skin and sclerotics.

SCHISTOSOMA MANSONI

Sambon, 1907

(*Manson's blood fluke*)

Geographical distribution. Egypt, East Africa, Belgian Congo, West Africa, Madagascar and South America.

Habitat. Adult worms are found in haemorrhoidal plexus of man. Eggs are found in the faeces and rarely in urine; larval stages are seen in fresh-water snails.

Morphology. ADULTS are very similar to *S. haematobium*. **Male.** It measures 10 to 12 mm by 1 mm. The ventral sucker shows pronounced wart-like tuberculation. The alimentary canal bifurcates at the level of the ventral sucker. It has 8 to 9 small testes. **Female.** It measures 12 to 16 mm in length. Ovary is anterior to the middle of the body.

Eggs measure 140-180μ in length by 60 to 70μ in breadth, oval, with lateral spine. Eggs are passed in stool with blood and mucus and are rarely found in urine. Miracidium is fork-tailed and may rarely escape in the lumen of the bowel.

Life cycle. It is similar to that of *S. haematobium*. DEFINITIVE HOST is man. ADULT WORM lives in the veins of lower part of the large intestine; eggs are passed in stools. INTERMEDIATE HOSTS. They are fresh water snail of the genus Planorbis, e.g., *Biomphalaria alexandrina* and *Australorbis glabratus*. Miracidium enters these snails of the family Planorbididae, and develops into sporocytes and cercariae. Cercariae penetrate the unbroken skin of man and **schistosomulae** enter the portal circulation. From there, they are carried to the liver, where they feed upon the portal blood and develop into the adult stage. They migrate against the blood stream and reach the capillaries of the sigmoidorectal plexus *via* the inferior mesenteric vein. At this site, the female lays eggs (oviposition), which finally pass through faeces. They rarely enter into the venus plexus of the urinary bladder.

Symptoms and pathology. Symptoms and pathological changes by *S. mansoni* are caused by inflammatory changes in the intestinal wall due to the lodgement of eggs in the haemorrhoidal veins near the rectum, the liver and the spleen, producing two types of lesions—**intestinal** and **visceral** bilharziasis, and not vesical lesions as in *S. haematobium*. **Cercarial dermatitis**, at the time of infection, may occur at the site of penetration.

INCUBATION PERIOD varies from 4-10 weeks, at the later part of which there may be diarrhoea, likely to be of toxic or irritative origin, associated with fever, anorexia, abdominal pain, or urticaria and pulmonary symptoms. **Oviposition** in the radicles of the portal vein begins about 6 to 8 weeks after infection.

INTESTINAL BILHARZIASIS. *S. mansoni* produces localising symptoms like abdominal pain and symptoms of dysentery with passage of blood, mucus and pus in the stools, but haemorrhages may be more marked, and prolapse of the rectum may take place with occasional intussusception.

The eggs are lodged in the venules of the submucosa and they escape into the mucosa of the intestinal wall and the lumen of the gut. They produce sign of irritation like that of a foreign protein, associated with inflammatory changes. The irritation is characterised by the formation of pseudotubercles around the egg-emboli, and formation of nodules due to cellular infiltration and proliferation of connective tissue. These **pseudotubercles** may form small abscesses due to necrosis followed by ulceration. Thickening of the mucosa and epithelial hyperplasia are followed by the development of papilloma, which may undergo carcinomatous changes. The whole digestive tract may be affected, as the worms are found in the whole portal system. Rectum and sigmoid colon are the sites of greatest damage.

Characteristic **sandy patches** appear in the intestinal mucosa due to calcification of the areas where eggs are deposited. Portal and retroperitoneal lymph nodes are enlarged.

VISCERAL BILHARZIASIS. The visceral form of the disease affects the spleen and the liver (*Egyptian splenomegaly*). It is manifested by splenomegaly and *periportal cirrhosis* in 2 to 3 years, showing ascites, oedema and haematemesis and, thus, the condition may resemble **Banti's syndrome**. Other organs may be affected by the localisation of egg emboli. There is anaemia, asthenia and marked wasting and death; jaundice is unusual.

SPLENIC ENLARGEMENT in 'Egyptian splenomegaly' is not only due to infiltration with eggs, but mainly due to portal venous congestion.

LESIONS IN THE LUNGS may be seen at necropsy in 33 percent of cases and 10 percent death is due to such a complication. Lung complication is often due to embolism by ova diverted from female flukes. They appear to be more severe in South America than in Egypt.

Laboratory diagnosis. Diagnosis is based on the finding of **eggs in faeces**, but these are often scanty and *concentration method* may be needed in light infections by sedimentation or centrifuging in 0.5 percent glycerine or water. In patients with pulmonary complications, eggs of *S. mansoni*, at times, may be found in sputum (Meira, 1942). Hatching method may be resorted to. **Rectal or intestinal biopsy** may be resorted to in the diagnosis and in assessing the effect of treatment. **Liver biopsy** is used as an aid to diagnosis. **Serological tests** are positive and more applicable to this than in *S. haematobium* infection.

Prophylaxis and Treatment are same as those described in *S. haematobium*.

SCHISTOSOMA JAPONICUM Katsurada, 1904

(*The oriental blood fluke causing Katayama disease*)

Geographical distribution. Japan, China (Yangtze Valley), Taiwan, Philippines, Celebes, and Thailand.

Habitat. Adult worms are found in: (1) portal radicles particularly of superior mesenteric, gastric, or other veins, (2) mesenteric veins (the ileocaecal region is usually involved), (3) intrahepatic portion of portal venous system.

Eggs are found in the stools and are infective to fresh-water snails, e.g., Oncomelania, in which larval development takes place. Adult worms are also found in the cattle, pig, dog, cat and horse.

Morphology. ADULTS. **Male** is 20 mm in length by 0.4 to 0.5 mm in breadth. Body is non-tubercular. It possesses 6 to 7 testes in a single file. **Female** is 12 to 20 mm in length by 0.3 mm in breadth. Ovary is central in position.

Eggs. They are 70-195μ in length and 50-80μ in breadth; typical spines are absent. They are rounded with a lateral knob-like thickening, or tubercle. In absence of spine and due to their roundness and heavy daily output, the eggs tend to be widely scattered in the body.

Life cycle. It is like that of *S. haematobium* and *S. mansoni*. The eggs are passed in water, where the miracidium infects various fresh-water snails of the genus Oncomelania and forms delicate finger-like sporocysts, which produce about 50 or more daughter sporocysts. The cercariae penetrate the skin and mucous membrane of man. The schistosomulae of *S. japonicum* are carried to the liver as in case of *S. haematobium*, where they live for 5-6 weeks for their development. They become sexually mature in the intrahepatic portion of the portal venous plexus, or in lower part of the ileum, caecum and the ascending colon. The females lay eggs, which are gradually extruded in the lumen and are evacuated with faeces.

Pathogenicity. *S. japonicum* causes *Katayama disease* of the Far East, causing intestinal or hepatic schistosomiasis, like those produced by *S. mansoni*. The symptoms of diarrhoea and dysentery are due to irritation caused by the passage of ova through the mucous surface and the symptoms of dysentery are more pronounced in case of *S. mansoni*.

Pathology. The essential lesions are associated with the formation of pseudotubercles in the intestinal mucosa, 0.5 mm in diameter. The lesions in case of *S. japonicum* are higher in the intestinal canal, when compared with *S. mansoni*, which affects the lower part of the large intestine producing symptoms of dysentery. **Microscopically**, in the centre of the pseudotubercle, eggs are seen surrounded by giant cells or a plasmodial mass, infiltration with eosinophils, mononuclear cells, and fibrosis in the periphery. As the lesion becomes old, eosinophils are replaced by fibrosis. When the eggs cannot escape in later stage of the disease, they pass into the liver, which is heavily involved. The spleen is also involved as a result of foreign material, elaborated by the worm, The pigment results from breakdown of haemoglobin, the food of the parasite. Therefore, main symptoms are those of diarrhoea, dysentery, cirrhosis, and splenomegaly.

(1) **Lesions in the colon:** (a) Thickening of mucosa, (b) papillomatous proliferation in the caecum; the polypoid mass may lead to intussusception through the anus.

(2) **Lesions in mesenteric glands** may resemble those of tuberculous infection. Retroperitoneal glands may be enlarged.

TABLE 11.5
CHARACTERISTIC FEATURES OF THREE SPECIES OF SCHISTOSOMA

	S. haematobium	*S. mansoni*	*S. japonicum*
Geographical distribution	Africa to Iran	Africa, South America	Far East
Main habitat	Urinary bladder	Colon, rectum and portal radicles	Intestine, and portal venous system
Male:			
Size	10-18 mm by 1 mm	10-12 mm by 1 mm	10-20 mm by 0.4 mm
Cuticle	Tubercular	Markedly tubercular	Smooth
Reunion site of intestinal caeca in the body	In the middle	In the anterior half	In the posterior fourth
Testes	4-5, large	8-9, small	6-8, medium
Female:			
Size	20 mm	12-16 mm	12-20 mm
Position of ovary in the body	Posterior half	Anterior half	Middle part
Ova bears:	Terminal spine	Lateral spine	Lateral tubercle
Ova found in:	Urine, rarely in faeces	Faeces, rarely in urine	Faeces only
Number of ova (daily)	20 to 30	1 to 4	50 or more

(3) **Pulmonary lesions.** Embolism occurs by blockage of vessels by masses of eggs.

(4) **Hepatic lesions.** Liver is hypertrophic, nodular and shows periportal or clay-pipe-stem cirrhosis. **Pigmentation** of the liver is due to deposit of haematin in the Kupffer cells. Haematin pigment is derived from digestion of blood liberated by the adult worm by its alimentary canal. Pseudotubercles are formed in the liver due to the escape of eggs, found on digestion of the liver with KOH solution. The *spleen* is fibrous, and congested due to absorption of toxic byproducts. Eggs may be scanty. But there is widespread deposit of haematin pigment.

(5) **Appendices epiploicae** are thickened and matted together.

(6) The **urinary bladder** is usually unaffected.

(7) The **brain** may be affected; induration or granuloma formation may be caused by the irritation of the eggs in the cortex. The symptoms are, like those of Jacksonian epilepsy, hemiplegia, blindness, cranial nerve injuries. These appear 2 to 6 months after infection. Mental deterioration and abnormalities may be detected by electroencephalography.

Clinical features (1) **Stage of invasion.** Cercarial dermatitis is seen at the site of entrance of cercariae. Six weeks later, Katayama disease occurs with remittent or intermittent pyrexia with rigor, urticaria, hepatic and splenic tenderness, leucocytosis (30,000 to 50,000 per cmm) with high eosinophilia (30 to 70 per cent).

(2) **Stage of deposition of eggs.** *Localised symptoms*: dysentery with tenesmus, and sometimes choleraic diarrhoea is seen.

(3) **Terminal stage.** Massive abdominal tumour resembling carcinoma or hypertrophied papilloma may render prolapse through the anus. Infiltration of buttocks with eggs, formation of fistula, massive induration of hypertrophied organs like the liver may occur. Ascites, appendicitis and pneumonia may occur as a result of deposition of eggs in lungs.

Laboratory diagnosis, Prophylaxis and Treatment are the same as for *S. haematobium.*

SUBORDER: DISTOMATA Zeder, 1800

Definitive stage is hermaphroditic; oral and ventral suckers are present. Reproductive organs are mostly or completely posterior to ventral sucker; a pair of **flame cells** are present in the miracidium. Certain member of digenetic trematodes classified as "distomes" probably have originated from "monostome" ancestors, while others from "amphistomes". Thousands of species of Distomata are parasitic in vertebrate hosts. Human representatives have been dealt in this chapter. (For description of **flame cell see Section II, Helminthology; also Fig. 11.2**).

SUPERFAMILY: FASCIOLOIDEA (Stiles and Goldberger) Faust, 1929

General characters. DEFINITIVE HOSTS are animals and human. ADULT **worms** are found in the intestine and biliary passages of herbivorous animals, and the **immature** ones at oviposition with a conspicuous unsegmented ovum. In water, miracidium develops within the eggs having X type of pigmented eye spots.

INTERMEDIATE HOSTS are fresh water molluscs. The miracidium passes through the stages of **sporocysts** and two or more generations of **radiae**, and free-swimming **cercariae** are liberated. They encyst on vegetations or in fish, and, after ingestion of cysts, they cause infection to the definitive hosts, sheep, or human.

Two species infect human—*Fasciola hepatica* (**liver fluke**) and *Fasciolopsis buski* (**intestinal fluke**).

FAMILY: **FASCIOLIDAE**

FASCIOLA HEPATICA Linnaeus, 1958

Geographical distribution. Cosmopolitan

Habitat. The ADULT is a parasite of herbivorous animals, like sheep, goat and cattle, and lives in the biliary passage. It is occasionally found in the liver of man.

Morphology (Fig. 11.7). ADULT. It is a typical trematode, flat, oval, leaf-like in appearance and

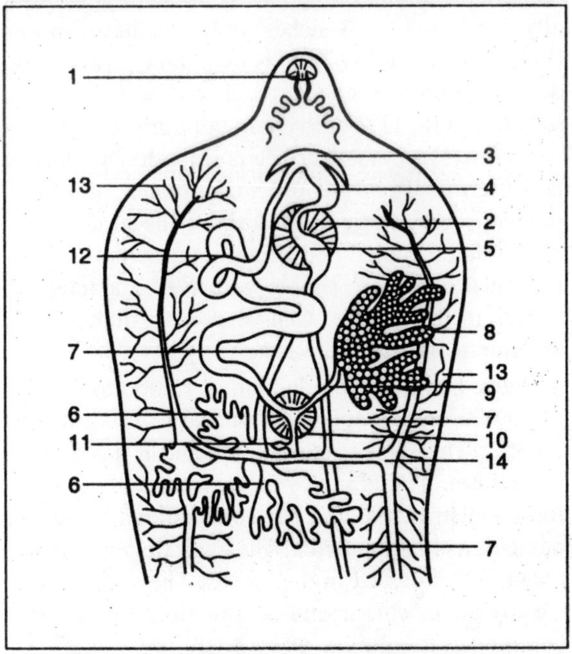

Fig. 11.7 Morphology of *Fasciola hepatica*
1. Oral sucker; 2. Ventral sucker; 3. Genital pore; 4. Cirrus pouch; 5. Seminal vesicle; 6. Testis; 7. Vas deferens; 8. Ovary; 9. Ovarian duct; 10. Shell gland; 11. Laurer's canal; 12. Uterus; 13. Vitelline gland; 14. Vitelline duct

brownish in colour; 3.5 cm in length by 1.2 cm in breadth. *Anteriorly*, it is characterised by a cone-shaped projection forming the **head** which carries the **oral sucker**, 1 mm in diameter. Its *constricted neck* is characteristic. **Acetabulum** (*ventral sucker*) is placed a little behind the anterior extremity and is larger than the oral sucker, being 1.6 mm in diameter. **Genital pore** opens immediately in front of the ventral sucker.

Eggs are operculated, 130 to 140μ in length and 80 to 90μ in breadth, brown and bile-stained. Each egg contains a large refractile, fertilised, unsegmented ovum, which lies in a mass of yolk granules. They can develop only in water, and **do not float in saturated solution of common salt.**

LIFE SPAN of the adult worm is 9-13 years in human, but it is about 5 years in sheep.

Life cycle. It occurs in two hosts. DEFINITIVE HOSTS are usually sheep, cattle and herbivorous animals, and rarely human. The adult worm lives in the biliary passage of these hosts.

Eggs are passed in stool along with bile from infected animal (sheep) or human. Inside the egg, the ciliated *miracidium* develops in about 2 to 3 weeks and the miracidium enters a suitable intermediate host.

INTERMEDIATE HOSTS are snails of the genus Lymnaea. In 2 to 6 weeks, the egg hatches out, a miracidium escapes in water, and enters into the snail. Inside the lymph spaces of snails the stages of **sporocyst**, two generations of *rediae* and *cercariae*, are completed in about 2 to 3 months. The mature cercariae emerge from the snail, swim around in water for a few hours and **encyst** as minute spherules (metacercariae) on aquatic vegetations, e.g., water-cress like *Nasturtium officinale*. They become infective to the definitive host (human or sheep) within 2 hours after encystment. The encysted cercariae or *metacercariae* are swallowed along with vegetables by herbivorous animals, and occasionally by human. Metacercariae excyst in the duodenum, migrate through the intestinal wall into the peritoneal cavity, penetrate the capsule of the liver, traverse its parenchyma, and ultimately settle in the biliary passage. They begin to liberate eggs in about 3 to 4 months.

Pathogenicity. IN SHEEP, it causes a fatal disease called "**liver rot**" with enlargement of the bile duct, cirrhosis of the liver and ascites.

IN HUMAN, it causes biliay colic, vomiting and diarrhoea. In Syria, it causes pharyngeal **fascioliasis**, colloquially known as "*halzoun*" i.e., suffocation due to swelling and congestion of pharynx from mechanical irritation.

Laboratory diagnosis. It is based on the finding of ova in stools. It is difficult, if not impossible, to distinguish ova of *Fasciola hepatica* from *Fasciolopsis buski*. Kamisaka (1930) stated that yolk granules of *F. hepatica* are clumped around the yolk cell nuclei. But in *F. buski*, they are equally distributed throughout the yolk cell. **Complement fixation test** is of doubtful value. If eggs are absent in stools, biliary drainage should be done to detect the eggs.

Prophylaxis. Sheep are the reservoirs. Therefore, eradication of the disease in sheep and herbivorous animals is one of the important measures to be adopted. Other measures are treatment of infected animals and destruction of molluscan hosts, as mentioned in *F. buski*.

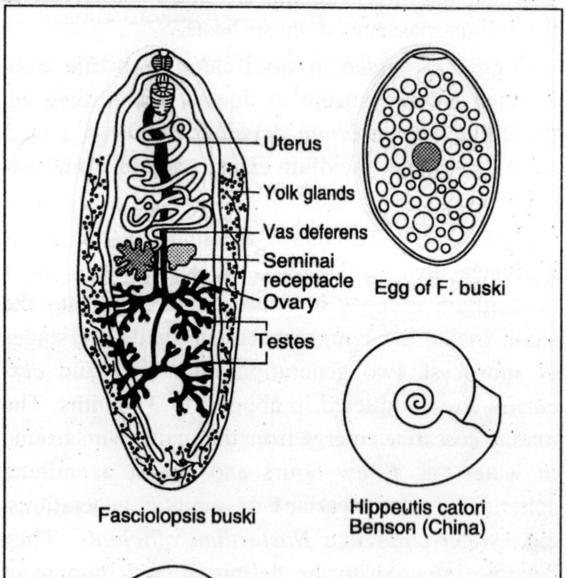

Fig. 11.8 Morphology and common intermediate snail hosts of *F. buski*

Treatment and **Prognosis**. In human infection, injections of **emetine hydrochloride** may show some beneficial results. A less toxic synthetic product **dehydroemetine** has been recommended (Lapierre, 1967). Prognosis is fair in light infection with less liver damage (see also **App. III**).

FAMILY: FASCIOLIDAE

FASCIOLOPSIS BUSKI

(Lankestar, 1857) Odhner, 1902

(*Giant intestinal fluke of man*)

Incidence. It varies from 5-50 percent of the population in the Far East.

Geographical distribution. Assam, Bengal, China, Taiwan, Indonesia, Vietnam, Thailand and other Far Eastern Countries.

Habitat. Adults are seen in the small intestine, specially doudenum of human and pigs. Eggs present in the faeces are infective to snails. The intermediate hosts are fresh-water snails of the genus Planorbis and Segmentina.

Morphology (Fig. 11.8). The ADULT is flesh coloured, flat and elongated; it varies in size, usually 5-7.5 cm (2 to 3 inches) in length and 12.5 mm (½ inch) in breadth; shape is oval. **Body**: The shoulder and anterior cone are absent (*c.f. Fasciola hepatica*; Fig. 11.7); covered with transverse spines ventrally. The dorsal surface is smooth. Oral sucker is subterminal and ventral. *Acetabulum* or **ventral sucker** is very large, 3 to 4 times the oral sucker. It is situated behind and adjacent to the oral sucker. **Intestinal caeca** are simple with two characteristic curves in the middle. **Genital pore** is immediately anterior to the ventral sucker.

Eggs. Daily egg production is 15,000 to 48,000, or 25,000 on average. Eggs are large 130-140μ by 80-85μ. The shell is clear, thick and it has a small operculum. The granules in the yolk cells are uniformly distributed, and not concentrated round the nucleus, as in *F. hepatica*. The eggs are not embryonated, when passed in the faeces. They are yellowish brown in colour and do not float in saturated common salt solution (**PL. Ap. II**).

LIFE SPAN is not more than 6 months in human.

Life cycle (Fig. 11.9). *F. buski* requires **two hosts** to complete the life cycle: 1. DEFINITIVE HOST is human, pig or dog. 2. INTERMEDIATE HOSTS are certain molluscan hosts of the genus Segmentina.

The *adult form* is found in the small intestine of man. Eggs are passed in the stool. Eggs hatch out to give ciliated miracidia in 2 to 3 weeks. They develop into sporocysts in 3 days and then into **radiae, daughter rediae** and **cercariae.**

Carcariae emerge from snails and metacercariae (encysted cercariae) are formed on the outer covering of water chestnut (*Trapa bicornis*). Infection of man occurs by ingestion of these raw, infected, water plants, where **encysted** cercariae are present. They pass through the stomach, become **excysted** in the duodenum and liberate young worms, which attach themselves to the wall of the intestine and develop into adult worms.

MORE IMPORTANT SNAIL HOSTS **(Fig. 11.8).** These are: ***Segmentina trochoideus*** in Assam, ***S. hemisphaerula*** in China, Taiwan and Japan, ***Hippeutis cantori*** (***S. schmackeri***) in China, and ***Gyraulus convexiusclus*** (***G. saigonensis***) in Vietnam, Philippines, Indonesia and India.

The PLANT HOSTS are water-chestnuts, namely, *Trapa bicornis* in India, *T. bospinosa* in Taiwan; *Eliocharis tuberosa* in South China and Taiwan; the water-caltrop *Trapa natans* in Canton, China; water-bamboo ***Zizania aquatica***, or water-hyacinth *Eichhornia crassipes* in Taiwan.

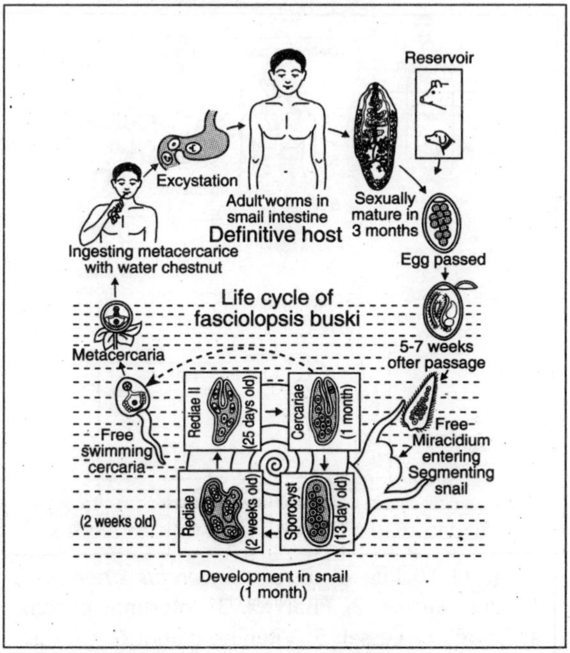

Fig. 11.9 Life cycle of *Fasciolopsis buski*

Epidemiology. Transmission occurs by the ingestion of metacercariae in fresh uncooked edible water plants. The infection is common due to peeling of the parasitised plant with teeth.

VECTORS. They are edible water plants like water caltrops, water chestnuts, which are most heavily infected, as they are grown in ponds and fertilised by night soil.

RESERVOIR HOSTS and CARRIERS are humens, pigs and dogs in Canton.

Clinical pathology. Blood. There is often leucocytosis with eosinophilia, up to 35 per cent. Occasionally there may be leucopenia with lymphocytosis.

Pathogenicity. The adult worm causes gastrointestinal irritation, nausea, vomiting, diarrhoea, ulcer; haemorrhage from bowels is common. General toxaemia and ascites may follow.

Laboratory diagnosis. It is based on the finding of:

(1) patient coming from an endemic area,

(2) adult worm in the stool after an anthelmintic or purgative. It is ***differentiated*** from ***F. hepatica*** by the absence of anterior cone in ***F. buski***. The eggs are passed in the stool and their differentiating ***features*** from those of ***F. hepatica*** have already been described.

Prophylaxis. ANTIORGANISM MEASURES. Prolonged storage of faeces or their treatment with quicklime will destroy the eggs in the night soil before it is disposed of as a fertiliser in the pond. Eggs, miracidia and cercariae in contaminated water are destroyed by quicklime 100 *parts per million* (100 p.p.m.) or copper sulphate (20 p.p.m.). Water plants (water chestnut) should be cooked or immersed in boiling water for a few minutes before consuming them. ANTIVECTOR MEASURES are based on destruction of snails by use of copper sulphate (20 p.p.m.) in ponds.

Treatment. Tetrachlorethylene, thymol, or hexylresorcinol acts specifically.

One should handle severely toxaemic cases very carefully, as death may result due to cardiac failure, following therapy.

Prognosis. The *prognosis* is good in the early diagnosed and lightly infected cases. The parasite disappears spontaneously within 6 months, if reinfection is avoided.

SUPERFAMILY: OPISTHORCHIOIDEA
Vogel, 1934 *emend.* Faust, 1949

ADULTS are medium or small-sized flukes, often spinose with poorly developed musculature with or without "eye spot" in adult stage; testes behind ovary;

cirrhus pouch lacking, metraterm and ejaculatory duct unite to form the common genital tract.

Eggs are small, thick-shelled, operculated. Miracidia are fully developed when oviposition occurs, but hatch only following ingestion by appropriate mollusc of the genus Melania and Bythinia. Cercariae develop in simple rediae without ambulatory appendages; pleurolophocercous or parapleurolophocercous "eye spots" and rudimentary acetabula, but without stylets and having 2 or 3 rows of short, hook-like spines above the mouth. Cercariae encyst in fishes; metacercariae are the sources of infection for the final host. Adults are found in the intestine and biliary tract of human, dog, cat etc.

Two families are known: (1) Family: Opisthorchiidae and (2) Family: Heterophyidae.

FAMILY: **OPISTHORCHIIDAE**

These are medium-sized flukes living in the biliary passages of man and fish-eating animals. The parasites of man belong to two genera, namely:

1. Genus Clonorchis—*C. sinensis*
2. Genus Opisthorchis—*O. felineus*

SUPERFAMILY: *OPISTHORCHIOIDEA*

FAMILY: *OPISTHORCHIIDAE*

CLONORCHIS SINENSIS

(Cobbold, 1875) Looss, 1907

SYNONYMS: *Clonorchis endemicus* Baelz, 1883; Chinese liver fluke.

Geographical distribution. Far East, *viz.*, China, Japan, Korea, Taiwan, Indonesia.

Incidence. It is related to eating raw fish. In south China, eggs of *C. sinensis* are found in the stools of over 10 per cent of the population. In Central China 75 to 100 per cent cats and dogs are infected, but incidence of human infection is low. In Japan, human infection is 6 to 40 per cent. The incidence is found to increase with age.

Habitat. Adults are found in the biliary tract of man, cat, dog, pig, rat, mouse, camel. Eggs are found in stools, and infective to snails.

Morphology. (Fig. 11.10). This is a medium-sized, elongated, flat, worm, infecting bile ducts of human, cat, dog, etc., causing obstructive symptoms. ADULT is 2 cm in length and 2 to 6 mm in breadth; cuticle is smooth without spine. The *oral sucker* is at the anterior end. The *ventral sucker* is little smaller than the oral sucker and situated at the junction of the anterior and middle third of the body. *Intestinal caeca* are simple and not branched, *testes* branched and lie in the posterior part of the body in the midline. *Genital pore* opens immediately in front of the ventral sucker.

Eggs. The fertile eggs are *yellowish brown* in colour due to staining with bile. They are operculated and possess a terminal hook-like spine at the abopercular end. They are ovoid but slightly narrowed where the operculum rests on a well-developed ring, and thus resembling an electric bulb.

They measure 27-35μm by 12-20μm, or 29μm by 16μm on average. The eggs are fully embryonated when discharged into the bile duct. The miracidium is asymmetrically organised in the egg. The eggs do not hatch out in water. They only hatch out after ingestion by the molluscan host. They do not float on saturated solution of common salt. Two types of infertile eggs may be passed without miracidium: (a) operculated eggs by young and old worms often passed after administering anthelmintics; (b) non-operculated eggs may be passed throughout of *Opisthorchis felineus* and *Heterophyes heterophyes*.

LIFE SPAN in man is 15 to 20 years.

Life cycle (Fig. 11.10). *C. sinensis* requires three hosts to complete the life cycle: 1. DEFINITIVE HOST is human, dog, cat, or pig. 2. INTERMEDIATE HOSTS:

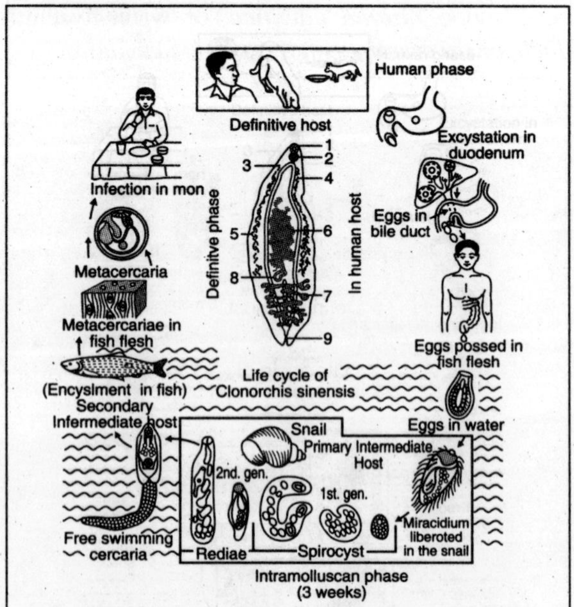

Fig. 11.10 Life cycle of *Clonorchis sinensis*. 1. Oral sucker. 2. Pharynx. 3. Intestinal caeca. 4. Excretory vessel. 5. Vitelline gland. 6. Uterus. 7. Testis. 8. Ovary. 9. Excretory vesicle

Primary—snail; Secondary—cyprinoids or other fishes.

PRIMARY INTERMEDIATE SNAIL HOSTS. They are of different species, namely, ***Parafossarulus manchouricus*** and ***P. manchouricus*** var. ***sinensis*** in China, Taiwan, Vietnam, Korea, Japan; ***Bulimus (Bithynia) fuchsianus*** in South China; and ***Alo inma longicornis*** and ***Hua ningpoensis*** in China.

Operculated egg passed in the stool contains a *miracidium*. The eggs containing the miracidia are ingested by, or they passively pass into, the **first intermediate host**, a *fresh-water snail*, where *miracidia* are liberated.

The **miracidium**, which is asymmetrically organised in the egg, hatches out in the midgut of the snail, penetrates its intestinal wall and escapes into vascular spaces, where it undergoes developmental stages as **sporocyst** (1st *generation*), **rediae** (2nd *generation*), and ***lophotrichus*** **cercariae** with *eye spots* and the *penetration glands*. They are liberated from the snail host in about three weeks. The free-swimming mature cercariae escape into water and, after a brief period of *free-swimming life* for 32 to 48 hours, it finds its **second intermediate host**, a *cyprinoid* or other fresh-water fish. The cercariae discard their tails and **encyst** in the scale or flesh of the fish. In South China, raw fish is considered to be a great delicacy by the epicures. When raw fish is ingested, the encysted metacercariae are ingested with raw fish by the definitive hosts and they **excyst** in the duodenum. The liberated **adolescariae** attach themselves in the region of the common bile duct. They enter through the biliary passage, make their way into the *ampulla of Vater*. They then migrate to the distal biliary passages, settle soon in the liver and attain maturity to adult worms in about a month's time and begin to pass eggs. Each adult worm passes 2,400 eggs daily.

Epidemiology. Infection takes place by eating uncooked fresh-water fish. The disease is prevalent more in South than in North China, depending on the habits of people ingesting raw, salted or pickled fish.

VECTORS. Fish cultivated in ponds (fresh-water) are vectors, as these ponds are contaminated with night soil.

RESERVOIR AND CARRIERS are dogs, cats, and pigs.

Pathogenesis and Pathology. The infection causes lesions producing a condition of clonorchiasis. The migration of the immature worm along the bile duct causes trauma to the bile duct epithelium by their suckers. The larvae of *C. sinensis* reach the distal bile ducts and as they mature, they initiate proliferation of an inflammatory reaction in the biliary epithelium with which they come in contact. This is followed by encapsulating fibrosis of the duct. Single exposure is of little clinical significance; whereas, repeated exposures provoke general involvements of the organ, when the lesions gradually extend to the larger ducts and gall bladder. Thus, after years of infection, there is an increasing tendency to pressure necrosis and **periportal cirrhosis**. The liver is enlarged and shows vesicle formation with thickening of the wall of the bile duct, containing the adult worms. The lesions are limited to the lobes of the liver. Twenty to 200 adult worms may be present on an average intensity of infection, but in heavy infections about 20,000 flukes may be present in the liver. The worm derives its nutrition from protein and glucose in blood in the peribiliary plexus and also from the mucus secreted by the epithelial cells. The adult worm cannot reach the gall bladder unless the cystic duct is dilated. Once it enters the gall bladder, it dies.

Symptoms. Mild infection does not show any symptom. Heavy infestation of the liver with *C. sinensis* causes chronic diarrhoea. There may be tenderness and enlargement of the liver, with oedema of the feet, ascites and general wasting. Recurrent jaundice due to the obstruction of the bile duct is sometimes present. The worm causes blocking of the biliary passage, and stagnation of bile favours cholangitis and bacterial infection, which causes death of the worm.

Complications like cholangitis, intrahepatic calculi formation and carcinoma may develop late in the disease; they are localised in their pathogenesis but may arise eventually to affect the whole liver. **Calculi formation** in intrahepatic bile ducts and associated clonorchiasis were found by Hou (1955).

Teoh (1963) reported eight out of 42 cases of **recurrent pyogenic cholangitis** in which there were inclusions of clonorchis ova as well as the adult flukes within the gall stones. Japanese investigators have also reported clonorchis and other parasites in calculi (Yamagata and Yaegashi, 1984). McFadzean and Yeung (1965) have described a group of cases of rare **acute suppurative cholangitis**. **Recurrent pyogenic cholangitis** have been reported in Hong Kong (Cook *et al*, 1954-55: Digby, 1930; Fung, 1961; Ong, 1962, Stock and Fung, 1962).

Acute pancreatitis has been reported as a complication of clonorchiasis in Hong Kong by McFadzean and Yeung (1966). and Clan and Teoh (1967). **Carcinoma of the liver** is often found in association with clonorchiasis in Hong Kong. Clonorchiasis has been strongly suggested to be an aetiologic factor particularly in **cholangiocarcinoma** (Ch'in *et al*, 1955).

Diagnosis. It is confirmed by finding of eggs in stools, which can hardly be differentiated from those of *H. heterophyes* and *O. felineus*. **Blood examination** shows: leucocytosis with marked eosinophilia up to 40 per cent. **Immunological intradermal test** (Chung *et al*, 1955, and Sawada *et al*, 1964), or **serological tests**, like *complement fixation* (Ruji, 1921), or *indirect haemagglutination* (Pacheco *et al*, 1960), and *precipitation reactions* (Yamagata and Yaegashi, 1964) are hardly necessary for diagnosis.

Prophylaxis. I. ANTI-ORGANISM MEASURES are: (1) Cooking of fresh-water fish, before eating. (2) Eggs die in putrifying faeces at 26°C in 48 hours. (3) Ammonium sulphate (one part of 0.7 per cent solution in 10 parts of faeces) kills the eggs in 30 minutes. (4) Eradication of snail host by molluscocides might injure the fish as well. (5) Prevention of pollution of water by human night soil or with faeces of reservoir hosts.

II. ADMINISTRATIVE MEASURES. (1) Serving of raw, inadequately cooked, dried, or pickled fresh-water fish should be prevented by legislation.

III. ANTIRESERVOIR MEASURES. Uncooked fish should not be fed to cat, dog and pigs.

Treatment. Injections of **sodium antimony tartrate** or tartar emetic 60 mg on the first day and then 120 mg on every alternate day I.V. up to a total dose of 1.3 to 1.8 g, alternately with arsphenamine, has either stopped the passage of eggs in stools, or this may be greatly effective in reducing the number of worms in the biliary passage and egg output in the faeces.

Chloroquin in daily doses of; 10.4 mg of chloroquin base daily per kg body weight for a period of 39 days has been recommended by Chung *et al*, (1955). The total dose may vary from 19.5 to 39 g.

Gentian violet (*Medicinal*). It is administered in keratin coated pills in doses of 0.06 g (60 mg) thrice daily before meals for one month. It cures the condition in early cases. It can be administered in 1 per cent solution in doses of 20 ml intravenously till a total dose of 6 g is reached.

At present, the use of **dithiazanine** *iodine* has been more effective (Komiya, 1966; Yamaguchi *et al*, 1962). **Hexachloroparaxylol** has been used with encouraging results (Chung *et al*, 1965; Kọmiya, 1966; Liu *et al*, 1965). Similarly, **hexachlorethane bentonite** has been found promising (Huang and McFadzean, 1965). **Hetol** (1, 4-bistrichloromethylbenzol) of Hoechst Pharmaceuticals is now being used and may emerge as superior to other remedies, if its toxicity proves to be low (Cho *et al*, 1966).

SUPERFAMILY: *OPISTHORCHIOIDEA*

FAMILY: OPISTHORCHIIDAE

OPISTHORCHIS FELINEUS

(Revolta, 1884) Blanchard, 1895

(*Cat liver fluke producing opisthorchiasis*)

Geographical distribution, Habitat and Epidemiology. *Opisthorchis felineus* inhabits the distal biliary and pancreatic tracts of cats, dogs, foxes and pigs in the Far East and Eastern Europe including Prussia (eastern part of Germany), Poland and Siberia, and Vietnam. Human is only accidentally infected by consuming raw fish. According to Chandler, 60 per cent cats were found to be infected in India; human cases were also found in India.

Morphology. It is a flat elongated, lanceolate fluke, 7 to 17 mm by 1.5 to 3 mm in diameter. The *anterior* end is tapering, and the *posterior* end is rounded. The *testes* are not branched. The *ovary* is slightly lobulated. Yolk glands lie in the middle third of the body. The shoulder at the margin of the opercular cap is not pronounced.

Egg is oval, slender, opeculated, measuring 30 by 11μm and has narrow and tapering ends. The egg is yellowish brown and contains an asymmetrical miracidium when passed in faeces.

LIFE SPAN is probably short.

Life cycle. It is like that of *C. sinensis*. PRIMARY INTERMEDIATE HOST is a snail *Bulimus tentaculate* or *Bythinia leachi* and the SECONDARY INTERMEDIATE HOSTS are fresh-water *cyprinoids*, like *Cyprinus carpio*, *Idus melantous*, or *Tinca tinca*.

DEFINITIVE HOSTS other than human, are dogs, cats, foxes and pigs. They act as RESERVOIR HOSTS.

Epidemiology. Transmission occurs by eating uncooked fish.

VECTORS are snail hosts and cyprinoid fish.

Pathology, Prevention and Treatment are like those of *C. sinensis*.

Harinasuta and Bunnag has obtained good results by administering **Hetol** (1, 4-bis-trichloromethylbenzol) in experimental hamsters. Also, they claimed that in human infection, the ova had disappeared in 3 weeks.

SUPERFAMILY: *OPISTHORCHIOIDEA*

FAMILY: HETEROPHYIDAE

These trematodes are small, egg-shaped parasites of the intestinal tract of fish-eating humans and animals like cats and dogs. They have rounded or slightly lobed ovary and testes; ovary is anterior to testes which are placed, side by side or obliquely, one behind the other. Genital sucker is present or absent.

There are two species parasitic to human: (1) *Heterophyes heterophyes*, (2) *Metagonimus yokogawai*.

HETEROPHYES HETEROPHYES

(Siebold, 1852) Stiles and Hassall, 1900

(*Chinese, Japanese and Egyptian intestinal flukes*)

Geographical distribution. Egypt, Japan, and China.

Habitat. Adults are found in the small intestine of man, dog, fox, cat and other definitive hosts. They also act as reservoir hosts.

Morphology. The ADULT fluke is minute (1 to 2 mm by 0.3 mm). It is greyish in colour, oval and spinous. It has 3 suckers: an *oral sucker*, *ventral sucker* near the middle of the body, and a *genital sucker* around the *genital pore*, posterior and lateral to the ventral sucker.

Eggs. The eggs are operculate and fully embryonated at oviposition, light brown, thick-shelled, measuring 29μm by 16μ and should be differentiated from those of Clonorchis by their broad ends, indistinct opercular shoulders and less well-developed posterior spine. The eggs are difficult to differentiate from these of ***M. yokogawai*** **(another intestinal fluke).**

Life cycle. *H. heterophyes* requires three hosts to complete the life cycle:

1. DEFINITIVE HOST is human, fox and cat.

2. INTERMEDIATE HOSTS. PRIMARY INTERMEDIATE HOST is a molluscan host, a marine or brackish-water snail, *Pironella conica* in Egypt and *Cerithidea cingulata* in Japan. The **free miracidium** passes through the stage of **sporocyst** within snail tissue developing into **rediae** for one or two generations, which ultimately lead to the stage of **cercariae**. The cercaria leaves the snail and becomes an **encysted metacercaria** in between the scales or flesh of the susceptible fish, the SECONDARY INTERMEDIATE HOSTS. These are brackish-water mullets *Mugil cephalus* and *Tilapia nilotica* in Egypt, and *Mugil japonicus* and Acanthoglobius species in Japan. Infection occurs by ingestion of infected raw mullets.

Pathogenicity. The infection with *H. heterophyes* causes heterophyasis in human. The worm lives in the **intestinal canal** and may cause *colicky pain* and *mucous diarrhoea*. At times the worm may be encysted in the tissue and eggs; in such cases eggs are not excreted in the faeces, but carried by lymphatics or blood, producing unusual manifestations.

Diagnosis. It is based on the finding of the eggs or adults in the stool.

Prophylaxis. It is prevented by avoiding eating raw or uncooked fish (mullets) in endemic areas.

Treatment. Tetrachlorethylene, hexylresorcinol or **bephenium hydroxynaphthoate** is given as in hookworm infestation with good results.

SUPERFAMILY: OPISTHORCHIOIDEA

FAMILY: HETEROPHYIDAE

METAGONIMUS YOKOGAWAI

Katsurada, 1912

Geographical distribution. Korea and Japan, Taiwan, China, Egypt and Bulkan states. *M. yokogawai* was the first species of Heterophyidae to be found in the Orient; it was discovered by Yokogawa in 1911 (Yokogawa, 1912) in the gills, scales and muscles of fresh-water fish in Taiwan.

Habitat. Small intestine of human and other definitive hosts like pigs, dogs, cats and the pelican bird.

Morphology. The ADULT is 1 to 2.5 mm in length and 0.4 to 0.75 mm in breadth.

Eggs measure 28μm by 16μm; oval, and operculated.

Life cycle. The worm requires three hosts to complete the life cycle.

1. DEFINITIVE HOSTS are human, pig, dog, cat, etc.
2. TWO INTERMEDIATE HOSTS are snails of the species Melania in which the miracidium passes through the stage of **sporocyst** and two generations of **rediae**. The **lophocercus cercariae** emerge from the snail. The SECONDARY INTERMEDIATE HOSTS are: fresh-water fish, *Plectoglossus altivelis*; a *salmonoid fish*, or a *cyprinoid fish*. In the flesh of the fish, cercariae are **encysted**. Infection of the definitive host occurs by ingestion of raw fish, containing the encysted cercariae.

Pathogenicity. *M. yokogawai* causes metagonimiasis associated with **mild diarrhoea.**

Diagnosis depends on the finding of characteristic eggs in the stool.

Treatment. It is same as that of *H. heterophyes* and ensures good prognosis.

SUPERFAMILY: TROGLOTREMATOIDEA

Faust, 1929 *emend.* 1937

These trematodes are of small to medium size and possess integumentary spines. The genital pore

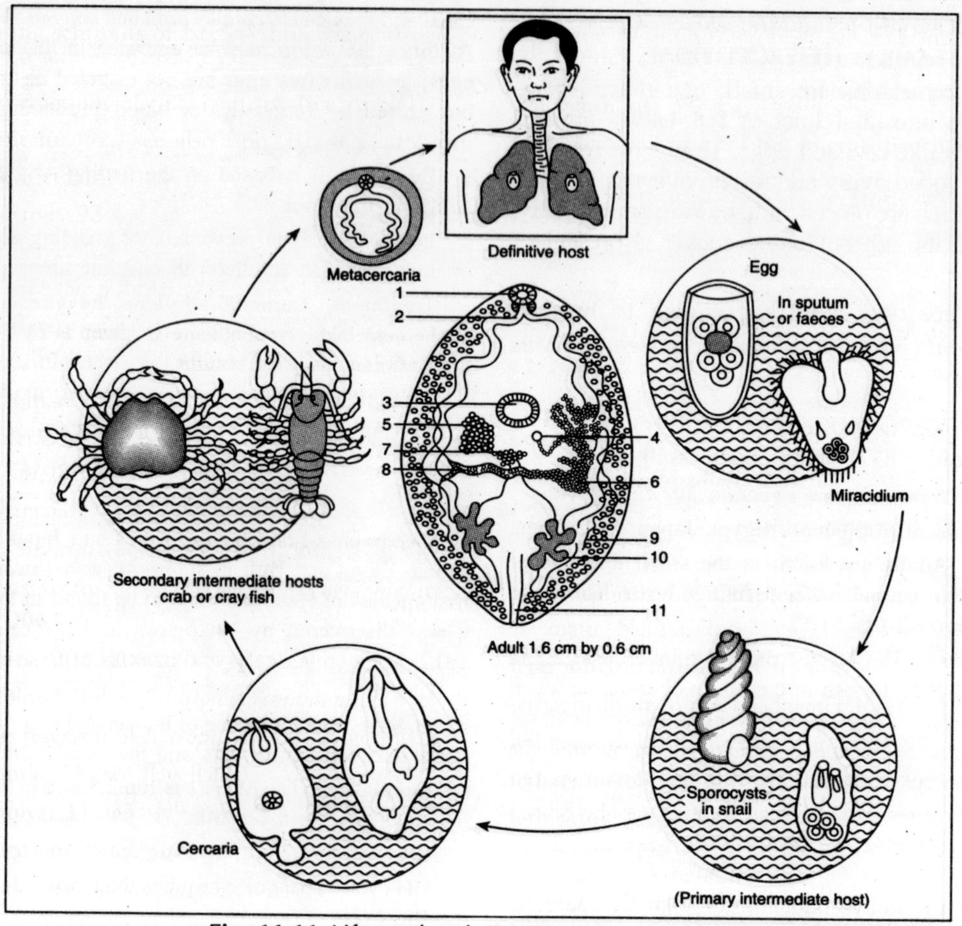

Fig. 11.11 Life cycle of *Paragonimus westermani*
1. Oral sucker. 2. Intestinal caeca. 3. Ventral sucker. 4. Genital pore. 5. Ovary. 6. Uterus. 7. Shell glands. 8. Vitelline duct. 9. Vitellaria. 10. Testes. 11. Excretory pore

lies behind the acetabulum; cirrus sac is absent. Vitellaria are highly developed, occupying the whole of the lateral field. The excretory vesicle is tubular or Y-shaped. The cercariae have knob-like tails and oral stylets; the miracidium is without "eye spots". The larval development occurs in two intermediate hosts, the first being a snail and the second one a crustacean, a crab, or a cray fish.

FAMILY: TROGLOTREMATIDAE

PARAGONIMUS WESTERMANI

(Kerbert, 1878) Braun, 1899

(The oriental lung fluke, producing pulmonary distomiasis, paragonimiasis or endemic haemoptysis)

Paragonimus westermani is a lung fluke of man and mammals, which is transmitted by eating uncooked crabs and cray fish, the secondary intermediate host of the parasite.

Habitat. The adult is usually found in cystic dilatations of the lung or bronchi of man, cat, pig and, occasionally, in the brain, liver or intestinal canal of human.

Morphology (Fig. 11.11, 1-11). It is a small fluke, reddish brown in colour and, when alive, constantly changes its shape. The cuticle is covered with simple or toothed spine. The ADULT worm is 8 to 20 mm in length and 4 to 8 mm in breadth; oval in shape and almost round on transverse section. *Ventral* sucker is relatively larger and lies near the centre of the body. *Testes* are lobed and situated in the posterior third of the body. The *ovary* is lobed, slightly larger than the testis and placed on the side of the midline just behind the sucker. The *uterus* is closely coiled and lies opposite the ovary. The *genital pore* is in the middle line immediately posterior to the ventral sucker.

Eggs are 85μm, oval and yellowish brown with flattened operculum which is widest towards the opercular end, where it shows a distinctly shouldered rim.

LIFE SPAN is probably several years.

Immunity. The infection is believed to confer partial immunity.

Life cycle (Fig. 11.11). *P. westermani* requires 3 hosts to complete the life cycle:

(1) DEFINITIVE HOSTS are human and domestic animals, like cat, dog and pig. There are two INTERMEDIATE HOSTS (1) The PRIMARY INTERMEDIATE HOST is usually fresh water snails of certain species of Thiaridae like *Semisulcospira libertina*. (2) The SECONDARY INTERMEDIATE HOST—is a cray fish or crab.

IMPORTANT SNAIL HOSTS are *semisulcospira libertina* and other species in China, Taiwan, Korea, Japan; *Hua amurensis* in China and Korea *Thiara (Tarebia) granifera* and *Brotia obliquegranosa* in Taiwan (Brotia and Melania are synonyms of Semisulcospira); *Pomatiopsis lapidaria* in North America.

The operculated eggs are voided in cystic pockets of lungs and are coughed out in the expectorated sputum or passed in faeces after swallowing of the sputum. In water, the egg completes full embryonation in about 20 days at an optimal temperature of 27°C and a ciliated embryo comes out with a sudden fall of temperature. The eggs cannot stand desiccation. A ciliated free-swimming miracidium escapes from the operculated egg in 4 to 7 weeks.

The miracidium swimming in water, enters the snail host of the genus Hua, Thiara or Semisulcospira. In the soft tissue of the snail, the miracidium passes through the stages of sporocyst and 2 generations of rediae (mother and daughter). Each redia contains about 20 cercariae with rudimentary knob-like tails and anterior stylet in about 90 days. The cercariae are relatively inactive and survive in water only for 24 to 48 hours. They finally penetrate the articulations and encyst in the crustacean host, a crab or a cray fish, the secondary intermediate host. The body of the cercariae is 225μ by 80μ and covered with spines. The tail, which is also spined, is very short and rudimentary. Inside the crustacean host, **metacercariae** are formed. They become encysted in the liver, heart, gills of crabs, and in the muscles and viscera of cray fish. Human becomes infected by eating the metacercariae in uncooked crabs and cray fish. They excyst in the intestine, when the cyst-wall is dissolved by the gastric juice and the adolescariae are released in the duodenum. They pass through the intestinal wall into the peritoneal cavity and, in 3-4 days, migrate upwards to penetrate the diaphragm and enter into the pleural cavity. They then penetrate into the lung tissue in about 20 days after infection and get encysted in a capsule near the bronchi and become mature in 5-6 weeks. The eggs are discharged into the bronchioles and coughed out with the sputum, and if the sputum is swallowed, adolescariae are with the faeces as well.

The adolescariae may remain in the peritoneal cavity for a long period or may enter and leave the liver and then become lodged in other organs.

Epidemiology. Transmission in human occurs by taking infected crab or cray fish—in the Far East. They are often eaten uncooked or pickled. In water, the metacercariae are killed at 55°C for 5 minutes.

RESERVOIR HOST. Natural mammalian hosts other than man may act as reservoir hosts. They are tigers, lions, foxes, wolves and domestic animals, like dogs, cats, goats, pigs, etc.

VECTORS. They are the crustacea, the secondary intermediate hosts.

Symptoms. The onset is gradual but pulmonary symptoms may start suddenly with fever and haemoptysis (endemic haemoptysis). Four groups of symptoms have been described: (1) general, (2) pulmonary, (3) abdominal, and (4) cerebral.

GENERAL SYMPTOMS are fever with enlargement of the lymph nodes (axillary and inguinal), or occasionally with ulceration and muscular pain.

PULMONARY SYMPTOMS are chronic cough, which becomes worse in the morning with rusty or purulent sputum, and haemoptysis which is slight but may be severe. There may be signs of pneumonia or tuberculosis. Pleural effusion and empyema may occur.

ABDOMINAL ORGANS. They may produce symptoms of pain in the abdomen with diarrhoea or enlargement of the liver.

BRAIN. In the brain, the encystment of mature flukes may produce Jacksonian epilepsy, or other symptoms of brain tumours and that of space-occupying lesions, which end fatally.

Pathology. Small, brown cystic spots in lungs, resembling tubercles, contain one or more flukes and about 13,000 eggs are coughed out everyday. They form cysts, which have fibrotic walls surrounded by congested, oedematous or collapsed lung tissues with inflammatory changes. Each cyst contains the worm, blood and tissue fluid containing eggs and **Charcot-Leyden crystals**. Four types of lesions may occur: (1) nonsuppurative, (2) suppurative, (3) tuberculoid (caseating), and (4) ulcerative. In a bronchus, the cyst may be lined by the epithelium.

Flukes may be found in other organs like the liver, intestine, skin, testes, muscles, and brain, where they form "**tunnelled tumours**".

CLINICAL PATHOLOGY. There is lymphocytosis with a total leucocyte count of 15,000 per cmm. Eosinophilia is absent. *Complement fixation test* is sometimes employed with success in paragonimus infection.

Diagnosis. Residence in an endemic area is suggestive of infection. Examination of sputum and faeces reveals operculated eggs and Charcot-Leyden crystals.

Complement fixation test is necessary when the eggs cannot be detected in cerebral or abdominal lesions.

As a mass screening test for paragonimiasis, the **intradermal test** with VBS (veronal-buffered saline extract of adult *P. westermani*) has been widely used with over 90% positivity (Yokogawa and Tsuji, 1962).

Prophylaxis. ANTI-ORGANISM MEASURES depend chiefly on the avoidance of eating uncooked crabs or cray fish. Immersion of these crustacean hosts in brine does not kill the metacercariae.

ANTIRESERVOIR and ANTIVECTOR measures depend on the elimination of mammalian reservoir hosts or snails, but this is not a practical method.

Treatment. Emetine may be administered in doses of 60-65 mg intramuscularly for 10-12 days and it is considered by some as curative. It is definitely effective in reducing the number of worms causing the infection. Emetine when combined with *sulphonamide* causes more rapid decrease of the eggs in the sputum than by emetine alone.

Chloroquin. The adult dose is 0.15 g of the base, twice daily for 2 months or longer (130 days), totalling a dose varying from 1.10 to 2.63 gm per kg body weight. It diminishes the number of ova in the sputum. No side effects are observed. *Postmortem* examination of such cases dying of intercurrent diseases may show dead worms in the lungs, brain and abdominal viscera.

Bithionol. It is 2, 2-thiobis (4, 6-*dichlorophenol*) derivative and administered in doses of 40 mg per kg body weight on alternate days for 15 days. One or two courses of treatment is required (Kang *et al*, 1963; Yokogawa *et al*, 1961, 1962, 1963). Side-effects are mild and transient, e.g., nausea, vomiting, diarrhoea and abdominal pain.

Removal of patients from endemic areas is recommended.

FAMILY: *TROGLOTREMATIDAE*

GENUS: TROGLOTREMA Odhner, 1914

(*GR. TROGLO*—hollow; *Trema*—orifice)

TROGLOTREMA SALMINCOLA

It is a nonpathogenic incidental parasite of human. The disease in dogs has been recognised for many years in the Pacific northwest of North America. Dogs are the common natural host but the disease has been found in ranch-raised foxes (Donham *et al*, 1926). *Experimentally*, the coyote has been infected (Donham and Simms, 1927). The **primary intermediate host** is the snail, *Goniobasis plicifera silicula*, limited to the area of the Pacific Coast between Northern California and Western Washington. The **free-swimming cercaria** becomes attached to and later develops into **metacercaria** which **encysts** primarily in the kidneys of salmon or trout, the **secondary intermediate host**; the **definitive host** being a dog or a fox, which harbours the flukes in their intestine.

The infected animals (dogs and foxes) develop a generalised hyperplasia of the mesenteric and pelvic lymph nodes and occasionally of the bronchial and sub-mandibular lymph nodes. Cordy and Gorham (1950) implicated an intracellular, rickettsia-like organism as aetiologic agent of the disease in animals. These animals presented a clinical syndrome of severe dysentery, hyperpyrexia and depression of sensorium, occasionally with convulsions and purulent conjunctival discharge. This symptomatology has never been reported in human. **Histopathologically**, numerous coccobacillary bodies were seen within the cytoplasm of the proliferating reticular cells. So the organism has been given the name *Neorickettsia helmintheca*, assuming that it belongs to the Rickettsia family, and it is not arthropod borne, but "(other) invertebrate borne", like the usual rickettsial organisms (Philip *et al*, 1953, 1954).

Treatment. The oleoresin of **aspidium** is an efficient anthelmintic. **Tetrachlorethylene** has been tried with success.

SUPERFAMILY: *ECHINOSTOMATOIDEA* Faust, 1929
FAMILY: *ECHINOSTOMIDAE*
GENUS: *ECHINOSTOMA* Rudolphi, 1809 *emend*, Dietz, 1910
(*Species*: *E. ilocanum*, E. revolutum, *E. lindoensis, etc., producing echinostomiasis or echinostomatosis*)

General considerations. About 11 species of Echinostomes are at present known belonging to the family Echinostomidae. *E. lindoensis* has also been found in India (Dube & Dube, 1967). Brug and Tesch, while examining stool of 96 persons living on the shore of Lake Lindoe district of Central Celebes, found in 46 specimens the operculated eggs of some trematode which agreed in particular to *Echinostoma ilocanum* (Garrison, 1908). The adult worms, however, were not produced for examination. Sandground and Bonne (1940) subjected the same population to anthelmintic therapy and obtained a large number of adult echinostomes, which were found to be *Echinostoma lindoensis*. It was described by Dube and Dube (1967) in Mangalore in a male child of 5 years, resident of South Kanara district, Mysore State, India.

Habitat. They inhabit the intestine of man in Lake Lindoe area in Central Celebes, Mangalore and Mumbai.

Morphology. (**Fig. 11.12.1**)—The worm measures from 8 to 13 mm by 1 to 1.3 mm. The *circumoral* collar bears 37 spines, the five arranged in a regular circle excepting ventral ones, set in a horse-shoe-shaped *anterior disc* on each side, which show some irregularity in arrangement. There is a great uniformity in the size of all collar spines on any individual specimen. The third ventral spine of the group is usually the largest, which occupies the internal collar of the lappet. The average measurement is as follows: Oral sucker–0.24 to 0.36 mm in diameter. Acetabulum 0.8 to 0.94 mm in diameter. Circumoral collar–0.40 mm. Largest spine–60μ by 18μ (average 52μ by 15μ). Both dorsal and ventral surfaces are beset with rows of spines, more prominent anteriorly and becoming smaller and more widely spaced posteriorly. Spination extends only to the region of the second testis. There is a long *oesophagus* and *intestinal caeca* which reach almost to the posterior extremity. The *vitellaria* extend from the tail end to near level of the posterior rim of the acetabulum. The testes are always lobed, often deeply (**Table 11.6**). The *ovary* is oval in shape with the largest axis measuring 4-5 mm.

Eggs (**Fig. 11.12—2 and 3**). In a wet coverslip preparation, the eggs measure 83μ to 116μ in length by 58 to 69μ in width. They have a slightly greenish tinge, with a thick shell with operculum at one end. The operculum is faint, inconspicuous and could not be perceptible at all in some cases, but a little pressure on the coverslip opens up the operculum. The nucleus of ovum is prominent and surrounded by heavily laden yolk cells. The eggs mature in water in 6 to 15 days and hatch MIRACIDIA (Tubangui and Pasco, 1933). Miracidia hatch out on about 12th day when faecal suspension is incubated in distilled water at 37°C. They measure 115μ by 45μ and morphological features are the same as in the case of other species of Echinostoma.

Life cycle (**Fig. 11.12**). The **miracidium** has short, active life until it dies or enters the viscera of the primary intermediate host, where it metamorphoses into mother **rediae, daughter rediae** and finally **cercariae** in 40 to 50 days. The *larval development* of redia and cercaria was found in natural infection of a small planorbid *Anisus*

TABLE 11.6

MORPHOLOGICAL DIFFERENCES OF SPECIES OF ECHINOSTOMA

	E. lindoensis	*E. ilocanum*	*E. malayanum*	*E. revolutum*
Spines	37	51	43	Like those of *E. lindoensis*
Testes	Deeply lobed	—	—	Simpler, oval
Cirrus sac	Never extends back to the middle of acetabulum	—	—	Extends back to the middle of acetabulum
Epidemiologically	Distinct species	—	—	—

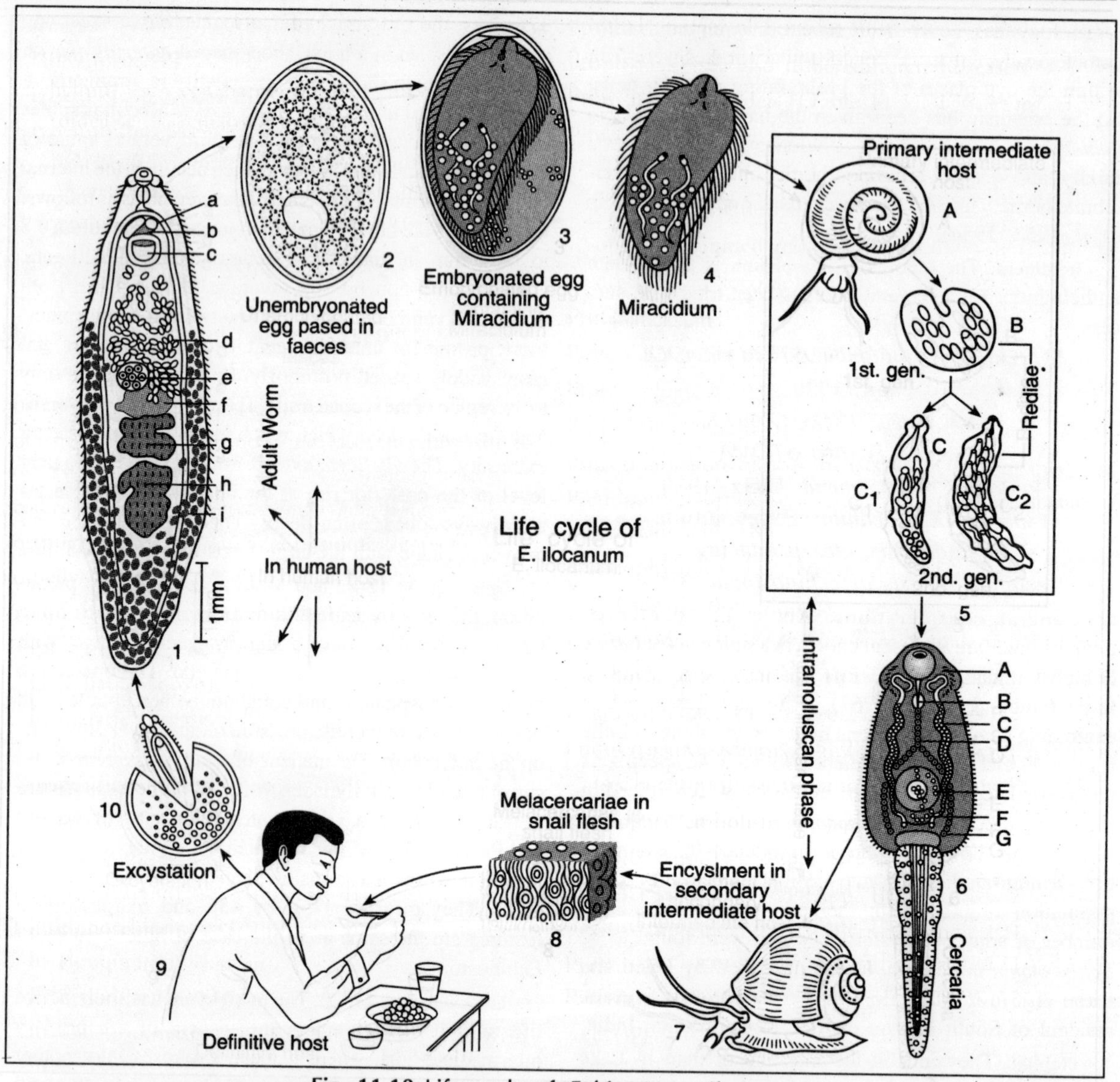

Fig. 11.12 Life cycle of *Echinostoma ilocanum*

1. Anatomy of adult *E. ilocanum* (Ventral view). *a.* Genital pore. *b.* Cirrus sac. *c.* Acetabulum. *d.* Uterus. *e.* Ovary. *f.* Shell gland. *g.* and *h.* Testes. *i.* Vitelleria. 2. Immature egg from faeces. 3. Embryonated egg with miracidium. 4. Free-swimming miracidium enters the primary intermediate host. 5A. Primary intermediate host. 5B. 1st generation redia. 5C. 2nd generation rediae (C_1 and C_2). 6. Cercaria, *A.* Collarette. *B.* Pharynx. *C.* Cystogenous glands. *D.* Oesophagus. *E.* Acetabulum. *F.* Genital primordia. *G.* Intestinal caecum

sarasinorum (*the primary intermediate host*) and metacercariae were found in several Pulmunate snails, e.g., *Viviparous javanicus* var. *rudipellis* in Java, and large species of *Pila conica* in the Philippines, and also the mussel *Corbicula lindoensis* (*Boll*)–the *secondary intermediate host* in the Celebes. These mussels formed a regular part of the diet of Lindoe population and so constituted the infective agent for human. It is interesting to note that in India also the infestation is found in the members of nonvegetarian families and fresh-water snails, which form a part of their diet, though infrequently.

Experimentally, ingestion of mussels by human resulted in the production of characteristic adult worm (Sandground and Bonne, 1940). Rats and mice have also been infected by the same workers. The worms are spontaneously expelled a few weeks after attaining maturity.

This description is based on Dube and Dube, who described it for the first time in India in a child aged 5 years.

Symptoms. They are referred to different systems: (*a*) *Respiratory System*: Atelectasis, idiopathic respiratory distress syndrome, pneumonia. (*b*) *Digestive System*: Thrush, diarrhoea, meconium peritonitis. (c) Biliary and *Vascular System*: Hyperbilirubinaemia (*jaundice*), kernicterus in different age groups, inspissated bile syndrome, neonatal hepatitis, haemorrhage in the newborn.

Diagnosis. The diagnosis depends on the finding and identification of eggs in the stools.

Treatment and Prognosis. Oleoresin of ***aspidium*** is specific, but **tetrachlorethylene** is the drug of choice. The *prognosis* is good.

SUBORDER: AMPHISTOMATA
(Rudolphi, 1801) Bojanus, 1817

SUPERFAMILY: PARAMPHISTOMATOIDEA
Stiles and Goldberger, 1910

Paramphistomatoidea is characterised by large, well-developed acetabulum, which occupies a position behind the reproductive organs and there may be ventral pouch or disc. They are chiefly parasitic to herbivorous animals. The parasites which infect man are:

FAMILY: PARAMPHISTOMATIDAE

GENUS: *WATSONIUS* Stiles and Goldberger, 1910.

SPECIES: *W. watsoni*.

This is a rare organism found pathogenic to man. Only one case was reported in early 20th century.

FAMILY: GASTRODISCOIDAE

GENUS: GASSTRODISCOIDES Lieper, 1913.

GASTRODISCOIDES HOMINIS
(Lewis and McConnel, 1876)
Leiper, 1913

Geographical distribution. Bengal and Assam in India, Cochin-China, Malayasia and Indian immigrants to British Guiana.

Incidence. It is highest in children, in whom 40 per cent may be infected in the endemic areas of Assam. It is also common in Cochin-China, British Guiana and Kazakhistan.

Habitat. The adult worms are found in the large intestine (caecum and ascending colon) of man, pig and Napu mouse deer.

Morphology. (Fig. 11.13). *G. hominis* is pea-like, pyriform in shape, dorsally convex and 5-8 mm by 3-5 mm in diameter. It is pink, when fresh. The cuticle is smooth. It has two suckers (amphistome) at opposite ends of the body. The anterior conical portion contains the oral sucker at the anterior end; the posterior hemispherical portion is hollowed out ventrally and forms a concave disc. The acetabulum is post-terminal on the ventral surface. The internal structures conform to the general structures of a trematode. The egg are ovoid (PL. IX; This Ch. & PL. 11.1 AP-II, 11), operculate and measure 150-170μm by 60-70μm at their widest dimension. They are unembryonated when passed in faeces. They mature in 16-17 days at 29°C, when **miracidium** is hatched out, which infects snails as **intermediate hosts** (Buckley, 1939; Le Roux, 1958).

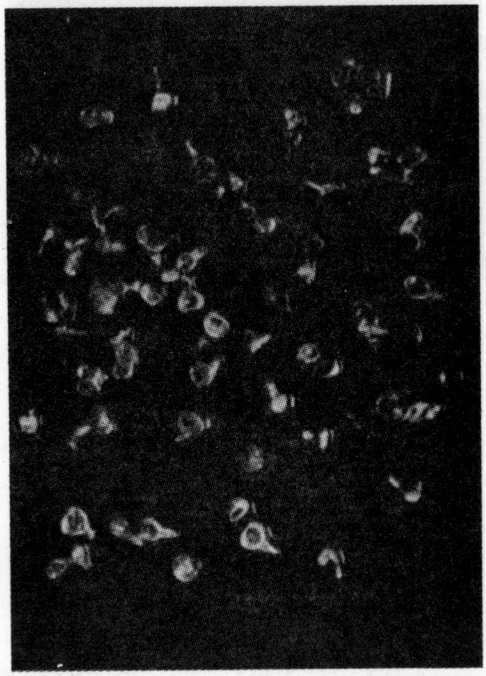

Fig. 11.13 *Gastrodiscoides hominis* (adult worms) See the anterior conical (pointed) portion, and the posterior disc-like sacular part (from natural specimen)

Life cycle. It is not definitely known, but cercariae probably encyst as metacercariae in aquatic vegetations after emerging from the snails.

DEFINITIVE HOSTS other than man are pigs and Napu mouse deer.

RESERVOIR HOSTS are pigs (Verma, 1954), but it occurs in human in absence of pigs.

Pathogenicity. A diarrhoea in human. □

CHAPTER

12 PHYLUM: NEMATHELMINTHES

SYNONYM: ASCHELMINTHES
(Grobben 1910) Hyman, 1951
CLASSES: NEMATODA & NEMATOMORPHA

Nemathelminths (roundworms) include not only true roundworms or nematodes (Class: Nematoda), but also "horse hair" worms or hair snakes (Class: Nematomorpha). The "hair snakes" have few species and rarely parasitise man. The acanthocephala (thorny-headed worms), a Class coordinates with the Nematodes and Nematomorpha in the phylum Nemathelminthes, are now regarded to belong to a distinct phylum.

CLASS: *NEMATOMORPHA*

The members of this group are characterised by a degenerated intestinal tract in adults; the body cavity is lined by mesothelium having a proboscis in the first larval stage. The species of human interest are as follows:

SUBCLASS: *GORDIACEA*
Von Siebold, 1848

Gordiid worms or "hair snakes" (adults) are found in fresh water with larval stages in insects. Accidentally ingested by man, they may be passed in the stools and actively migrate out in the anus or mouth, or rarely passed *per urethrum*.

TERMS USED IN THE DESCRIPTION OF NEMATODA

ALAE. These are cuticular, wing-like expansions, either caudal or cervical.

AMPHIDS. These are a pair of supposedly olfactory receptors at the anterior end.

APHASMID. Without caudal chemoreceptor, e.g., *Trichinella spiralis*, *Trichuris trichiura*.

BUCCAL CAPSULE. The part which constitutes the oral cavity.

CLOACA. It is found in male nematodes only and contains the terminal parts of the rectum and genital duct.

COPULATORY BURSA. This is an umbrella-like cuticular expansion present round the cloaca of the male worms of the superfamily Strongyloidea, supported by rays of stouter tissue.

ECDYSIS (pl. ecdyses; GK. *ecdysis*—I strip off). It is moulting—the act of getting out of the cuticula of the previous stage.

FILARIFORM LARVA. A larva having a filariform oesophagus, which is long and not dilated posteriorly.

LARVA. It is an intermediate developmental stage between an egg and an adult.

MICROFILARIA. A larva discharged by an adult filaria.

OVIPAROUS. This is applied to a female which lays eggs.

PAPILLAE. These are minute knob-like protuberances of the cuticle in the neighbourhood of the mouth or anus.

PHASMID. Nematodes with caudal chemoreceptor (special sensory organs) situated on minute papillae behind the anus, e.g., *Ascaris lumbricoides* and others.

RHABDITIFORM LARVA. A larva having a rhabditiform oesophagus, which is short and dilated posteriorly into a bulb.

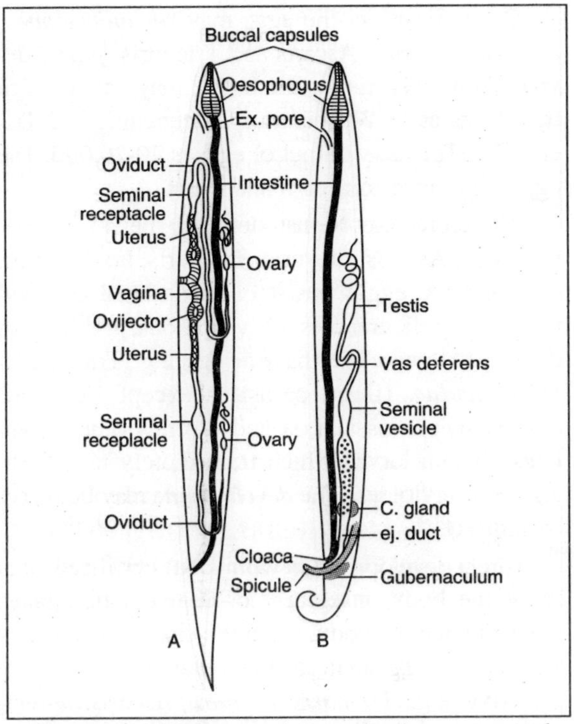

Fig. 12.1 Digestive and reproductive system of a nematode. A–female; B–male

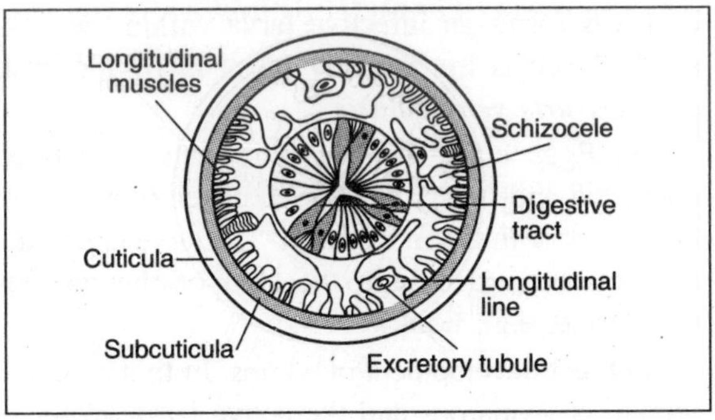

Fig. 12.2 Cross-section of *Ascaris lumbricoides*; □ 16

VIVIPAROUS. This implies to a female which gives birth to larvae.

CLASS: NEMATODA

General characters. (1) The Nematodes are elongated, unsegmented, cylindrical or filiform worms having a body cavity in which the organs lie (Fig. 12.1). (2) They are bilaterally symmetrical but with a triradiate symmetry at the anterior end (Fig.12. 2). (3) Their sizes vary greatly, the smallest being less than quarter of an inch as in *T. spiralis* or *Strongyloides stercoralis*, but the largest may measure up to 100 cm (40 inches) as in the case of the female *Dracanculus medinensis*. The body is covered with a tough, resistant cuticle. (4) The alimentary canal is complete with mouth and anus at opposite ends of the body. (5) The body wall consists of longitudinal muscle fibres and the body cavity is an unlined *pseudocoele*. (6) They have no circulatory or respiratory organs. (7) Excretory organs are simple. (8) Nerve rings around the oesophagus connect with the 6 anterior nerves and 6 or more posterior nerves or cords. (9) They are sexually differentiated. The males are smaller than the females.

ALIMENTARY CANAL. The alimentary canal is complete and the oral cavity (mouth) begins at the anterior part.

Mouth. In the primitive free-living nematodes the mouth is surrounded by three lips, 1 dorsal and 2 lateroventrals. This is retained in Ascaris, Oxyuris and Strongyloides. In filaria parasite, there is no lip. In some of the strongylata, the mouth has been highly modified into a buccal capsule, supplied with cutting ridges, teeth or lancets. The mouth leads to the alimentary canal, which ends in the anus, a short distance proximal to the posterior end. The *alimentary canal* consists of an oesophagus and an intestine. The *oesophagus* has a chitinised triradiate lumen surrounded by muscles and gland cells. Sometimes, as in Oxyuris (Enterobius), the oesophagus enlarges into a bulb (rhabditiform) provided with valves.

The **intestine** is a flat or cylindrical tube, often straight and lined by a single layer of cells (Fig. 12.1). In strongyloides, it is lined by 18-20 cells but, in Ascaris, there are about million cells. At the posterior end, there is a chitinised rectum. In **females**, there is a separate anal opening; whereas, in the **males**, the intestine and reproductive organs open in a common cloaca.

THE NERVOUS SYSTEM consists of a dorsal, a ventral and four lateral longitudinal trunks with transverse commissures. The circumoesophageal ring constitutes the nerve centre, from which longitudinal nerve trunks go forward and backward. The nerves terminate in all organs and specially in the *sensory papillae*.

Special receptor or sensory organs. There is a pair of laterally placed supposedly olfactory receptors called *amphids*, or lateral organs in the cervical region of all nematodes. There are also tactile pa-

pillae about the mouth, a pair in the neck region of many forms, called **deirids** and paired caudal and genital papillae of many males. In species without caudal glands, there is a minute pair of lateral postanal **phasmids**, which are caudal *chemoreceptor organs*. These differ from ordinary tactile papillae in having canals connected with gland-like structures.

REPRODUCTIVE ORGANS. The nematodes are sexually differentiated (**diecious**). The males are smaller than the females and the posterior end of the body is coiled ventrally; whereas, in the females, they are tapering.

The female genital system (Fig. 12.3A) consists of a single tube (Trichuris) or a bifurcate tube (Oxyuris, Ancylostoma), which is differentiated into ovary, oviduct, seminal receptacle, uterus, ovijector, vagina and vulva. The vagina opens on the ventral surface of the worm near the middle of the body or near the mouth. Ova are fertilised in the seminal receptacle and the shell is secreted in the first part of the uterus, where eggs are stored.

The male genital system (Fig. 12.3B) consists of a single, long coiled or convoluted tube differentiated into testis, vas deferens, seminal vesicles, and ejaculatory duct, which opens with the intestine into a common cloaca. Accessory copulatory apparatus consists of one or two unsheathed spicules with or without a gubernaculum; a **copulatory bursa** may be present in some species. The immature (amoeboid rather than flagellate type) spermatozoa are passed into the females.

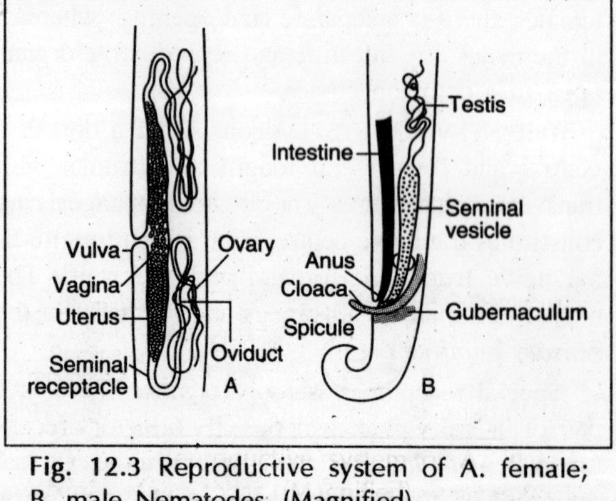

Fig. 12.3 Reproductive system of A. female; B. male Nematodes. (Magnified)

On oviposition, the eggs may be *undeveloped*, as in hookworms, Ascaris and Trichuris; *partly* developed in Oxyuris; or the larvae may hatch out in the uterus as in Wuchereria, Dracunculus and Trichinella. The daily output of eggs is 20-20,000. The eggs may have thin or thick shells.

Therefore, the Nematodes may be: (1) **oviparous**, e.g., Ascaris, Oxyuris, Trichuris, hookworms, etc.; and the eggs consist of a fertilised cell and numerous yolk granules, (2) **viviparous**, giving birth directly to larvae. They have no egg, e.g., Trichinella, *Dracunculus*, filaria parasites except Loa, and (3) **ovoviviparous** in Loa and Strongyloides when eggs contain larvae which immediately hatch out, e.g., Strongyloides. The *development* may be direct or indirect.

Direct development of worms. (a) Fertilised eggs leave the body unsegmented. Segmentation takes place outside the body, when the embryonated eggs within the egg shell mature outside and become infective, e.g., *Trichuris trichiura, Ascaris lumbricoides.*

(b) Eggs leave the body in a segmented condition and forms an infective larva within the egg-shell, which is immediately taken in by the host, e.g., *Oxyuris vermicularis.*

(c) Eggs leave the body in partly segmented condition and full grown larvae develop outside in the faeces or in the moist earth. The larva enters the host by boring through the skin or the mucous membrane, e.g., hookworms.

Indirect development of worms. In this case, the female is **viviparous** and the active larva grows in an intermediate host, wherefrom infection in man takes place. The intermediate host is a mosquito in case of *Wuchereria bancrofti*. It is to be noted that, in this nematode, the larvae do not multiply within the body of the mosquito host. Cyclops are intermediate hosts in case of *Dracunculus medinensis* and larval development takes place in the cyclops, when they become infective to man.

SPAN OF LIFE. It is variable in different nematodes. It is 4 to 8 weeks for *Trichinella spiralis*, 3 months for *Oxyuris vermicularis*, one year for *Ascaris lumbricoides*, 2 years for *Dracunculus medinensis* and 5 years for *Ancylostoma duodenale*.

LOCOMOTION. It occurs by alternate shortening and elongation by muscular action aided by elasticity of the cuticle. They attach by their buccal capsule as in Ancylostoma, by penetration of the attenuated anterior part of the body as in Trichuris, or by penetration of the mucosa by the female as in Strongyloides.

NUTRITION. It depends on the habitat of the parasite. Nutrition is obtained from the tissue fluids, intestinal contents, or blood. Metabolism is chiefly anaerobic and reserve of glycogen and fat may be seen in some phases of development.

Life cycle. (1) The nematode parasites typically pass the life cycle in one host except for the somatic nematodes of the superfamilies Filarioidea and Dracunculoidea, where two hosts are necessary. (2) The development of the larval stage occurs outside the host except in Strongyloides in which the complete cycle may develop in one host. (3) The larvae mature in the egg after passage outside the body, and fully embryonated eggs containing the larvae of intestinal parasites, when ingested by the host hatch out in the intestine, as in cases of *Ascaris lumbricoides*, *Trichuris trichiura* or *Oxyuris vermicularis*. (4) The eggs of hookworm may hatch out in faeces, and develop in moist earth to an infective stage (filariform larva). The larva then penetrates the skin or mucous membrane, and is carried by the venous channel to the right heart. The larvae migrate to the bronchioles by penetrating the lung capillaries. They then enter the air passage, and migrate to the intestine. In the case of Strongyloides, there is also an additional free-living adult stage outside the body. In *Trichinella spiralis infection*, the larvae are encysted in the muscles of pigs and rats, and after ingestion, the larvae hatch out and mature in the intestine of the definitive hosts, e.g., man, pig, or rat, as the case may be.

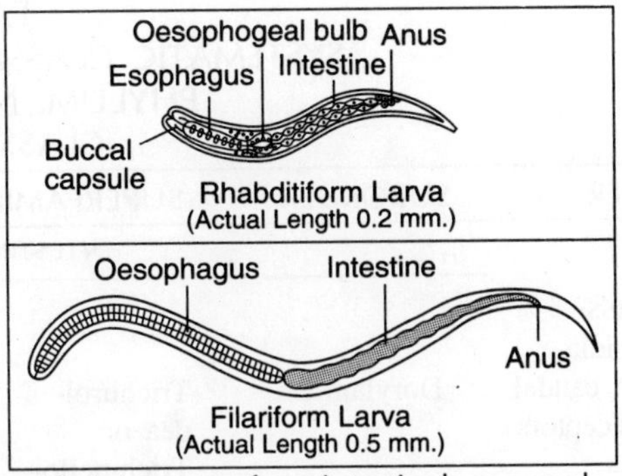

Fig. 12.4 Larvae of an intestinal nematode

During the development of the larva, several moults or ecdyses take place. In some worms, the **rhabditiform stage** develops, characterised by enlarged posterior oesophageal bulb. This finally develops into a **filariform larva** with a cylindrical oesophagus, which is the infective form of hookworm and strongyloides infection (Fig. 12.4).

Epidemiology. Transmission of nematodes may occur to human beings by various methods. The modes of transmission are tabulated in Table 12.1.

VECTORS. These are mosquitoes and blood-sucking flies in filarial worms, and cyclops in *Dracunculus medinensis*.

RESERVOIRS. Man is the only and most important reservoir host in some species; pigs are the

TABLE 12.1

MODES OF TRANSMISSION OF NEMATODES

Ingestions embryonated egg	Inhalation of infected dust containing embryonated eggs	Penetration of skin or mucous membrane by filariform larva	Ingestion of mature larva	By the bite of blood-sucking insects
A. lumbricoides	*A. lumbricoides*	*A. duodenale*	*T. spiralis* (Pork)	Somatic nematodes belonging to the superfamily Filarioidea, e.g., Wüchereria, Acanthocheilonema, Onchocerca, Mansonella, Loa and Dirofilaria
T. trichiura	*O. vermicularis*	*N. americanus*	*D. medinensis* (infected cyclops with drink)	
O. vermicularis		*S. stercoralis*		

TABLE 12.2
SYSTEMATIC CLASSIFICATION OF NEMATODES
PHYLUM: NEMATHELMINTHES
CLASS: NEMATODA

ORDER	SUBORDER	SUPERFAMILY	FAMILY	GENUS	SPECIES
		INTESTINAL NEMATODES			
SUBCLASS: Aphasmidia (without caudal chemoreceptors) Enoplida	Dorylaimina	Trichuroidea or Trichinelloidea	Trichinellidae	Trichinella	*T. spiralis*
			Trichuridae	Trichuris	*T. trichiura*
SUBCLASS: Phasmidia (with caudal chemoreceptors)	Rhabditina	Rhabditoidea	Strongyloididae	Strongyloides	*S. stercoralis*
	Strongylina	Strongyloidea	Strongylidae	Oesophagostomum	*O. apiostomum*
			Ancylostomatidae	Ancylostoma	*A. duodenale*
				Necator	*N. americanus*
		Trichostrongyloidea	Trichostrongylidae	Trichostrongylus	*T. colubriformis*
					T. orientalis
	Ascaridina	Oxyuroidea	Oxyuridae	Oxyuris	*O. vermicularis*
		Ascaridoidea	Ascarididae	Ascaris	*A. lumbricoides*
				Toxocara	*T. canis, T. cati*
		SOMATIC NEMATODES			
Spirurida	Spirurina	Filariodea	Onchocercidae	Wuchereria	*W. bancrofti*
				Brugia	*B. malayi*
				Onchocerca	*O. volvulus*
				Acanthocheilonema (Dipetalonema)	*A. perstans*
					A. streptocerca
				Mansonella	*M. ozzardi*
				Loa	*L. loa*
				Dirofilaria	*D. imitis*
		Spiruroidea	Gnathostomatidae	Gnathostoma	*G. spinigerum*
			Thelaziidae	Gonglyonema	*G. pulchrum*
	Camallanina	Dracunculoidea	Dracunculidae	Dracunculus	*D. medinensis*

important reservoirs in *Trichinella spiralis* infection.

CARRIERS. Usually infected human beings are the carriers.

Classification. The class Nematoda is classified as shown in Table 12.2.

Diagnosis. INTESTINAL NEMATODES are diagnosed *directly* by finding of (a) ova in the stool, or (b) adult worms after administration of anthelmintics. In case of SOMATIC NEMATODES, the diagnosis is based on the finding of larvae in blood or adults in tissues. *Indirectly*, eosinophilia helps in the diagnosis of all nematodes.

Immunity. Some immunity is produced by tissue nematodes with production of hypersensitivity. Complement fixing and skin sensitising antibodies

TABLE 12.3
DIAGNOSIS OF INTESTINAL NEMATODES BY EXAMINATION OF THEIR OVA

Ova or larva coloured or not	Species	Saturated solution of common salt
(*a*) **Coloured** (bile stained) eggs in stool	*Ascaris lumbricoides*	Float (only the fertilised one)
	Trichuris trichiura	Float
(*b*) **Colourless** (i) eggs in stool	Hookworms:	
	Ancylostoma duodenale	Float
	Necator americanus	Float
(ii) Larvae in stool (occasionally present)	***Oxyuris*** *vermicularis*	Float
	Strongyloides *stercoralis*	Float
(iii) Eggs in perianal region	*Oxyuris vermicularis*	Float

may develop in the host. Most of them give group reactions for related species, but some may be species specific. Immunity against infection is practically of no value.

SUBCLASS: APHASMIDIA
ORDER: ENOPLIDA
SUBORDER: DORYLAIMINA
SUPERFAMILY: *TRICHINELLOIDEA* Hall, 1916

In this group, the body of the worm is divided into two distinct parts, viz., a hair-like or filiform anterior, and a stout posterior part. Oesophagus is more or less degenerated and consists of a narrow channel leading into a column of large cells. The intestine is cellular. The female possesses a single ovary. The superfamily comprises two genera of medical importance. These are: (1) Trichinella (*T. spiralis*) and (2) Trichuris (*T. trichiura*) under the family Trichinellidae.

FAMILY: TRICHINELLIDAE

TRICHINELLA SPIRALIS

(Owen, 1835) Railliet, 1895

(*The Trichina worm producing trichinosis*)

General consideration. The genus Trichinella is characterised by smoothness of the adult worm. The male is rarely seen and lacks in spicule and copulatory sheath; the female is *viviparous*. *Trichinella spiralis* is a nematode parasite of rats and pigs, transmitted to man, when man eats uncooked or inadequately cooked infected pork containing the larvae. The symptoms in man are due to migration of larvae in the body through blood, while the adults remain in the small intestine of man.

Incidence. Epidemics may occur in localised areas after ingestion of pork from a common source. The incidence is as high as 16 per cent in the U.S.A. but it is 3 per cent in the U.K. as detected at autopsy series. Many infections are mild and not detected during the life time. The infection in rats has been found to be 5 per cent, but it is 1 per cent in pigs in the U.K.

Habitat. Adult worms live in the small intestine of pig, rat and man. Larvae are encysted in the striped muscles of the body.

Geographical distribution. It is common in Europe and America. It has also been reported from some parts of China, Africa and Syria. It is rare in India.

Morphology. ADULT. It is the smallest nematode of man. The male measures about 1.5 mm in length by 40 to 60μ in diameter. The genital organ consists of a cylindrical testis, which lies in the *posterior third* of the body. The *vas deferens* opens through the seminal vesicle in the terminal cloaca. The *cloaca* is guarded by the large, conical fleshy lappets. *Spicules* are absent. The female is longer than the male, measuring 3 to 4 mm in length and 0.06 mm in diameter. The ovary is posterior and opens *via* receptaculum seminis, uterus, vagina and the vulva at the *anterior fifth* of the body. The female is viviparous and gives birth to embryos instead of eggs.

LIFE SPAN. The adult male dies shortly after fertilisation. The life span of the female is about 4 to 8 weeks and that of the larvae is 8 to 12 months, but survival of the larva for 30 years in man, and 10 years in pigs have been recorded.

Immunity. Immunity against the development of the adult or survival of the larva may follow previous infection in rats.

TABLE 12.4
DIFFERENCE BETWEEN MALE AND FEMALE *T. SPIRALIS*

Male	Female
1. About 1.5 mm in length and 40-60μm in breadth	About 3-4 mm in length and 60μ in breadth
2. No spicule; cloaca evertible and guarded by a pair of ear-like terminal papilae	Viviparous. Vulva close to the anterior extremity

Life cycle (PL. 12.I). It is primarily a disease of rats, from which pigs and men are infected. The life cycle is passed in one host, namely, rat, pig or human. Although one host serves as both definitive and intermediate host, the life cycle is completed in two hosts. The worm is most commonly found in rats, in which infection occurs by ingestion of muscles of other rats. Pigs get the infection by eating infected rats. Man is infected by eating under-cooked or **uncooked infected pork. Adult worms** live in the small intestine of human. Infection takes place by eating uncooked striated muscles of a pig, containing **encysted larvae** (PL. 12.II). **Infective larvae** after ingestion grow into male and female adults in the intestine of human within 48 hours. The adult worms become sexually mature and after fertilisation, larvae are liberated in another 24 hours. The male dies immediately after **fertilising** the female. The **larvae** pass into the mucous membrane of the small intestine. They gain entrance to the circulation *via* the lymphatics, capillaries of venules. The larvae pass through the liver and lungs and escape into the general circulation in greater number from the 9th to 14th day. They develop chiefly in **striated muscles**, where they coil up followed by **encystment**. The peak invasion occurs on the 10th day when clinical manifestations occur. The larvae are mature and become infective after 16 days in case of pigs and rats. The encapsulation of the larva is complete in a month or so and calcification occurs in 6 months. Each adult female liberates about 1,500 larvae. The larvae—which are about 500μm by 250μm—are carried to different parts of the body by the blood stream. A larva is provided with a *spur* at the anterior end, which helps it in boring through the capillaries to the muscles richly supplied with blood, namely, the *diaphragm*, *tongue*, *thoracic* and *eye muscles*, where they become encysted. Larvae which do not reach the muscle die within a period of 6 weeks.

The cysts are small, 800μ by 300μ, ellipsoidal in shape and lie in the long axis of muscle fibres (PL. 12.I). The encysted larvae remain infective for 10 to 30 years, but the larvae may eventually die and then the cyst-wall is calcified. The encysted larvae develop into adult worms, when the mature larvae are taken by another host, e.g., human, rat or pig. The same process of development occurs either in human, rats or pigs and the encystment of larvae in the muscles continues. The cycle continues from rat to rat, rat to pig, or pig to human by eating infected muscles containing encysted larvae.

Pathogenicity. In majority of cases, the infection does not show any manifestation due to the presence of the adult worms in the intestine. The clinical conditions produced by *T. spiralis* in man is known as **trichinelliasis**, also called *trichiniasis* or *trichinosis*.

Symptomatology. The severity of the disease depends upon the number of viable larval cysts ingested. Three **clinical types** of the disease are known. (I) **Asymptomatic** or subclinical trichinosis. This is manifested only by eosinophilia in peripheral blood, usually discovered by chance during an epidemiologic study.

(II) **Oligosymptomatic**. There is one presenting symptom, e.g., fleeting facial or palpebral oedema, or muscle pain of the *torticollis* type and *lumbago*, or transient *diarrhoea*.

(III) **Polysymptomatic** trichinosis: This type may be categorised into (i) mild, (ii) moderate and (iii) severe.

After ingestion of the infected pork, three stages may be recognised clinically: (1) **Stage of incubation** (The intestinal phase): During this period the larvae grow as adult males and females, and the latter begin to discharge the larvae into general circulation. The symptoms are chiefly gastrointestinal, comprising enteritis, petechiae or ulceration of the mucosa. (2) **Stage of Invasion of Larvae**. This commences from the 7th to the 10th day, the peak being on the 10th day after infection. This goes on for about 6 weeks. This is clinically manifested by remittent fever, myositis, urticarial rash, eosinophilia and leucocytosis often attended with fatal toxaemia. This is followed by the (3) **Stage of recovery**. Depending on the severity of the case the course varies. It is about 2 weeks in mild cases but may take about 6-8 weeks in severe cases, when the larvae are encysted in muscles and tissues.

PLATE 12.1
LIFE CYCLE OF *TRICHINELLA SPIRALIS*

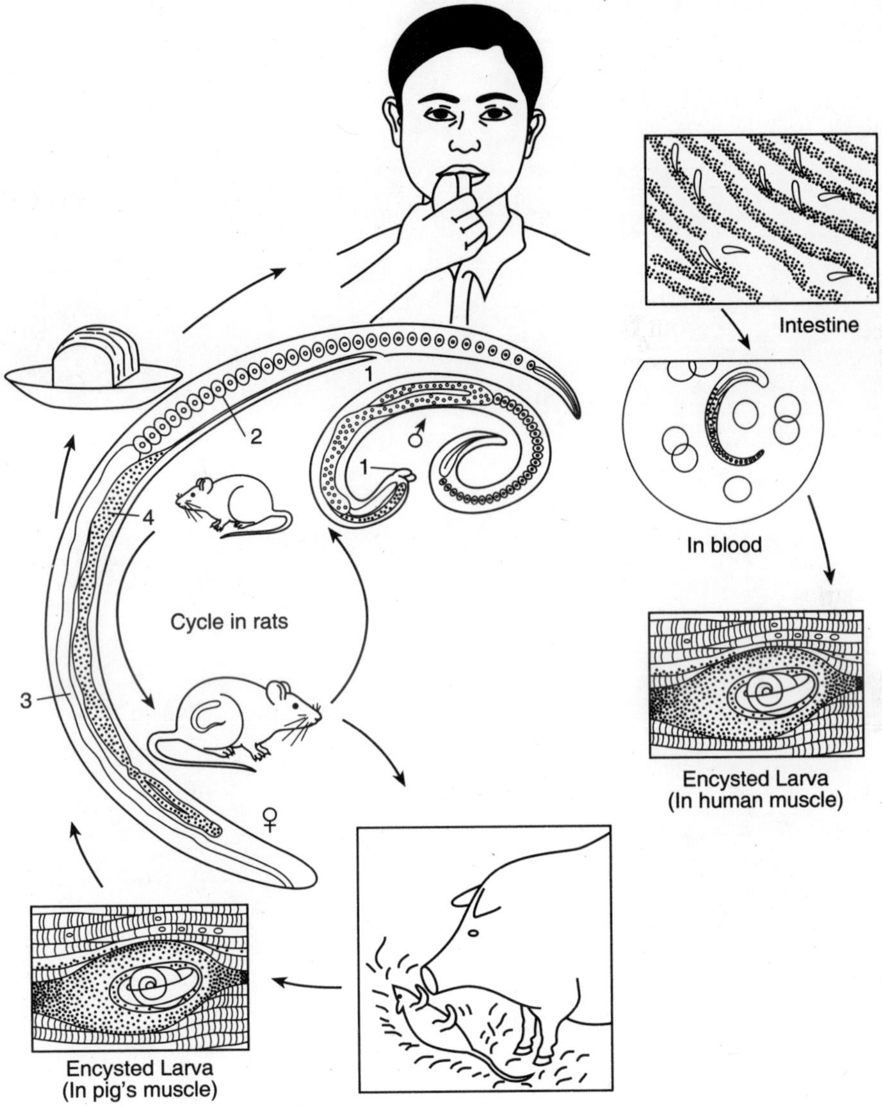

Life cycle of *Trichinella spiralis*
Female: 1. Vulva. 2. Oesophagus. 3. Intestine. 4. Uterus.
Male: 1. Two ear-like papillae posteriorly

PLATE 12.II

ENCYSTED LARVA OF TRICHINELLA

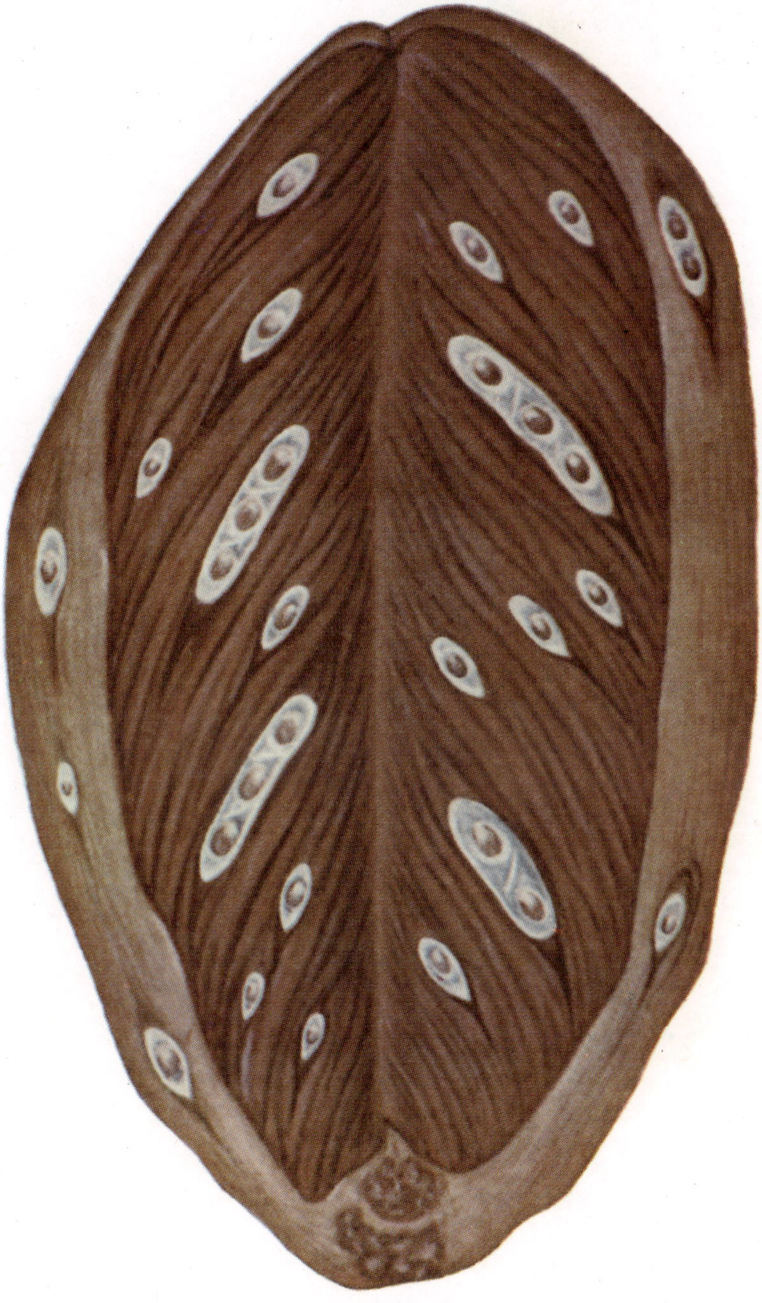

A large number of larvae of Trichinella spiralis are seen encysted within pork meat after incision of the muscle belly.

Pathology. DIGESTIVE TRACT. After the 3rd day of infection, up to the 2nd week, there is **acute catarrhal enteritis** associated with gaseous distension and dilatation of the bowel. In some areas, the wall of the intestine is *thin* and transparent due to *distension*, while in others it is *thickened* by *oedema*. The serosa is lustureless and shows punctate haemorrhages. Peyer's patches become prominent.

Microscopically, the villi are swollen, straight and show marked axial vascular **congestion**. They are covered by a thick layer of mucus, where there are numerous free or partially **embedded adult worms** in the mucosa (Askanazy, 1950; Gould, 1943; Ribas-Mujal, 1955; Stryker, 1946). In more severe cases, there is marked **desquamation** of the villi epithelium and marked **necrosis** of the vertex of the villi. The **secretory activity** of the 'crypt' cells is markedly increased. There is oedema and diffuse eosinophilic infiltration of the lamina propria.

The parasite never pierces the muscularis mucosa (Romanovitch, 1912). It is noteworthy that no author has described any foreign body reaction around these parasites unlike in cases of other parasites. Stryker points out that there is no leucocytic exudate around the parasite, which suggests that the female worm does not remain totally anchored to the mucosa but migrates and is occasionally located in the intestinal chyme. Hence, it is possible, that liberation of migrating larvae is not continuous (Ribas-Mujal, 1971). The intestinal changes are not due to direct mechanical irritation of the parasite (Hemmert-Halswick, 1934), but they are secondary to the presence of toxic or metabolic products originating either in the parasites, or in the altered mucosa.

STRIATED MUSCLES. The **diaphragm** is the muscle most often parasitised, followed by the lingual, the masseters, the intercostal, the extrinsic ocular muscles, the laryngeal and the paravertebral muscles. Selective affinity for different muscles is probably related to the degree of glycogen content in a particular muscle (Flury, 1913), or this may be governed by the degree of activity of a muscle, e.g., intensity or continuity of muscular activity, which may be accompanied by greater vascularisation (Lewis, 1928a, b); so, there is more marked involvement of the muscles related to respiration and mastication.

The migrating larvae possibly abandons the blood capillaries when reaching muscle, and penetrates a muscle fibre, where development and encystment follows. A few hours after larval penetration, the sarcoplasm of the affected fibre becomes homogeneous or acquires a grumous appearance due to disappearance of the cross-striations indicating **myofibrillar lysis**.

At first, there is **basophilic degeneration** of the muscle fibres and a **hyaline capsule** is formed with *leucocytic infiltration* followed by *fibrosis*. The sarcoplasm becomes basophilic (with basic stains), or it acquires intense argentophilia with ammoniacal silver (Gross-Bielschowsky's method). If myofibrillar impregnations with silver carbonate (Hortage method) are employed, the parasitised fibres do not take the stain in contrast to the uninvolved fibres (Ribas-Mujal, 1950).

The **basophilia** is due to the *fatty acid* and *lactic acid* produced by the parasite which impregnates the fibre (Flury, 1913). The first alterations appear in the zones adjacent to the parasites and extend rapidly throughout the fibre (Nevinny, 1927). This observation was confirmed with the **electron microscope** by Fasske and Themann (1961), who observed that the classically described *homogeneous appearance* corresponds to a *dissolution of the rhabdomyofibrils* accompanied by the *loss of* the typical linear *distribution* of the **muscular mitochondria** and by the appearance of small vesicles filled with a material lacking in electronic contrast. These vesicles are dilated portions of the **endoplasmic reticulum**; the characteristic submicroscopic arrangement of the normal sarcoplasm is lost. Toward the 5th day after penetration of the muscle fibre, there is involution of the tubular and *vesicular dilatations* of the **endoplasmic reticulum** and the appearance of a numerical increase of the **mitochondria** (Ribas-Mujal & Rivera-Pomar, 1968). With these changes the nuclei of the muscle fibres show typically and consistently a marked proliferation (Fiedler, 1864) and a vesicular (cystic) transformation accompanied by an increase in volume of the muscle fibre and a **nuclear displacement** towards the axis of the fibres. Later on, the nuclei undergo **pyknosis**. The phenomenal events of the **hyperplasia, hypertrophy** and **vesiculation** of the nuclei of the muscle fibres have been attributed to "**adaptive nuclear hyperplasia**" (Ribas-Mujal, 1950) like that in case of *Sarcocystis lindemanni*. HENCE THE ESSENTIAL CHANGE IN THE STRIATED MUSCLE IS ONE OF BASOPHILIC DEGENERATION, HOMOGENEOUS APPEARANCE FOLLOWED BY HYALINE CAPSULE FORMATION, PLASMA CELLULAR INFILTRATION, FIBROSIS AND PARTIAL REGENERATION WITHIN 15 MONTHS. FOREIGN

BODY GIANT CELLS MAY BE PRESENT. CALCIFICATION MAY OCCUR IN THE CYSTS WITHIN 6 MONTHS, WHICH COMMENCES FROM ONE POLE OF THE CYST. CALCIFIED CYSTS CONTAINING LARVAE MAY RETAIN THE INFECTIVE POWER.

HEART. Larvae may reach the heart muscle during migration, where it may cause areas of *interstitial infiltration* (myocarditis), *fragmentation* of the muscle fibres with *fatty degeneration*. *Perivascular leucocytic infiltration* may occur and produce thrombosis.

CENTRAL NERVOUS SYSTEM. In the brain, the larvae may produce leptomeningitis, granulomatous nodules in the basal ganglion around the migrating larvae, chiefly in the subcortical white matter of the cerebrum or cerebellum. There is generalised hyperaemia, or perivascular infiltration in the cortex. These are due to the presence of larvae, or allergic reactions.

EYE. There may be injection of the conjunctiva, or choroiditis.

OTHER ORGANS. Lungs, liver, or kidneys may show signs of inflammation or oedema. Peripheral blood may show eosinophilia up to 50 per cent or more in the second week, with leucocytosis, which is the *most single important finding* for the correct approach to the diagnosis (Gould, 1945).

Clinical diagnosis. Gastrointestinal disturbances, fever, like 'flu', with rheumatic or typhoid pain, and orbital oedema after a pork meal, are very suggestive. Respiratory, cardiac, ocular or meningeal symptoms are often added. Subungual haemorrhages are almost diagnostic.

Laboratory diagnosis. MUSCLE BIOPSY. The easy and correct method of diagnosis is to demonstrate the encysted larva in the muscle by biopsy. The optimum time for muscle biopsy is the fourth week after appearance of symptoms. The following methods may also be helpful for diagnosis:

STOOLS. Recognition of adults or larvae is rare in the diarrhoeic stools.

BLOOD. Larvae may be rarely found in the blood smear, spinal fluid or mother's milk during the stage of migration. A leucocytosis with an eosinophilia up to 50 percent or more is present in the 2nd or 3rd week but the latter may persist slightly (7 percent) for several years.

SEROLOGICAL TESTS. At present three serological tests help in the diagnosis of trichinosis: (1) Bentonite flocculation (BF) test which is of sufficient sensitivity to measure active infection (Kagan, 1965; Norman *et al*, 1963) but it is not adequate for testing lightly infected pigs. (2) The complement fixation (CF) test appears earlier than the third week; whereas, the BF test becomes positive after the 3rd week, but BF titres rise rapidly and drop slowly.

1:2,500 is found in 90 per cent cases in fourth to ninth week. It is occasionally positive in CSF. Agglutination of latex particles, coated with trichinella antigen (Innella and Redna, 1959) becomes positive in trichinelliasis.

IMMUNOLOGICAL TESTS

(1) Fluorescent antibody (FA) test is the only procedure, which is adequate in pigs infected with less than one larva per gram of muscle (diaphragm) tissue. Evaluation of FA test for trichinosis was done by

TABLE 12.5

TABLE SHOWING A COMPARATIVE STATEMENT OF SEROLOGICAL TESTS IN DIFFERENT PARASITIC INFECTIONS IN HUMAN

Human infection	Bentonite flocculation: No. positive / No. tested	Bentonite flocculation: Percent Positive	Fluorescent antibody: No. positive / No. tested	Fluorescent antibody: Percent Positive
Trichina	38/39	97	25/27	93
Echinococcus	0/28	0	2/7	29
Filaria	0/25	0	0/19	0
Schistosoma	0/34	0	3/26	12
Ascaris/Toxocara	0/21	0	1/21	5

Sulzer & Kagan., 1967. It is almost as specific as BF test. According to Labzoffsky *et al*, (1964), BF test is the most sensitive of several tests in detecting early infection.

(2) **Intradermal test**. The test becomes positive with **Bachman's antigen**, which is prepared by extracting trichinella larvae from infected laboatory rats. After injection of antigen, 0.02 ml in a dilution of 1:3000 into the skin, it produces an erythematous irregular wheal, 6 cm in diameter in 15-20 minutes. The reaction is specific, when the antigen dilution 1:10,000 is used. It is positive in 80-90 per cent cases of infection after the third week.

(3) **Precipitation test**. A simple **precipitation ring test** is performed where a dilution of 1:100 of the antigen is used which is overlaid on the serum to be tested, allowing it to stand for 30 to 70 minutes. A whitish ring if formed at the interphase, the test is considered positive.

The precipitin and intradermal tests are regarded to be highly specific and more useful than biopsy. But according to Kagan (1960), these tests have to be carefully evaluated.

HISTOPATHOLOGY. See before, under pathology, microscopic findings.

XENODIAGNOSIS (Beck, 1953). Beck performed it in 100 human diaphragms. He first examined the samples microscopically and then fed the material to uninfected albino rats, which were sacrificed a month or more later. The method was particularly recommended for survey work to detect viable larvae.

X-RAY EXAMINATION. This is useful when the encysted larva is calcified.

DEMONSTRATION OF MIGRATING LARVAE IN PERIPHERAL BLOOD. During the period of muscular invasion, there is possibility of recovering migrating larvae in peripheral blood. The volume of blood obtained by puncture is mixed with 10 volumes of 3% acetic acid (Staubli, 1905), or 0.1N hydrochloric acid (Gould, 1945) to cause haemolysis. The centrifuged sediment is examined immediately for the presence of larvae, which is positive in severe infections around 3rd and 4th week of parasitism.

Treatment. As there is no chemotherapy for trichinosis, treatment is purely symptomatic by administration of sedatives and analgesics. If early diagnosis is made, anthelmintics and frequent saline purgatives may be administered. This may remove the unembedded female, and reduce the intensity of infection and symptoms. Small doses of cortisone have been reported to be useful (Magath, 1956). Martinez-Fernandez (1965) confirmed the action of **thiabendazole** (2, 4-thiazolbenzimidazole) and *methiridine* (a pyrimidine derivative), introduced by Campbell (1961) and Janitschke (1962), respectively. He found effective action of methiridine on intestinal adult parasite during the first 2 weeks; in later stages, it destroys a portion of the migrated larvae in the muscle, or else prevents their development.

With *thiabendazole* an almost total reduction in the number of encysted larvae during the first week of infection, and a lessening of their action during the course of the 2nd and 3rd weeks have been observed. The effects of *thiabendazole* are more favourable and constant with repeated and moderate doses, than with a single high dose administration. Stone *et al*, (1954) have used *thiabendazole* in the dosage of 2 mg orally twice daily, with encouraging results.

FAMILY: TRICHURIDAE

TRICHURIS TRICHIURA

(Linnaeus, 1771) Stiles, 1901

(Producing trichuriasis in man)

SYNONYM: *Trichocephalus trichiurus* **Blanchard, 1895**; Whip-worm.

Geographical distribution. All over the world.

Habitat. The adult worm lives in the large intestine of man, specially the caecum and vermiform appendix.

Morphology. ADULT. The adult worm is whip-like in shape. It is about 30-50 mm long. Anterior three-fifths of the worm resemble the lash of a whip, and hence the name; the posterior two-fifths are thick (**Fig. 12.5**). The anterior thin part remains buried in the intestinal mucosa.

ALIMENTARY TRACT. The mouth is simple and the whip-like anterior extremity consists of a long simple, cellular oesophagus, which is a minute channel with a single column of secretory cells. It opens into the anterior thin part of the worm into the midgut. The *anus* is terminal.

GENITALIA. The **male** has a long saccular, tubular *testis*, which runs forward from the posterior part of the narrow anterior portion of the body, wherefrom the *vas*

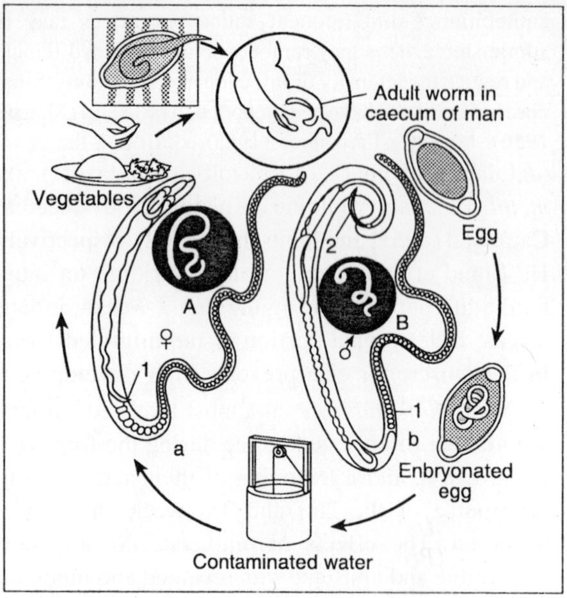

Fig. 12.5 Life cycle of *Trichuris trichiura*
A. Female; and B. Male.
a. Adult female. 1. Vulva, b. Adult male.
1. Oesophagus. 2. Spicule

deferens leads posteriorly to the *cloaca* via the *ejaculatory duct*. There is a single lanceolate spicule 2.5 mm long protruding through a retractile penile sheath having a bulbous termination covered with numerous recurved spines. The **female** has a sacculate *tubular ovary*, which runs forward from the posterior end for over half the thick part of the body. The *oviduct* then runs posteriorly and opens into the *uterus*, which, in its turn, runs forward to open into the vulva through a short *vagina*. The *vulva* is situated on the ventral surface of the anterior end of the thick part of the body. Males are differentiated from females as shown in **Table 12.6**.

Eggs. The ova are barrel-shaped and triple-shelled measuring 54μ by 22μ. The outermost shell is bile-stained. There are bipolar, unstained, intralaminar prominences, which appear like mucoid plugs (Faust and Russell, 1964).

LIFE SPAN of the adult worm in man is many years.

Life cycle (Fig. 12.5). There is no intermediate host but a change of host is necessary to continue the new life cycle. *Eggs* (unsegmented) are non-infective, but those containing larvae are only infective to man. The egg develops by segmentation, which occurs slowly. In about 3-5 weeks or longer after the passage of the eggs in the faeces, the infective larva in moist soil develops inside the egg-shell without *ecdysis* or hatching of the *embryonated egg* in the soil. In a temperate climate, it may take a longer period (10-12 months); in dry condition embryonation may be prevented. *Egg-shell* is thick and the embryo may lie latent in it for 5 years.

When the embryonated eggs containing **larvae** are ingested by human hosts with food and water, the shell is digested by the digestive juice and larvae are liberated through one pole. They emerge in the small intestine and penetrate the villi, where they lie coiled and develop in about a week. They then re-enter the lumen and reach the mucous membrane at the site of its adult attachment. They become sexually mature in about three months, from the time of ingestion of the embryonated egg, when the females begin to lay eggs. Eggs are passed in the faeces. The cycle is thus repeated.

Pathology. With light infection, no obvious pathological changes of bowel has been recognised. However, moderate infection may cause mild catarrhal changes of the large bowel with or without small subepithelial haemorrhages. With heavy worm load, there appears eosinophilic and lymphocytic infiltrate with restriction up to muscularis mucosae. The lymphoid follicles are enlarged which may confer pressure necrotic effect to the adjacent cells.

Epidemiology. Infection occurs by ingesting embryonated eggs in soil, or by contaminated food, raw vegetables and infected water.

TABLE 12.6

DIFFERENCES BETWEEN MALE AND FEMALE *T. TRICHIURA*

Male	Female
1. About 3-4 cm long	Longer than male (4-5 cm)
2. Posterior end is coiled	Posterior part straight or slightly curved
3. Has a single terminal spicule	No spicule

RESERVOIR HOST AND CARRIERS. Human is the only reservoir host, although closely related, but not identical species occur in different animals, e.g., pig, sheep, ox, rabbit, etc.

Clinically, in light or moderate infections, the symptoms appearing vague which includes headache, nervousness, insomnia, anorexia, etc. With increasing worm load, there may be gastric or right iliac pain, vomiting, abdominal distension, fever, etc. Mild eosinophilia is usually associated.

With heavy worm load, there may be marked mucous diarrhoea and the stool sample may be streaked with blood, or even frankly bloody. There may be dehydration, emaciation and weakness prevailing, diffuse abdominal pain, tenesmus and even rectal prolapse. There is associated anaemia in trichuriasis, the cause of which is not clear. However, Askanazy (1896) demonstrated iron containing pigment in the intestinal epithelium of *T. trichiura*.

Laboratory Diagnosis. The diagnosis solely rests on the finding of ova in the stool during routine examination, or by salt floatation method. The presence of 133 to 300 ova per gramme of stool indicates one worm present in the bowel. The presence of 15 worms or more in the intestine indicates a significant infection.

Prophylaxis. The ANTIPARASITIC MEASURES consist of: (1) proper disposal of night soil; (2) prevention of eating uncooked vegetables and fruits, and of (3) drinking contaminated water.

Treatment and Prognosis. Tetrachlorethylene, hexylresorcinol, or other drugs useful against hookworm disease may be used. But all the worms are not removed, as they fail to reach the worm in sufficient concentration to be effective. Latex of fig trees (*Ficus glabrata* and *F. doliaria*), which is "leche de higueron" in Central America and Northern part of South America, are administered in doeses of 60 ml in an empty stomach. The active principle is ficin, a *proteolytic enzyme*. The latex is not active, unless kept in a cold atmosphere. No purgative is required. This treatment removes about 75 per cent of worms.

Maldonado (1965) has shown that Monopar (Stilbazium iodide of Burroughs Wellcome Co., New York) in daily single dose of 500 mg (2 capsules) for 2 days, cures the infection. The dose is standard irrespective of weight of the patients.

Mebendazole ("Mebex": *Cipla*). The drug is claimed to be highly effective. The adult dose is 100 mg (1 tablet) orally, twice daily for 3 consecutive days. Cases of reinfection may be tried with this drug.

With reinfestation, it is difficult to cure the disease as the worm may live for many years. Myers *et al* (1958) proved that, with single infection the worms die within 3 years.

PHASMID NEMATODE PARASITES OF HUMAN

SUBCLASS: *PHASMIDIA*

ORDER: *RHABDITIDA*

SUBORDER: *RHABDITINA*

SUPERFAMILY: *RHABDITOIDEA*

GENUS: **STRONGYLOIDES** (Grassi, 1871)

STRONGYLOIDES STERCORALIS

(Bavay, 1876) **Stiles** and Hassall, 1902

(Producing strongyloidosis or strongyloidiasis in human)

General consideration. *Strongyloides stercoralis* is a parasite of the small intestine of man, which may undergo sexual multiplication either in the intestine or outside the body. It is specially found to be prevalent and frequent in the tropics. It has two forms—the parasitic, and the free-living form.

Incidence. It may exceed 25 per cent of population in the tropics and the highest incidence is often seen in children.

Geographical distribution. The worm is commonly found in Brazil, Cochin-China and other tropical countries.

Habitat. The adults (both male and female) are *primarily* found in the lung. *Secondarily*, the females lie buried in the mucosa of jejunum, and the males are found free, though rarely in the lumen of the small intestine.

Larvae—and not eggs—are passed in human stool. Infective larvae are found in the latrine, contaminated soil and water. Warm, moist soil is necessary to complete the life cycle of the free-living form outside the body.

Morphology. There are two kinds of the adult worm: (a) the parasitic form, and (b) the free-living form. Free-living generation is the basic life cycle of the parasite, which is constantly present in warm climates, where moisture and abundant faecal matter in the soil favour *"free-living existence"*.

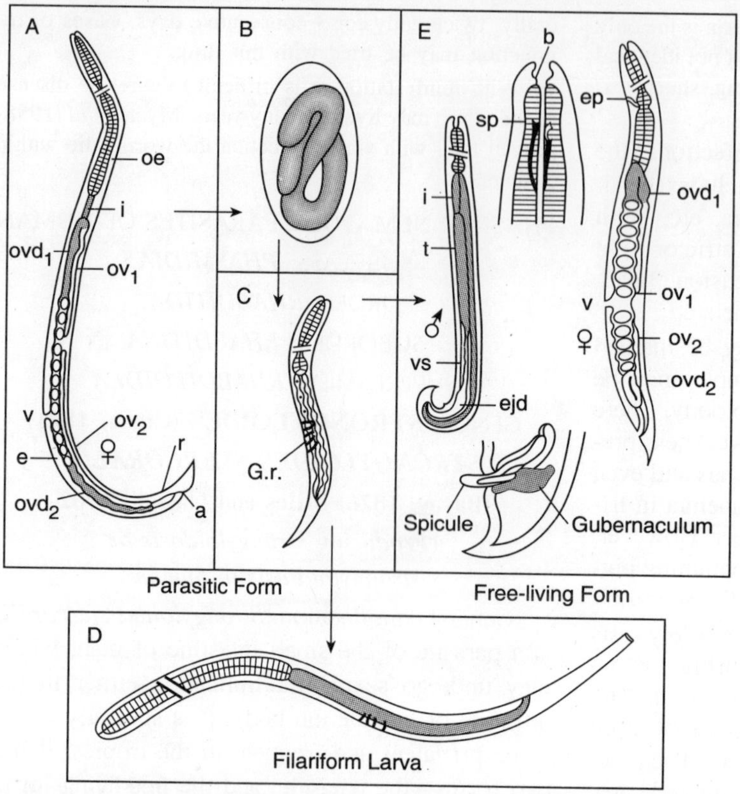

Fig. 12.6 *Strongyloides stercoralis*. A. Parasitic female; oe-oesophagus; i-midgut; ovd_1-anterior oviduct; ov_1-anterior ovary; ov_2-posterior ovary; v-vulva; e-egg in utero; ovd_2-posterior oviduct; r-rectum; a-anus. B. Egg. C. Rhabditiform larva; G.r.-genital rudiment. D. Filariform larva. E. Free-living male and female in soil; b-buccal cavity; sp-buccal spears; ep-excretory pore; t-testis; vs-seminal vesicle; ejd-ejaculatory duct

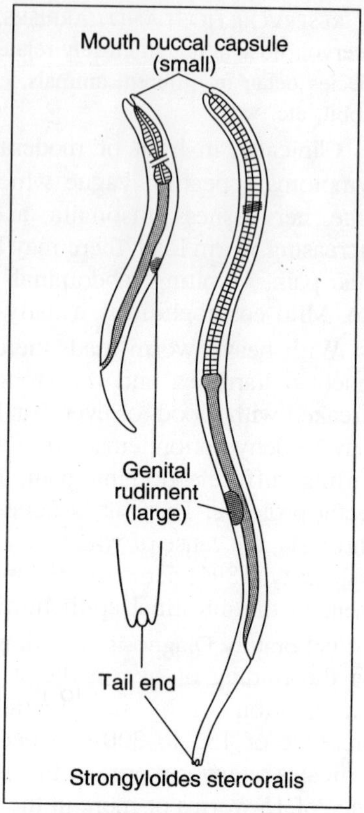

Fig. 12.7 Larvae of *S. stercoralis*; left—*rhabditiform*; right—*filariform*

THE PARASITIC FORM

ADULTS. The **parasitic male** is seldom seen and its morphology is not definitely known. The parasitic males are more often found in the lungs than in the intestine. They are *not tissue parasites* and *do not penetrate* the epithelium. They are soon **expelled** with the faeces.

The **parasitic females (Fig. 12.6A)** are colourless, transparent, slender and filiform. They are 2.2 mm by 0.075 to 0.3 mm with a finely striated cuticle. The posterior end is pointed. The anterior end is thin, a short buccal cavity and four indistinct lips.

ALIMENTARY TRACT. In the **female**, the *oesophagus* is cylindrical and extends through the anterior one-third of the worm, where it is continuous with the midgut. The ventral *anus* opens a short distance anterior to the posterior end.

GENITALIA. The vulva opens ventrally at the junction of the middle and posterior third of the body; from this a pair of uteri extend anteriorly and posteriorly to become the oviducts, which are joined by cylindrical ovaries. A number of 6-8 eggs lie in the uterus.

Eggs. The eggs are oval, thin-shelled transparent and measure 50μm by 30μm. They are segmented at the oviposition in the mucosa. They hatch out in a few hours to form **rhabditiform larva**, and this stage is passed in the human faeces.

FREE-LIVING FORM

ADULTS. The female (rhabditiform) is shorter than the parasitic female and measures 1 mm by 0.06 mm **(Fig. 6D.E)**. The cuticle is smooth. The rhabditoid male is broad, short and measures 0.7 by 0.04 mm. Its posterior end is tapering, pointed and ventrally curved. There is no caudal ala, but there are two **spicules** and a **gubernaculum**.

ALIMENTARY TRACT. In both sexes the **oesophagus** is *rhabditiform*.

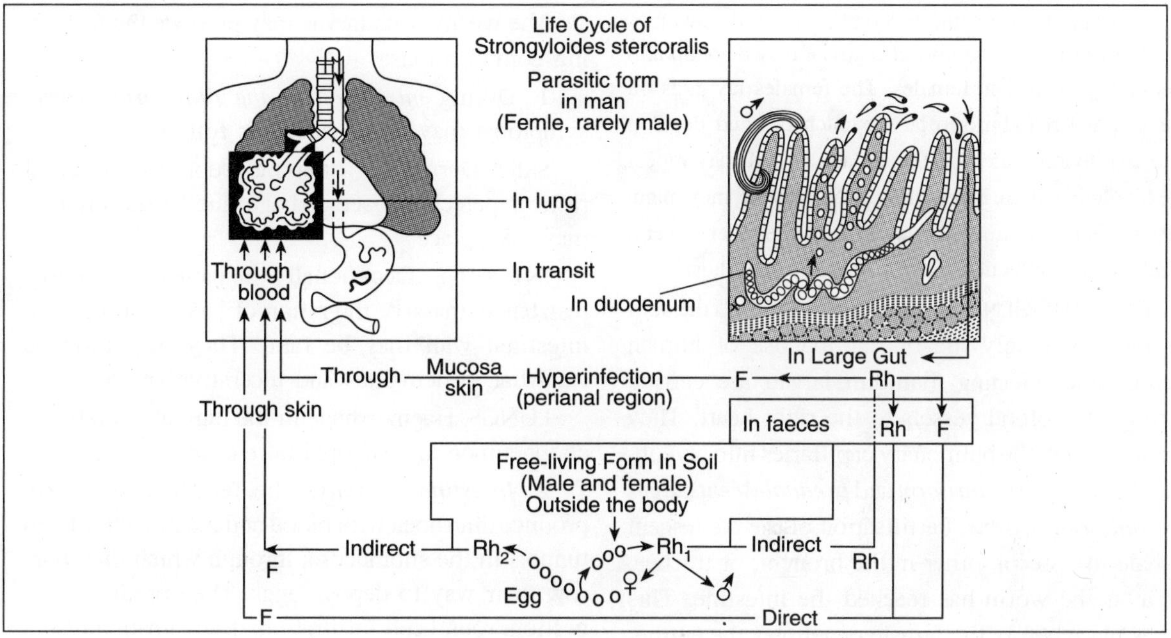

Fig. 12.8 Life cycle (direct and indirect) of *S. stercoralis* (parasitic and free-living). Rh—rhabditiform larva; F—filariform larva infective to man. Rh_1—first generation and Rh_2—2nd generation rhabditoid larvae. The free-living life may continue indefinitely

GENITALIA. The cylindrical testis in the *male* lies in the middle third of the body and opens by the seminal vesicle and ejaculatory duct into the cloaca. In the *female*, the genitalia resemble those of the parasitic female.

Eggs. The fertilised female deposits eggs, which are partially embryonated. The eggs are transparent, oval, thin-shelled and measure 70 by 40μ.

LIFE SPAN in man is unknown as auto-infection may occur. But it is estimated to be about 5 years. The free-living form lives for a few days.

Life cycle (Fig. 12.8). The adult **parasitic female** of *S. stercoralis* lives within the serpiginous tunnels of the mucosa of the small intestine. **Parasitic males** are rarely seen. The partially embryonated (segmented) eggs are laid by the parasitic female in the submucous tissue of the small intestine. They become ***mature*** and ***hatch out*** within a few hours to **rhabditiform** larvae (Fig. 12.7), as found in the lumen of the small intestine, are passed in the faeces. As they are deposited on the soil, they feed on organic debris and **metamorphose** in a short time into **filariform** larvae (Fig. 12.7), which is infective to man and may remain viable in soil for a few weeks.

FREE-LIVING GENERATION. The developmental stages are seen outside the body in the case of free-living form: (1) *Indirect development*, and (2) *Direct development*.

1. **Indirect development of larvae.** Under conditions of moisture and temperature in the tropics, the *rhabditiform larva* matures in 24-30 hours into free-living sexual generations of males and females. After fertilisation, the female lays second batch of approximately 60 eggs, which hatch out into *rhabditiform larvae*. These are hardly distinguished from those produced by parasitic females. After 3-4 days, they become *filariform* and may infect human by penetrating the skin, and migrate like the larvae of the parasitic form.

2. **Direct development of larvae.** Rhabditiform larvae undergo metamorphosis and directly develop in 3-4 days into *filariform larvae* on the surface of the moist soil; the sexual phase being absent. A rhabditiform larva produces a single filariform larva after moulting.

The filariform larvae are infective, but may remain in the moist soil for several weeks under optimum conditions.

Variation. Under optimum conditions of the development of worms, the rhabditiform larvae may develop into free-living males and females. The females lay eggs on the soil and rhabditiform larvae hatch out and develop into free-living male and female adults and may repeat the free-living phase indefinitely. Alternatively, they might develop into filariform larvae. These die after several weeks unless infection takes place in a new host.

PARASITIC GENERATION. PENETRATING the skin or less commonly the buccal mucosa of human beings, the **infecting filariform larvae** are carried through the blood vessels to the right heart. They break through the pulmonary capillaries into alveoli, develop into *post-filariform* and *preadolescent stages* to *adolescent worms*. Fertilisation of the adolescent **female** may occur either in the bronchi, or trachea, or after the worm has reached the intestine. This takes place before the female penetrates the epithelium of these organs, because **rhabditoid adult parasitic males** are not tissue parasites. They are voided in the faeces after a brief stay in the body. But in the case of parastrongyloides (a parasite of shrew), the **male is filariform** and is a *tissue parasite* like the female. In the bronchi or trachea, some of the adolescent females—after entering the columnar epithelium—oviposit, but others pass to the epiglottis and are swallowed. After reaching the small intestine, they migrate into the submucosa, mature and begin to deposit eggs in the tissues. The incubation period is about 28 days.

AUTO-INFECTION OR HYPERINFECTION (**Fig. 12.8**). In heavily parasitised weak patients, the **rhabditiform larvae** from the parasitic female may develop into infective, dwarf **filariform larvae** in the bowel. By penetration of the perineal or the perianal skin, the *filariform larvae* might enter into the circulation and finally reach the intestine *via* lungs as in the parasitic form. The rhabditiform larvae in constipated stool may develop into filariform larvae within the colon and produce internal **auto-infection** in a similar way (**hyperinfection** of Faust).

Pathogenicity. Infection by *S. stercoralis* is known as strongyloidiasis or strongyloidosis.

The worm or its larvae may produce the following complications:

1. During *migration of the filariform larvae*, symptoms may be produced as follows:

SKIN. Dermatitis, creeping eruptions, urticarial rash or petechial haemorrhage due to **sensitisation** may take place.

INTESTINE. Occasionally in patients with low resistance, massive migration of larvae through the intestinal wall may be fatal. They may produce catarrhal, oedematous and ulcerative enteritis.

LUNGS. Haemorrhage in the lung alveoli, bronchopneumonia, eosinophilia, etc. may occur.

2. *Intestinal lesions*. The female adults may produce diarrhoea with blood and mucus. They form tunnels in the submucosa, through which they burrow their way to deposit eggs. They produce congestion, round cell infiltration, desquamation of the epithelium and sometimes haemorrhage.

Blood may show *leucocytosis* with marked *eosinophilia*.

Epidemiology. TRANSMISSION. Infection occurs by contact of the skin with soil contaminated with filariform larvae, but infection may occur through the mucous surface, or an auto-infection may occur from the perianal or perineal region or through the colon.

Laboratory diagnosis. The DIRECT METHOD of diagnosis is by the recognition of living or dead rhabditiform larvae in the faeces. In light infection and in chronic cases, *concentration method* with 33 percent zinc sulphate may be needed (see **Appendix II**).

Dwarf filariform larvae may be present in the faeces, if auto-infection is occurring. Larvae are occasionally found in the sputum, urine or duodenal fluid obtained by intubation. If infected stools are allowed to stand for at least 30 hours, free-living forms may be recognised.

SEROLOGICAL AND IMMUNOLOGICAL TESTS. (a) *Intradermal*, and (b) *Precipitation tests* with extracts of filariform larvae have been carried out successfully.

Prophylaxis. It is similar to those for hookworm infection.

Treatment. Dithiazanine has been used as a *specific anthelmintic* for strongyloides infection. Gentian violet (medicinal) has been found to be specific. Hetrazan may also be tried in doses of 2 mg per kg body weight, thrice daily for 3 weeks.

Thiabendazole has been found to be effective (Cuckler and Mezey, 1966) with a cure rate of 85%, when a single dose of 50 mg/kg body weight is administered (Coura, 1963; Chaia and Cunha, 1963).

Mebendazole ("Mebex": *Cipla*). The adult dose is 200 mg (2 tablets) orally, twice daily for 3 successive days.

IMMUNOPATHOLOGICAL RESPONSE AS RELATED TO PROGNOSIS

In human no known specific response to Strongyloides has been demonstrated (Sheldon, 1937). Repeated experimental infections render dogs and cats partially immune. Arthus type of skin reactions, haemagglutinin titres in the sera, and degranulation of mast cells of immune animals by the specific Strongyloides antigen have been reported (Coldgrabber & Lewert, 1965). Fatal cases of strongyloidiasis due to chronic infection with altered immunity, or with treatment with immunosuppressive drugs have been referred in the literature (Cruz *et al*, 1966); Rivera *et al*, 1970; Rogers & Nelson, 1966).

The parasitic disease and the immunosuppressive drugs, e.g., cortisone, brings about alterations in the immune mechanism by disturbing the *immunologic balance* between the host and the parasite. Such alterations allow for increased virulence and pathogenicity on the part of the parasite. Heavily infected chronic cases with *hyperinfection, dissemination of the parasites* throughout the body and *failure of eosinophilic response* may be fatal. Patients from endemic areas with altered immunologic response, and also under immunosuppressive therapy, should be carefully handled, as they are prone to develop hyperinfective and disseminated stages of the disease, which may prove fatal, if not adequately treated early in its course.

SUBORDER: *STRONGYLINA*

SUPERFAMILY: *STRONGYLOIDEA*

(Weinland, 1958) Hall, 1916

The members of this group possess (i) well-developed buccal capsule, (ii) copulatory bursa in the male round the cloaca, and (iii) eggs with transparent shell and segments at the time of oviposition, which hatch out in the faeces and develop further in the moist earth.

FAMILY: ANCYLOSTOMATIDAE (having teeth or plates in the buccal cavity).

A. (i) TWO PAIRS OF TEETH—*Ancylostoma duodenale* (Dubini, 1843) Creplin, 1845, the Old World species.

(ii) ONE PAIR EACH OR SMALL MEDIAN and LARGER OUTER TEETH—A. *braziliense*; Gomez and Faria, 1910.

(iii) THREE PAIRS OR TEETH—*A. caninum* (Ercolani, 1859) Hall, 1913.

B. With cutting plates—*Necator americanus* (Stiles, 1902) Stiles, 1903; American or the New World hookworm.

FAMILY: STRONGYLIDAE—lacking teeth or cutting plates, e.g., *Oesophagostomum apiostomum*, which infrequently infects man.

FAMILY: *ANCYLOSTOMATIDAE*

GENUS: ANKYLOSTOMA AND NECATOR

(*Gk. Ankylos*—curved, hooked; *Stoma*—mouth)

The members of this group are hook-like and hence called hookworms. They posses a well-developed buccal capsule containing teeth or cutting plates.

The male possesses a bursa copulatrix, a membranous tubular expansion at the posterior end supported by rays

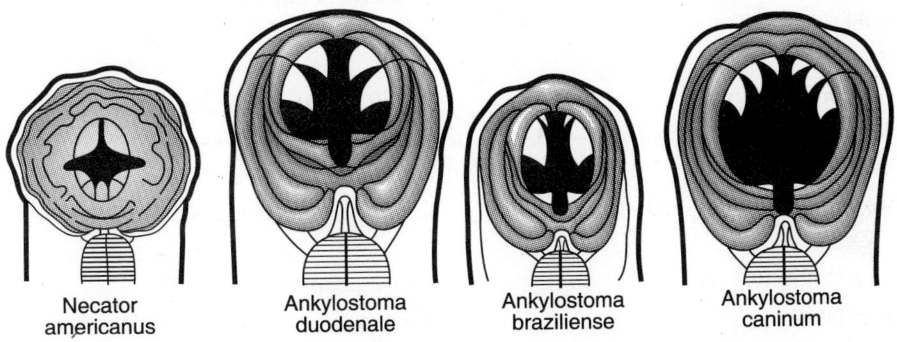

Fig. 12.9 Differentiating characters of buccal capsules of hookworms

or ribs of stouter tissue and a pair of spicules. Two species of this groups are pathogenic to man.

1. *ANCYLOSTOMA DUODENALE* **(Dubini, 1843) Creplin, 1845**, the Old World species. They are characterised by two pairs of teeth ventrally arranged in the buccal capsule and a pair of dorsal plates.

2. *NECATOR AMERICANUS* **(Stiles, 1902) Stiles, 1903**, the New World species. It is characterised by four chitinous plates in the buccal capsule—two ventral and two dorsal ones. They are characterised by a cervical (dorsal) bend at the anterior extremity. Both sexes are cylindrical, white, grey or reddish in colour. Eggs are oval and colourless and segmented either at the time of oviposition, or when they are passed in the faeces.

OTHER MEMBERS of this family are: (a) *A. braziliense* having one pair of small median teeth and a pair of outer teeth and is a parasite of dogs or cats in Brazil, and (b) *A. caninum*, a parasite of dog. It has a wide buccal capsule to accommodate 3 pairs of ventral teeth which is the diagnostic character of the species. The filariform larvae of both may cause **creeping eruptions** in human, by penetrating the skin. The characters of the buccal cavity are shown in **Fig. 12.9**.

HOOKWORM DISEASE
(*A. DUODENALE* AND *N. AMERICANUS*)
(*Producing ankylostomiasis and necatariasis in man*)

Geographical distribution. They are found in tropical and sub-tropical regions on either side of the equator (36°N to 30°S), where humidity and temperature are favourable.

Ancylostoma duodenale is prevalent in the Old World; whereas, *N. americanus* is a New World species; the latter is common in Assam and in South India. The disease is prevalent in Southern United States, West Indies, Northern part of South America, Egypt, China and Pacific Islands. In India it is most prevalent in the Sub-mountainous regions of the Himalayas, like Darjeeling and Assam, the Punjab and Uttar Pradesh; other regions affected are East and West Coasts of India, Sri Lanka (Ceylon) and Myanmar (Burma).

The disease is common amongst labourers who walk barefooted on damp soil. Miners and tea-garden labourers are prone to this infection. Ancylostomiasis is due to parasitism caused by *A. duodenale* and *N. americanus*. A mild infection produces a condition associated with anaemia and debility. Warm, moist condition favours transmission of the disease.

Morphology (PL. 12.III) of both the species is considered together in **Table 12.7**.

ADULT WORM. Adult hookworms are cylindrical, greyish white nematodes, but when freshly passed, pinkish brown in colour due to the ingested blood. They are tapering anteriorly and slightly curved and hook-like and hence the name. The **males** measure 8 to 11 mm in length whereas **females** range from 10 to 13 mm. The cuticle is smooth with fine transverse striations. They have 2 lateral

TABLE 12.7

DIFFERENCES BETWEEN *A. DUODENALE* AND *N. AMERICANUS*

A. duodenale	*N. americanus*
1. Size—Longer and thicker than *N. americanus*	Shorter and thinner than *A. duodenale*
2. Teeth—Present, 2 pairs ventrally	Absent but 2 cutting plates present
3. Head—Curvature of head in the same line with the body	Dorsiflexed and abruptly curved
Male:	
Size—8 to 11 mm by 0.4 mm	7 to 9 mm by 0.3 mm
Copulatory bursa—Total number of rays—13 Dorsal ray is tripartite	Total number of rays—14. Dorsal ray is deeply indented; each division bifurcates (bipartite)
Spicule—Two in number, long and slender	Long, slender, united and terminate in a barbed end
Female:	
Size—10 to 13 mm by 0.6 mm	9 to 11 mm by 0.6 mm
Posterior tip—spined	No spine
Vulva—Situated behind the middle of the body (posterior half)	Situated in front of the middle (anterior half) of the body

cervical papillae just behind the nerve ring at about the level of the middle of the oesophagus.

ALIMENTARY TRACT. The buccal capsule is well-developed and opens slightly dorsally and is provided with teeth or cutting plates to help its attachment to the intestinal mucosa. The oesophagus is cylindrical, about one-sixth the length of the worm. The intestine is straight and opens at the posterior end.

GENITALIA. In *males*, a single testis lies along the intestine, leading to the *seminal vesicles* through *ejaculatory duct* into the *cloaca*. The copulatory bursa is membranous, reinforced by *rib-like rays*. There are two bristle-like spicules (2 mm in length) within the bursa, and the cloaca opens into it.

In **males**, in the case of *A. duodenale*, the copulatory bursa consists of 3 lobes, one dorsal and two lateral. The dorsal lobe containing one single dorsal ray and 2 large externodorsal rays. The two lateral lobes contain 5 pairs of rays (3 pairs lateral and 2 pairs ventral). The caudal bursa is seen to be open by the naked eye. The dorsal ray of the copulatory bursa is split up less than half of its length. The spicules are not united. In the case of *N. americanus*, the dorsal ray is split deeply up to its base, and the spicules are fused to form a barb. The caudal bursa is closed as seen by the naked eye.

In **females**, the posterior end is cone-shaped. The paired vaginae lead from the vulva anteriorly and posteriorly into the oviducts and then to long, slender, coiled ovaries. The vulval opening is posterior to the middle of the body in *A. duodenale*; whereas, it is situated anterior to the middle of the body in *N. americanus*. The anus is sub-terminal.

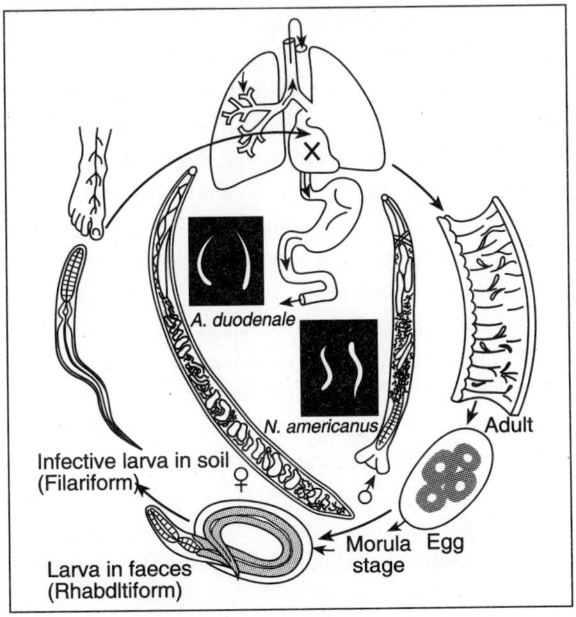

Fig. 12.10 Life cycle of hookworms

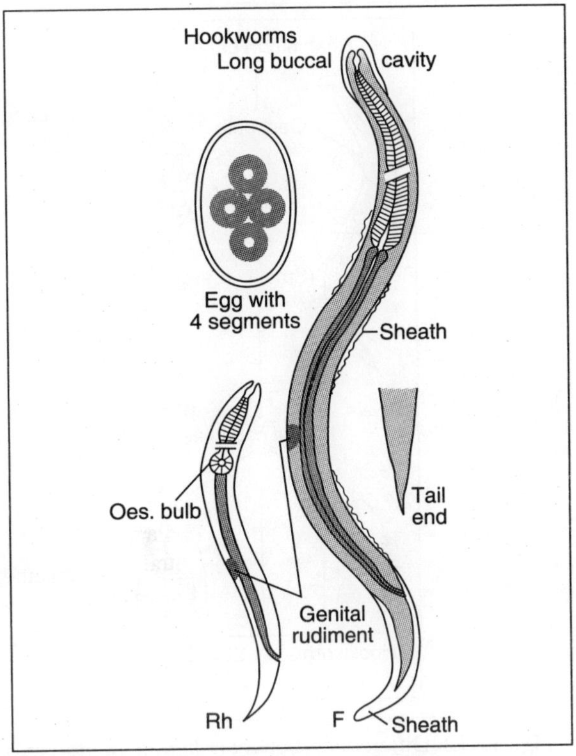

Fig. 12.11 Egg and larvae of hookworms

Eggs measure 56-76μm by 35-40μm; oval in shape. When passed by the worm the eggs are unsegmented. In a fresh specimen of stool, they contain 2 to 8 cells but usually only four granular cells are seen inside the egg capsule with a clear, thin egg-shell (**Fig. 12.11**). They are **colourless** and never bile-stained. There is a **clear space** between the egg-shell and the ovum. Eggs can live long in water. They float on saturated solution of common salt (PL. AP. II). About 25,000 eggs are passed daily by an adult female of *A. duodenale* but 10,000 by that of *N. americanus*.

LIFE SPAN in man is **6-8** years in case of *A. duodenale*, but it is **4-5** years in case of *N. americanus*. In the former case, it has been traced up to a maximum of 9 years.

Life cycle is the same for both species (Fig. 12.10). The worm requires one host to complete its life cycle and the DEFINITIVE HOST is man. Development of infective larva occurs outside the body. *Infection* may occur in two ways:

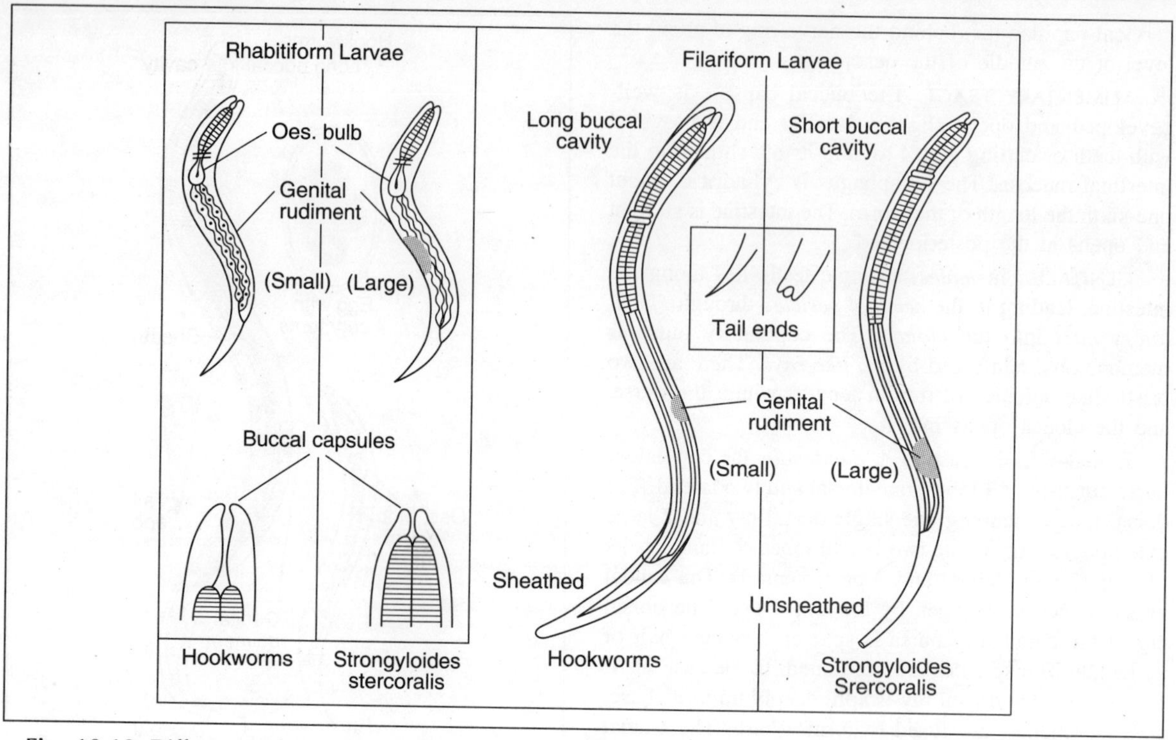

Fig. 12.12 Differences between larvae of hookworms and *S. stercoralis*

1. Through the skin.
2. Through the mouth, accidentally, by drinking water containing *filariform larvae*.

The former is the more important and commoner route of infection.

So, the infective form is the filariform larva.

DEVELOPMENT OF EGGS. Four-segmented eggs are generally passed by the human host in faeces and are not infective to man until they develop into filariform larvae outside the body, where they develop in the *free-living phase*.

RHABDITIFORM LARVAE. Eggs passed in stool, develop rapidly under favourable conditions of moisture and temperature at 25° to 35°C. Eggs develop into a blastomere consisting of 8, 16 and 32 cells and larvae hatch out in 24 to 48 hours, after their excretion in stool. The newly hatched larvae are 250μ by 17μ and are called rhabditiform larvae. This is the *first stage rhabditoid* larvae which has a long, narrow buccal chamber, a *bulbous oesophagus*, occupying the anterior third of the digestive tract, a short rectum and a small genital primordium (Fig. 12.10, 12.11 & 12.12), and feed voraciously. After 3 days of feeding, and growth, the larva sheds its cuticle, and a *second stage rhabditoid* grows to a maximum length of 0.5 to 0.7 mm, by 0.023 mm (23μ).

FILARIFORM LARVA (Fig. 12.10, 12.11 & 12.12). Between 5th and 8th day, the *mouth is closed* and it becomes *a non-feeding filariform larva*, the third larval stage, losing the *bulb-like swelling of the oesophagus*. This is the infective stage, which develops in 7 to 10 days after the ova are passed in stool. In this the old cuticle, which acts as a protective sheath is retained. The larvae now pass through a *resting phase*, when they cease to take any food but remain actively motile and can crawl up the grass blades and migrate a few centimetres. At this stage, they are relatively resistant and remain alive for about 2 months in damp soil, provided moisture is maintained, as they cannot withstand desiccation.

DEVELOPMENT IN HUMAN HOST (PL. 12.IV). As the body of the human host comes in contact with contaminated soil, larvae enter the skin as people walk barefooted, or work with bare hands. The larvae *burrow through the unbroken skin* or *hair follicles*

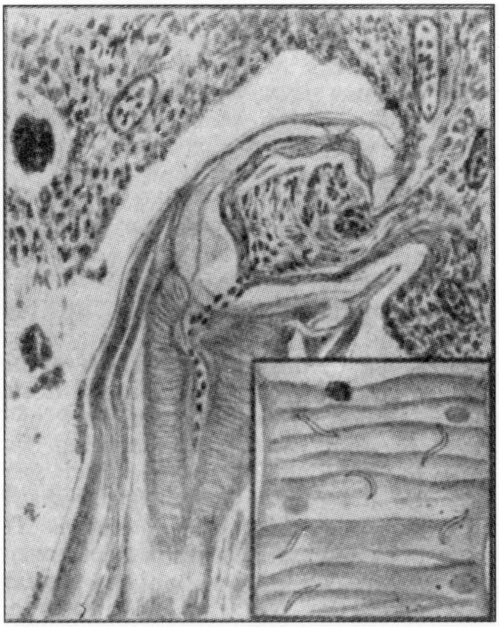

Fig. 12.13 Attachment of hookworm to human jejunum. Note how blood is sucked in by the powerful oesophagus. Inset—Hookworm on the wall of the jejunum showing haemorrhagic lesions

after *shedding* the *cuticle*, which is retained up to the time of penetration of the skin. On entering the subcutaneous tissue, they find their way through **lymphatics** or **venules** of the skin to **reach** the **right side** of the **heart** and lung capillaries, by the third day after infection. They then **penetrate** the walls of the capillaries and **enter** the **lung alveoli** and are carried up the bronchi and trachea to the intestine in about one week. The **third moult** occurs during this migration with the formation of a *temporary buccal capsule*, bearing four small teeth. The larvae feed and grow until about 4 mm in length, and then the **4th moult** occurs in the duodenum. The worm becomes *sexually mature* in three to four weeks. The interval between the time of skin infection and the first appearance of eggs in the faeces is about six weeks.

Epidemiology. Infection occurs by the entry of filariform larvae through the skin or rarely by the ingestion of larvae with contaminated food or drink. Therefore, defaecation near dwelling places, fields or gardens may become the most important source of infection.

REINFECTION (**Super-infection**). The problem of reinfection requires consideration. In an endemic area, reinfection is constantly occurring and new broods of worms are being added, replacing the old broods. Undoubtedly, patients acquire **resistance to reinfection** provided they receive proper nutrition after the primary infection.

Aetiology. The worms may produce **"hookworm disease"** when the infection is pronounced (53%), or they may produce a **"carriers of worms"** stage. The parasites attach themselves on to the mucous membrane of the jejunum and feed on the epithelium and leave punctate bleeding area (**Fig. 12.13** and **PL. 12.IV**). Test for **occult blood** is, therefore, positive in stool (Benzidine reaction).

The pathological effects are due to the degree of **anaemia** which, again, depends on: (a) the worm load (each female worm being represented by 50 eggs per gm of faeces), and (b) nutritional condition of the host. The latter is, however, the deciding factor in most cases. But ordinarily, anaemia is proportional to the intensity of infection. Low or moderate worm loads are carried by the host without symptoms. One hundred *N. americanus* or 20 *A. duodenale* **do not cause any clinical symptom**; but severe symptoms are produced when the worm load is 500 in the former and 100 in the latter. In case of nutritional deficiencies, however, the critical figures for the load is much lower.

According to Darling, 12 worms are responsible for the loss of 1 per cent (0.14 g) of haemoglobin. It has been estimated that, when *A. duodenale* is recently established in the intestine, the average **loss of blood** per day per worm **is 0.67 ml**, and most of this amount is pumped out through the gut, and the remaining escaping from the sides of the attached head. Moreover, Necators, which are established in the intestine, do not extract more than 0.2-0.5 ml blood per diem. It was also observed that, although blood is sucked by the worms, plasma forms the main source of nutrition, as RBCs pass out practically unchanged in the lumen of the host's intestine, wherefrom only iron may be absorbed (Fig. 12.13 and **PL. 12.IV**).

Nutritional deficiency in relation to anaemia. Anaemia depends on the nutritional condition of the patient. The chronic blood loss cannot be compensated by a faulty diet and a low iron intake. It has been observed that **anaemia can be easily combated** by people **who take high protein diet**, or **anaemia can be easily cured by administration of iron** even without any specific anthelmintics. Deficiency of iron causes **hypochromic microcytic anaemia**; whereas, **macrocytic** anaemia is produced by deficiency of either intake or absorption of vitamin B_{12} and folic acid.

Clinical Pathology. The infection produces severe anaemia and the blood picture varies according to the type of anaemia. This may be: (1) **Microcytic hypochromic**, or (2) **Macrocytic hyperchromic**, or (3) **Dimorphic** (Macrocytic hypochromic).

HAEMOGRAM. Microcytic hypochromic anaemia is often of secondary type due to chronic loss of blood. In these cases, the *colour index* is as low as 0.7 or may fall down to 0.5; *MCV* and *MCHC* are below normal. Occasionally *normoblasts* are present. The *reticulocyte count* is less than 3%. Polychromatophilic cells appear. *Van den Bergh reaction* is negative. It may be cured by iron therapy alone.

Dimorphic anaemia showing *macrocytic hypochromic* blood picture with high MCV and low MCHC has been reported by Chatterjee and Dasgupta (1963). This is due to combined deficiency of iron, vitamin B_{12} and folic acid.

Macrocytic anaemia is due to deficiency of the intake, or absorption of vitamin B_{12} and folic acid from the gastro-intestinal tract. It is seen in patients living on borderline diet, poor in animal protein, as in the case of labourers. PERSONS WHO LIVE ON BALANCED DIET SELDOM DEVELOP SEVERE ANAEMIA EXCEPT IN CASE OF HYPER-INFECTION.

There is *decrease of plasma protein* and plasma albumen with *increase of globulin* and reduction of colloidal osmotic pressure. Plasma volume increases (hydraemia in anaemia) and there is an increase in the *eosinophil count* (10 to 20%) with proportionate decrease of neutrophils. In chronic cases, eosinophilia is less evident.

Causes of anaemia: (1) Chronic blood loss is due to punctiform haemorrhages from jejunal mucosa, where hookworms lodge. Each worm sucks 0.67 ml of blood per day, but those which have been in the intestine for months do not extract more than 0.2-0.5 ml blood per day. Blood sucking is essential for consumption of oxygen and glucose. Oozing persists at the site of previous bites. A secondary anaemia is, therefore, the chief pathological condition due to blood loss. (2) Depression of the haemopoietic system, especially the bone-marrow, by deficient intake of protein, or (3) Deficient absorption of vitamin B_{12} and folic acid. (4) Interference with absorption from the villi. Iron absorption is deficient, and there is diminution of iron storage in the liver as in chlorosis. (5) Invasion of blood by haemolytic streptococci present in the ulcers.

Pathogenesis. Pathogenesis is divided under four heads: (1) Cutaneous (*cutaneous larva migrans* or *creeping eruption*, and *ground itch*).

(2) Migration of larvae in the lungs. (*Visceral larva migrans*).

(3) Lesions of the small intestine produced by adult worms (PL. 12.IV).

(4) Effects produced by anaemia.

GROUND ITCH. *At the site of penetration*, they often produce a condition of "ground itch". This appears as a papule and is soon followed by vesicle formation with secondary infection and oozing dermatitis.

CREEPING ERUPTIONS (PL. 12.IV). These are produced by infection caused by filariform larvae: of canine (*A. caninum*), feline or possibly human strains of *A. braziliense*, and occasionally of *N. americanus* and *A. duodenale*. The larvae produce *serpiginous tunnels* in the stratum germinativum, with corium as the floor. The lesions are erythematous to begin with, and then vesicular. Larvae proceed from several millimetres to few centimetres per day with local eosinophilic and round cell infiltration around the tunnel. The abandoned part of the tunnel becomes dry and crusty. The movements of the larvae cause intense pruritus and scratching—with subsequent pyogenic infection. The lesions may be single or multiple, often on feet or hands. Previous infection sensitises the skin and makes the inflammation intense.

Lesions produced during migration through the lungs. The migrating larvae may produce a condition of local leucocytic infiltration by eosinophils, pneumonitis, haemorrhagic lesions, bronchitis or bronchopneumonia. In general, pulmomary lesions are less severe than one accompanying ascariasis or strongyloidiasis.

Lesions of the intestine (PL. 12.IV). Duodenum and jejunum show raw surface with punctiform haemorrhagic areas, where worms are attached (See PL. 12.IV).

Pathological effects of anaemia. *Stomach*. A condition of achlorhydria or hypochlorhydria is met with in hookworm disease. *The liver* may be enlarged with a tinge of jaundice and often shows fatty changes with deposit of haematoidin pigment. MICROSCOPY reveals toxic degeneration of parenchyma cells of the liver with deposits of haemosiderin granules and also free iron (positive Purssian blue reaction). *Kidneys* show fatty changes and nephro-

PLATE 12.III
DIFFERENCES BETWEEN *A. DUODENALE* AND *N. AMERICANUS*

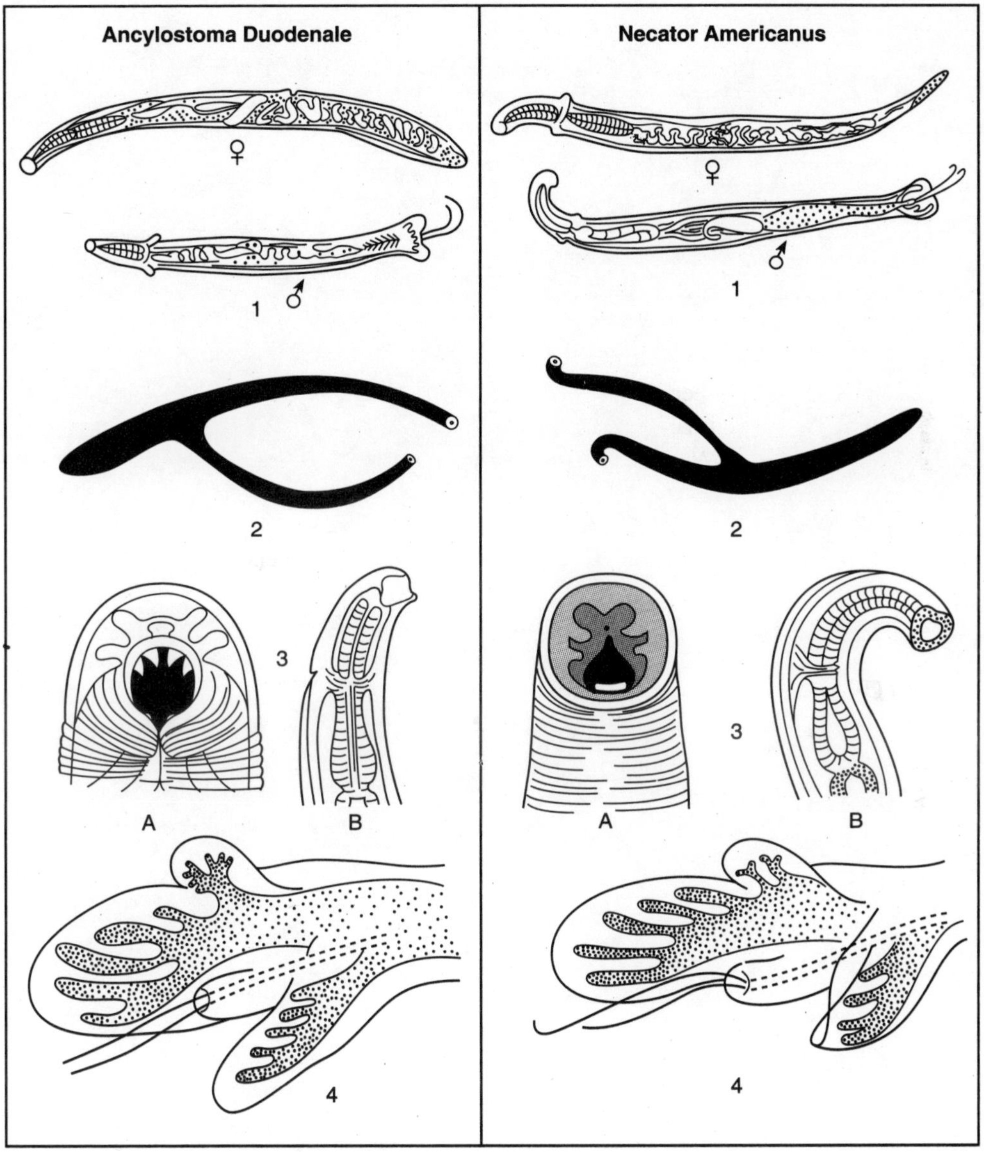

1.	Adult (male and female)	1.	Adults (male and female)
2.	In copulation	2.	In copulation
3 A.	Two pairs of teeth ventrally	3 A.	Two cutting plates ventrally
B.	Curvature of head in the same line with that of the body	B.	Head abruptly curved, dorsiflexed
4.	Copulatory bursa: dorsal ray division is shallow, tripartite Spicules: two, separate	4.	Coputatory bursa: dorasl ray is deeply indented, bipartite Spicules: two, fused and hook like at the tip

PLATE 12.IV

MANIFESTATIONS OF HOOKWORM DISEASE

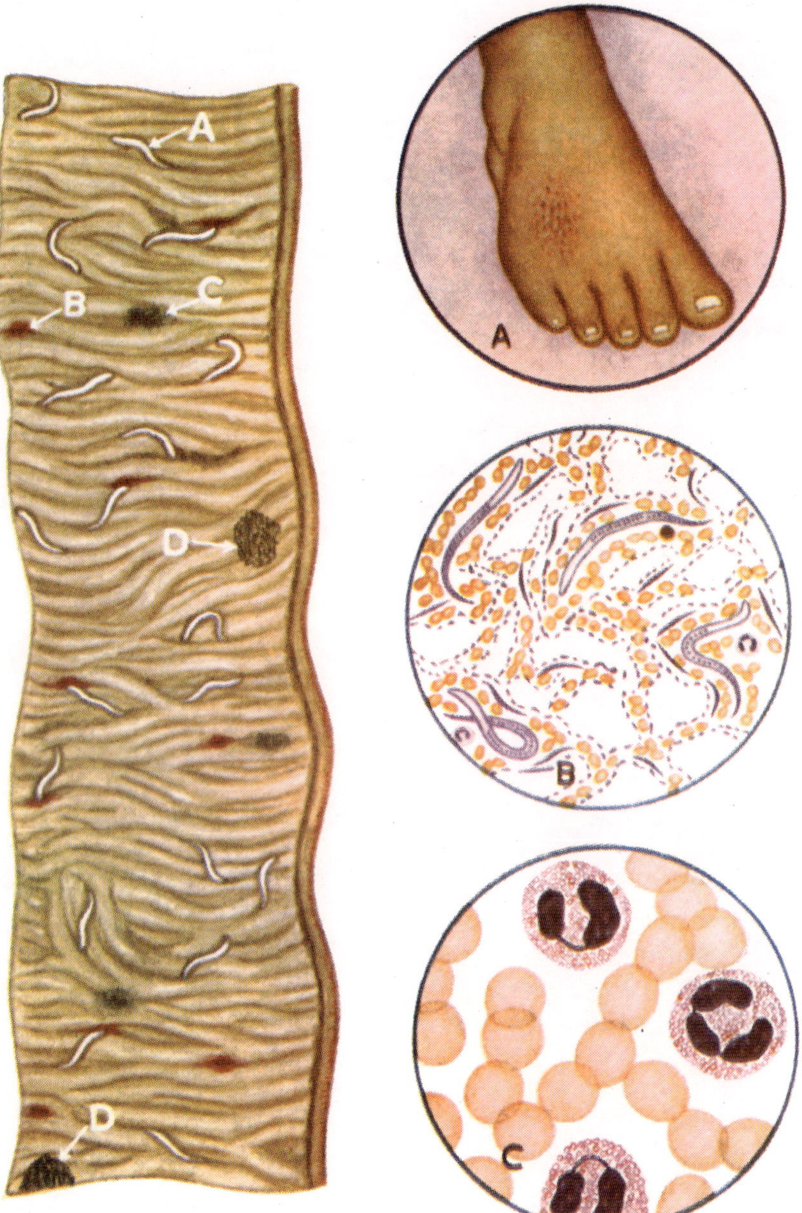

Right—A Ground itch and creeping eruption causing ankylostomal dermatitis. B. Microscopic appearance of ankylostomal pneumonia. C. Peripheral blood picture in ankylostomiasis (invasive stage); three eosinophils are seen.

Left—Gross pathology of the intestine in ankylostomiasis. A. Worms are seen free on the intestinal wall. B. Recent punctiform haemorrhagic areas during and after sucking of Blood. C. Greyish black old punctiform haemorrhagic areas (due to iron-sulphide formation). D. Intestinal lymph nodules (Peyer's patches) are seen

sis. *Bone marrow* often shows a normoblastic reaction and yellow marrow is transformed into a red formative bone marrow. *The heart is* dilated and shows marked fatty degeneration. *Spleen* is not enlarged.

Oedema of subcutaneous tissues or effusion into serous cavities is due to hypoproteinaemia resulting in reduction of colloid osmotic pressure.

Clinical features. Presence of a few worms in the intestine does not produce any clinical manifestation and sometimes several hundred worms may be harboured with a few clinical symptoms. Therefore, it is important to differentiate between "**hookworm infection**" and "**hookworm disease**".

Clinical cases are classified as **mild, moderate** and **severe** according to the degree of infection. Mild cases may act as carriers.

CRYPTIC OR MILD CASES. In these cases, symptoms are lacking. Such cases are of no clinical importance and may be considered as carriers. They are rather of epidemiological importance.

MODERATE CASES. In moderate infection, symptoms are less marked with appreciable blood compensation. There is "heart burn" and flatulence. Epigastric pain, when present, is relieved by eating bulky food. Low grade intermittent fever with lassitude may be present at times. Vasomotor disturbance, dyspepsia, palpitation, breathlessness and haemic murmur are common.

SEVERE CASES. Pale skin with **muddy complexion** and **puffiness of face** are characteristic. **Microcytic hypochromic anaemia** is marked and it is associated with oedema round the ankles, dead-white conjunctivae, and **flabby, "blotting paper tongue"** which is often pigmented.

Physical and mental lassitude is pronounced and some cases show a peculiar **geophagy** (ingestion of clay).

Pot-belly appearance is typical in children.

Puberty may be delayed with stunted growth. Repeated abortions and miscarriage are common in severe cases, and there is heavy maternal and infantile mortality. In the **terminal stage**, there is increasing anaemia, oedema, diarrhoea. Death is due to cardiac failure, oedema and anaemia.

Indirect evidences show that "the demand for a great circulating blood volume in the vital areas leads to reduction of the volume of the peripheral blood flow" and hence the marked **skin pallor**.

A correlation is often seen between advanced hookworm disease and nephrosis with manifestations of oedema, albuminuria and hypoproteinaemia. There is a tendency to compensate for the loss of haemoglobin by augmented vital capacity of lungs and increase of oxygen tolerance of the tissue cells, but without any circulatory compensation for reduced oxygen-carrying capacity of blood. While diastolic blood pressure remains normal, the systolic pressure is diminished.

Laboratory diagnosis. History of "ground itch", creeping eruptions of hookworm origin, pulmonary symptoms due to migration of larvae are helpful.

A. DIRECT METHODS comprise as follows: (1) The *microscopic examination of stools* will show the eggs of hookworm. Intensity of the infection can be judged by the enumeration of the eggs present in a gram of stool. The **concentration method** may be utilised with advantage (See **Appendix II**).

(2) *The diagnosis of the species* is not possible from the morphological features of the eggs. Therefore, specific diagnosis of hookworm infection, i.e., whether it is caused by *N. americanus* or *A. duodenale* will depend on the real finding of the adult worms. This is usually done by macroscopic examination of stool after an anthelmintic. This finding is confirmatory.

B. INDIRECT METHODS. (1) Examination of blood helps to determine the type and degree of anaemia.

(2) Eosinophilia is usually 10 to 20 percent. It is specially high in the invasive stage, when it may reach even up to 60 percent.

(3) Evidence of occult blood and presence of Charcot-Leyden crystals may be present in stool. Rhabditiform larvae of hookworm may be occasionally seen in constipated stool, or in *samples held too long* before examination. When only rhabditiform larvae are present, strongyloidosis is to be suspected. In hookworm infection, both eggs and larvae are present, but mixed infection may also be present with *S. stercoralis* as shown in **Fig. 12.12**.

Immunopathology. Any effective immunity is possibly directed against the larvae. Antiserum of laboratory animals to Necator larval injection has *inhibited respiration of infective larvae*. Several *bands of precipitation* by agar gel diffusion method have been reported by

Desowitz (1962), when the sera of infected patients were tested against larval or adult hookworm extracts. Some **cross-reactions** have been observed in precipitating antigens common to both Necator and Ascaris. A saline extract of infected larvae has been used in **tanned-red-cell** (TRC) **agglutination** test (Soulchy and Gilles, 1965).

Prophylaxis–(1) **Mass treatment**. This is the only method by which patients and carriers could be reduced in a community.

(2) Proper disposal of night soil is important to prevent pollution of soil.

(3) Prevention of **spread of larva** by proper sanitary measures. Practice of defaecation in the field should be abandoned. **Borehole latrine** should be introduced in villages. The life of infective larvae is about 6 weeks in free state in the soil. They can migrate to the surface from a depth of 90 cm (36 inches). Therefore, destruction from the surface is rather difficult.

(4) Common salt—when intimately mixed with soil—may act as a disinfecting agent.

(5) **Personal prophylaxis** is possible by wearing boots and gloves while working in the garden.

Treatment. Treatment of hookworm disease can be classified under two heads:

(A) SUPPORTIVE TREATMENT. This is administered in the form of salts of iron, such as **ferrous sulphate** or **gluconate** or **carbonate**, or **iron ammonium citrate**. At first, ferrous sulphate may be administered in doses of 1 gm per day till haemoglobin is raised to 10 gm, and then in doses of 0.5 gm per day. In macrocytic anaemia, intramuscular injection of vitamin B_{12}, folic acid and high protein food are helpful.

(B) SPECIFIC TREATMENT. The previous methods of removing hookworms by **chloroform, thymol, oil of chenopodium and carbon tetrachloride** have been replaced by several new drugs, which have proved efficacious, and at present **mebendazole** (**Mebex**: *Cipla*) and **bephenium hydroxynaphthoate** (**Alcopar**: *Burroughs Wellcome*) are the drugs of choice, because of their efficacy and safety.

Tetrachlorethylene. The established dose for tetrachlorethylene is 0.1 to 0.13 mg/kg of body weight (Jung and McCroon, 1960). It should be administered in an empty stomach, early in the morning, and the recommended adult dose is 4 ml in capsule, or 0.2 ml per year of apparent age in children. The easier method of administration is to mix the drug with a saline purgative (saturated solution of sodium or magnesium sulphate mixed by vigorous shaking) and administered in a single dose. This method of administration is found to be more effective than when given in capsules. The drug undergoes rapid deterioration in the tropics with evolution of phosgene gas, which renders the drug worthless as an anthelmintic. In the absence of alcohol and absorbable oils, tetrachlorethylene does not produce any appreciable damage to the liver.

Contraindications. The drug should not be used in pregnancy, dysenteric conditions, hepatic, renal, or cardiac disorders.

Merits and demerits. With the course of treatment, 66 per cent cases of Necator, and 25 per cent of Ancylostoma infections are cured. But with a second course of administration, 10 days after the first medication, 85 and 55 per cent cases are cured, respectively, as evident by examination of stool for ova. The worms are expelled in a stunt condition due to saline purgative. The drug has no effect on the migratory activity of the worm. Therefore, in a mixed infection of ancylostomiasis and severe ascariasis, the drug should not be used without deworming for ascariasis first (see ascariasis). The drug temporarily inhibits the egg-laying capacity of the female hookworms. Re-examination of stool is, therefore, done 10 days later.

Bephenium hydroxy-naphthoate (**Alcopar**: B. W. & Co.). It is available in dispersible granules in containers of 5 gm equivalent to 2.5 gm of the bephenium base (Jung and McCroon, 1960). It is given as a suspension in about 50 ml of a sweet liquid in a syrupy base. It is effective both in ancylostomiasis and necatariasis, and can be administered in ancylostomiasis concurrent with ascariasis. No purgation or dietary restriction is necessary, but no food is given for at least an hour before the drug is administered, in order to ensure maximum contact between the drug and the parasite. The dose for adults is 5 gm of the salt; children's dose is proportionately reduced. For children under 2 years or under 9 kg (20 lbs) in weight, half the above dose is recommended. In patients with persistent diarrhoea, three doses as above may be given if necessary in one day between meals. The dose may be vomited out, and this is why it is administered in a syrupy base. The drug has no side-effect except loose motions, nausea or vomiting.

Oil of chenopodium. The dose is 1 ml in capsules. For children, 1 minim per year of apparent age is administered. A saline purgative is followed 2 hours later. *Contraindications*. It should not be used in pregnancy, dysenteric conditions, hepatic, renal, or cardiac disorders.

Hexylresorcinol (crystoids). It is a true vermicide and administered in hard gelatin capsule (0.1 or 0.2 gm), because it produces necrosis of the buccal mucosa and oesophagus, if it comes in contact with the mucous surface.

The adult dose is 1 gm (0.2 gm × 5 capsules) given in subjects over 16 years of age. For 12-15 years 0.1 gm, 10-11 years 0.6 gm, or 0.2 gm for each 2 years of age.

The capsules should be swallowed and not chewed. The drug is given in an empty stomach in the morning following a light meal in the previous night. Although a post-purgative is not necessary, a saline purgative helps expulsion of the worms. No food is given for 5 hours after the capsules. The drug may be repeated after 3-5 days, if the eggs are still present in the stool. It is effective against *ascariasis* and *ancylostomiasis* but it is more effective against *N. americanus* than *A. duodenale*.

Cashew-nut shell extract. The dose for an adult is 6 g (in capsule). For children of 10-14 years, the dose is 4-5 g, and between 5-9 years, it is 2.5 to 3.5 g. A saline post-purgative is administered 2 hours later.

Cardol. The dose is the same as that of cashew-nut shell extract. There is practically no contraindication to its use.

In a mixed heavy infection of ascaris and hookworms, either the former is treated first, or a drug **effective against both ascaris and hookworms** are used, e.g., *oil of chenopodium hexylresorcinol, cashew-nut·extract*, or *cardol*, or a combination of drugs may be used as follows:

(a) Combination of *tetrachlorethylene* 2.7 ml and oil of *chenopodium* 0.3 ml is the dose for adults. For children, the dose is 0.6 ml of the above mixture for each year of age.

(b) **Neobedermin** (Bayer) is a combination of *ascaridol* and *tetrachlorethylene* and can be safely administered for **mixed ascaris and hookworm infection**.

(c) **Hydroxylene capsules**, each containing *hexylresorcinol* 0.1 g and *tetrachlorethylene* 0.3 ml, can be administered in adult doses of 10 capsules, or 1 capsule for each year of apparent age. The drug is also satisfactory for oxyuriasis when administered in repeated doses, but vomiting may occur as a side-effect.

Mebendazole ("**Mebex**": *Cipla*). The drug has been claimed to be effective, the adult dose being 100 mg (1 tablet) orally, twice daily for 3 consecutive days.

TEST OF CURE. Stools should be examined 10 days after the administration of the drug and subsequently also for the ova.

ANCYLOSTOMA BRAZILIENSE

Gomez de Faria' 1910

This is the smallest of the species of Ancylostoma. The buccal capsule is characterised by its small orifice and the ventral dental plate contains a pair of small median teeth and a pair of larger outer teeth. The **male** measures 7.75 to 8.5 mm by 0.35 mm in diameter. The **females** are 9-10.5 mm by 0.375 mm. The bursa of the male is small but distinct, as broad as long, and is supported by short sturdy rays. The **rays** are not readily distinguishable from those of *A. duodenale*, but they are comparatively smaller than the latter.

Life cycle is the same as *A. duodenale*.

Pathogenicity. Human host is unsuitable for its development. Therefore, the larvae wander over the skin causing **creeping eruptions** in man. This is common in Southern States of America. The adult worm has occasionally been recovered from the stools in the case of mixed *A. duodenale* or *N. americanus* infection in human, along with *A. braziliense*.

ANCYLOSTOMA CANINUM

(Ercolani, 1859) Hall, 1913

(The dog hookworm)

It is a common parasite of the dog and hence called the dog hookworm. It is distributed all over the world. The buccal capsule has a large orifice containing 3 teeth in the paired ventral plates, the outermost being the largest and the innermost being the smallest.

The life cycle is the same as that of *Ancylostoma duodenale*. The infective filariform larvae may produce **creeping eruptions** in human.

SUPERFAMILY: *TRICHOSTRONGYLOIDEA*

Cram, 1927

The members of this group have reduced mouth, and with buccal capsule rudimentary or lacking. The body is slender, but bursa copulatrix conspicuous. The most important human representatives are members of the genus Trichostrongylus.

TRICHOSTRONGYLUS SPP.

SUBORDER: *RHABDITINA*

FAMILY: *TRICHOSTRONGYLIDAE*

GENUS: *TRICHOSTRONGYLUS*

(Producing trichostrongyloidosis or trichostrongyloidiasis or trihostrongyliasis in man)

General consideration. These parasites commonly affect the digestive tract of herbivorous animals throughout the world and affect the bovine, ovine or carpine industry in some countries. There are more than 32 species of Trichostrongylus, of which at least eight have been reported as incidental pathogens in man (Biocca *et al*, 1960; Lie Kian, 1947; Orsuru, 1962; Skrjabin *et al* 1960; Stewart, 1949; Travassos, 1937). The more frequent human pathogenic species are *Trichostrongylus colubriformis* and *T. orientalis*.

Incidence. Stoll (1947) estimated that Trichostrongylus species constitute a worm burden for 5.5 million human beings, almost exclusively natives of Asia and Russia. Because of its usually silent clinical course and the fact that the eggs and the very early larval stages may be confused with those of hookworm, the infection has been named as "**Pseudohookworm**" **disease** (Markell, 1968).

Habitat. Adult worms inhabit the small intestine of herbivorous animals and human throughout the world.

Geographical distribution. It is worldwide; Assam in India (Maplestone, 1941); reported from Brazil (Campos *et al*, 1963), Peru (Tejda and Burstein, 1964) and Chile (Naghme, 1965).

Morphology. The adult worms are hair-like, thin and delicate. They measure 0.5 to 1 cm in length with a minute, unarmed *head*, lack a distinct buccal capsule, and having a conspicuous *ventral notch* in the cervical region, where the *excretory pore* opens. The **males** have a *copulatory bursa* with long lateral and ill-developed dorsal rays. The copulatory *spicules* are brownish, stout and sculptured differently at the posterior end, which are useful in *differentiating* several species. In the **female**, the paired generative tubules open through a common vulva, which is situated a short distance behind the anterior half of the body.

Eggs. The eggs resemble those of hookworm, but are longer and narrower with more pointed ends varying from 73 to 115μ by 40μ in width. They are hyaline-shelled. The eggs are usually discharged in the morula stage of embryonation and—under favourable conditions of moisture and temperature—may hatch in the ground within twenty-four hours. Unlike the eggs of hookworm, those of Trichostrongylus are remarkably resistant of environmental changes. The hatched larvae are of **pseudo-rhabditoid** type with a long capillary, pre-oesophageal cavity, an oesophagus with a long, ovoid, anterior portion, a constricted portion behind the oesophageal nerve ring and a typical posterior bulbous swelling. At the anal region, they have a noticeable dorsal bend. The postanal portion is attenuate and terminates in a minute knob.

Life cycle. There are three free-living larval stages with 2 ecdyses (moulting). The hatched larvae pass through three-free-living stages, until they become third stage infective larvae in a minimum period of 60 hours. Only one host is required to complete its life cycle.

The **semifilariform** infective third stage larvae may enter through the intact skin; however, the more frequent portal of entry is by *ingestion* as a contaminant in vegetation. The ingested larvae attach themselves to the duodenum and jejunum with the minute head embedded in the mucosa, and within 25 days attain sexual maturity.

Pathology and Symptomatology. The primary lesion is essentially produced by, maturing and adult worms caus-

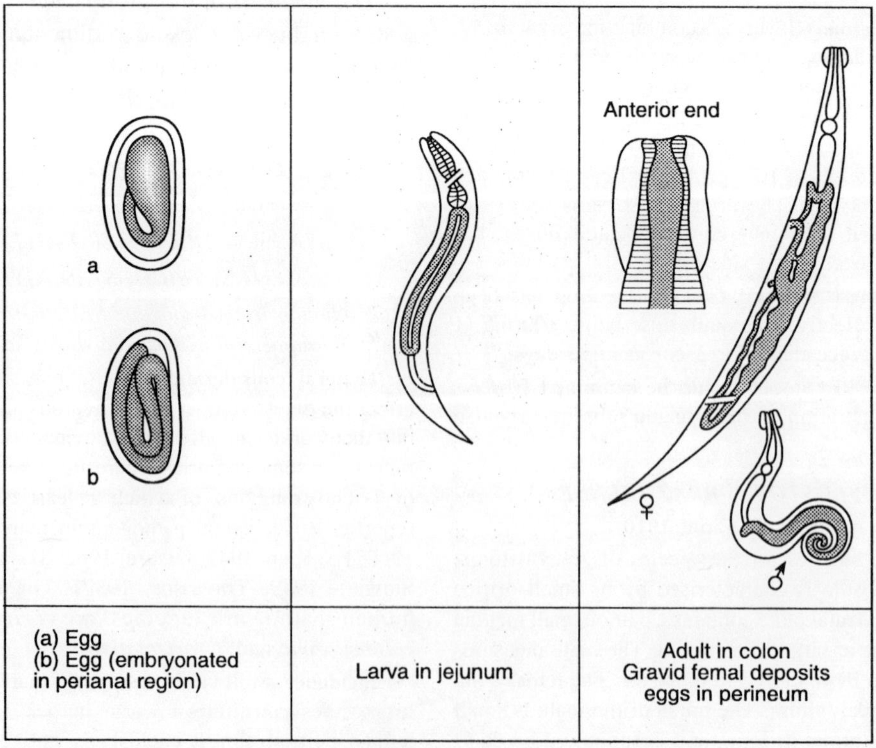

Fig. 12.14 Eggs, larva and adults (male and female) of *Oxyuris vermicularis*

ing traumatic damage to the intestinal mucosa; as is evident by the presence of desquamation, hyperaemia and haemorrhage. However, it takes several hundred worms to provoke clinical symptoms characterised by vague intestinal disturbances like occasional diarrhoea, and emaciation, dry skin, transient eosinophilia to a maximum of 10 per cent (Lie Kian, 1947). The adult worms are blood-suckers, hence, mild anaemia may be associated with the infection.

Diagnosis. Identification of eggs in the faeces or bile (Maki *et al*, 1954), or culturing faeces with powdered animal-charcoal and recovering the typical larvae is essential. These larvae must be differentiated from those of hookworm and Strongyloides. The eggs of Trichostrongylus are readily concentrated by brine (Lane, 1924) and zinc sulphate techniques (Faust 1938, 1939; see **Appendix II**).

Treatment and Prognosis. Trichostrongylus is highly resistant to tetrachlorethylene—so repeated failures of this drug in treating hookworm infection should suggest that one is dealing with trichostrongyliasis. **Bephenium hydroxynaphthoate** and **1-bromo-β-naphthol** were found to be effective in Japan (Otsuru, 1962) and Brazil (Campos *et al*, 1963). **Thiabendazole** is also *effective*, but sometimes may cause serious side-effects. **Mebex** may be tried with efficacy.

Prognosis is excellent.

OXYURIS VERMICULARIS

Lamark, 1816

SUPERFAMILY: OXYUROIDEA **Ralliet, 1915**

GENUS: OXYURIS or ENTEROBIUS **Leach, 1944**

GK. *Oxys*—sharp; *oura*—tail

GK. *Enteron*—intestine; *Bios*—life

SYNONYM: *Enterobius vermicularis*

(Linnaeus, 1758) Leach, 1853

General consideration. *Oxyuris vermicularis* is a small nematode parasite of the caecum and large intestine of man; the gravid females come down to perianal region, where they lay eggs. **Auto-infection** is the rule. They cause perianal irritation and nervous changes in children but often the symptoms are negligible or absent.

Geographical distribution. Its distribution is world-wide (cosmopolitan).

Habitat. The adults inhabit the caecum and vermiform appendix, where they are attached or occasionally encysted in the mucosa. The gravid females migrate, when the eggs are developed down the intestine to the anus and the adjacent skin—specially at night—to lay eggs in the perianal region. Occasionally, they might migrate into the vagina, female urethra or bladder, or enter into the peritoneal cavity via the Fallopian tubes.

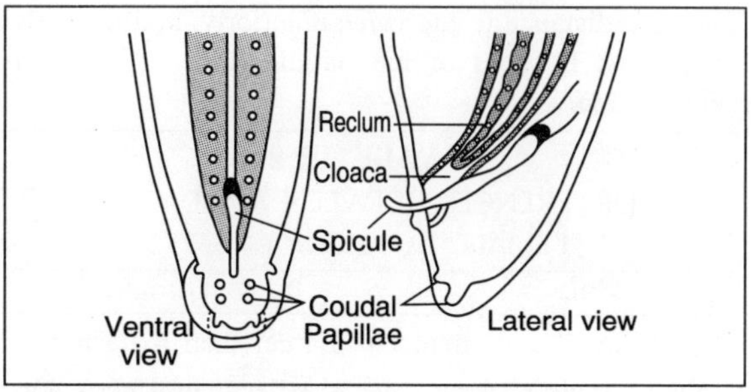

Fig. 12.15 Posterior end of the male *Oxyuris vermicularis*

Incidence. In communities, the incidence may be 50 percent of the population, but in school-going children, it may be even 80 percent. The highest incidence is seen in congested urban areas, institutions, or in large families. The infection brought by a child may spread to other children and adults of the family.

Morphology. *Oxyuris vermicularis* is a nematode with finely striated cuticle. *The oral end* lacks a true buccal capsule, but it has three lips with a dorsiventral bladder-like expansion of the cuticle (Beaver, 1952).

ALIMENTARY CANAL. The *oesophagus* is short and has a posterior bulb and joins the intestine. The *anus* is at the junction of the middle and posterior thirds of the body in the female (**Fig. 12.14**). The **male** is about 5 mm by 0.2 mm and is rarely found. It is coiled ventrally; at the posterior end it is blunt. It has a copulatory *spicule* without a gubernaculum. The attenuated bursa is called "Caudal ala", supported by a pair of anterior pedunculated papillae. There are also 3 pairs of more median *postanal sessile papillae* and a pair of sessile papillae lateral to the anterior pedunculated pair (**Fig. 12.15**). The **female** is longer and has a straight body with a tapering posterior end. It is 8-13 mm by 0.3-0.5 mm. In a gravid worm, the uteri are tremendously distended with eggs, varying in number from 4,672-16,888 with an average of 11,105; the uterus practically fills the entire body.

GENITALIA. The **male** has a single tubular testis, two seminal vesicles, ejaculatory ducts leading into the cloaca. It has a sharply curved conspicuous terminal copulatory spicule 70μ long, but lacks a gubernaculum. The reduced bursa called the *caudal, ala* is supported by a pair of anterior vesicular or pedunculated papillae, and a pair of posterior papillae. The **female** has anterior and posterior *oviducts* and *uteri leading* into the *vagina*, which extends for some distance to the *vulva* anteriorly, and the vulva opens just in front of the middle third of the body (Fig.12. 14).

TABLE 12.8
DIFFERENCES BETWEEN MALE AND FEMALE *O. VERMICULARIS*

Male	Female
1. Very small and smaller than female (3-4 mm × 0.2 mm)	Larger than male but smaller than a hookworm (8 to 12 mm × 0.6 mm)
2. Posterior end—coiled	Posterior end—tapering and straight

Eggs. The fully embryonated eggs measure 50 to 60μ by 16 to 25μ, oval, **colourless** (not bile-stained) and **plano-convex**, i.e., one side is flat and the other convex. The shell is composed of a hyaline membrane, and a shell proper composed of 2 layers of chitin and an innermost layer of embryonic lipoid. The eggs are rarely found in the faeces, as they often stick to the perianal region where they become embryonated containing a coiled tadpole-like larva

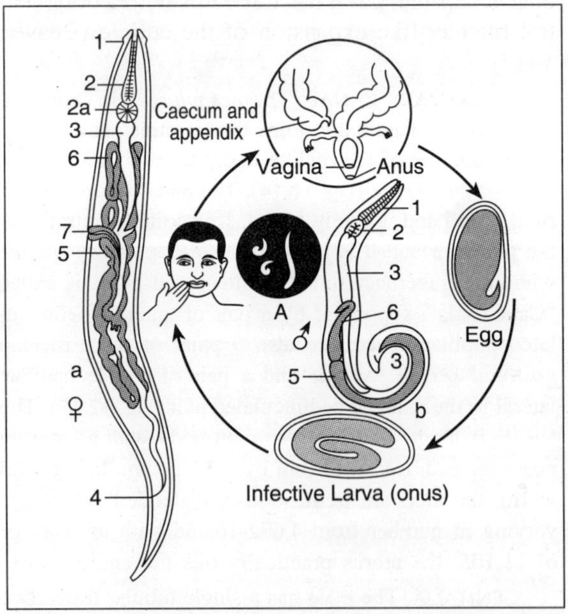

Fig. 12.16 Life Cycle of *Oxyuris vermicularis* Thread worm: A. Adult worm. a. Gravid female. 1. Cervical alae. 2. Oesophagus. 2a. Bulb of oesophagus. 3. Intestine. 4. Anus. 5. Ovary. 6. Uterus. 7. Vulva. b. Male. 1. Oesophagus. 2. Bulb of oesophagus. 3. Intestine. 4. Spicule. 5. Seminal vesicle. 6. Testis

and is **infective** after 36 hours. They are readily picked up on a piece of cellophane rolled over the perianal region with the help of **NIH swab** (See Appendix II). The infective larvae may survive outside the body for 4 to 5 weeks at 14°-18°C. Eggs are relatively resistant to antiseptics.

LIFE SPAN is short; the adult females live for 37-100 days and the male is short-lived.

Life cycle (Fig. 12.16). The life cycle is complete in one host due to direct infection caused by the infective larvae and, therefore, no intermediate host is necessary. Eggs are not infective until larvae develop in them. When the infective first-stage larvae containing eggs are swallowed by man, the tadpole larvae (140-150μ by 10μ) hatch out in the duodenum and are set free. They pass down the small intestine, and enroute moult twice lodging in the crypts of jejunum and upper segments of ileum. In the caecum, the adolescent worms become attached to the mucosa and, in 15 to 43 days after the ingestion of the larval stage within the eggs, they become adult. The **gravid females** release their attachment to the bowel wall and migrate freely in the lumen of the large intestine. They pass to the colon and crawl to the anus and lay eggs in the **perianal** and **perineal** regions at night. The eggs have an albuminous coating, which help them to adhere to the skin and the mucoid material, causing the **characteristic itch**. Each egg further develops into a tadpole-like larva in the egg shell and this is hastened by favourable temperature and moist condition of the perianal skin, where the eggs rest on the flat surface. In 6 hours in presence of oxygen, the egg develops into an **infective first-stage larva** within the egg-shell and survives in this condition for a variable period. The eggs may adhere to clothes or bed linen. The infective larvae may survive in the egg-shell outside the body for 2-3 weeks at 17°-20°C, or 4-5 weeks at 14°-18°C.

Infection. The FOREMOST SOURCE of infection is due to scratching of the perianal region, when the eggs contaminate the **fingers** and **nails**. When **contaminated fingers** are put into the mouth, or **food contaminated** with infected fingers is ingested, infection occurs and the cycle repeats (**Fig. 12.16**).

SECONDLY. Persons sleeping in the same bed, or living in the same room may become infected.

The eggs dislodged from linen are mixed up with the dust of the room and get into the mouth, or the inhaled eggs settle in the posterior part of the pharynx and, thereafter, swallowed by the host. **Retrofection** is possible, in which eggs laid on the perianal skin develop into infective (embryonated) eggs, which hatch out on the anal mucosa, and the hatched larvae then migrate up into the bowel and develop into the adult form in the colon. There is, however, no evidence of **internal autoinfection**.

Epidemiology. In the house, the eggs may be found in the dust, door, clothes and lavatories. Damp condition, a temperature of 26°C with minimal ventilation, are optimal for their survival. Eggs survive in the dust for 3 weeks, such dust may cause only mild infection; heavy infection takes place in children, when they infect their hands by scratching the perianal region. By this means 100-1,000 eggs may be ingested at a time.

Pathogenesis. The attachment of the worm may cause mild inflammatory lesions of the mucosa and this may be aggravated by bacterial infection causing haemorrhage, small ulcers or submucosal abscess. That Oxyuris may cause appendicitis is uncertain and not important. However, worms may be found in the gross specimen or histological section (Dey, 1974). The worms which migrate to the perianal skin to oviposit cause distressing irritation and excoriation of perianal and perineal regions by scratching, and this may sometimes cause insomnia, symptoms of dysentery, or **vulvovaginitis** in children. The peritoneum may be reached through the bowel-wall, or through the Fallopian tube in females causing **pseudotuberculous inflammation**. There is a rise of **eosinophil** count (10 per cent) in children in most of the cases.

Laboratory diagnosis. It consists of (i) the detection of adult worms, and (ii) demonstration of eggs. (iii) Eosinophilia is only an indirect evidence.

The ADULT WORMS are passed in the stool as usual or after a purgative or enema. This is often detected by the patient or his relatives. The worms, specially the gravid females, may be found in the perianal region during the time of itching at night.

EGGS. The eggs from the perianal region, on bed sheets or garments, can be easily demonstrated by **NIH swab** (for details, see **Appendix II**). Oviposition in the caecum is exceptional and, in that case, eggs may be demonstrated in the stool either by direct smear, or by concentration method. **The eggs float in saturated solution of common salt.**

Prophylaxis. Human is the only host of *O. vermicularis*. The eggs resist desiccation and may contaminate clothes, bedding, and also the house dust, which might infect by inhalation. Thus the eggs may maintain a constant source of infection in homes and institutions. The infection is common in children due to their insanitary habits, and itching the anus due to the irritation. Therefore, the treatment of cases is the most useful method of control, provided reinfection is prevented.

Treatment. The most valuable present day chemotherapy consists of anthelmintics containing piperazine salts like citrate, adipate, tartrate, hexahydrate, etc. These are specific and many preparations are available. *Doses* are determined according to the age of the patient.

The drug is administered for 7 days in doses not exceeding 50 mg per kg body weight (as mentioned in ascariasis). According to White and Scopes (1960), a single dose of the combined drug, namely, **piperazine phosphate** and **calcium senoside** (see treatment of ascariasis) will effect a cure rate of 97 percent. This mode of treatment replace the 7 days' course, which may be repeated at an interval of 7 days, if required.

Tetrachlorethylene. The dose is the same as for hookworm infection.

Gentian Violet (Medicinal). Adult dose is 60 mg (1 gr) three times a day before food for 8 days, followed by a rest for one week, and then the course is repeated. For children, a daily dose of 10 mg for each year of apparent age should be administered. The tablets are swallowed and chewed. The drug is stopped, if there is nausea, vomiting, or abdominal cramps. Relapses are frequent, unless all the members of the house are treated at the same time. Measures to prevent reinfection are essential for the success of chemotherapy. Hygienic measures should be adopted. **Ammoniated mercury ointment** [10 gr (600 mg) to one ounce] or **petroleum** jelly should be appiled over the perianal region everynight before retiring. Re-examination of the whole stool for ova is done one month after the course of treatment, and NIH anal swab is taken for 6 or 7 consecutive days, early in the morning before toilet.

Pyrivinium pamoate is considered to be highly efficient for single dose therapy (Beck *et al*, 1959).

Mebendazole ("**Mebex**": *Cipla*). The drug has a potential therapeutic value, the adult dose being 100 mg (1 tablet) orally for 1 day. This is a single dose treatment.

Prognosis. Prognosis is favourable after periodic treatment. Uncomplicated oxyuriasis is never fatal.

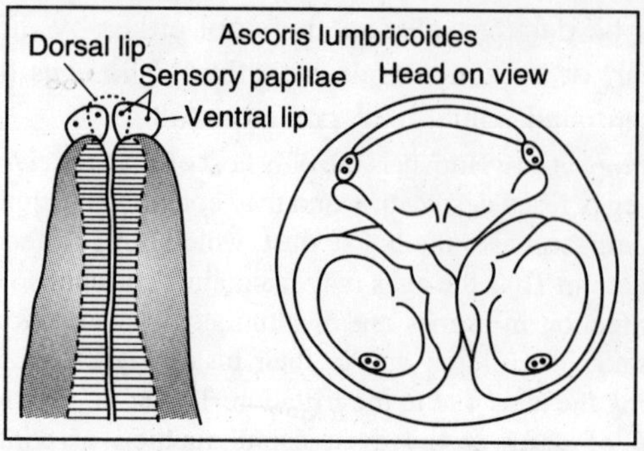

Fig. 12.17 Left—Anterior end of *A. lumbricoides* (similar in both male and female) Right—Head-on view (after Yorke and Maplestone)

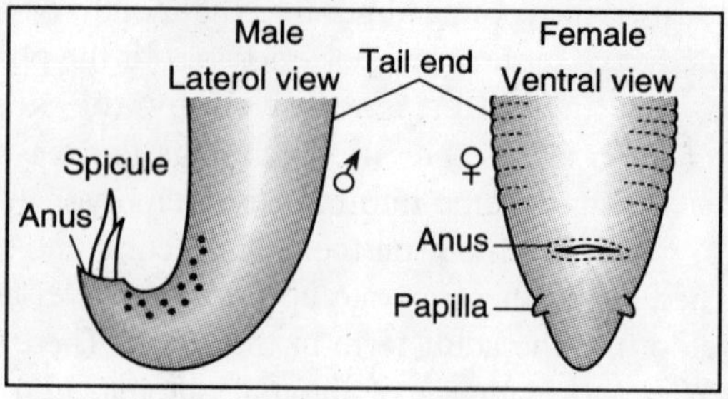

Fig. 12.18 Posterior ends of *A. lumbricoides* (male and female)

ASCARIS LUMBRICOIDES

Linnaeus, 1758

SUPERFAMILY: ASCARIOIDEA

GK. *Askaris*—an intestinal worm

(*Giant intestinal roundworm, causing ascariasis*)

General consideration. Ascaris lumbri*coides* is the common roundworm of man. They inhabit the small intestine of man and cause abdominal pain and digestive disturbances. Wandering adults may cause serious illness and the migrating larvae produce pulmonary lesions and eosinophilia, known as **Loeffler□s syndrome** discovered by Loeffler (1932).

Geographical distribution. It is found all over the world, i.e., cosmopolitan in distribution.

Habitat. Adults are found in the intestine of man, specially in children. Similar species are found in gorilla, larger apes, and pigs, but they are not identical. Experiment with porcine strains have failed to infect man so far.

Incidence. The incidence of ascariasis may be very high in rural areas with poor sanitation (80 per cent or more). It is most frequent in children and often limited to some families.

Morphology. They are the largest intestinal nematodes, white, cream or flesh-coloured, cylindrical, tapering at either ends, but somewhat more attenuated at the posterior end. *Lateral lines* can be seen as a pair of whitish streaks along the entire length of the body. *The mouth* is provided with 3 conspicuous lips—two ventral and one dorsal and finely denticulate. Each lip on its lateral margins has a pair of sensory papillae (Fig. 12.17). Centrally located amongst the lips is a small, triangular *buccal cavity*. The cuticle is finely and transversely straited.

The **male** is smaller than the female, 150 to 300 mm by 2-4 mm in diameter, and curved ventrally at the posterior end. *The posterior end* is conical in the female, *the anus* opens subterminally on the ventral aspect in the form of a transverse slit (Fig. 12.18). Distal to this are the **papillae**. Near the vulva, the worm has a narrow band, called the *vulval waist*.

The **female** measures 200-350 mm by 3-6 mm in diameter, but there is a great variation in size.

ALIMENTARY CANAL. The mouth opens into a cylindrical muscular oesophagus, 12 mm long. The simple tubular intestine opens at the *anus in the female*, and

TABLE 12.9

DIFFERENCES BETWEEN MALE AND FEMALE *A. LUMBRICOIDES*

	Male	Female
SIZE	Smaller than females, 15-20 cm (6-8 inches)	Longer than males, about 30 cm (12 inches)
POSTERIOR END	Coiled	Tapering
GENITAL OPENING	At the posterior end near the anus. Two spicules present corresponding to penis	Vulva at the junction of anterior and middle third. No spicule present
PAPILLAE	Pre- and post-anal—multiple	Post-anal—one pair

cloaca in the male at the base of the caudal cone (Fig. 12.18).

GENITALIA. In the **male**, the genitalia consists of a single, long, tortuous tubule, made up of *testis, vas deferens* and *ejaculatory duct* coiled at the posterior part of the body and opens at the cloaca, which is subterminal. A pair of pointed *spicules* equal in size and 2-3.5 mm in length is situated in a pocket, dorsal to the genital tubule. Occasionally, rudimentary *caudal alae* are seen.

In the female, there are tortuous, tubular, paired *ovaries, oviduct, seminal receptacles, uteri* leading to the vagina, the last one opening into a small *vulva* ventrally, near the junction of the anterior and middle thirds of the body. The tubules are coiled in the middle and posterior thirds of the body, and are several times longer than the entire length of the worm.

Eggs are either ovoid or elliptical and **bile-stained**. They measure 50 to 70μ by 40 to 50μ. Egg shell is thick and transparent and covered on the outer side by an albuminous envelope, which is mammillated. Fertilised eggs contain the unsegmented granular embryo. The **infertile egg** is elongated (90μ by 40μ) and contains a disorganised attenuated ovum and yolk granules of various sizes instead of a fertilised ovum. The egg is **bile-stained** and the shell is thick with an irregular albuminous coat. It does not float on saturated salt solution (see **Appendix II**).

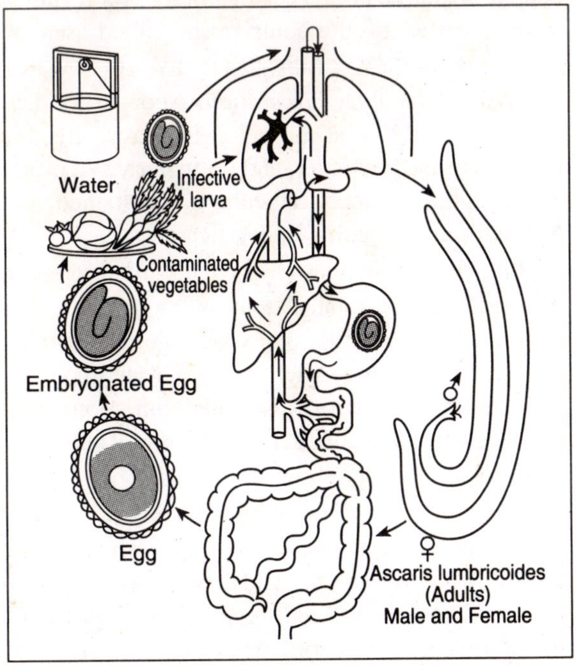

Fig. 12.19 Life cycle of *Ascaris lumbricoides*

A gravid *A. lumbricoides* may contain 27 million ova and the average output is 200,000 per day.

LIFE SPAN of an adult ascaris is 10-12 months and that of an egg is 3-7 years.

Life cycle (Fig. 12.19). The adult worm lives in the intestine of man. No intermediate host is necessary to complete the life cycle.

EGGS. Fertilised unsegmented ova are passed in the faeces. They are not infective.

Development in soil. The development of ovum takes place outside the human host under suitable temperature (22°-33°C) and moisture. A **first stage larva** forms by segmentation of the ovum about a week after the passage of the egg. This is followed by the first moulting after another week without hatching and a fully developed **second stage rhabditiform infective larva** forms within the egg-shell three weeks after the passage of the egg. In moist, loose soil with moderate shade, the infective larvae may remain alive for 3 years or more. Direct sunlight or a moist temperature above 70°C kills them.

Pathogenesis and Pathology. Human acquires infection by the ingestion of eggs containing embryonated **second stage infective larva** in food, drink, or raw vegetables. Infection by ingestion of eggs frequently takes place by contamination of hands with soil. Eggs may be carried with dust and contaminate uncovered food, or the dust may be inhaled and swallowed from the pharynx. When fully embryonated eggs are swallowed, the gastric juice cannot kill the embryo due to the presence of thick egg-shell. The egg-shell is softened by the digestive juice in the duodenum, where the enclosed larvae are stimulated to activity, and emerge through a rent in the shell. They are 250μ in length by 14μ in diameter and show a club-shaped oesophagus (*rhabditiform*), which is about a quarter of the length of the body. This is the **first moult**. The larvae then reach the small intestine, enter the portal circulation by burrowing through the wall of the small intestine or mesenteric lymphatics.

MIGRATION OF LARVA. Through mesenteric lymphatics or hepatic venules, larvae reach the right side of the heart. They then escape through the pulmonary artery into the lungs. Here, after a sojourn of several days, they break-through the alveolar wall. During this sojourn, they **moult twice** (2nd and 3rd moult) on the 6th and 10th day, respectively. This ***blood bath*** is necessary for this development, and the process is complete in 10-14 days. Larvae now burrow through lung capillaries and alveolar walls to reach the bronchioles. Larvae next travel up the bronchus and are coughed up, adhere to the oesophagus, from where they are swallowed. They now attain an average length of 1.5 mm, and acquire resistance to gastric juice by the time they reach the stomach. After passing through the stomach, they reach the intestine and those which survive, undergo metamorphosis to the **fourth moult** (between the 25th and 29th day). The worms now localise in the upper part of the small intestine. They begin to grow into adult worms and become sexually mature. The interval between the infection and oviposition takes about 60-75 days, and the fertilised eggs are passed in the faeces at least two months after the ingestion of the infective larvae.

ABERRANT CYCLE. In massive infestation the larvae may escape into the mesenteric lymph nodes *via* lymphatics and the peritoneal cavity, wherefrom, the larvae may reach the lungs by entering the liver and piercing the diaphragm in 6-7 days. The larvae reach the lungs *via* circulation in 18-24 hours. The aberrant larvae **might** gain entrance to general circulation *via* the left heart in different organs, like the brain, spinal cord, kidneys and other organs, and get lost or destroyed, provoking tissue reaction. They might be passed in the urine or through the placental filter to the foetus.

Immunopathology. The granulomatous response to the presence of Ascaris eggs has been studied extensively and it is now generally accepted that the granulomatous process represents an attempt by the host to sequester and localise materials of low solubility (Rich, 1951). Enhanced inflammatory reaction observed by injecting Ascaris eggs into sensitised animals is suggestive of a **delayed type of hypersensitivity**, which is operative in the genesis of the granuloma (Lichtenberg and Mekbel, 1962). Relation of such hypersensitivity reaction to the protective immunity of the host is unknown, and it has been reported that injections of *nonviable Ascaris eggs will not protect the host*, against challenge infections (Crandall and Arean, 1965).

The **hypersensitive reactions**, asthma, angioneurotic oedema, urticaria, etc., observed during the course of larval migration after infection, are indicative of a previous exposure to Ascaris (or its fluids as in experimental animals; Barry and O'Rourke, 1964; Girges, 1934). The antibody responsible for the immediate skin reaction is the **atopic reagin** (antibody), which can be demonstrated by Prausnitz-Kuestner (P-K) reaction. Johansson *et al*, (1968) discovered higher levels of **IgE** (immunoglobulin E; –E for epsilon chain) in Ethiopian children harbouring Ascaris, than in Swedish children free from this disease. The level of IgE drops to normal, after the infected children became free of the parasite, after treatment.

Epidemiology. TRANSMISSION is common by ingestion of food contaminated by hands with soil or by dust containing eggs. Lack of personal cleanliness and poor nutrition, favour the infection. Vegetables and water may contain scanty eggs and this method of infection is unusual. Faeces, when used as fertiliser in gardens, may be an important source of infection.

Clinical manifestations. The infection of *A. lumbricoides* produces a condition of ascariasis, producing various clinical manifestations. They may be conveniently divided into following groups:

1. Symptoms produced by **migrating larvae**.
2. Symptoms (a) due to **adult worms**, and (b) or **allergic manifestations** (*sensitisation*) as a result of **toxin** liberated by the adult worm, called **ascaron**.

1. SYMPTOMS PRODUCED BY MIGRATING LARVAE. *Pulmonary circulation.* About 6-12 days after infection, larval migration in heavy infection is characterised by fever, and pulmonary symptoms like cough, dyspnoea, asthenia, blood stained sputum with eosinophilia, and urticaria.

Bronchopneumonia may develop in children, in whom it may be fatal. Patchy pulmonary consolidation, or pneumonitis and eosinophilia constitute **Loeffler's syndrome.** Allergy may play an important role in its production. Repeated infections may produce chronic pulmonary symptoms. The blood-tinged sputum may show the presence of larvae.

Effect in general circulation. Rarely larvae may escape into general circulation by passing beyond the pulmonary capillaries, and they may pass through the capillaries of different organs of the body, e.g., the brain, eye, spinal cord, heart and kidneys. In the brain and eyeball, they may give rise to transient symptoms of meningitis, epilepsy, retinitis and palpebral oedema. The liver may be enlarged.

2a. SYMPTOMS DUE TO ADULT WORMS. When a few worms are present, they may not usually cause any symptoms at all. In case of moderate infections, children may suffer from ill-health resulting in physical and mental retardation. This may be due to spoliative action of ascarids, in which the host is deprived of nutrition. Death may occur in poorly nourished children who develop convulsions.

General symptoms. The adult worms in the small intestine produce general discomfort, nausea, vomiting, anorexia, colicky pain, digestive disturbances, perverted appetite and pyrexia. The nervous symptoms in children are irritability, nose pricking, disturbed sleep with grinding of teeth and occasionally there may be convulsions, meningism or hemiplegia.

Ectopic ascariasis. The worms may migrate through the stomach and may be *vomited out* or may pass through the mouth or nose, or even accidentally enter through the air passage and *block* the rima glottidis, causing *suffocation* or enter the bronchus. The wandering worm may enter the lumen of the appendix causing appendicitis (PL-12.V), *obstruction of common bile duct* or the *ampula of Vater causing cholecystitis, ascending cholangitis* (PL-12.VIII), obstructive jaundice or *acute haemorrhagic pancreatitis*, etc. If it can reach higher up, it may produce liver abscess. Wandering adults may cause perforation of intestine—specially through an ulcer causing peritonitis (PL-12.VI), or *salpingitis*.

Mechanical effect. A large number (200-300) of adult worms may cause intestinal obstruction specially in children or they may be responsible to produce intussusception.

2b. SYMPTOMS DUE TO SENSITISATION. The metabolites of Ascaris—both during the period of biological incubation and after the worms mature in small bowels—may produce sensitisation phenomenon or allergic manifestations of skin (urticaria), nose (rhinitis), lungs (bronchial asthma), intestinal tract (diarrhoea) of eye (conjunctivitis with photophobia, etc.), or even haematuria.

The irritant action caused by *A. lumbricoides* is due to liberation of ascarin, or ascaron, or ascarase by the adult worm from its body fluid of the nature of *primary albumose*, a proteose; particularly seen in laboratory workers, who may develop such sensitisation by handling worms, or due to emanations (secretions).

Complications (PL. 12.V to VIII). 1. Peritonitis may be caused by ova of *A. lumbricoides* (showing cross-section of ova and cellular infiltration, PL. 12.VI).

2. *Ascaris lumbricoides* may infest in the caecum and the appendix.

3. *Ascaris lumbricoides* and *Oxyuris vermicularis* in the lumen of the small intestine may cause obstruction (PL. 12.V and VII).

4. *Ascaris lumbricoides* in the biliary passage and liver may cause hepatobiliary disturbances (PL. 12.VIII).

Laboratory diagnosis. This depends on *direct evidence* of the presence of adult worms or their eggs in faeces. *The indirect evidences* are not dependable and are of academic interest only. Therefore, one is to rely mainly on direct evidence.

DIRECT METHODS. (1) Finding of adult worm. The adult worm may occasionally pass spontaneously per anus, or a vagrant (wandering) worm may be vomited out or may pass through the nares. Worms may be expelled after an effective anthelmintic. Worms may be detected perchance by X-ray examination, which is hardly paractised for this purpose only. *A. lumbricoides* within 4-6 hours after a barium meal, may offer an opaque string-like shadow.

(2) Finding of eggs. This is done by direct examination of a fairly thick suspension of faeces in saline, but concentration by floatation method (see Appendix II) is always preferable. It should be noted, that *infertile eggs* do not float at the surface of the saturated solution of common salt. When only a few male worms are present, the diagnosis can only be confirmed by the passage of worm after an anthelmintic. Sometimes, microscopic examination of bile, obtained by duodenal intubation, may reveal ascaris eggs.

(3) Larvae may be found in the sputum during their migration in the lung.

INDIRECT METHOD. Eosinophilia may indicate the worm infection, but in case of *A. lumbricoides*, it is seen in the migrating or larval stage. Eosinophilia often disappears with localisation of the worm in the intestine.

Dermal reaction. Skin scratch test with ascaris antigen (immunological skin reaction) is often found to be positive, but the results are variable.

Prophylaxis. ANTIPARASITIC MEASURES are: (1) *proper disposal* of night soil. (2) *Washing of hands*, and raw vegetables before eating. (3) *Mass treatment* of children, but this is ineffective on account of reinfection. (4) *Education* of children on hygienic measures in the schools.

Treatment. Chemotherapy can remove the adult worms effectively. Many drugs have been successfully used. Drugs used are varied.

Santonin. Dose for adults is 180-200 mg (3 grs). For children between 7-14 years, the dose is 120 mg (2grs) and for children from 1-6 years 10 mg (1/6 gr) per year of age. The drug is administered in the morning combined with calomel, and is followed in 3 hours by a saline purgative rendering it relatively nontoxic. But this treatment only removes 25 per cent of the worms. The vision is sometimes transiently yellow coloured. The reexamination of faeces is done 10 days later for ova.

Hexylresorcinol is a drug of choice. It is relatively nontoxic and a single course of treatment may remove 90-100 per cent of worms; 70-80 percent cases are dewormed by a single dose and 90-98 per cent by the second course. The doses are same as those for hookworm disease.

Diethylcarbamazine (**hetrazan**, or **banocide** of Burroughs Wellcome). For adults, it is used in doses of 20 mg per kg body weight daily in invided doses, for 4 to 7 days; for children the dose is 6 mg per kg body weight per day in 3 divided doses for 7 days. There is no specific treatment for larvae in the lungs. The stool should be examined on different occasions during a period of 10 days, after the course of treatment is complete to ensure cure.

Oil of chenopodium. The dose is the same as for hookworm infection. Santonin can be combined with oil of chenopodium, and administered in doses already mentioned (see also treatment of Hookworm disease).

Piperazine derivatives. Various preparations of piperazine are available; namely, antipar elixir, antipar chewing tablets, entacyl (BDH), helmacid (Glaxo). There are various salts of piperazine, namely, citrate, adipate, tartrate, etc., the doses being calculated on the basis of piperazine hexahydrate. Single dose therapy is followed by a post-purgative. Alternatively, divided doses may be administered in doses not exceeding 50 mg of piperazine hydrate per kg of the body weight per day for 4 days, morning and evening. This treatment has the advantage that no preliminary preparation or post-purgative is necessary.

Single doses are 2 gms for those between 14 to 23 kg (30-50 lbs) body weight, 3 gms for 23 to 46 kg (50-100 lbs) body weight, and 3.5 gm for body weight over 46 kg (100 lbs) of piperazine hydrate. It is administered orally. The single dose therapy may be followed 12 hours after by a mild saline purgative. Of 26 cases of Swartzwelder *et al*, (1955), there was one failure, 2 cases with 98 and 97 per cent egg reduction, respectively, and 23 cures. Side-effects are nil.

Mebendazole ("**Mebex**": *Cipla*). It has been proved to be effective in a dose of 100 mg (1 tablet) daily for 3 successive days.

GENUS: *TOXOCARA* Stiles, 1905
TOXOCARA CANIS
(Werner, 1872) Johnston, 1916

This is the dog ascarid and very rarely infects man. Young pups may be infected after their birth and often die from the infection. The **males** are 4-6 cm and **females** 6.5 to 10 cm long. In addition to 3 ascarid lips, they have *cervical alae*. The perianal papillae in males are characteristic. The eggs are *subglobose*, pitted superficially, and measure 85 by 75 microns. THE LIFE CYCLE is like that of *A. lumbricoides* with larval stages, but the larvae cause visceral larva migrans in human beings.

TOXOCARA CATI (Schrank, 1788)
Brumpt, 1927

This is the common ascarid of domestic cats but may rarely infect man. The **males** are 4-6 cm and **females** 4-12 cm long. They have characteristic ascarid lips and a pair of broad, lateral *cervical alae*. The perianal papillae in males are diagnostic.

Eggs are thin-shelled, delicately pitted and measure 60-70 microns in diameter.

Life cycle is like that of *A. lumbricoides*. They cause little symptoms in feline hosts but cause visceral larva migrans in human beings.

LARVAE MIGRANS

Certain **nematode larvae**, after entering an unnatural host, or under unfavourable conditions in the natural host, may not complete their usual sojourn for localisation in the normal abode, and become arrested in the host's tissue or viscera—to cause **larva migrans**. According to the portal of entry, they may produce: (i) **Cutaneous larva migrans** or *creeping eruption*. It is produced by entering through the skin, and such lesions may be produced by the infective stage larvae of *A. lumbricoides*, and *A. caninum* (see before). (ii) **Visceral larva migrans** , on the other

PLATE XI. 12.V

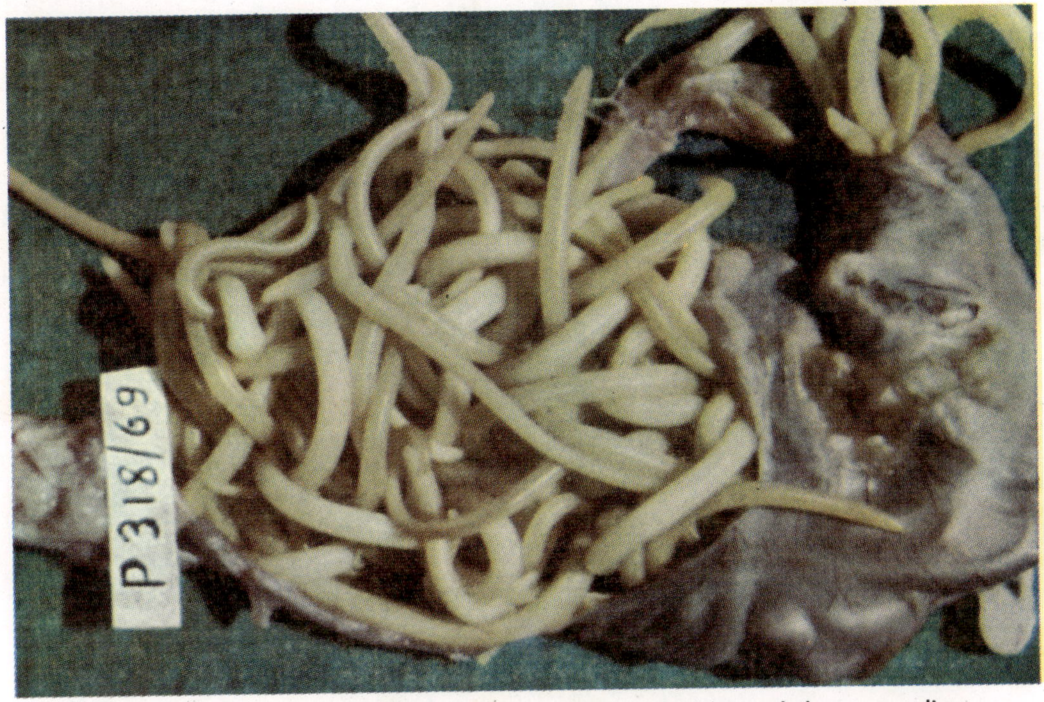

Roundworm (*A. lumbricoides*) mass in the caecum and the appendix produced intussusception and intestinal obstruction.

(Courtesy, Prof. R. K. Gadgil).

PLATE XI. 12.VI

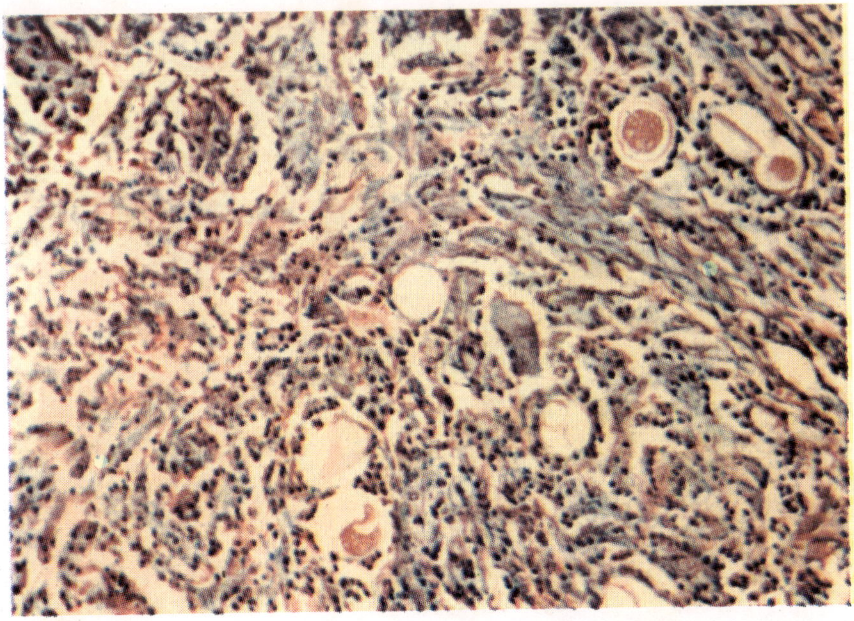

Microscopical appearance of peritonitis caused by perforation of the bowel by *Ascaris lumbricoides*. A few ova are seen in the section along with cellular infiltration and giant cell formation; *H & E* × 400.

PLATE 12. VII

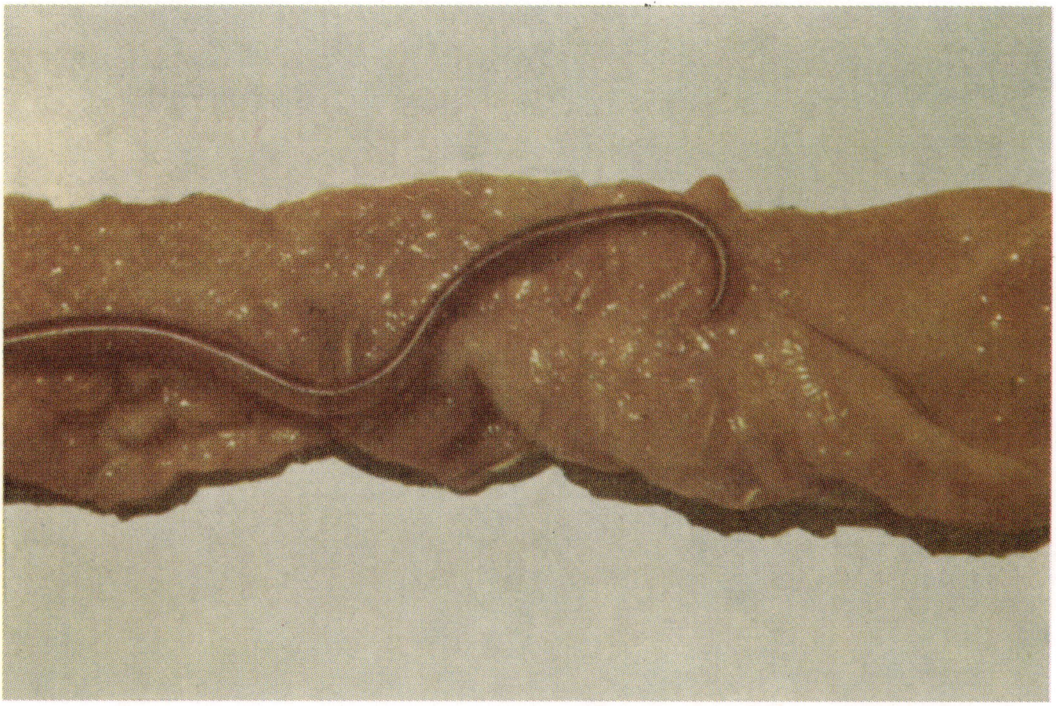

Ascaris lumbricoides and *Oxyuris vermicularis* in the small intestine.
(Courtesy, Prof. R. K. Gadgil).

PLATE 12. VIII

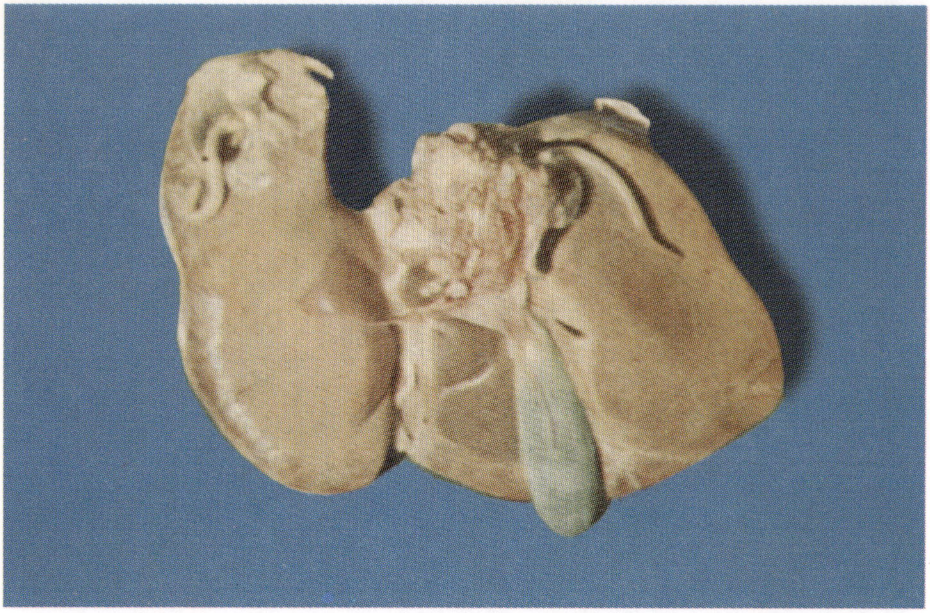

Roundworm in the biliary passage and liver caused obstructive jaundice and ascending cholangitis

TABLE 12.10

EVALUATION OF SPECIFICITY & SENSITIVITY OF BENTONITE FLOCCULATION (BF) TEST WITH ASCARIS AND TOXOCARA ANTIGENS (AFTER KAGAN AND NORMAN, 1970)

Human infection	ANTIGENS			
	Ascaris		Toxocara	
	No. positive / No. tested	Percent Positive	No. positive / No. tested	Percent Positive
Ascaris-Toxocara	14/21	66.7	8/21	38.1
Normal control	1/24	4.2	1/24	4.2
Filaria	2/23	8.7	14/23	60.9
Echinococcus	3/19	15.8	0.19	0.0
Trichina	4/33	12.1	7/33	21.2

hand, is caused by infective larvae, when they enter by the oral route.

VISCERAL LARVA MIGRANS

This is due to entry of nematode larvae to extra-intestinal viscera of unnatural or incompatible host, or under unfavourable conditions in the natural host, provoking **granulomatous lesions**. This common specific agent is *Toxocara cenis*, the dog ascarid, but in some cases *T. cati*, the cat ascarid may be responsible. When the eggs containing the infective larvae are ingested by incompatible host—like human or mouse—the eggs hatch out in the upper level of the small intestine and the freed larvae gain entrance to mesenteric venules or lymphatics. Thus they are carried to *extra-intestinal viscera*. In the capillaries of the liver and less frequently of those of lungs, brain, eyes or other viscera including muscles, the larvae are attacked by host cell reaction, forming **granulomatous lesions** containing *eosinophils*, *macrophages* and *giant cells*, effectively blocking their migration (Smith and Beaver, 1953, Nichole, 1956a). In later stage there may be *abscess formation*, when polymorphonuclear leucocytic reaction may be observed. Within 24 hours after infection, it is possible to discern **epithelioid** and **multinucleated giant cell formations** in these foci; these cells become arranged in pseudotubercles at a later stage. Peripherally, there is formation of a *fibrous capsule* by **fibroblastic proliferation** limiting the **granuloma** from the adjacent tissues, which is infiltrated by **plasma cells, lymphocytes** and **mast cells**. There may be resorption of the necrotic and inflammatory material in the centre of the granulomas, leaving an intact larva, encased in a thick *connective tissue hyaline capsule*; in this condition the larvae may remain alive for a long time. In the unnatural host, they do not undergo further moulting and remain **encapsulated**, for weeks or months. *T. cains* and *T. cati* entering the extra-intestinal viscera, cannot complete their life cycle *via* lungs back to the intestine, and at least larvae of *T. canis* do not mature in the human intestine. In case *A. lumbricoides* infects the incompatible host, the larvae usually complete migration to lung, but on arrival in the small intestine, they are rapidly evacuated through faeces. Other agents causing visceral larva migrans are:

(i) Internal autoinfection in *Strongyloides stercoralis*.

(ii) Infection with filarial larvae, specially by *Dirofilaria conjunctivae*.

(iii) Infection with Spiruroid larva of *Gnathostoma spinigerum*.*

Symptoms. The condition is common in children. The clinical picture varies from an asymptomatic stage or persistent eosinophilia (Smith and Beaver, 1953), with or without constitutional symptoms to one of **hypereosinophilia, hepatomegaly, cough or asthma**, cardiac dysfunction, **nephrosis, fever, hyperglobulinaemia**, cerebral lesion, pseudotuberculous eye lesions, depending on the site and number of granulomas.

* Many cases of tropical eosinophilia have been explained on this basis

Diagnosis. According to Nichols (1956, a, b), the diagnostic criteria in visceral larva migrans caused by *T. cains*, *T. cati*, *A. lumbricoides*, hookworms and *S. stercoralis* depend on the histological characters to identify the larvae in the granuloma in the biopsy or autopsy material. Toxocara larvae are always rhabditoid (second stage); those of *T. canis* measure 290-350μ by 14-120μ and those of *T. cati* are narrower, 12-16μ in breadth. *Advanced second stage larvae* of *A. lumbricoides* resemble those of Toxocara, but the *third stage larvae* are longer and broader (550-650μ by 24-26 microns). The third stage filariform larvae of hookworms measure about 530-700μ by 23μ and those of *S. stercoralis* measure about 500μ by 16μ,

Serological tests for the diagnosis of visceral larva migrans (VLM) are less satisfactory. Two antigens—extracts of *Ascaris lumbricoides* and *Toxocara canis* are employed. In spite of considerable cross-reactivity, a relatively specific diagnosis may be reported on the basis of the difference in titres produced by the two antigens. A combination of two tests—**haemagglutination** (HA) and **bentonite flocculation** (BF)—are most often used and sera reacting in one test are usually reactive in both. But **differential agglutination titre** (DAT) may contribute some information. The tests are difficult to interprete and evaluate; false negative reactions are a problem in Ascaris-Toxocara infections, and sera of both may be negative serologically. A high titre is indicative of present infection, or previous experience for the parasite. The diagnosis of VLM has been discussed by Kagan *et al* (1967, 1968), and Jung and Pacheco (1960).

The HA and BF tests are usually performed and a titre of 1:400 or higher in HA, or 1:5 or greater in the BF test is considered diagnostic. The sensitivity is not over 66% and specificity is poor.

Control. Periodic deworming of household cats and dogs by anthelmintics may be used to safeguard young children from exposure to these larvae (Smith and Beaver, 1953).

Treatment and Prognosis. There is no specific therapy, but **hetrazan** may be used with good effect, may be along with corticosteroids when indicated (in case of marked eosinophilia). □

CHAPTER

13 SOMATIC NEMATODES

PHASMID NEMATODES (CONCLUDED)

Somatic nematodes are those worms whose adults live in the tissues of human.

Adult worms of this group are Filariae and Guinea worm. They are parasites of the lymphatic system and subcutaneous tissues of man, respectively. They are long and **thread-like**. The females are longer than males and **viviparous**. Few are *ovoviviparous*. **Filarial worms** complete their life cycles indirectly in an intermediate host—a mosquito—which transmits microfilaria in human blood. In the mosquito, the immature larvae undergo **metamorphosis** and the infection is transmitted by the *mosquito to man*—the **definitive host**. Incidentally, man acts as the *reservoir host*.

In the case of **guinea worm**, the adult deposits her larvae in small, cutaneous ulcers, wherefrom larvae escape in water. The larvae ingested by **cyclops** develop in them. Cyclops act as the **intermediate host**. Man acquires infection by ingestion of infected cyclops.

Classification. The order Spirurida are phamid nematodes, comprising two suborders—Spirurina and Camallanina. The former contains 2 superfamilies:

I. SPIRUROIDEA. Adults are filiform to robust worms, mouth without lips or 2 or more pseudolips, surrounding the buccal cavity. Human representatives are *Gnathostoma spinigerum*, *Gongylonema pulchrum*, etc.

II. FILARIODEA. Filiform worms with simple mouth, circular or dorsiventrally elongated, and surrounded by papillae. Males are with or without caudal alae. The family Acanthocheilonematidae contains 2 subfamilies; Acanthocheilonematinae and Dirofilarinae. The former comprises: *Wuchereria bancrofti*, *Brugia malayi*, *Onchocerca volvulus*, *Acanthocheilonema perstans*, *A. streptocerca*; the latter (Dirofilariae) contains *Dirofilaria* spp. and *Loa loa*.

The suborder Camallanina comprises the superfamily Dracunculoidea. They are long cord-like worms, the females much longer than the males. The mouth is pore-like, surrounded by the inner circle of 4-6 papillae, and the outer circle of double papillae, and amphids posterior to the lateral papillae. Oesophagus and intestine are attenuated; the vulva is near the anterior part of the body, which atrophies before maturity; uteri divergent; viviparous; larvae typically **rhabditoid**. Human representative is *Dracunculus medinensis* (**Table 13.1**).

SUPERFAMILY: FILARIOIDEA
(Weinland, 1858) Stiles, 1907

The superfamily Filariodea includes nematodes, adults of which live in the tissue or body cavity of vertebrate hosts. They are 2-10 cm in length except the female of onchocerca, which is 20 to 40 cm. The females are longer and produce partially embryonated eggs (viviparous):

The ADULT WORM has a mouth without lips, a cylindrical oesophagus without a bulb and a simple intestine attenuated posteriorly. The caudal alae are often lacking and spicules are unequal and dissimilar.

KEY TO ADULT FILARIAE

Cuticle—smooth:

1. Head without cuticular appendage—*W. bancrofti*, *Br. malayi*.

2. Head with cuticular appendage—*A. perstans*.

Cuticle—not smooth:

1. Cuticle with annular oblique thickening—*O. volvulus*.

2. Cuticle with minute warty thickening—*L. loa*.

Larvae. The eggs at the time of oviposition contain uncoiled embryos. These embryos are delicate, snake-like minute larvae called **microfilaria**. If the egg membrane is elongated and retained a sheath forms and the larva is called **sheathed**; but, if the egg-shell ruptures, a naked embryo is liberated and it is then called **unsheathed**.

Morphology of microfilariae. (Fig. 13.1). It varies from 100 to 300μ in length. Some are *sheathed* (a delicate membrane, which *Mf. malayi*, *Mf. loa*; others are *unsheathed*.

Anterior end is rounded off and has a stylet.

Clear spots seen in the embryo are: (i) Nerve ring, (ii) anterior V spot (rudimentary excretory pore). (iii) posterior V spot (tail spot) or anal pore (Fig. 13.1).

Genital cells. There are four prominent cells in the posterior third of the body, one of which (Fig. 1–8(1)) lies anterior to the remaining three G cells (Figs. 1–8(2-4)).

Innenkorper of Fulleborn or Central (internal) body of Manson extends from the anterior V spot to genital (G) cell (Fig. 1–7).

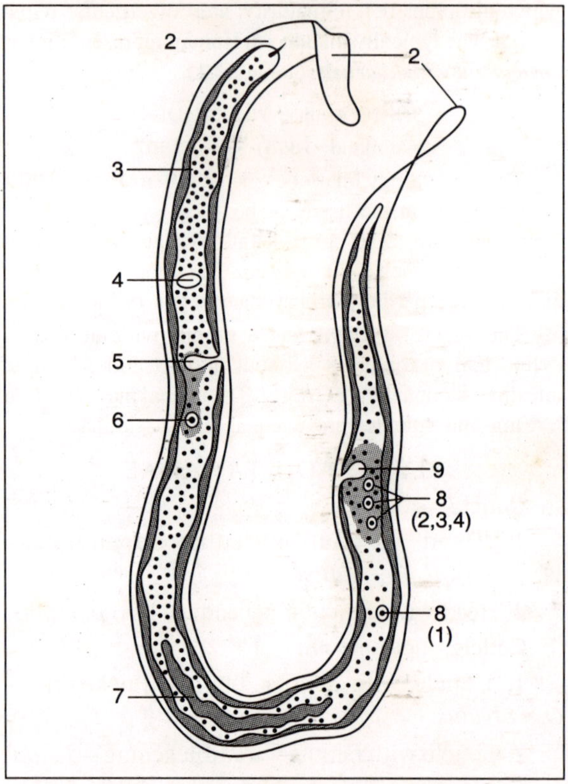

Fig. 13.1 Structure of a microfilaria.
1. Sheath. 2. Stylet. 3. Somatic cells. 4. Nerve ring. 5. Excretory pore (V spot). 6. Excretory cell. 7. Internal body. 8. Genital or G. cells. 9. Anal pore.

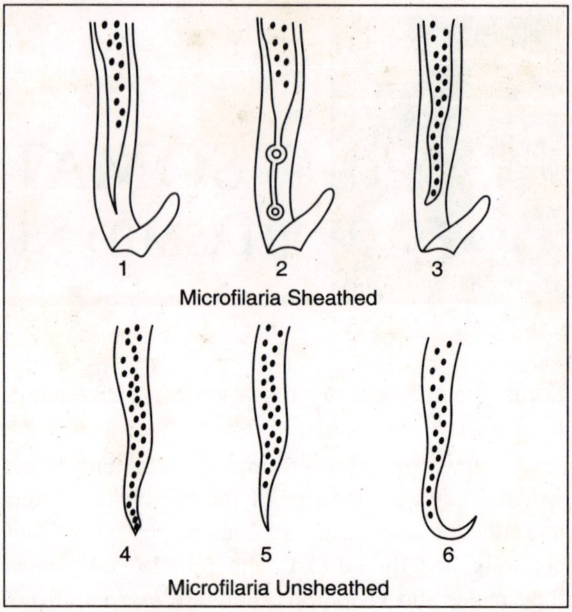

Fig. 13.2 Diagnostic characters from the posterior extremity of microfilaria. **Sheathed**: 1. *Mf. bancrofti*. 2. *Mf. malayi*. 3. *Mf. loa*. **Unsheathed**: 4. *Mf perstans*. 5. *Mf. ozzardi*. 6. *Mf. volvulus*.

Nuclei represent rudimentary intestine. They run from the head to the pointed tail, occupying the whole length and width of the body of the larva. The nuclei may extend up to the tip of the tail as in *Mf. loa* and *Mf. perstans* (Figs. 2–3 & 3 & 4)). But they do not extend up to the tip as in *Mf. bancrofti, Mf. malayi, Mf. oxxardi* and *Mf. volvulus* (Figs. 2–1, 2, 5 & 6).

Diagnosis of species is made by the study of the larval forms (microfilariae), as adult are rarely obtained.

CLASSIFICATION OF MICROFILARIAE ACCORDING TO THEIR CHARACTERS AND HABITAT (Fig. 2 Table 2).

I. MICROFILARIAE WITH SHEATH:

Sheath projects beyond the rounded end anteriorly, and pointed tail posteriorly. Differentiation is made by the extent and arrangement of nuclei at the tail end–whether they are up to the tip, or run short of the tip of the tail.

MICROFILARIA OF:

(i) *W. bancrofti*—Nuclei not up to the tip; (ii) *Burgia malayi*—2 terminal nuclei; (iii) *L. loa*—Nuclei up to the tip (Figs. 2–1, 2 & 3, respectively).

TABLE 13.1

ORDER: *SPIRURINA*
SUBORDER 1: *SPIRURIDA*
SUPERFAMILY I: *Filarioidea*; FAMILY: *Onchocercidae*

Species and distribution	Adult, habitat, etc.	Microfilaria, characters, habitat, pathogenicity to man, etc.
SUBFAMILY: ACANTHOCHEILO-NEMATINAE OR ONCHOGERCINAE		
Wuchereria buncrofti (Tropical regions)	Lymphatics and lymph nodes typically, below the diaphragm, superficial abscesses, retroperitoneal tissues	Sheathed: nocturnal periodicity except in the South Pacific ones: in blood: pathogenic
Brugia malayi (India, Malayasia, China)	Same as above but in lymphatics above the diaphragm	Sheathed: partial nocturnal periodicity: in blood: pathogenic
Acanthocheilonema perstans (Tropical Africa, South America)	Serous cavities, mesentery and parietal peritoneum	Unsheathed: non-periodic: in blood: pathogenicity doubtful
Acanthocheilonema streptocerca (Tropical America)	Skin and subcutaneous connective tissues	Unsheathed: on skin: non-pathogenic
Onchocerca volvulus Central America, Tropical Africa)	Subcutaneous connective tissues (nodules) and lymph spaces	Unsheathed: rarely in blood stream through subcutaneous lymphatics: pathogenic
Mansonella ozzardi (West Indies and Tropical America)	Mesentery, retroperitoneal tissue, lymphatic varices of skin	Unsheathed: nonperiodic: in blood: pathogenicity doubtful
SUBFAMILY: DIROFILARINAE		
Loa loa (Central Africa)	Skin and subcutaneous tissues, migrating in connective tissues	Sheathed with diurnal periodicity: in blood: causes calabar swelling
*Dirofilaria immitis** and allied species e.g.,	Heart of dog	Not definitely known
D. conjunctivae, D. repens, D. magalhaesi, D. louisianensis	See footnote	Rarely pathogenic to man
SUPERFAMILY II. *Spiruroidea*; FAMILY I. *Gnathostomatidae*		
Gnathostoma spinigerum	Adults in cats, dogs, hogs, etc.	Immature adults are in skin and subcutaneous tissues of neck causing creeping eruptions, breast abscesses, etc.
SUPERFAMILY II. *Spiruroidea*; FAMILY II. *Thelaziidae*		
Gongylonema pulchrum (Gullet worms)	Mucosa and submucosa of buccal cavity	Larvae in cockroaches and other insects. Migrating maturing worms cause irritation
SUBORDER II. *Camallanina*; SUPERFAMILY; *Dracunculoidea*; FAMILY; *Gnathostomatidae*		
Dracunculus medinensis	Female: subcutaneous tissue of lower limbs specially. Male: in retroperitoneal tissues (rarely seen)	Larvae in water; infect cyclops subcutaneous inflammation, blebs, ulcers

* *D. immitis* "cruel filaria or dog heart worm" and *D. repens* are filariae of dog. The latter is a natural parasite of dogs almost all over the world. Man is an inappropriate host for Dirofilaria infection. *D. repens* was found as a single male in the nodule of lower eyelid of a female patient in erstwhile USSR. *D. conjunctivae* was found in a nodule in the eyelid of a human subject as immature adult. *D. magalhaesi* in the left ventricle of a boy and *D. lousianensis* in the inferior vena cava of a female patient. *D. conjunctivae* is allied to *D. repens*; whereas there may be varieties of *D. immitis*. It seems probable that mosquitoes are the intermediate hosts of *D. conjunctivae* and others, as they are for *D. immitis* and *D. repens*

II MICROFILARIAE WITHOUT SHEATH:

(a) In blood: MICROFILARIA OF: (i) *Acanthocheilonema perstans*—Nuclei up to the tip; (ii) *Mansolella ozzardi*—Nuclei not up to the tip (Figs. 2–4 & 5).

(b) In skin lymphatics: (i) *Onchocerca volvulus*—Nuclei not up to the tip; tail curved and pointed (Fig. 2–6).

The life cycle is passed in 2 hosts; namely, man and blood sucking insect. The larvae, while circulating in peripheral blood or tissues, are ingested by blood sucking insects. The microfilaria completes process of metamorphosis into first and later into more advanced larval stages. The mature larvae pass into and down the haemocele to the labium and escape into the body through the host skin, when the insect takes its next blood meal.

The species of filariae parasitic to man are:

Wuchereria bancrofti (Bancroft's filaria). Adults inhabit the lymphatics, often *below the diaphragm*; microfilariae are sheathed with nocturnal periodicity except in the South Pacific. They are found throughout the warm climates. The species of South Pacific which lacks periodicity are designated as *W. pacifica* by Manson-Bahr (1951).

Brugia malayi (Malayasia filaria). Adults are in the lymphatics often *above the diaphragm*; microfilariae are *sheathed* with partial nocturnal periodicity. They are found in India, Sri Lanka, Malayasia, Eastern Asia, South Eastern Pacific islands, etc.

Onchocerca volvulus (Convoluted filaria). Adults are found in subcutaneous nodules. The microfilariae are *unsheathed* and found in cutaneous lymphatics and rarely in blood stream. They are found in tropical Africa and central part of America.

Acanthocheilonema perstans (Presistent filaria). Adults are found in the body carivites. Microfilariae are *unsheathed* and non-periodic; found in Tropical Africa and Tropical America.

Acanthocheilonema streptocerca. Adults are found in the skin and subcutaneous tissues. Microfilariae are *unsheathed* and non-periodic; found in tropical Africa.

Mansonella ozzardi. Adults are found in body cavities. The microfilariae are unsheathed and nonperiodic. They are found in Tropical America.

Loa loa (loa worm). The adults are found migrating in cutaneous and subcutaneous tissues. Microfilariae are *sheathed*, exhibiting diurnal periodicity; found in Tropical Africa.

WUCHERERIA BANCROFTI

(Cobbold, 1877) Seurat, 1921

GENUS: WUCHERERIA

(*in honour of Dr. O. Wucherer,* 1877)

Geographical distribution. It is common in the tropics, and subtropical regions, especially in South China, Sri Lanka, Pacific Islands, West Indies. The filarial belt is indicated around the earth at the equator and also a zone 30° South to 35° North latitude. In India, it is prevalent chiefly in the region of the South-East coast line including Bengal.

Habitat. ADULTS inhabit the lymph nodes, where they lie coiled or in lymphatics of the trunk and extremities and the retroperitoneal tissues, or in superficial abscesses.

MICROFILARIA occurs in lymph vessels and appears in the peripheral blood at midnight (nocturnal periodicity).

INFECTIVE LARVAE develop in certain species of mosquitoes, usually *Culex fatigans*, and remain in their mouth parts.

Morphology. Adults are smooth, creamy white, thread-like transparent nematodes. The head end is slightly thicker and rounded than the tapering tail end. It has 2 rows of 10 small sessile papillae. The cuticle is smooth with fine transverse striations and the posterior end of the female is finely tuberculated. The male measures about 40 μm by 0.1 μm and the female 80-100 μm by 0.25-0.30 μm. The male and the female remain coiled together.

TABLE 13.2

DIFFERENTIAL CHARACTERS OF MICROFILARIAE

Nuclei	Sheathed (periodic)		Unsheathed (nonperiodic)		Found in
			Tail end: round	Tail end: pointed	
Upto tip of the tail	Present	Absent	Present	Absent	
	B. malayi	*W. bancrofti*	*A. perstans*	*M. ozzardi*	Blood
	L. Loa		*A. streptocerca*	*O. volvulus*	Skin

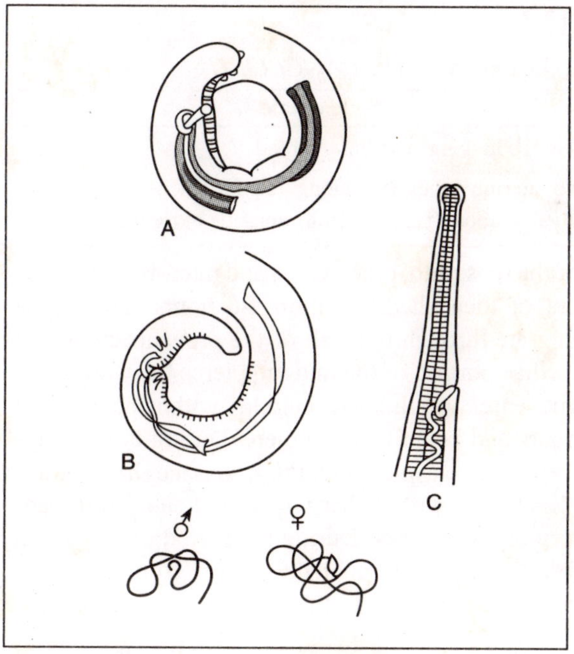

Fig. 13.3 A. Tail end of male *W. bancrofti*, showing the papillae on narrow alae, spicules and a crescentic gubernaculum.

B. Tail end of male *W. malayi.*

C. *W. bancrofti*—anterior end showing bulbous head and position of the vulva.

Lower: male and female of adult *W. bancrofti.*

(After Maplestone)

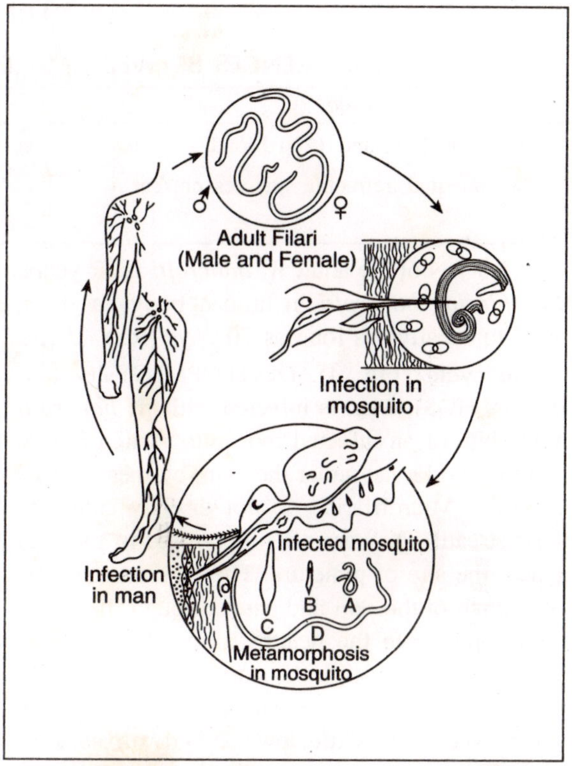

Fig. 13.4 Life cycle of *Wuchereria bancrofti.* A. Microfilaria out of sheath. B. Quiescent state. C. Motile stage. D. Infective stage.

GENITALIA. **In the male**, the posterior end is curved ventrally and 12-15 pairs of sessile papillae are present on the ventral surface. There are two unequal spicules, which are 0.2 and 0.6 μm in length, respectively, with a crescentic gubernaculum (Fig. 13.3A).

In the female, a short vagina opens at the vulva about 1 mm away from the anterior end.

Two ovaries lie at the posterior end of the worm leading to two oviducts and two uterine branches, which coil back and forth along the greater part of the body to fuse before opening into the vagina (Fig. 13.3C). In the uteri, the eggs and microfilariae are coiled within the ovoid membranes, which measures 38μ by 25μ. Near the vulva, microfilariae are crowded and liberated with the sheath. The females are viviparous, giving birth to larvae.

MICROFILARIA. *Mf. bancrofti* are thread-like organisms, 244-296μ by 7.5-10μ in diameter. The anterior end is pointed. It has a hyaline sheath, which is much longer and project beyond the extremities of the embryo, so that the larva can move to and fro within it. This represents the chorionic envelope of the egg. The cuticle is striated. It shows somatic cells or nuclei all over the body except at the tail end. At the cephalic end, there is a space free from granules called the cephalic space and thus differing from those of *B. malayi* and *L. loa.* The following structures are present, from front rearward, in all microfilariae, namely, the nerve ring, the excretory pore (V spot), excretory cell, genital cells 1, 2, 3, and 4, and the anal pore in the column of the body (Fig. 1). Their relative position helps in accurate specific identification. The central internal body of Manson (**Innenkorper of Fulleborn**)* extends from anterior V spot to the genital cell [Fig. 1–8(1)]. The tail end, which is diagnostic, is straight and sheathed. Terminal cells do not fill the tail end up to the tip (Fig. 1–1).

---

* This body is rich in PAS positive glycogen, which gradually disappears as the larva matures

TABLE 13.3

DIFFERENCES BETWEEN MALE AND FEMALE *W. BANCROFTI*

Male	Female
25 to 30μ long and 120μ broad	80 to 100μ long and 230μ broad
Two unequal, refractile spicules present	Two uterine tubes run along the length of the body. Vulva is about 1.2 mm from anterior extremity

LIFE SPAN of the adult *W. bancrofti* is 17 years. *Microfilariae bancrofti* in human body has been found to be alive as long as 70 days (Rao, 1933).

Life cycle (Fig. 4). DEVELOPMENT IN THE HUMAN HOST. Man is infected with *W. bancrofti* by the bite of an infected mosquito, which injects the infective larvae under the skin, by means of its proboscis. Microfilariae do not directly enter the blood stream. They are often deposited in pairs, at or near the site of puncture. They are attracted by the **warmth of the skin** and enter through the puncture, or **penetrate** the healthy skin. The infective larvae, after penetrating the skin through the puncture by their active movement, enter the lymphatic system, where they settle down and grow to an adult stage. The worms are usually harboured in the inguinal, scrotal or abdominal lymphatics. The male and female are found entangled in a mass and there they mate. The male fertilises the female and the gravid female discharges microfilaria within 14 to 18 months. The adult infective worms are tightly coiled up in lymphatic vessels or in nodular dilatations of lymphatic trunks. The viviparous female living in the lymph nodes and spaces gives birth to young microfilariae. The sheathed microfilariae pass to the circulation *via* the lymph node (lymph spaces) if they are not obstructed. They pass through the thoracic duct or right lymphatic duct to the venous system, right heart and pulmonary capillaries, wherefrom they enter into the circulation at night in case of **periodic variety** (diurnal or nocturnal). In the nonperiodic variety, they are capable of living in the peripheral blood for a considerable time without any metamorphosis.

DEVELOPMENT IN MOSQUITO VECTORS. It has been estimated that, there may be 30 microfilariae per μ1, whereas, 1-3 per μ1 are optimal for infection of the mosquito (intermediate host) and more than 5 per μ1 is fatal to the mosquitoes. In the stomach of the mosquito, blood clots, and microfilariae come out of their sheaths within 2-6 hours. The larvae migrate through the wall of the proventriculus and cardiac portion of the midgut, pierce the wall of the gut, enter the **thoracic muscles** within about 4-17 hours and begin to grow there. During next 2 days they assume a ***quiescent, thick*, sausage shaped** form (124-250μ) with a sharp, **spiky tail** and a rudimentary digestive tract. During the period of 5th to 6th day, the tail has atrophied to a mere stump, the first cuticle is shred off, the larvae grow rapidly to measure on average 250μ by 25μ and the subterminal caudal papillae appear. By the 10th or 11th day usually in the tropics, the second ecdysis occurs and larvae rapidly elongate and mature to **filaform larvae** (1.4 to 2 mm by 18-23μ). The metamorphosis is complete by now, and the larvae become *actively motile* and **infective**. The larvae now **migrate** from the thoracic muscle to the **head region** through the *haemocele* and enter the muscular labium (proboscis). They pass to the human skin through the flexion of the proboscis at the time of blood meal, being helped by the drawing up of the proboscis. It is to be noted that there is no multiplication of larvae in the mosquito. There may be several larvae coiled up, waiting for an opportunity to infect by the mosquito bite. The time taken for **complete development** of microfilaria in the mosquito varies from **10-21 days**, depending on the atmospheric humidity and temperature and also the species of the mosquito. The optimal temperature is 26°C and over 90 per cent relative humidity.

Epidemiology. The TRANSMISSION depends on: (1) density of population; (2) efficient vector and suitable tropical climate, and (3) breeding places in endemic areas.

The microfilariae rate may be as high as 20-30 per cent or more and mild clinical manifestations, like hydrocele (10-15 per cent) and severe manifestations, like elephantiasis (less common) may develop. These subjects are carriers and act as RESERVOIR HOSTS.

MOSQUITO VECTORS. Important mosquito vectors of *W. bancrofti* belong to more than 50 species of Culex, Aedes, Anopheles and mansonia (Mansonioides). The common ones are:

The disease is transmitted by *Cules fatigans* in most parts of the world, namely, India, Sri Lanka, South China. Indonesia, Philippines, Celebes, Maldive islands, Egypt, East Africa, West Indies, Guyana, Brazil, North Australia and New Hebrides; *Aedes aegypti* in West Africa, Congo, West Indies and *Aedes scutelaris* in South Pacific islands causing non-periodic *filariasis*. Anopheles species are found scattered all over the world. *A. subpictus*, *A. rossi*, *A. vagus*, *A. sundiacus*, *A. varunia*. etc., in India. *A. hyrcanus* var. *nigerriums* and *A. funestus* in tropical Africa, *A. darlingi* in Brazil and Guyana, *A. farauti* in New Guinea, Solomon islands and New Hebrides and *A. barbirostris bancrofti* in S. W. New Guinea. *Culex fatigans* breeds in water containing organic matters. The adults remain in the house and bite at night. The infection rate may be about 20 per cent. The cycle in non-periodic variety of filaria does not develop in *C. fatigans* or *Aedes aegypti*.

Symptoms. The infection of *W. bancrofti* causes filariasis, which is characterised in its early stage by irregular fever, often periodic, lymphangitis with lymphomatosis (enlargement of lymph nodes) and thickening of skin. When the condition becomes chronic, it gives rise to obstructive symptoms, like elephantiasis. Some authorities hold that acute symptoms are not due to liberation of microfilariae in blood, but due to **associated** secondary **streptococcal infection** and **absorption** of **allergen** from the worm.

The symptoms caused by *W. bancrofti* depends on several factors, e.g., (1) individual tolerance to the parasite; (2) the dose of infective larvae injected by the mosquitoes; (3) number of infected bites; (4) site of bite and location of the parasite, and (5) possibility of supervening streptococcal infection.

Pathogenesis. The infection caused by *W. bancrofti* produces symptoms of filariasis. The term is not accurate, as it means symptoms produced by any organism of the superfamily Filarioidea with or without pathological changes. Therefore, it is proper to use the term **Wuchereriasis**. The symptoms are produced by the adult worm—either dead or alive producing **lymphangitis**. Therefore, larvae circulating in the blood does not produce any symptom. Some authorities hold that acute symptoms are not due to liberation of microfilaria in blood, but due to ***associated secondary streptococcal infection***. The causes of lymphangitis are: (1) mechanical irritation, (2) liberation of toxic fluid by the females during parturition; (3) absorption of toxic products or allergens by the disintegration of the dead worm; (4) secondary streptococcal infection may produce additional inflammatory changes.

Pathology: LYMPHANGITIS. If living immature or adult *W. bancrofti* are present in *afferent lymphatic vessels*, the parasites create a response of RE cell proliferation to engulf or absorb the worms (Michael, 1944). The lining of the vessels becomes thickened, stratified and roughened with deposit of fibrin on the surface of the endothelium. The wall of the vessel becomes oedematous with heavy infiltration of **eosinophils**, if the reaction is severe. Within the lumen of the vessel, *histiocytes, epithelioid cells, lymphocytes* and often *foreign body giant cells* appear. This, with deposit of fibrinous threads, produces **endolymphatic obliteration**. At the same time, *perilymphatic changes* of similar type constrict the walls of the vessels. The worm is thus strangled, unless it can migrate into the damaged lymph channel.

In many highly reacting patients, the immature filariae escape from the blocked channel to produce similar reaction at new sites. But in mildly reacting patients, the growing worms migrate freely through the lymphatic channels, until they become sexually mature and mate. Then the fertilised females discharge microfilariae in lymphatics. The parturition is asociated with local tissue reactión, causing acute or subacute manifestations of **filarial lymphangitis** and **lymph-noditis**. The initial tissue responses are due to the parasites and their metabolic products, showing infiltration with **eosinophils**, but the supervening infections with *Streptococcus haemolyticus* and *Staphylococcus aureus* are probably responsible for subsequent inflammatory changes—specially in chronic cases, when the secondary organisms may produce inflammatory reactions with infiltration of neutrophils.

IN THE CHRONIC STAGE—as the adult worms are gradually confined by obliterative endolymphangitis—they die, become absorbed and impregnated with calcific deposits. The degenerated worms may also provoke cellular reactions. With the death of the worm, microfilariae soon disappear from peripheral blood. But persons living in endemic areas are repeatedly infected. Elephantiasis is specially seen in hyperendemic areas along the South-East coast line of India, but it is rare in Bengal. This is explained by: (1) repeated infections of multiple lymph channels, (2) endolymphangitis of the proximal portion obstructing the lymph flow, (3) dilatation of the distal part of the lymphatics and lymph stasis, (4) infection, (5) inability to establish adequate collaterals through the hypertrophied tissues.

LYMPHATIC OBSTRUCTION. Attacks of lymphangitis are often recurrent. Such repeated attacks may lead to lymphatic obstruction, which is brought about by the following causes:

(*a*) **Mechanical obstruction**. Adult worms—alive or dead—cause obstruction to the lymph flow by mechanically blocking the lumen. A single worm or a batch of worms act as an embolus and may be responsible for occlusion of the lymphatic channel.

(*b*) **Obliterative endolymphangitis**. Lymphatic vessels become obliterated as a result of repeated lymphangitis and endothelial proliferation and inflammatory thickening of the walls (**obliterative endolymphangitis**).

(*c*) **Fibrosis of the afferent lymphatic vessels**. The lymph node draining a particular area may undergo inflammatory changes, *allergic* in nature, with **eosinophilic cellular reaction, giant cell** formation and ultimate **fibrosis**. These changes may be due to irritant action of the dead adult worms or toxins liberated by them. This may be due to persistent destruction of microfilariae in the lymphatic sinuses by RE cells.

RESULTS OF OBSTRUCTION (**Lymph statis**). **Elephantiasis**. When a large number of worms block the majority of the lymph channels, elephantiasis results. This develops only after repeated infections for several years. The condition is seen in the leg, scrotum, penis, vulva, arms and, rarely, in the breast, due to **obstruction** of the regional groups of lymph nodes. In 95 per cent of cases, the parts drained by the inguinal group of lymph nodes are involved and symptoms are due to obstruction of this group of nodes. The affection of the axillary group is of much rarer occurrence.

Pathological effects: With the increase of fibrosis and obstruction of lymph flow, the lesions extend distally, and, with repeated filarial reinfections, the obstruction becomes more extensive to produce lymph varix, varicose lymph nodes and elephantiasis commencing from the dependent parts.

(i) The **oedema** causes hyperplasia and hypertrophy of subcutaneous tissue due to chronic lymphatic obstruction. Microfilaria is often absent in blood, and eosinophilia is not marked in chronic cases.

(ii) **Varicosity of groin lymph nodes**. This condition is often associated with *lymph scrotum*, *chylous ascites* or *chyluria*. The inguinal lymph nodes are enlarged, hard and fibrotic in a bed of distorted *varicose lymphatics* and often mistaken for a femoral hernia. Puncture of the node may reveal microfilaria.

(iii) **Lymph varix** (dilatation of lymphatics) is due to *varicosity of inguinal* and rarely *axillary lymphatic vessels*. Similar changes in the spermatic cord produce varicocele.

(iv) **Chylous exudation** into various serous sacs gives rise to *chylous ascites, chylocele* and rarely *chylothorax* and *chylopericardium*. This is due to obstruction of lymphatics near the *receptaculum chyli* caused by the pressure of *inflamed paravertebral lymph nodes*.

(v) **Chyluria** is produced by the escape of chyle with urine due to the rupture of lymph **varicocele** in the wall of the *urinary tract*, pelvis of the kidney, ureter or bladder, resulting in **chyluria**. Such rupture in the intestine produces chylous diarrhoea. *Lymph scrotum* follows, when the rupture of the lymphatics occurs in the scrotal skin.

ALLERGY. Allergy is produced by the product of disintegration of the dead worm and is responsible for inflammatory changes in the obstructed lymphatics and lymph nodes. In sensitised individuals, allergy is often associated with **urticaria, exfoliative dermatitis** observed by the authors, **eosinophilia** and swelling of the lymph nodes (lymphomatosis). Lymph noditis is characterised by oedema, hyperplasia of RE cells and a local eosinophilia. There is a reaction of **foreign body granuloma**. The filariae lie in the sinuses surrounded by macrophages, eosinophils and foreign body giant cells. As the worms die, they become calcified and block the lymph channels permanently.

SECONDARY BACTERIAL INFECTION. It is usually of streptococcal origin. The conditions developing due to the infection are: (*a*) Lymphangitis, (*b*) Lymphnoditis; (*c*) Epididymoorchitis, (*d*) Funiculitis, (*e*) Hydrocele due to recurrent epididymoorchitis.

Filarial abscess of skin, subcutaneous tissue of limbs, pelvis of the kidney, inguinal and axillary lymph nodes, retroperitoneal tissue and spermatic cord are due to *Staphylococcus aureus* infection.

LYMPH NODES. When the worms are *in the lymph nodes*, afferent lymphatics become hypertrophied with varices, which may extend to the deeper parts of the lymph nodes. There is formation of masses of eosinophils rapidly surrounding the worm. Lymph follicles are oedematous, and intact centres show rapidly dividing cells. The essence of the lesion starting from endothelial hyperplasia, initiated by RE cell activity, which constitutes the cellular granulation, progresses to proliferative granulation followed by fibrocytic repair. This determines the degree of degeneration of filariae caught in the lymph node. The *filarial granulation tissue* is very characteristic and almost pathognomonic (Michael, 1945). Microscopically, the early lesions show a central core of necrotic tissue, surrounded by a radiating zone of *proliferating endothelial cells, epitheloid cells, foreign body giant cells, fibroblasts* and a *peripheral dense infiltrate of eosinophils*. Death and absorption of the trapped parasite is either in the lymph node or lymphatic, which is associated with (*a*) fibrosis, replacing the former cellular infiltrate, and (*b*) disappearance of the cardinal diagnostic criteria.

Diagnosis. The diagnosis of Bancroft's filariasis depends on Direct methods of finding microfilaria in: (i) peripheral blood, (ii) lymphatic exudate in the lymph varix, (iii) calcified lymph node detected by X-ray. Indirect methods are (i) eosinophilia in peripheral blood, and (ii) immunological tests, like *complement fixation,* and *intradermal tests* using antigen from *Dirofilaria immitis*.

MICROFILARIA. For finding of microfilaria in the peripheral blood, midnight sample is suitable for periodic variety. Microfilariae seen in the wet preparation under the low power objective exhibit a characteristic movement (*wriggling*). Though motile, they move within the area enclosed by their sheath. The morphology is best determined in stained preparations. When this method fails, a concentration method may be used by examining the centrifuge deposit of about 2 ml of blood collected from a vein; RBCs are lysed by adding a few ml of 2 percent acetic acid or with 10 ml of 2 percent formalin. A few coverslip preparations may be examined for this. Similarly, other fluids and exudates may be examined. Fallacy in finding microfilariae are: (i) they *may not be found in elephantiasis* due to the lymphatic obstruction; (ii) after *inflammatory obstruction* of lymphatics by streptococcal endolymphangitis, or (iii) due to the *death of the adult worm*.

The adult worms should be searched for in excised nodes, where male and female worms may be seen entangled. *Calcified worms* may be found by X-ray examination.

IMMUNOLOGICAL TESTS

The reactions are group-specific, not species-specific. The antigen is prepared from any of the filarial worms, namely, *Dirofilaria immitis* of dog, *Setaria equina* of horse, or *Letomosoides carinii* of cotton rats. Intradermal test.* An extract of *D. immitis* (1:8,000 dilution of saline extract of the worm) is used. A dose of 0.01 ml is injected intradermally. Immediate reaction takes place characterised by doubling of the diameter of the wheal in 10-15 minutes. Although it is a group reaction, positive reaction is found in 100 percent suspected cases of *W. bancrofti* in biological incubation period and Michael (1944) obtained positive reaction in 87.3 percent of 307 known cases of the disease.

* Mode of preparation of antigen: Antigen can be prepared from any true filaria worm but the best yield is obtained from the living *D. immitis*, which should be freed of blood and should then be dried and separated from lipoids; again they should be thoroughly dried, pulverised and diluted with physiological salt solution in the proportion of 1 to 200 parts by weight. This is the stock solution of antigen for intradermal test

SEROLOGICAL TESTS

Complement fixation test may be carried out with same antigen. The antigen used is prepared from *Dirofilaria immitis* and this antigen is routinely used in **Haemagglutination** (HA) and **Bentonite flocculation** (BF) tests. The test is fairly sensitive, but specificity is not satisfactory (Kagan *et al*, 1963; McQuay, 1967). In *Loa loa* and *Onchocerca volvulus* infections, titres are high, but infection titre is very low as a rule with *Acanthocheilonema perstans* infection. Kagan and Norman, and others evaluated and found that 27 (73%) out of 37 filariasis sera were positive by the above tests.

Prophylaxis. It depends on: (1) Anti-organism measures, (2) antivector measures, and (3) personal prophylaxis. All campaigns must be planned at least for 5 years.

ANTIORGANISM MEASURES. Treatment of carriers with diethyl carbamazine (**hetrazan**) will reduce the risk of vectors getting infected. A mass treatment with 100 mg for adults and 50 mg for children for 7 days has shown considerable reduction in incidence (80 per cent) and intensity (90 per cent) of microfilaria in blood. As an alternative, hetrazan in doses of 5 mg per kg body weight once daily for 5 days may be administered for mass treatment. A year later, 60 per cent of the persons treated are free from microfilaria. Infective larvae and immature adults are treated with **para-melaminylphenyl stibonate** (MSb).

ANTIVECTOR MEASURES. Insecticides against adult mosquitoes that rest in the houses as in malaria are effective. DDT (dichlorodiphenyl trichlorethane) to give a surface distribution of 100-200 mg per sq. foot or 3-6 oz. per 100 sq. foot; or BHC (benzene hexachloride—gammexane to give 10-20 mg per sq. foot is effective as a suspension of wettable powder. In South Pacific islands rat-eaten coconuts are the important breeding places. Therefore, anti-rat measures are applicable there, by putting rat bands on coconut trees.

PERSONAL PROPHYLAXIS. It consists of such measures as protection against mosquito bites.

Prolonged administration of certain antimonials and arsenicals kill circulating microfilariae, eventually inhibiting their production. It is uncertain whether they kill adult worms, unless treatment is prolonged beyond the limit of practicability.

Treatment (Antifilarial chemotherapy). *Specific*. Diethylcarbamazine kill circulating microfilariae. Its prolonged use may kill the adults and eventually inhibits the production of embryos. **Suramin** is more specific than arsenic or antimony.

DIETHYLCARBAMAZINE, a piperazine derivative is used under various trade names—*hetrazan, banocide, naterine, herogen*, etc. is specific for microfilaraemia and is the drug of choice. Tablets are available in doses of 50 mg. The dose is 2 mg per kg body weight thrice daily after meals for a period of 3 weeks. The dose may be extended for a longer period if necessary for killing the adult worms. The drug is nontoxic and has little side-effects like nausea, anorexia, headache, fever, lymphnoditis, epididymitis, orchitis, but they pass off soon. If the reactions are severe, the drug may be stopped. Sometimes allergic manifestations are seen due to the liberation of protein from the breakdown products of the dead adult worms.

MEL W. It is a water soluble form of Mel B, a *trivalent arsenical compound*. It can be administered intramuscularly. It is issued in doses of 0.1 gm and administered for 3 or 4 successive days. It causes the death of the worm with reduction of microfilaria in blood. The drug deserves more extensive trial to work out its efficacy and toxicity.

ANTIMONY COMPOUNDS. The *trivalent antimony compounds* of **lithium antimony thiomalate** (anthiomaline) is used in daily doses of 2 ml up to a total of 60 ml. The drug is toxic and may sometimes show severe reaction.

Sodium stibogluconate and *methyl glucamine antimoniate* have also given good results. The doses are same as administered in Kala-azar.

SYMPTOMATIC (SECONDARY) TREATMENT is to be undertaken along with specific treatment. In acute condition of lymphangitis, or other antibiotics may help in these cases, followed by a course of mixed vaccine containing streptococci—100 million, and staphylococci—500 million per ml in graduated doses of 0.1 to 0.8 ml. **Diaminodiphenyl sulphone** (DDS) in a single dose of 50 mg daily together with haematinics and vitamin B complex for 3-6 months, has been found to be effective.

For chyluria, rest in bed is essential to relieve orthostatic pressure. Fat-free diet, restriction of fluid, and use of purgatives may help greatly in controlling chyluria.

NON-PERIODIC VARIETY OF *W. BANCROFTI*

This form of filaria is universally seen in the Pacific Islands including Philippines. In this, the microfilariae and the adults are morphologically similar to *W. bancrofti*, but the microfilaria is present in peripheral blood by day and night. The microfilaria does not readily develop in *Culex fatigans* as in the case of microfilaria of the periodic variety of *W. bancrofti*, but they readily develop in *Aedes polynesiensis* (syn. *Aedes scutellaris*), a mosquito peculiar to Pacific Islands. (Polynesia includes Fiji, Samoa, Tokelau, etc.).

TABLE 13.4

EVALUATION OF SENSITIVITY AND SPECIFICITY OF THE SEROLOGICAL TESTS FOR THE DIAGNOSIS OF FILARIASIS (AFTER KAGAN AND NORMAN, 1970)

Human infection	Serological Tests: HA		BF	
	No. positive / No. tested	Percent Positive	No. positive / No. tested	Percent Positive
Filaria	27/37	73.0	24/37	64.8
Normal sera	4/84	4.8	10/84	11.9
Ascaris/Toxocara	6/22	27.3	8/22	36.4
Trichina	15/43	34.9	23/43	53.5

The non-periodic variety often produces elephantiasis of arms. Glandular enlargements are specially associated with non-periodic Pacific variety, and, in this, there is enormous enlargement of the epitrochlear node with fibrosis.

BRUGIA MALAYI

(Producing Malayan filariasis)

SYNONYM: *Wuchereria malayi* (Brug, 1927)

Rao and Maplestone, 1940

Geographical distribution. Malayasia, East Indies, South China, Indonesia, Sri Lanka, India.

Habitat. Adult male and female live in dilated lymphatics.

Morphology. ADULT is similar to *W. bancrofti*. The male measures 22 to 23 mm by 0.08 mm, and the female, 55 mm by 0.16 mm. Female is about the same size as that of *W. bancrofti*, but the male differs from *W. bancrofti* in that the spicules and the tail papillae are more delicate, and the transverse corrugations on the stout portion of the spicules are not prominent as in *W. bancrofti* (Rao and Maplestone, 1940).

MICROFILARIAE (*Mf*), first described by Brug (1927) are smaller in size than *Mf. bancrofti* (175 to 250μ in length by 6μ in breadth). They are distinguished from *W. bancrofti* by the presence of: (1) secondary kinks along the body, (2) the broader cephalic space, (3) two stylets at the anterior end. (4) two terminal discrete nuclei at the tip of the tail (Fig.. 2,—2), and (5) easily visible excretory pore and cells.

Life cycle. Two hosts are required to complete the life cycle:

1. Definitive host is man.

2. Intermediate host is mosquitoes of the Genus Mansonia and certain species of Anopheles. Other stages of life cycle are like those of *W. bancrofti*, but the larval development takes place by 2 moults in the thoracic muscles of the mosquito, when the infective form appears in the labium in 6-12 days. Transmission is like that of *W. bancrofti*.

LIFESPAN of the adults is the same as that of *W. bancrofti*.

RESERVOIR OF INFECTION is man, but domestic animals like dogs and cats may act as reservoirs, in whom sheathed microfilariae like those of *W. malayi* have been found in these animals in India and Malayasia.

Pathogenicity. It causes *lymphangitis* and *elephantiasis* of upper extremities. *Genital organs* involvement is unknown.

Diagnosis. This is done by finding of microfilariae in the peripheral blood. Microfilariae are more often found in the late stage of the disease than those in case of *W. bancrofti* infection, but the larva count is often higher in this case than that in *W. bancrofti*.

Prophylaxis. It is similar to that of *W. bancrofti* except that the transmission takes place by Mansonioides mosquito. Water plants like pistia, water hyacinth and swamp grass are necessary for the growth of Mansonioides, and clearing of these plants from ponds will eradicate the mosquitoes.

A selective weed-killer phenoxylene 30 (sodium and ammonium salts of methyl phenoxyacetic acid) may be used diluted with 1:300 parts of water and this may be sprayed on vegetations at about 100 gallons (450 litre) per acre.

Treatment. It is similar to that of *W. bancrofti*. During hetrazan treatment, febrile reaction for the first 2-4 days is common, but this may be more severe in *B. malayi* than in *W. bancrofti*. Therefore, antihistaminic drugs may be used during the first few days.

ONCHOCERCA VOLVULUS (Leukart, 1893)

Raillet and Henry, 1910

GENUS: *ONCHOCERCA* Diesing, 1841

Onchocerca volvulus causes an infection, transmitted by flies of Simulium species. The adults form nodules in the subcutaneous tissues (Fig. 5A) and the embryos, which are unsheathed, may cause skin and eye lesions, sometimes producing blindness.

Geographical distribution. Tropical Africa, Central America.

Habitat. They are found in lymph spaces, tissues and subcutaneous nodules over the ribs, axillae, popliteal space or the elbow. In America, they are usually seen in the subcutaneous tissues around the scalp. The nodules contain at least one male and one female parasite.

Morphology. Adults are whitish nematodes. At the anterior end, there are 8 small papillae in 2 circles including a large lateral pair. The cuticle shows conspicuous ring-like thickenings (Fig. 5B).

Male measures 3 cm in length and 0.15 mm in diameter.

Female is 30 to 50 cm in length and 0.4 mm in diameter. It is **ovoviviparous.**

GENITALIA. **In males** the posterior end is curved with a number of perianal and caudal papillae, and two unequal spicules (Fig. 5C). In **females**, the vulva opens about 9.85 mm away from the anterior end. The *uterus* is bicornuate. The **eggs** are within egg membranes, but larvae escape out of the sheath.

Embryos. Microfilariae of *O. volvulus* are found in the puncture fluid from a nodule or cystic swelling and do not escape in blood. They are 150 to 370μ by 17μ. The embryos have no sheath and the nuclei do not extend up to the tail end, which is hooklike (Fig. 2—6).

LIFE SPAN of *O. volvulus* in man is for many years.

Life cycle. It requires two hosts to complete the life cycle:

1. DEFINITIVE HOSTS is man.

2. INTERMEDIATE HOST. Microfilariae of *Onchocerca volvulus* develop in a biting fly of the genus Simulium. They are hunch-backed nematocera fleas, which breed in well-aerated rapidly flowing water. The infection rate is about 5-30 per cent in endemic areas. Larval development occurs in simulium in 7 days and only a few larvae are found in each simulium. In the thoracic muscle 2 ecdyses occur and the 3rd **(filiform) stage** is infective.

Pathogenicity in man. The incubation period is about one year. Adults and microfilariae of *O. volvulus* cause small painless nonsuppurative, cystic tumours, 3-25 mm or more in diameter—in the axillary and popliteal spaces and other areas. They rarely suppurate, but contain many microfilariae. They have been claimed to produce *elephantiasis* in Congo by lymphatic obstruction. From the scalp, they may penetrate into the tissue of the eye and cause irritation of the eye with lachrymation, punctate keratitis, iritis, retinitis, optic atrophy and other complications. In Sudan, it has been incriminated to produce blindness—"Sudan blindness". These are due to the presence of adult worms and microfilaria, but allergy may develop in some cases.

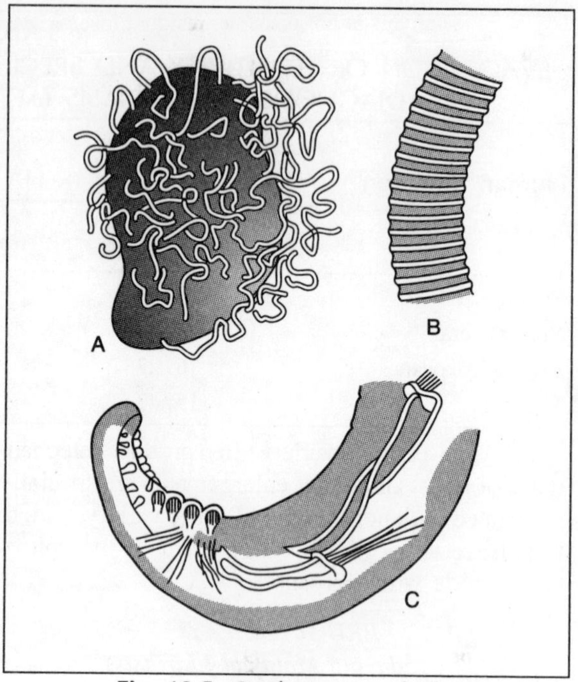

Fig. 13.5 *Onchocerca volvulus*
A. A subcutaneous nodules showing strangled worms inside (After Brumpt). B. Body showing annular thickenings. C. Tail end of male showing spicules and papillae (B & C—after Fulleborn)

Diagnosis. (1) By finding microfilaria in fluid from the cyst or in shaving of the skin. (2) Adult worms are present inside the excised nodules. In the ocular lesions, microfilariae may be seen by slit lamp microscopy. (3) Eggs may be seen accidentally due to puncture of the uterus of the adult female, while trying to obtain the fluid. Puncture of the worm in the nodule causes severe allergic reactions. Therefore, *biopsy* and not puncture is indicated for finding of the adult. Blood shows **eosinophilia. Immunological reactions**—like *intradermal* and *complement fixation tests* with onchocerca antigens—are positive, but they are of little practical value, when compared with the demonstration of the parasite.

Prophylaxis. ANTIPARASITIC MEASURES depend on chemotherapy and excision of the nodule and this reduces the transmission rate.

ANTIVECTOR MEASURES. Application of concentrated DDT to give a final dilution of 2 parts per million for 30 minutes is effective against *Simulium neaver*. For eradication of the vector, this may be repeated every 14 days for 3 months until the last surviving adult has laid her eggs. When this is not possible, residual insecticides from aircraft may be used on vegetations on which simulium rests near the water. The dose is 200 to 400 gm of DDT per acre in 5-10 percent solutions in oil on alternate days for 3 weeks. BHC (Gammexane) may be similarly used to give a final dilution of 1.5 mg per litre (1.5 parts per million).

PERSONAL PROPHYLAXIS should be observed against bite of simulium flies.

Treatment. Specific drugs—**naphyride sodium (Suramine)** 1 gm is injected; this kills the adult worm. *Hetrazan* in maximum doses of 0.1 to 0.2 gm per kg body weight administered daily over a period of 2-3 weeks destroys the microfilaria quickly, but it is slower in action on adult worms. Excision of the nodule is always indicated as the source of infection is removed by it. The puncture may set up *allergic reactions*.

ACANTHOCHEILONEMA PERSTANS

(Manson, 1891)

Railliet, Henry and Langeron, 1912

SYNONYMS: *Filaria perstans*, **Manson, 1891**, *Dipetalonema perstans* **(Manson, 1891) York** and **Maplestone, 1926.**

This is a nonpathogenic parasite of man transmitted by the bite of an infected midge—Culicoides species.

Geographical distribution. Tropical Africa and South America.

Habitat. ADULT WORMS are found in the subcutaneous connective tissues. The *microfilariae* are often found in the blood of local people of the Gold Coast of West Africa.

Morphology. ADULT. The cuticle is smooth.

The **Male** measures 4.5 cm in length and 0.07 mm in breadth and has an incurved tail with caudal papillae and spicules.

The **Female** measures 7 cm in length and 0.13 mm in breadth with two triangular appendages at the extremity giving a bifid appearance. The vulva ends 0.6 mm away from the head end. The are **viviparous.**

The MICROFILARIA has sheath (Figs. 2—4). They are 200μ by 4.5μ; posterior end is blunt. **Tail** is filled completely with **terminal nuclei**. They have no periodicity. They are found in the peripheral blood of human subjects (10 per μl) and tend to be more numerous **at night**.

LIFE SPAN is not known.

Life cycle. *A. perstans* requires two hosts to complete the life cycle:

DEFINITIVE HOST is man. INTERMEDIATE HOST is a midge (waterfly) of the genus Culicoides. Rest of the life cycle is like that of other filaria.

Pathogenicity. It is not known, as infection causes no symptoms.

Treatment. Hetrazan is ineffective. A higher dose than usual (10 mg per kg body weight) may be partly effective against adults, but with little effect on microfilariae.

MANSONELLA OZZARDI

(Manson, 1897) Faust, 1929

(In honour of Sir Patrick Manson)

This is a **non-pathogenic parasite** of man transmitted by the bite of infected culicoides species. The filaria is of no clinical importance. It is limited to the Western Hemisphere, e.g., West Indian islands and South America. The adults live in the body cavities of man (mesentery and subperitoneal tissue). The **adult females** are 70 mm by 0.25 mm. The **adult male** is unknown. The cuticle is smooth. It has 2 fleshy lappets at the posterior end. The *microfilariae* are present in blood. They are small—200 by 4.5μ. They are unsheathed, nonperiodic. The tail is sharply pointed and the **nuclei do not extend up to tip** of the tail (Figs. 2—5). LIFE SPAN is not known. **Incidence.** 25-40 percent population have been found to harbour the worm in endemic areas. Infection does not occur, as it does not harm the body in any way. **Life cycle.** The intermediate host is a midge, *C. furens* in St. Vincent (West Indies), but it is *C. paraensis* in Argentina (South America). Larvae assume the propagating or transmitting form in 8 days in the midges and five percent of the midges have been found infected in nature. **Pathogenicity.** No pathogenic effect is seen in man. **Diagnosis.** By recognition of characteristic microfilariae in blood. **Treatment.** It is not necessary, as there is no infection or disease. Hetrazan is ineffective.

LOA LOA (Cobbold, 1864) Castellani & Chalmers, 1913

GENUS: *LOA* **Stiles, 1905**

(A West African name for the eye worm)

Geographical distribution. West Africa and a part of Central Africa.

Habitat. The adult worm is found in the subcutaneous connective tissue and in the subconjunctival tissues. The microfilariae enter the blood stream and remain there.

Morphology. ADULTS. The worm is cylindrical and transparent. The head end is truncated and has a ring of 6 papillae just behind the level of the mouth. Cuticle in both sexes is covered with smooth transparent, cuticular bosses except at the extremities. (Fig. 6A).

The **male** is 3 cm in length and 0.35 mm in diameter. It has a coiled tail. The posterior end has narrow caudal alae, 8 pairs of perianal papillae and a pair of copulatory spicules (Fig. 6B)

The **female** measures 6 cm in length and 0.4 mm in diameter. It is **ovoviviparous**.

MICROFILARIAE are diagnosed by examining the tail, which is curved. They are sheathed 300μ by 6-8.5μ. The nuclei extend up to the tip of the pointed tail (Figs. 2—3). They appear in the peripheral blood in the **daytime**, and is, therefore, called *Microfilariae diurna*.

LIFE SPAN of the adult worm may be as long as 15 years or more.

Periodicity. Diurnal periodicity of this microfilaria is characteristic from dawn to dusk, and there is no change of periodicity with change of habit of the host. The maximum number of microfilariae occurs in 5-6 hours about noon, when 40 microfilariae per μl may be present in the blood.

Life cycle. Two hosts are necessary to complete the life cycle:

1. DEFINITIVE HOST. Natural definitive hosts are man and monkeys.

2. INTERMEDIATE HOST is the biting **horseflies** of the genus Chrysops. Developing forms appear in the gut and muscles of certain biting horseflies, e.g., *Chrysops dimidiata* and *Chrysops silacea*. Other stages of life cycle are like those of *W. bancrofti* in the *mosquito*. The infective larvae reach the mouth part of the horsefly, when they become infective to man.

RESERVOIR HOST. Simian hosts may serve as reservoir of infection in addition to man.

Pathogenicity. The incubation period is 3-4 years. Adults cause **loasis** or *calabar swelling* in various parts of the body in man; the lesions are itchy, but the itch is transient. Red swelling generally appears over a joint, or face, and **calabar swelling** may occur without microfilariae in blood, but occasionally they may appear. This is due to poor microfilaria output by females whose development is partially inhibited by the immunity resulting from repeated reinfections. There is **eosinophilia** and **leucocytosis**. After entering the body of the human host, the worm migrates in the subcutaneous connective tissue with a predilection for creeping in around the eyes. During the migration, it causes "*calabar or fugitive swelling*", which subsides in 2 to 3 days. This is likely to be due to **allergic reaction** of **filarial toxin**. Microfilariae are seldom found during the stage of *calabar swelling* and diagnosis is made by the history of swelling and high eosinophilia. Anaemia is often present.

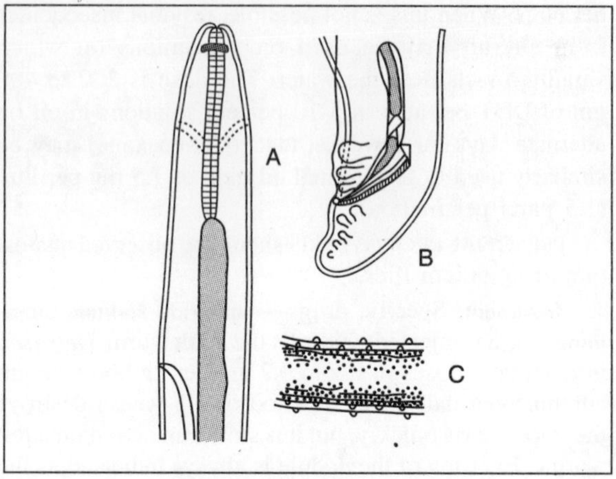

Fig. 13.6 *Loa loa*

A. Showing the muscular and the glandular parts of the oesophagus and the position of the vulva.
B. Tail end of the male with narrow alae, papillae and copulatory spicules.
C. A part of the body showing dewdrop-like warts on the cuticle along the lateral lines.

Diagnosis. A mid-day sample of blood is examined for *Mf. loa*, keeping in mind that microfilaria of *W. bancrofti* may also appear in the daytime. Repeated examinations are necessary, as the microfilariae are scanty. The microfilaria may be present in only 20-30 percent of cases. An adult may be seen under the conjunctiva. **Eosinophilia** may be present.

Complement fixation and **intradermal tests** with Dirofilaria antigen are often positive. The antigen gives group reactions rather than a specific one and is of little specific diagnostic value.

Prophylaxis. It depends on: Antivector measures against Chrysops, and PERSONAL PROTECTION against bites of the infected horse-flies. ANTIPARASITIC MEASURE consists of mass treatment with chemotherapy.

Treatment. Specific chemotherapy is carried out by administration of **hetrazan**, which rapidly destroys microfilariae and the adults, in doses of 6 mg per kg body weight daily, in 3 divided doses. During the first 2 days, fever and allergic manifestations may occur, which are controlled by antihistaminic drugs. After 6 months, complement fixation test may be negative, although intradermal test remains positive. □

CHAPTER

14 SOMATIC NEMATODES

DRACUNCULOSIS

SUPERFAMILY: DRACUNCULOIDEA
FAMILY: DRACUNCULIDAE
GENUS: **DRACUNCULUS**
DRACUNCULUS MEDINENSIS
(Linnaeus, 1758) Gallandant, 1773
SYNONYMS: *Fullebornius medinensis*
Leiper, 1926, Guinea or Medina worm

Dracunculus medinensis is the **longest nematode** of man and the **female** wanders in deeper tissues and then appear in the subcutaneous tissues of the lower extremities. Infection of man takes place by ingestion of **cyclops**, in water containing the infective larvae. It is a crustacean host. *Clinical manifestations* are due to emergence of the female through the skin, and secondary bacterial infection of the track in the tissues.

Incidence. It is found mostly in adults and 90 per cent may belong to the age group near 30 years. It is rare under the age of 4 years. High incidence of onset is noticed from May to September with the peak at July, which is the warmest month in the rainy season in Rajasthan, when the larvae are incubated most rapidly in the cyclops. The incubation period is 8-12 months.

Geographical distribution. In India, Hyderabad and Rajputana; in North Western region of Pakistan; in tropical and subtropical Africa, Arabia, South America and West Indies.

Habitat. **Adult female** is found in subcutaneous tissue, especially **round the ankle** and intermuscular connective tissues of lower extremities.

Adult male resides in the retroperitoneal connective tissues and dies shortly after copulation. It is calcified or absorbed in the tissue.

Morphology. ADULTS have a rounded head, terminating in a thickened chitinous shield containing the triangular mouth and papillae.

ADULT MALE is rarely seen; it is small and about 1.2 to 2.9 cm by 0.4 mm.

ADULT FEMALES are 50 to 120 cm in length and 1.5 mm in breadth, cylindrical milky white in colour with slightly tapering end; the tip of the tail is curved forming a chitinous hook, called anchoring hook, which is said to maintain her hold during extraction. The mouth is terminal and surrounded by several pairs of papillae (Fig. 7).

GENITALIA. *Male organs*. The anus opens 0.25 mm proximal to the coiled posterior end. They have 4 pre-anal and 6 postanal papillae and two almost equal spicules 0.5 to 0.73 mm long, supported by a gubernaculum 0.2 mm long (Fig. 14.1).

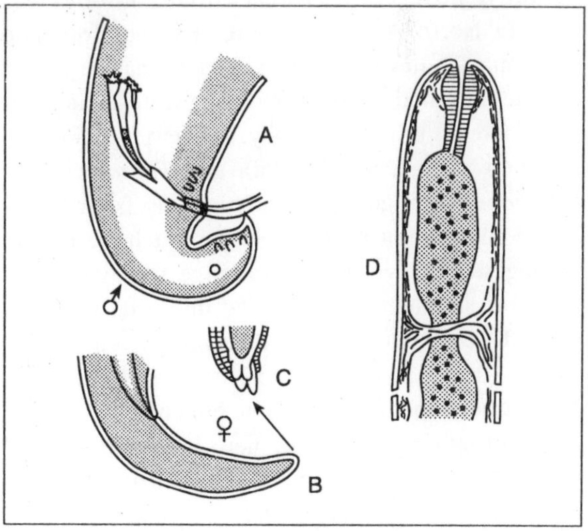

Fig. 14.1 *D. medinensis*
A. Tail end of male. B and C. Tail end of female. D. Head end of male, showing small anterior muscular, and a posterior glandular constriction at the nerve ring (after Moorthy, 1931)

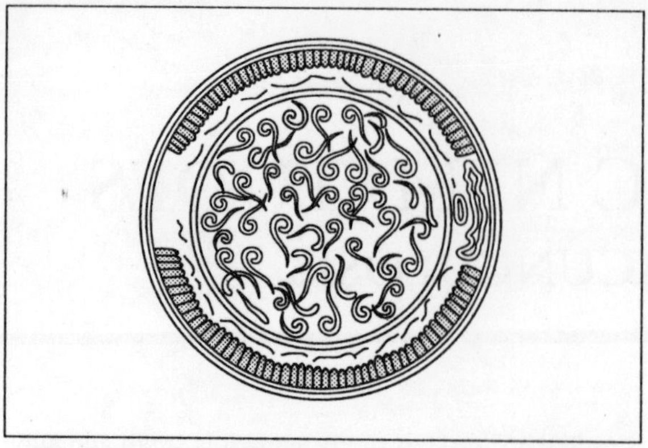

Fig. 14.2 Cross-section of guinea worm, showing the uterus with embryos; × 25 (after Leuckart)

Female organs. The vulva is near the middle of the body; it is nonfunctioning. The intestine in a gravid worm atrophies behind the oesophagus. The uteri are coiled, paired, distended with a large number of larvae and occupy the greater part of the body (Fig. 2). They are **viviparous**.

The EMBRYOS are unsheathed, **rhabditoid**. They are 500 to 750μ in length and 15 to 25μ in diameter; the cuticle is finely striated. They are coiled up with a long tapering tail.

Life cycle (Fig. 3). Man is the most important definitive host, but it has been found in dogs and cats. In North America, where it is not found to infest man, it may be found in other animals. Cyclops are the **intermediate host**, having greatest diameter in the anterior third of the body. *Mesocyclops leukarti* is found in Rajasthan (India), and *Thermocyclops nigerianus* in Nigeria. **Larvae** escaping from ulcers in the foot or leg near the ankle, reach water and are **ingested by cyclops**, Larvae ingested by cyclops enter the stomach, penetrate the intestinal wall and **enter the coelomic cavity** of the cyclops, where they **moult**. After 2 moults on the 7th-8th and 12th day, respectively, the larvae become **infective** by the **21st day**. During first moulting, there is loss of striated cuticle with the development of a delicate enveloping sheath 2 or 3 days later. Soon after this, it becomes **tightly coiled** and inactive without any inclination to quit the cyclops and **remains as such** in cyclops up to 4 months. Usually 3-6 larvae are seen in each cyclop, as a number more than that causes death of the cyclops. **High atmospheric temperature** is necessary for the development of the larvae. As many as 35 per cent of cyclops in India may be infected (Lindberg, 1946 a, b).

The **definitive host** is man.

Infection in man occurs *via* drinking water, containing the infected cyclops. The digestive juice destroys the cyclops without affecting the larvae. The larvae are now very active and after the *final moult*, penetrate through the wall of the intestine and proceed towards the retroperitoneal tissue, where they become adults after a period of eight months to one year. The male probably dies after fertilisation and is often found calcified in the retroperitoneal tissue. *It is also possible that females do not require fertilisation to produce a viable progeny.*

However, the fertilised female usually **migrates through** the **femoral canal** and Hunter's canal, reaches the medial side of the knee and **passes downwards** to the leg round the ankle joint and appears on the surface (**geotropic**). As a result of its *toxic secretion*, lymph collects under the epidermis and a **vesicle** forms with a gelatinous bed. It is usually 5-7 cm in diameter with indurated margin near the ankle or the sole of the foot, but it may be found in arms, trunk, buttock, scrotum or near the knee joint or near the angle of the jaw. The bed eventually breaks and an **ulcer forms**. The granulation tissue at the floor of the ulcer acts as a barrier against secondary infection.

At the base of this ulcer, there is a minute pore through which the worm protrudes its head end and causes a *reflex discharge* of fluid, which is at first clear and, later, **milky**. It contains a large number of embryos ejected from the prolapsed uterus. Major

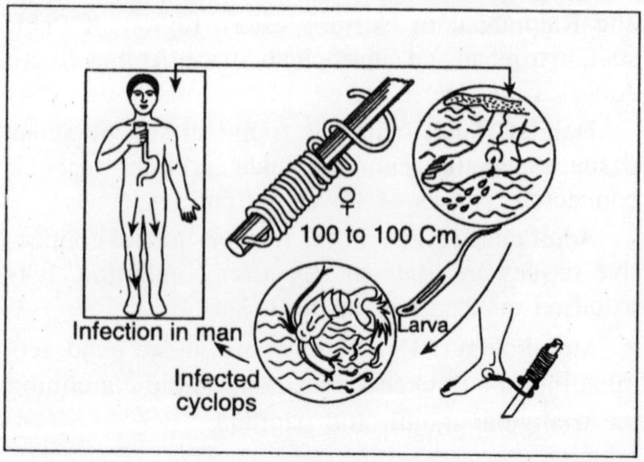

Fig. 14.3 Life cycle of *Dracunculus medinensis*

part of the body of the female worm is occupied by the uterus. Whenever it comes in contact with cold water, numerous coiled up larvae escape due to contraction and prolapse of the uterus. *D. medinensis* is *viviparaous* and segmentation of eggs takes place within the uterus, before larvae escape. In the course of a fortnight the worm empties through the ulcer spontaneously, or aided by gentle, gradual traction. If, however, undue traction is applied, the worm might give way with liberation of embryos in the subcutaneous tissues causing **serious inflammatory changes** and **cellulitis** with *secondary infection.*

Pathogenicity in man. It is produced as follows:

(1) Toxic histamine-like substances are liberated by the female guinea worm as soon as she starts migration, causing profound allergic symptoms. It is characterised by erythema, urticarial rash, nausea, vomiting, diarrhoea, severe dyspnoea, giddiness and syncope associated with marked eosinophilia. This is followed by the appearance of the worm under the skin associated with blister formation, which bursts and the larvae are discharged after coming in contact with fresh water.

(2) Premature liberation of embryos in the tissue causes irritation and inflammation. This happens particularly when the female worm is torn at the time of its extraction prematurely.

(3) Septic infection is caused by secondary bacterial infection. *Staphylococcus aureus* and *Streptococcus pyogenes* are responsible for producing cellulitis, abscess and other septic complications. This is due to secondary organisms from the surface, which contaminate the tissue during the progress of retraction of the worm.

Laboratory diagnosis. Diagnosis may be arrived at by:

(1) Finding of the **adult female** on the skin surface forming a blister or an ulcer.

(2) The finding of a dead **calcified worm** under X-ray. This gives a beaded cord-like appearance—when near the surface.

(3) Finding of the **embryo**. This is done in the laboratory by putting a drop of cold water on the ulcer. After a few minutes, a little quantity of milky fluid is pipetted off. Embryos will be seen under 2/3 inch low power objective.

(4) Blood examination showing **eosinophilia**.

(5) Allergic **(immunological)** skin test. This is done with an antigen, which is an extract of Dracunculus, prepared from the dried worm in physiological saline. The dracunculus antigen is injected **intradermally** in a dose of 0.1 to 0.25 ml and, in positive cases, a wheal of 2 to 3 cm in diameter with pseudopodia develops in 24 hours. The test is positive in 85 percent of cases in Nigeria.

Prophylaxis. ANTIPARASTIC MEASURES. Infected persons should not be allowed to bathe and wade in water for drinking purposes. Persons must be taught not to drink water of step-wells. They should use water of draw-wells (tubewells) for drinking purpose.

ANTIVECTOR MEASURES. (1) *Introduction of fish* in ponds is advisable to consume cyclops (Moorthy and Sweet, 1936).

(2) *Use of chemicals*—hyperchlorination. Use quick lime (1:1,000); copper sulphate or perchloride have been used to disinfect well water. Application of wettable DDT (10 parts per million) in pond water may be used for household purposes, and this greatly reduces the infection rate.

PERSONAL PROTECTION. Boiling water and straining with thick cloth will retain the cyclops.

GENERAL MEASURES. These include education of the community regarding transmission of the disease and other preventive measures.

Treatment. No specific chemotherapy has been discovered for the treatment of dracunculosis, but **hetrazan** may be used as prophylactic and curative. According to Rousset (1952), large doses of hetrazan—orally—kill the adult worms, and the developing stages of the worm are destroyed, when the drug is administered prophylactically. It is given about 3 and 6 months after the period of transmission in doses of 0.5 gm and 0.3 gm daily, respectively, for 10 days. The drug may be administered 2-3 times a year (when the transmission occurs during the whole year), avoiding side-effects which are frequent. Maximum doses are to be used when adult worms are present.

EXTRACTION OF THE WORM. Gradual traction takes about 15 to 21 days (minimum 2 days) to get the whole worm extracted.

The methods of extraction are:

(*a*) 1:1,000 *perchloride of mercury*, when injected locally, kills the worm. The worm is then extracted. (*b*) Chloroform, or 1:1,000 of *acriflavine* lotion, has been similarly used. (*c*) 2 gm of *phe-*

nothiazine (finely powdered) mixed with 0.35 gm of *lanoline* and 15 ml of sterile *olive oil* is introduced, and the emulsion is put into a 60 ml bottle. It is autoclaved at 115°C for 30 minutes. The part is anaesthetised with procaine (novocaine) and a dose of 20 ml of the emulsion is injected in the central part and neighbourhood of the worm. The site of infection is gently massaged for 5 minutes after injection. In 5 to 7 days the worm dies and can be extracted.

ALLERGIC SYMPTOMS. Adrenaline 0.5 to 1 ml hypodermically prevents acute allergic reactions and *antihistaminic drugs* may be tried in less severe cases. Other steroids like β-methasone, dexamethasone are also helpful to combat this.

SECONDARY INFECTION. In cellulitis—1:400 *chinosol*, or 1:1,000 *acriflavine* may be injected locally. Antibiotics are also useful. □

REFERENCES

Lindberg, K. (1946a). Enquete epidemiologique Sur la dracunculose dans un village de Deccan (Inde). *Bull. Soc. path. Exot.* 39, 303-318.

Lindberg, K. (1946b). Dracunculose dans l'etal de Djodhpour. (Radipootana), Inde. *Bull. Soc. path. Exot.* 39, 318-328.

Moorthy, V. N. (1938). A redescription of *Dracunculus medinensis* Velsch. *J. Parasitol.* 23, 220-224.

Moorthy, V. N. and Sweet, W. C. (1936). A Biological method for the control of dracontiasis. *Ind. med. Gaz.* 71, 565-567.

Rousset, P. (1952). Essai de prophylaxie et de traitment de la dracunculose par la notezine en Adrar. *Bull. Med. Afr. occid. franc.* 9, 351-568.

CHAPTER

15 SOMATIC NEMATODES

GNATHOSTOMIASIS

ORDER: SPIRURIDA
SUBORDER: SPIRURINA
SUPERFAMILY: SPIRUROIDEA
FAMILY: GNATHOSTOMATIDAE
GENUS: **GNATHOSTOMA (Owen, 1836)**

GNATHOSTOMA SPINIGERUM

(*Producing gnathostomiasis*)

Greek: *Gnathos*—jaw; *Stoma*—mouth

SYNONYM: *G. siamense*
(Levinson, 1890) Rallient, 1893

Historical consideration, Geographical distribution and Epidemiology. *G. spinigerum* was first described by Owen from gastric tumours of a tiger, following which it has been described in domestic and wild cat, the leopard and the dog in China, India, Japan, the Malayasia and Thailand (Siam). Yoshida (1931, 1932) discovered *G. nipponica* in Japanese mink, which was erroneously diagnosed as *G. spinigera* (verified by Miyazaki, 1954).

Human cases have been reported from Thailand (Castens, 1934; Daengsvang, 1938, 1939, 1949; Daengsvang *et al*, 1964; Leiper, 1909; Levinson, 1890; Prommas and Daengsvang, 1934); from India (Datta and Maplestone, 1930; Dey and Dey 1969; Maplestone, and Bhaduri, 1937; Mukherji and Bhaduri, 1945; Sen and Ghosh, 1945); from Vietnam and Philippines, (Chanco *et al*, 1956); from Japan (Ando, 1957, Miyazaki, 1960) and from Australia (Heydon, 1929). Possibly all human infections have occurred with the immature worms in the subcutaneous tissue.

Thailand is the world's most important endemic area of heaviest infection in both human and reservoir hosts (Daengsvang *et al*, 1964). The disease is being diagnosed with increasing frequency in Japan (Miyazaki, 1960). However, consumption of **inadequately processed fish flesh** *containing* the encapsulated **third stage larvae** is usually responsible for human **gnathostomiasis**. At one time it was thought that the disease occurred more in females than in males. In the majority of Daengvang's cases, most of the infected people had cats in their homes. Fermented flesh of the fish *Ophiocephalus straitus* in Thailand, a fermented fish delicacy colloqually called **"Sashime"**, the raw fish tidbits of Japan, contribute to the possible source of infection in fairly large population.

Morphology. The ADULT WORMS vary in length from 11 to 25 mm for *males* and 25 to 54 mm for *females*. In smaller hosts, they are considerably reduced in size. They are reddish, stout, coloured and relatively transparent nematodes with a subglobose cephalic swelling separated from the rest of the body by a cervical constriction. The worms are curved at both ends ventrally. The anterior half of the body is covered with leaf-like spines, which are broader and tridentate sharply behind the cervix (neck), but narrower and highly pointed towards the equator region. The posterior half of the cuticula is aspinose. The cephalic portion of the body is covered with 4 to 8 transverse rows of sharp, recurved hooks (Fig. 15.1). The mouth is guarded by a pair of conspicuous fleshy lips. Four conspicuous cervical glands are arranged symmetrically around the oesophagus. They fuse in pairs

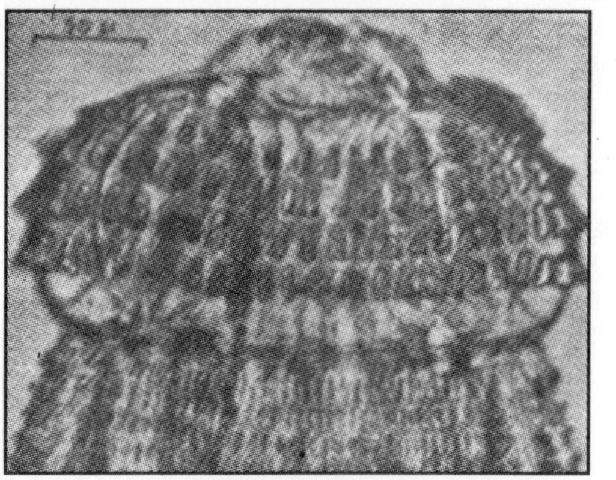

Fig. 15.1 Showing the cephalic bulb of the second stage larva of *G. spinigerum* provided with 4 rows of single-pointed spines, developing in the primary intermediate host, a cyclop

and open through two ducts perforating the lips. The **male** has a pseudobursa, provided with 4 pairs of perianal nipple-shaped papillae. In **females**, the vagina is long and is anteriorly directed. The other genital tubules are paired.

Eggs are ovoidal, transparent, superficially pitted, and measure 65 to 70μ by 38 to 40μ (Fig. 15.2). They have a mucoid plug at one end and unembryonated when laid, which actively enters the first intermediate host, cyclop, gets metamorphosed and becomes embryonated.

Pathogenesis and Life cycle. Gnathostome is not a fully adapted parasite in human being and produces lesions in the subcutaneous tissue and somatic musculature as it migrates through these tissues. Abscess formation may be provoked by the early and the advanced larval stage in the course of the disease. In nature, the ADULT parasites are found in the stomach of cats, dogs and felines like the tiger (Owen, 1936), and the leopard (Mitter, 1912). Ova passed in the faeces hatch in water (Heydon, 1929), forming free-swimming **first stage larvae** after about 7 days. The minute copepod crustacean host, the cyclops, ingest the larvae to develop the latter into the **second stage larvae** in course of 7 to 14 days (Prommas and Daengsvang, 1933; Refuerzo and Garcia, 1938). This is the **first infection** and the cyclops is the PRIMARY INTERMEDIATE HOST. The second stage larva is characterised by the presence of a cephalic bulb having four rows of single-pointed spines (Fig. 15.1).

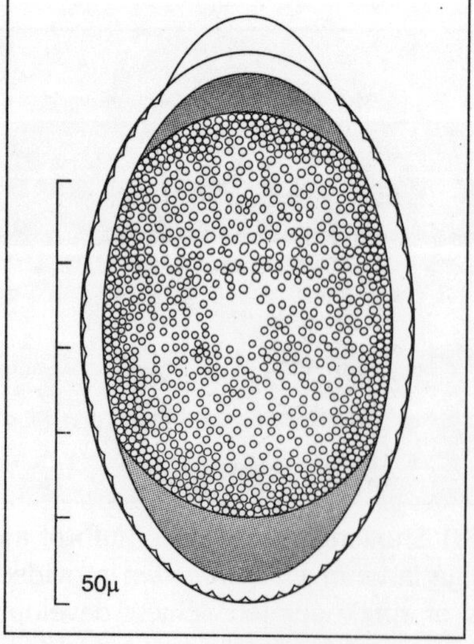

Fig. 15.2 Diagrammatic representation of fertilised unsegmented ova of *G. spinigerum*

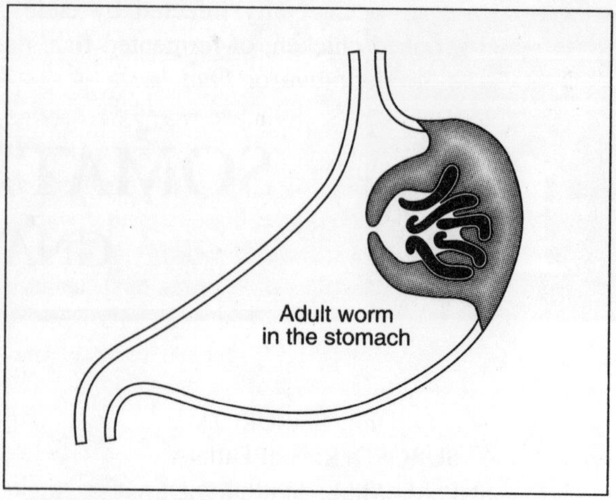

Fig. 15.3 Adult *G. spinigerum* causing tumour (swelling) in the digestive tract of definitive host and live there for sometime. This is gnathostomiasis interna, posterior portions of five parasites are seen protruding into the lumen of the tumour, the wall of which is formed by hyperplastic gastric mucosa

Infection of the (*first*) SECONDARY INTERMEDIATE HOST occurs in selected fresh water fish (**second infection**; second larval host) of the genera Ophiocephalus, Ciarius, Glossogobias, etc.—eels, frogs and snakes, which feed on cyclops harbouring mature second stage larvae (Africa *et al*, 1936a, b; Daengsvang and Tansurat, 1938; Pro-b; Daengsvang and Tansurat, 1938; Prommas and Daengsvang, 1936). Migration of larvae takes place after penetration of the stomach wall of the host (commonly a fish). Growth, development, and the final **encystment** of the **"third stage larvae"** in skeletal muscle takes place in course of a month or longer. Infection may occur in the domestic chicken fed on infected offal or fish-flesh when it becomes another SECONDARY (*Second*) INTERMEDIATE HOST (Miyazaki, 1960; Miyazaki and Kikuchi, 1954). Apart from chicken, other animals may act as *secondary intermediate host*, either experimentally or naturally infected, e.g., other fish-eating birds, freshwater crustaceans other than cyclops, amphibians, reptiles, other fishes as well as some mammals like rats, mice, guineapigs, rabbits, weasles and pigs. In the secondary intermediate host, reencystment occurs in the skeletal muscle. The DEFINITIVE HOST like cat and dog usually becomes infected by eating raw, infective flesh.

Human—when accidentally infected by eating inadequately-cooked chicken, or fermented fish, or pork—acts as the **definitive** or *final host*.

IN RESERVOIR HOSTS, the adult worms are coiled inside tumours of the digestive tract and is referred to as **gnathostomiasis interna** (Fig. 15.3). Such condition has not been described for the human host; immature worms occur in the peripheral tissues of the latter and the condition is called **gnathostomiasis externa**, which includes the development of abscess pockets, indurated nodules with abscessed centres, and the formation of deep cutaneous or subcutaneous tunnels in which the worms are migrating (**"larva migrans"** causing "*creeping eruption*").

Histopathologically, the worms are usually found in the region between the epidermis and the dermis (*stratum basale*). There is infiltration of large number of eosinophils, lymphocytes, neutrophils and plasma cells. **Histochemically**, a *haemolytic factor* (Shimizu, 1957)—*acetylcholine-like substance*—and a *proteolytic enzyme* (Metsuda, 1959) have been demonstrated in parasites, or in fluid containing their metabolic products. These substances are thought to be responsible for the toxicity of infection and help in the penetration through the tissue. Extracts of third stage larvae, adult parasites and their metabolic products are highly antigenic, and with them, **Shwartzman** and Arhus phenomena can be elicited in guineapigs (Yamanaka, 1958).

Symptomatology. The onset of symptoms reportedly occurs in course of 24 to 48 hours of ingestion of infected food (Kitamura, 1952) in the form of nausea, salivation, vomiting, flushing, pruritus, urticaria, upper abdominal pain and discomfort. At the first contact or experience with the parasite, there may be striking eosinophilia ranging up to 90 per cent in association with leucocytosis. Pain and tenderness in the right hypochondrium may signal penetration of the liver associated with mild abnormalities of liver function. Within the next few weeks, migration of the larva within the abdominal or the thoracic organs or the peripheral tissues may provoke brief, sharp pains indicating the localisation of the larvae. At times by mistake, it may be suggested as an acute abdominal episode, like cholecystitis and pulmonary symptoms like tuberculosis, even on radiological report. Usually the migrating larva finds its way to the subcutaneous tissue within one month. The common sites of subcutaneous localisation are the head, upper extremities, chest, abdomen and thighs.

Diagnosis. Non-migrating variety of the infection must be differentiated from furunculosis or other localised bacterial processes, while the migrating type of the infection is to be differentiated from migrating larvae of hookworms and cutaneous myiasis; in both types, specific diagnosis can be made only after the worms have been removed and their characteristic features discovered. Other cutaneous lesions are caused by larvae of *Paragonimus westermani* and spargana of *Diphyllobothrium mansonoides*, which should be considered in the differential diagnosis, especially in areas, where geographical distribution of three parasites overlap. However, a clinical course characterised by painless subcutaneous migratory oedema, recurring intermittently, is pathognomonic of gnathostomiasis.

IMMUNOLOGICAL TEST. Gnathostome **skin test** antigens have been developed, and used successfully in Japan (Egashira, 1953; Yamaguchi, 1952). In this, cross reactivity with *P. westermani* infection does not occur. Passive transfer of gnathostome antibodies has been demonstrated by *Prausnitz-Kuestner reaction* (Yamanaka, 1958).

SEROLOGICAL TEST. A serum **precipitin** reaction has been described (Furuno, 1959; Kita, 1957; Yamaguchi, 1951, 1952). After successful extirpation of the parasite, the serum precipitin test becomes negative, while the intradermal test becomes positive.

PERIPHERAL BLOOD. In peripheral blood, there is **leucocytosis** with a rise of **eosinophils** to a level up to 90% may give some hint for the diagnosis.

Prevention. Effective prevention is best achieved by excluding poorly cooked fish or chicken from the diet in endemic areas.

Treatment. There is general agreement that unequivocal cure is not usually effected by any of the available drugs. **X-ray treatment** has proven unsatisfactory (Uozumi, 1959). **Ultrasonic disintegration** of the parasite *in situ* is under investigation (Punyogupta). **Surgical Excision** is difficult because for the small size of the parasite, its mobility, and its non-differentiating coloration from the tissue. However, when the position of the parasite can be affirmed with reasonable certainty in a site feasible for **excisional biopsy**, *surgical treatment* is the treatment of choice. There may be failure in this, as the parasite being stimulated by the procedure, moves to hide away into the adjacent tissue.

CHAPTER 16

SECTION III

MEDICAL ENTOMOLOGY

ARTHROPODS AND MOLLUSCS OF MEDICAL IMPORTANCE

Medical parasitology is intimately associated with members of the Phylum Arthropoda; while some of them act as *carriers* or *vectors* of parasitic diseases; there are yet others which act as *ectoparasites*. A brief review of them is necessary to appraise their importance in relation to transmission of diseases, as they affect human hosts in one or other of the following ways:

1. Insects are often pests of man, because they produce lesions by *mechanical trauma*; the lesions may be secondarily infected; or by their bite or stings they may infect substances which are normally harmless but to which a subject may be *sensitised* due to a previous exposure; e.g., *Cimex lectularious*, commonly known as bed bugs.

2. They may invade the skin and produce skin lesions due to the irritation, e.g., *Sarcoptes scabei*—the itch mite. Following this, a secondary streptococcal infection may occur causing impetigo contagiosa. They might often *sensitise* infants and children and produce *eczematous* lesions.

3. Many insects act as biological vectors of diseases. (a) The pathogenic organisms undergo cyclical development in arthropods with multiplication of the parasite, e.g., plasmodia show formation of sporocysts (sexual multiplication) in many species of Anopheles mosquitoes. (b) Common flies (*Musca domestica*) may act as mechanical vectors by carrying organisms like *Vibrio cholerae* on their feet or wings and may contaminate food by sitting on it; or (c) in another case, it might infect food by defaecation or regurgitation of cysts of *E. histolytica*, which they ingested earlier. The cyst remains unaltered in the fly gut in this case. (d) Pathogenic organisms sometimes undergo developmental changes without multiplication; e.g., microfilaria in mosquitoes, or (e) organisms (bacteria) may multiply in an arthropod vector without any change in form, e.g., *Pasteurella pestis* multiplying within the rat flea *Xenopsyla cheopis*.

PHYLUM: ARTHROPODA

These are invertebrates having *bilaterally symmetrical* body composed of *joined segments*; a *chitinous* exoskeleton, which covers the body with paired and *joined appendages* arising from the body segments. Body consists of head, thorax and abdomen. The body cavity is fully, developed with a mouth and anus. Their *vascular system* is dorsal and *nervous system* ventral to the alimentary tract. They are sexually differentiated and are classified as:

I. Class: Insecta. The body consists of head, thorax and abdomen. The head carries one pair of eyes, antennae and mouth parts. The thorax carries 3 pairs of legs and hence called *hexapoda*. They have typically two pairs of wings, but may have one pair of wings, or no wing at all. Metamorphosis is complete, e.g., *mosquito*.

II. Class: Arachnida. These are *ticks* and *mites* having four pair of legs in adult state: the head, thorax and abdomen are fused together. The head and thorax in *spiders* are fused together to form a Cephalothorax and the other segment forms the abdomen.

III. Class: Crustacea. (a) **Cyclops:** These are aquatic animals with gills, 2 pairs of antennae and at least 5 pairs of legs. They have cephalothoracic and abdominal segments, and they act as intermediate host of *Diphyllobothrium latum*, *Dracunculus medinensis*, *Gnathostoma spinigerum*, etc.

(b) **Crabs, cray-fish and lobster:** They act as secondary intermediate hosts of *Paragonimus westermani*, a lung fluke.

IV. Class: Chilopoda (Centipedes). These are *worm-like animals* with *numerous* legs; one pair of legs arising from each segment of the body.

V. Class: Diplopoda (Millipedes). Usually harmless; only one species acts as an intermediate host of the rat tapeworm *Hymenolepis diminuta*.

CLASS: INSECTA

Hexapoda

The body of hexapoda is divided into three segments, namely the head, thorax, and abdomen. There are three pairs of legs on the thorax; one pair of antennae on the head. Abdomen is usually composed of 9 segments and the terminal one is modified as the genital organ at the caudal end. Metamorphosis is complete, except in lice.

Key to medically important insects

One pair of wings with straight proboscis—
Diptera (Flies, mosquitoes)

Body laterally compressed, having no wing—
Siphonaptera (Fleas)

Body flattened dorsiventrally, having no wing—
Anoplura (Lice)

Proboscis joined and flexed, ventrally placed and having typically two pairs of wings—
Hemiptera (True bugs).

ORDER I: DIPTERA

Diptera have one pair of membranous wings, and a posterior pair which is modified into knob-like balancer or halters. The mouth parts are usually adapted for sucking or piercing. The proboscis is straight. Abdominal segments are 4 to 9 in number.

Metamorphosis is complete—usually in 4 stages, namely, *egg, larva, pupa* and *imago* or the *adult* stage.

SUBORDER I: *Nematocera*
SUBORDER II: *Brachycera*
SUBORDER III: *Athericera* (Orthorrhapha, Cyclorrhapha).

SUBORDER I: NEMATOCERA

Antennae are long, slender and composed of six to sixteen segments. Mouth parts can pierce the skin of man. Only the females bite and often transmit diseases.

FAMILY I. *Culicidae*: mosquitoes
FAMILY II. *Psychodidae*: sandflies, moth (flies)
FAMILY III. *Simuliidae*: buffalo gnats, black flies
FAMILY IV. *Ceratopogonidae*: biting midges.

FAMILY: CULICIDAE

Mosquitoes

The subfamily Culicinae of the family Culicidae is of medical importance. This is divided into tribes—Anophelini (genus—Anopheles), and Culicini (genera—Culex and Aedes). Mosquitoes are small, slender diptera; typical antennae consists of 14 to 15 segments, wings are long and narrow, and venations are characteristic.

The *female mosquitoes* are *blood—suckers* and transmit diseases, but the males live on vegetables or fruit juice. There are four genera which are of medical importantce.

CLASSIFICATION OF MOSQUITOES

FAMILY: Culicidae: SUBFAMILY: Culicinae
TRIBE I: *Anophelini;*; GENUS: Anopheles
TRIBE II: Culicini; GENUS: Culex; SUBGENUS: Culex
GENUS: Mansonia; SUBGENUS: Mansonioides
GENUS: Aedes; SUBGENUS: Stegomyia.

Life cycle of mosquito. There are four stages of development of a mosquito, e.g., egg, larva, pupa and imago or the adult stage. Under favourable conditions, the life cycle is completed in 10 to 12 days in the tropics. Eggs are laid on the surface of water singly (Anopheles) or in rafts (Culex). As they develop into larval stage, they come to the surface of water to take air for their respiration. After some days the larva develops into pupa. The *larva* lives on organic matters; the *pupa* does not take any food. Pupa next develops into *Imago* or adult stage and fly in the air. *Males* live on vegetables or fruit juice, but *females* feed on blood, which is required for laying their eggs.

Anopheles. These are usually spotted-winged mosquitoes. Unlike Culicini, the females have palps as long as the proboscis. They prefer to breed in ponds, streamlets and in paddy fields, where the water is clear. The eggs are single, solitary and float with the help of air-floats. The larvae have rudimentary breathing tubes. They lie parallel to the surface of water (Fig. 15.1). Hairs on the abdominal segments are palmate. Many adult females are vectors of *malaria* and *filaria*.

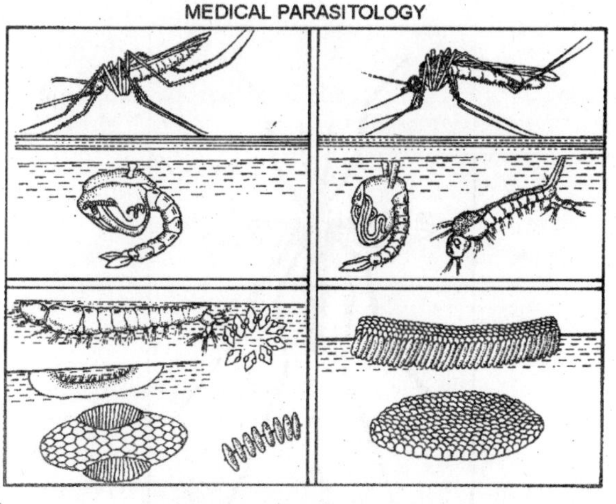

Fig. 16.1 Difference between Anopheles and Culex mosquitoes

Culex. These are common brown house mosquitoes and breed in water polluted with organic matters, e.g., cesspools, drains, sullage water, etc., and also in ponds. The eggs are seen in the form of *siphon tube* and rest near the surface of water in an angular fashion (Fig. 15.1).

Culex fatigans is the chief carrier of *Wiichereria bancrofti* and causes filariasis in India and other tropical and subtropical regions.

FEMALES. Both Anopheles and Culex possess *pilose hairs* in the antennae.

MALES of both species possess *plumose hairs* in the antennae.

Mansonioides. *Mf. malayi* undergoes metamorphosis in these mosquitoes and also in some species of Anopheles. The breeding habits of Mansonioides differ from those of *Culex fatigans*. The eggs, which are spindle-shaped, are deposited on the submerged leaves of certain water weeds (pistia, water hyacinth, and swamp grass). The *larva* and *pupa* pierce the root tissue of the aquatic plants and attach their *breathing siphons* to the roots to obtain oxygen from the internal air cavities.

Aedes. These are house mosquitoes and commonly breed in small collections of water in various parts of the house, e.g., tin cans, tree holes, bamboo stumps, coconut shells. They are ornamented with silvery scales and the *species A. aegypti* has a *lyre*-like shiny-silvery mark on the scutum (Fig. 15.2). They are avid biters and bite throughout the day—specially in the morning and in the afternoon. They do not fly to a long distance. *A. aegypti* is responsible for transmission of *yellow fever* and *dengue*. Dengue is also transmitted by the bite of *Stegomyia fasciata. A albopictus* is responsible for the transmission of dengue in Philippines and in the Far East. *A. scutellaris* transmits *filaria* and *dengue* in Australia and in Philippines. Some species are responsible for transmission of *equine encephalomyelomyelitis*.

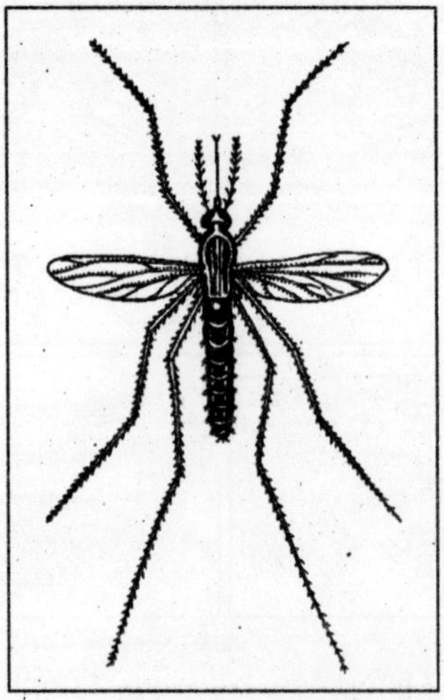

Fig. 16.2 Aedes aegypti (Female)

FAMILY: PSYCHODIDAE (*Sandflies*)

GENUS: PHLEBOTOMUS (Vein cutter)

The genus is characterised by their wings raised over the abdomen at an angle of 45° when the adult is at rest. The body and wings are covered with hairs. The antennae are long and hairy and consist of about 10 segments. Palpi are 4 in number, joined and longer than the head.

Sandflies are the vectors of visceral and cutaneous leishmaniasis. They belong to the genus Phlebotonus. *Leishmania donovani* is transmitted by *Phlebotomus argentipes* in India (Fig. 15.3) and *P. chinensis* in China, *P. major* and *P. papatasii* and *P. sergenti* transmits *L. braxiliensis. P. papatasii* is responsible for the transmission of sandfly or papatasii fever, kala-azar and oriental sore in the Mediterranean region.

The females are blood-suckers and bite at night. They cannot fly a long distance and cannot rise more than a (few feet) metre or two above the ground level. They live in dark corners of the house, crevices of dark damp rocks and remains of buildings. They often breed in dung heaps. The females lay about 50 eggs once in its life time. The eggs pass through the stages of larva and pupa before attaining the imago form. The life cycle is complete in 4 to 8 weeks. The females suck blood before laying eggs. They occasionally feed a second time to deposit a second batch of ova. They have been kept alive in captivity for 45 days.

Control. Sandflies are usually controlled by spraying of 5 percent DDT in breeding places, which require extirpation.

FAMILY: SIMULIDAE

GENUS: SIMULIUM

These are black gnats or black flies, small, stoutly built with short legs. The antennae protrude like horns of an animal and consist of 11 joints; wings are scaleless with thickened anterior veins (Fig. 15.4). The females of the genus Simulium are voracious blood-suckers and transmitter of the human filaria *Onchocerce volvulus* in Africa and tropical America. The bite is followed by pain, itching and swelling.

FAMILY: CERATOPOGONIDAE (Chironomidae)

GENUS: CULICOIDES (Punkies)

These are commonly known as *biting midges*, and are mistaken for mosquitoes. The antennae are like those of mosquitoes with *plumose hairs* in the male, but *pilose hairs* in the female. The head is small, and concealed by the thorax. The mouth parts are suited for sucking. Wings

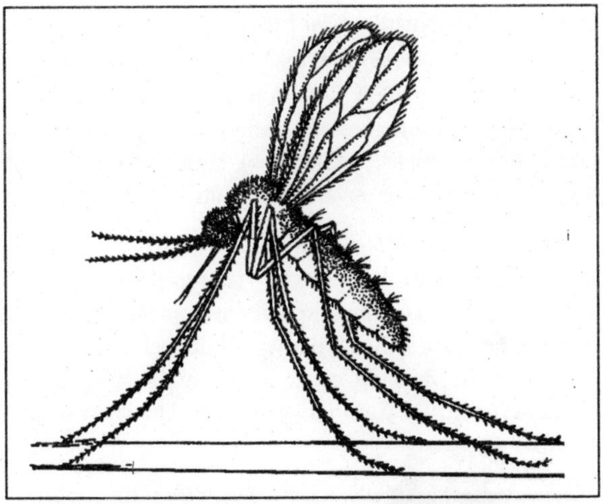

Fig. 16.3 Phlebotomus argentipes (female), the vector of *L. donovani*

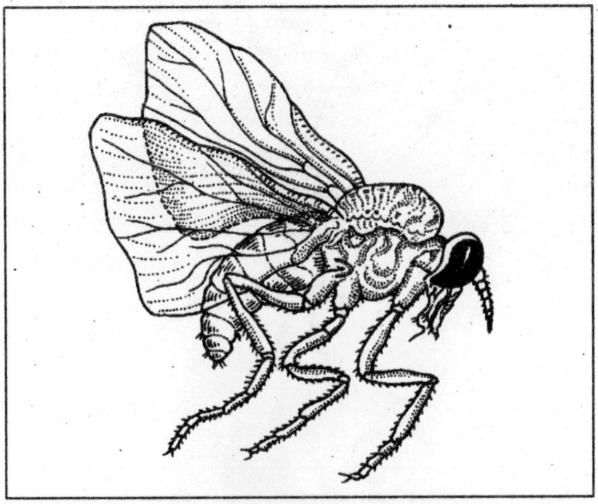

Fig. 16.4 Adult Simulium, the black fly

are hairy, but lacking in scales (Fig. 15.5). Culicoides are voracious blood-suckers and intermediate hosts of filarial worms, *Acanthocheilonema perstans. C. furens* is the intermediate host of *Mansonella ozzardi.*

SUBORDER II: BRACHYCERA

Out of seventeen families only one family is of medical importance. These are large or medium sized flies with robust bodies and large eyes. The antennae have three segments and the third joint is often annulated.

FAMILY: TABANIDAE

(Horse flies)

Members of the genus Tabanus have antennae with three segments, the third joint is annulated. They have a piercing and sucking proboscis projecting downwards; blood sucking habit is confined to females.

Members of the genus Chrysops have conspicuous markings on the wings. *Chrysops dimidiata* (Fig. 15.6), and *C. silacea* are intermediate host of *Loa loa. C. discalis*, the western deer fly, transmits *Francisella tubarensis*.

SUBORDER III: ATHERICERA

(Cyclorrhapha)

The members of the suborder are characterised by their antennae, which are short and consist of not more than three segments and the distal one bears a spine-like arista at its base. The are conveniently divided into biting and non-biting groups.

NON-BITING FLIES

The non-biting group of flies comprise of *Musca domestica* flies in the family Muscidae and several other families, larvae of which cause cutaneous myiasis.

FAMILY: MUSCIDAE

GENUS: MUSCA (Flies)

The family Muscidae includes the genus Musca and other important genera like Fannia, Stomoxys and Glossina. The last two are considered with *biting flies* (see later).

Musca domestica are typical representatives of the order diptera. They are common houseflies. They have dirty habits of sitting and feeding on human excreta, food, etc., and breed in horse manure and moist refuge like dung of domestic animals and other decaying animal and vegetable matters.

Life cycle (Fig. 15.7). The eggs are 1 mm in length and are laid in masses of 75 to 150 eggs. A single female can lay 21 batches of eggs in a single month after

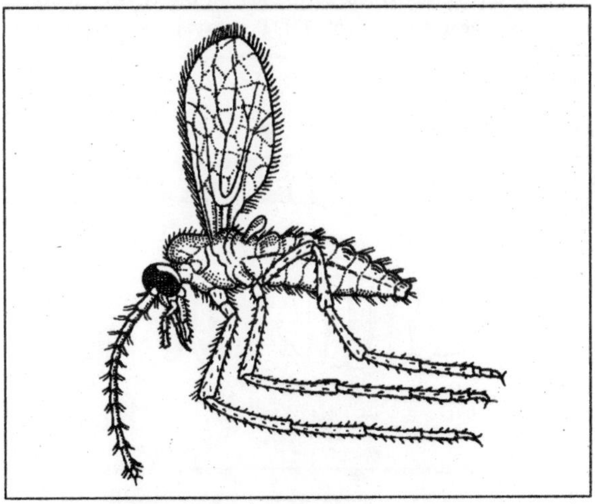

Fig. 16.5 Culicoides, a biting midge

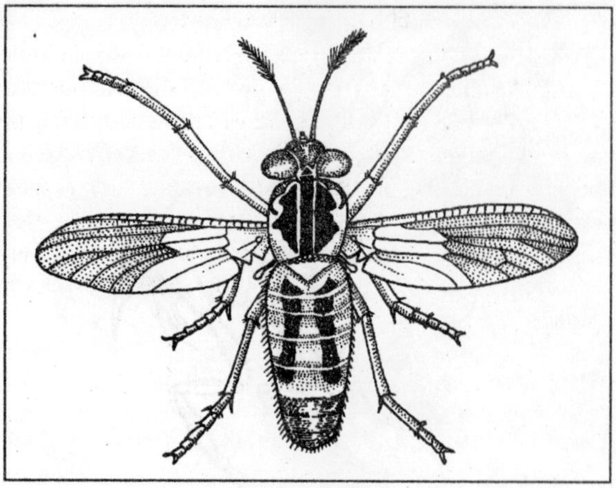

Fig. 16.6 *Chrysops dimidiata*

emergence. Depending on temperature, eggs develop into the larval stage in one to three days. They are seen as maggots and live on organic matter. They develop into pupae in one week. The pupa stage may last for about two weeks, whereafter, the imago or adult comes out. They are about 1 inch (2.5 cm) in length. They multiply enormously in the summer and feed indiscriminately on filthy matters and also on human food—thus food is contaminated. While they carry bacteria on their feet and wings, they also defaecate and vomit while taking food. Thus they also contaminate food. They are responsible for the spread of *zymotic diseases* like cholera, enteric fever, infantile diarrhoea, bacillary and amoebic dysenteries. In the last instance they carry the cysts of *E. histolytica.*

Control. Refuge should not be scattered indiscriminately. Covered refuge-can should be used in every house and the garbage, which furnishes an excellent breeding medium, should be burnt. DDT spray is very effective.

FAMILY: CALLIPHORIDAE
(Blowflies, etc.)

The following genera are included—Auchmeromyia, Cordylobia, Callitroga (Cochliomyia), Chrysomyia, Lucilia, Phormia (black bottle flies), Calliphora. Many of these larvae produce *myiasis* in man.

GENUS: AUCHMEROMYIA

These are commonly known as "Congo floor maggots" and *A. luteola* is a common species in tropical Africa. The flies are large, brownish yellow and deposit eggs on the floor of huts, sleeping mats, or dry and contaminated human excreta. They are active at night. The larvae cause external myiasis.

GENUS: CORDYLOBIA

C. anthropophaga is a large, brownish yellow fly and differs from *A. luteola* by possessing a narrower front and more rounded abdomen. The species is confined to Africa, where it is known as "Tumbu" fly. The eggs are deposited in polluted soil, or clothing with odour of perspiration. The larvae hatch in 24 hours and cause *non-migratory cutaneous myiasis.*

GENUS: CALLITROGA
(Cochliomyia)

C. americana and *C. macellaria* are of medical importance. These are screw worm flies of man and animals in Western hemisphere. The adults are metallic green in colour and are recognised by dark stripes on the thorax.

GELUX: CHRYSOMYIA

They are like Callitroga and medium-sized flies of bright metallic colour. The members of the genus are confined to Africa, America, Australia and Philippines. *G. bezziana* not only cause *myiasis* in sheep but also *in man.*

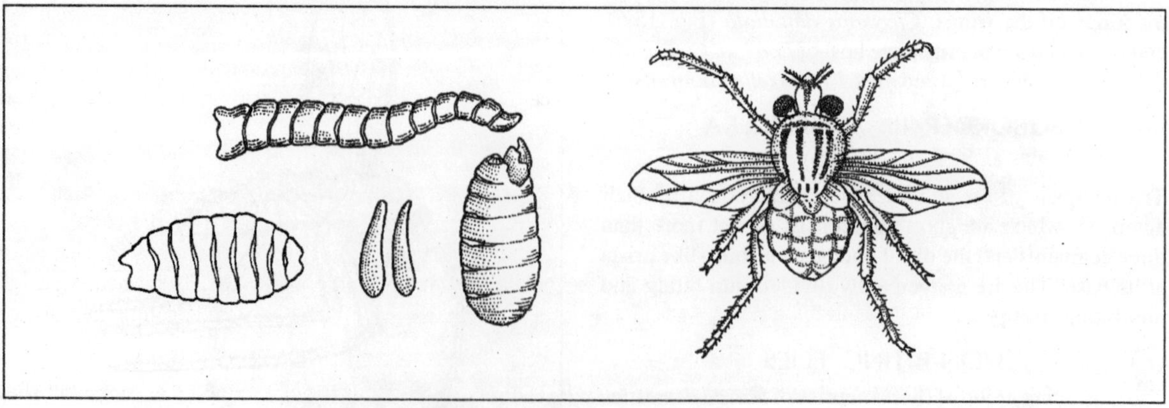

Fig. 16.7 *Musca domestica*
(a) Egg, (b) Larva, (c) Pupa, (d) Empty puparium, (e) Adult

GENUS: PHORMIA
(Black blowfly)

They are either shiny black or green in colour and differentiated from Lucilia by the prothoracic spiracle, which is orange rather than black. *P. regina*, normally breeding in decaying meat, may cause *traumatic myiasis* in man. This species is used in the therapy of osteomyelitis.

GENUS: CALLIPHORA
(Blue bottle flies)

They are large, about 10 to 15 mm long, and are popularly known as "*blowflies*" or *blue flies*. The body is blue in colour with a metallic lustre and the eyes are red.

They deposit eggs in exposed food or meat and decaying animal and vegatable matters, and on ulcers in animals or man causing *myiasis*.

GENUS: LUCILIA
(Green bottle flies)

They are small and are of the size of a housefly. The adults are metallic green in colour with yellow palpi. They have habits like those of Calliphora and often cause *intestinal* or *genitourinary myiasis*. Larvae of *S. sericata* are saprophagous and are used as surgical maggots for cleaning wounds.

Warble Flies

FAMILY: GASTEROPHILIDAE (*Botflies*)

Gasterophilus spp., also known as horse botfly or warble fly have worldwide distribution. They cause *intestinal myiasis* in horses. Eggs are laid on lips or legs of horse. The maggots are licked up, they migrate to the intestine and passed in the excreta several months later.

Maggots of some species can penetrate human skin producing cutaneous myiasis. The latter resembles creeping eruption caused by *Ancylostoma braziliense*.

FAMILY: OESTRIDAE
(Botflies)

GENUS: OESTRUS OVIS is the sheep botfly having a worldwide distribution. These are greyish brown flies, normally depositing hatched maggot on the heads of sheep or goats. They migrate into the nasal passages and sinuses.

In man, they invade the eyes causing severe pain, migrate through conjunctiva and produce an *ophthalmomyiasis*. They may also invade the nasal passages or the *pharynx* in man.

GENUS: RHINOESTRUX

Rhinoestrus purpureus is the *head botfly* of horses which may cause *ophthalmomyiasis* in man.

GENUS: HYPODERMA

Hypoderma bovix is the *cattle botfly*, or ox warble in the northern hemisphere. The *eggs* are deposited in the hairs of cattle, and the developing larva burrows through the skin and migrate to reach the skin of the back. Man is an abnormal host in whom the migrating larvae cause swelling and soreness of the organ they reach by their aimless migration (migration from knee to chin has been reported). When they appear below the skin, they can be readily removed.

GENUS: DERMATOBIA

This is a genus of flies of the family Oestridae found in tropical America. The larvae—called *Ver macaque* (later forms called *torcel,* or *berne*) of species *D. hominis*—sometimes cause *butaneous myiasis* with abscess formation. Their abdomen has a bluish cast on reflected light and the legs and face are orange yellow.

GENUS: FANNIA

F. canicularis is the chief cause of *intestinal myiasis* in Europe and is caused by ingestion of its larvae. It closely resembles house flies but is smaller. *F. scalaris* is a latrine fly.

GENUS: MUSCINA

The flies of the genus Muscina (*nonbiting stable flies*) are sometimes of medical importance as the larvae may cause *traumatic* or *intestinal myiasis*.

FAMILY: SARCOPHAGIDAE
(Flesh flies)

Sarcophaga spp. These are flesh flies, gery with chequered pattern of the abdomen and feed on filth. The maggots feed on animal excrement and decaying flesh. *Intestinal myiasis* is produced by *S. haemorrhoidalis* after ingestion of food contaminated with eggs or larvae. Some species prefer oviposition on wounds or nasal passages, but others prefer to do so on the vaginal orifice. The *maggots* can produce *gestrointestinal* or *cutaneous myiasis*. *S. dux* may cause *tissue myiasis*; *S. ruficornis* may be recovered from wounds; *S. fuscicauda* may cause extensive *traumatic myiasis* of the face.

GENUS: WOHLFAHRTIA. These are sarcophaga except that the chequer-board pattern of abdomen gives way to black spotting to most species. Various species cause *myiasis* of the *skin* and sense organs. They are *larviparous* and larvae are capable of penetrating unbroken skin.

FAMILY: HIPOBOSCIDAE

The members of this special group of degenerated flies, called sheep tick or *ked*, is represented by *Melophagus ovinus* (Linn), a wingless species, which feeds on blood of sheep and may be accidentally transferred to the hands of sheep handlers and crawl to the human body. The group is interesting in the sense that, somewhat like *Glossina*, the females retain the larvae till pupation. Melophagus is a proved *vector* of *Rickettsial* and *trypanosomal infection* in sheep.

Myiasis. Various maggots may produce myiasis. Maggots are footless and worm-like. They are segmented and have tapering anterior end. The posterior end is blunt and bears stigmal plates with spiracles. The shape and arrangement of these spiracles in stigmal plates are utilised for tentative identification of the larvae. For this purpose, a thin slice of the posterior end of maggot is removed and examined under a low power microscope for details. At the same time, living maggots are allowed to develop for the stage of pupa and adults on which the identification is based (Fig. 16.8).

Myiasis can be divided into 3 groups, namely: (a) *specific*, (b) *semi-specific* and (c) *accidental myiasis*.

Specific myiasis is produced by maggots, which are obligate parasites of the tissue: whereas, *semispecific myiasis* is produced by the maggots, which are facultative parasites.

Accidental myiasis is produced by the accidental ingestion of eggs or maggots in food or drink or by contamination of wounds. According to the tissue involved, myiasis is *classified as*:

(1) **Cutaneous myiasis.** The maggots burrow into the skin up to the stratum germinativum of the epidermis, where they may survive for months. In other cases, they migrate into the skin in a zigzag fashion, causing *cutaneous larva migrans*, resulting in furuncular swelling with intense itching. Cutaneous myiasis may be: (i) SUPERFICIAL—Caused by *Auchmeromyia luteola*. (ii) TYPICAL. (a) *Non-migratory*: *Cordylobia anthropophaga, Dermatobia hominis*. (b *Migratory*: *Gasterophilus* and *Hypoderma*.

(2) **Gastric myiasis** is due to the presence of the maggots in the stomach, producing nausea and vomiting. The maggots in the vomitus are used for diagnosis and identification.

(3) **Intestinal myiasis** may sometimes produce diarrhoea with passage of maggots in the faeces. *Gastrointestinal myiasis* is caused by Musca, Muscina, Sarcophaga, Fannia, *Pioplila casei*, Tubelera, etc.

(4) **Genito-urinary myiasis** causes dysuria, haematuria and pyuria. Maggots are spontaneously passed through the urinary tract. Genitourinary myiasis may also be migration of psychoda from the alimentary tract or by oviposition in the sexual aperture of *Fannia, Sarcophaga carnaria*.

(5) **Ophthalmic**—*Oestrus ovis, Rhinoestrus purpureus* (*nasalis*).

(6) **Miscellaneous**—*Callitroga americana, Chrysomya bezziana, Callitroga macellaria*, etc.

Traumatic myiasis (Flies attracted by wounds, ulcers and malodorous skin)—Sarcophaga, Wohlfahrtia, *Chrysomya bezziana, Callitroga macellaria*, Phormia, Lucilia, Calliphora, and Stomoxys (rarely).

FAMILY: OSCINIDAE

Eye gnats

The members of this family are minute flies of acalyptrate form, i.e., without axillary basal lobes to the wings; but with short antennae, having spheroidal third segment, an arista, essentially bare, short, dark-coloured, bare wings, and a glistening dark thorax and pale legs. In medically important species, mouth parts are able to minutely cut with fine incisions in granulation tissues or the delicate conjunctival epithelium carrying pathogenic organisms.

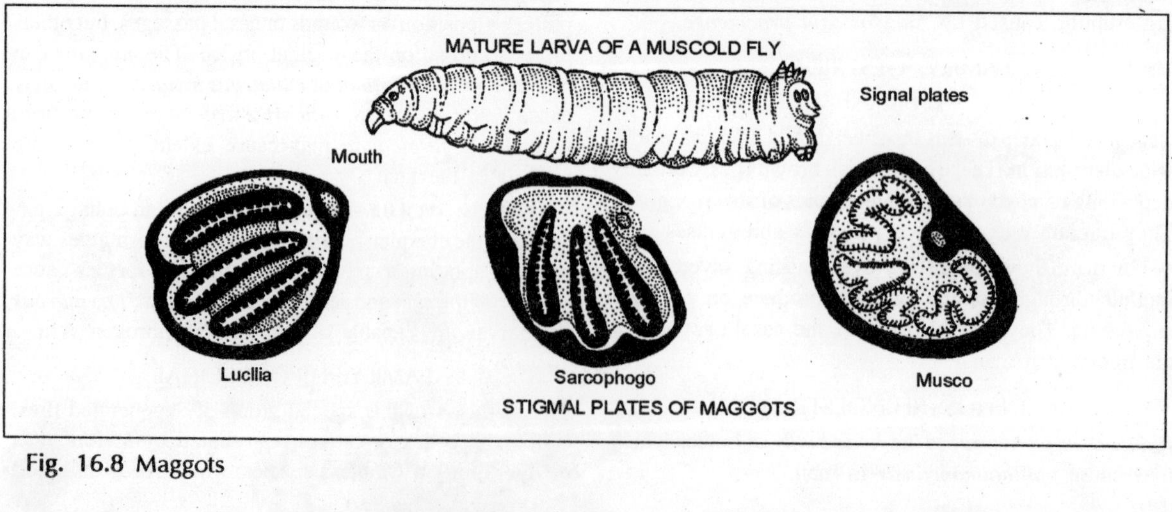

Fig. 16.8 Maggots

They have huge oesophageal diverticulum, and regurgitate blood, serum and exudate, which appear as numerous vomit drops "*fly specks*" within first 2-3 hours after a meal (Kumm, 1935). The life cycle requires 6-14 days. The flies breed in vegetables. urine and faeces.

Medically important species *Oscinis pallipes* feeds on conjunctival exudate (Egypt); *Siphunculina funicola* feeds on lacrymal secretions, exudates of wounds and granulation tissues (Yawn in India). *Hipplelates collulusor* (*syn. pusio*) feeds on blood, open wounds, sore mucous membranes, conjunctivae, and transmits eye infections (California). *Haemophilus* group of bacteria have been isolated from them, which may cause and transmit acute conjunctivitis (Davis and Pillman, 1950). Other species are *H. flavipes* (Texas, Florida, Georgia and Alabame) and *H. pallipes* (West Indies). They also feed on the exudate of domestic animals. They are strongly phototactic. Eye infection is treated successfully with streptomycin.

BITING FLIES

They have rigid chitinised labium, the piercing organ.

Tsetse flies. GENUS: GLOSSINA. These are dark brown or honey brown biting flies and not larger than the house flies. At rest they have their wings folded flat, one directly over the other, like the blades of a pair of scissors. They are characterised by bayonet-like proboscis in front of the head, consisting of a *labium* of *piercing type*. While biting, a hole is rasped into the skin by the pointed tip and the whole proboscis is plunged in. Both males and females are voracious blood suckers and they feed during the daytime.

SPAN OF LIFE is from 4 up to 8 months.

Life cycle. The females pass eggs from the ovary to the uterus, where they hatch out. The larvae are nourished by the milk glands, at the inner end of the uterus, and by oxygen from the atmosphere, and develop further. The posterior spiracle through which the larvae respire, are situated near the external os of the vulva.

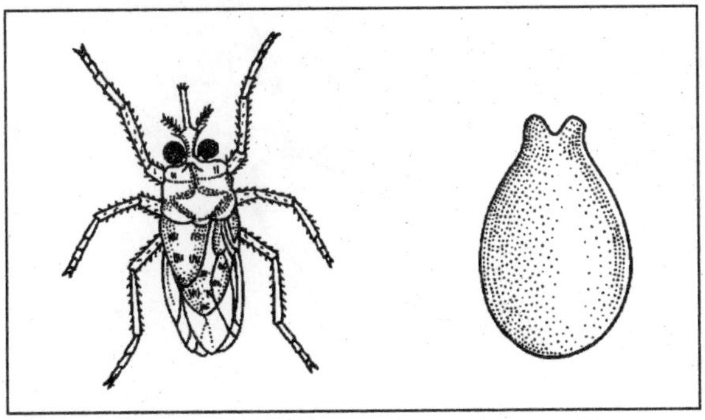

Fig. 16.9 Adult and Puparium of tsetse fly

Only one larva develops at a time and is given birth to every 10-12 days. The larvae are cream-coloured, but the posterior extremity is black. Near about the time of pupation, the larvae are deposited in the soil to a depth of a few centimetres only, and within a few hours pupate there in the shade, not too far from water source (*G. palpalis*). The larvae are identified by their peculiar shape. They have two caudal protruding knobs, on each of which a spiracle is borne.

Glossina are limited to the equatorial regions and transmit African trypanosomiasis (sleeping sickness). There are several species involved in transmitting the disease. *Glossina palpalis* lives along the water courses and near the lakes; it transmits *Trypanosoma gambiense* (Fig. 16.9, see Plate, CH. ZOOMASTIGOPHOREA).

Glossina morsitans prefers to live in the high savannah area and transmits *T. rhodesiense*. Both of them (*G. palpalis* and *G. morsitans*) are important vectors of *T. brucei* of animals also causing *naggna* disease of domestic animals in Africa. *G. tachinoides* and *G. swynnertoni* are of minor importance in transmission of trypanosomiasis. The former restricts itself to human habitations.

GENUS: STOMOXYS

Horse Fly

Stomoxys calcitrans or stable fly is the blood-sucking muscid fly, resembling a house fly. It is a mechanical vector of *T. gambiense, T. rhodesiense* and *T. evansi* (the last one being the causative organism of surra), *L. tropica*, and anthrax, tetanus, tularaemia and poliomyelitis.

ORDER II: SIPHONAPTERA FLEAS

(*Rat fleas transmitting plague belong to this group*)

Several families of fleas are recognised. Siphonaptera are small insects, laterally compressed, wingless, but with strong legs for jumping. Mouth parts are equipped with piercing and sucking mechanisms. Metamorphosis is complete in four stages.

The adults are identified by the following characteristics: (1) number of rows of spines in the abdomen, (2) presence or absence of eyes, and position of ocular bristles; (3) presence or absence of genal or pronotal comb and number of spines in them, (4) number of teeth in each, (5) the shape of the spermatheca, (6) structure of the mesopleuron, and (7) females larger than the males.

The EGGS are white, glistening and oval and about 0.5 ml in size. They are found in cracks of floors, under rugs or in the nests of their hosts.

The LARVAE are small, worm-like without legs and eyes. The body is white but the head is brown. They develop into the pupa stage in about a week. The PUPA is encased into a silken cocoon.

The adult emerges in about a week. The adults are medium to dark brown in colour. They are ectoparasites of mammal and bird. Besides transmitting diseases by their bites, they may produce severe dermatitis. When thirsty, they readily attack any warm-blooded animals.

Fleas act as vectors of plague and endemic (murine) typhus; they act as intermediate hosts of the dog tapeworm, *Dipylidium caninum*. Their bites often cause severe dermatitis in susceptible individuals. Fleas like chigoe or *Tungapenetrans* invade the epidermal tissues and produce dermatitis with secondary infections. Although various animals have fleas peculiar to them, they are not host-specific and, when thirsty and hungry, they may attack any warm-blooded animal. This habit increases their potentialities to transmit diseases to man.

Key to the medically important fleas (see Pl. XXXVII).

Fleas without Combs: Head is angular: *Tunga penetrans* (the *sandflea*); with ocular bristle below the eye: *Pulex irritans* (the *human flea*).

With Pronotal and Genal Combs: Without eyes: Ctenocephalides: *C. canis* (the *dog flea*), *C. felis* (the *cat flea*). With eyes: *Ctenopsyllus segnis* (the *mouse flea*).

Tunga penetrans (Chigoe). It is the *smallest flea* ever known (about 1 mm in length). It is also called sandflea, burrowing flea, the chigoe. Both males and females suck blood. In addition, the females burrow through the skin of mammals and feet of man, and lay eggs there. The wounds caused by them are very painful. Secondary infection may take place, causing tetanus and gas gangrene.

Treatment. The flea is surgically removed by needle and the wound is dressed aseptically.

Tyrophagus castellani. It occurs among copra worker causing *copra itch* in them. It also infests cheese and cereals.

Glycyphagus domesticus (*G. prunorum*) infests sugar, dried prunes and other fruits and may cause *grocer's itch*.

Pulex irritans is also called the human flea. It is cosmopolitan in distribution and found in the skin of man and dog, causing *flea dermatitis*. It may transmit *plague* and *endemic typhus*. It is found in Europe amongst the poorer classes of people, who sleep on the floor of insanitary houses. It is rarely found in rats. This is a wingless small insect, flattened laterally. The three pairs of legs are long and powerful and adapted for hopping.

Eggs. Eggs hatch out as worm-like larvae in 1 week followed by metamorphosis. The latter (larvae) forms cocoons and pupae, which become adult fleas and emerge from the cocoon. The metamorphosis takes about 3 weeks, depending on the temperature. They are found in Europe.

Lesions. The bite of the flea produces irritation causing a central blanching surrounded by a patch of hyperaemia. The older spots are petechial in appearance.

Zenopsylla cheopis is the tropical rat flea, specially found in India and other places; this species is primarily responsible for *transmission of plague* and *murine typhus*.

There is a number of species of Xenopsylla in rats—*X. cheopis, X. astia* and *X. braziliensis*. They are differentiated on the basis of antipygidial bristles and spermathecae, the peculiarities of the latter is shown in *PL. XXXVIII*.

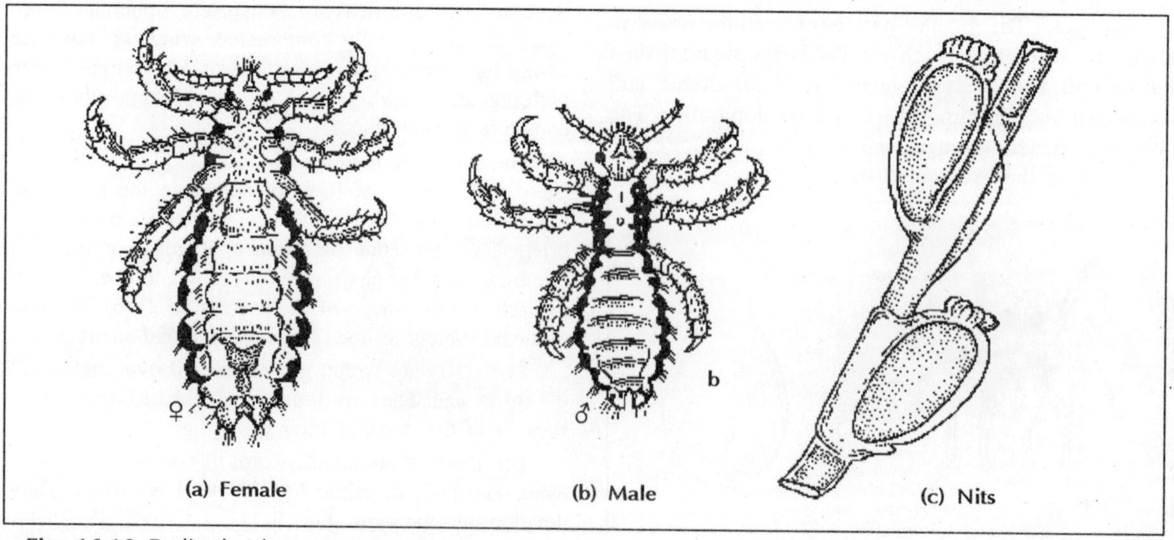

Fig. 16.10 Pediculus humanus capitis

Nosopsyllus fasciatus is the common flea of *Ratus norvegicus* in Europe and United States (brown rats); which attack man. It is a potent *vector* of *plague* and *typhus* fever among rats and mice.

Diamanus montanus and *Hoplopsyllus anomalus* are vector pf plague among wild rodents in California and Western States. They transmit sylvatic plague from squirrel to squirrel and to rats. They do not attack man.

Ctenopsyllus segnis (the *mouse flea*) and *C. felis* (the *cat flea*) readily attack man, and may sometimes transmit plague and endemic typhus in USA. *C. segnis* occasionally attacks man in America and Europe. They transmit plague among rodents.

Control. Fleas in their adult and larval stages are susceptible to DDT. Animals like dogs or cats may be treated with DDT powder. Repeated bathing with 3 percent solution of cresol is efficient. Benzene hexachloride (BHC, gammaxene, etc.) is more effective than any of the above. Benzene hexachloride acts on arthropods as a *contact position*, and as a *fumigant*—it kills them by *paralysis*. The action spray remains effective for shorter time.

ORDER III: ANOPLURA LICE

Pediculi are generally known as lice. They are external parasites of man and are found in various parts of the body, according to which they have been named *Pediculus humanus capitis* (head louse; Fig. 16a, b); *pediculus humanus corporis* (body louse; Fig. 16a, b); *Phthirus pubis* (crab louse; Fig. 16c).

Pediculi are wingless insects, flattened dorsiventrally with a pear-shaped head, a proboscis and two joined antennae, and a pair of compound eyes behind the antennae. They have three pairs of legs, each ending in claws. They are blood-sucker of mammals. They are 2-3 mm in length. The males are half to two-thirds the size of the females. The metamorphosis is incomplete.

Ova or *nits* are corn-shaped with a chitinous envelope. They are operculated (Fig. 16c). The operculum opens at the time of hatching of larva and the young louse emerges through it. Nits are deposited on hair or clothing, attached by a gelatinous substance derived from the genital opening at the time of laying eggs.

The eggs hatch out in 5 to 7 days without any metamorphosis. The larvae mould three times and become adults in about a week.

Phthirus pubis (crab louse). They look like a crab. They are 1-2 mm in length and nearly as broad as long. Head is impacted on the thorax. The first pair of legs is extremely slender. Antennae are prominent. Thorax carries three pairs of legs.

TABLE 16.1

DIFFERENCES BETWEEN *PEDICULUS CAPITIS* AND *PEDICULUS* CORPORIS

Pediculus humanus capitis	*Pediculus humanus corporis*
SIZE—Smaller	Larger
BODY—Deeply pigmented	Pigmentation absent
ABDOMINAL SEGMENTS—Marked indentations between successive segments	Rounded, with shallow indentations
ANTENNAE—Short and broad	Long and slender
LEGS—Shorter and stouter	Relatively slender and longer

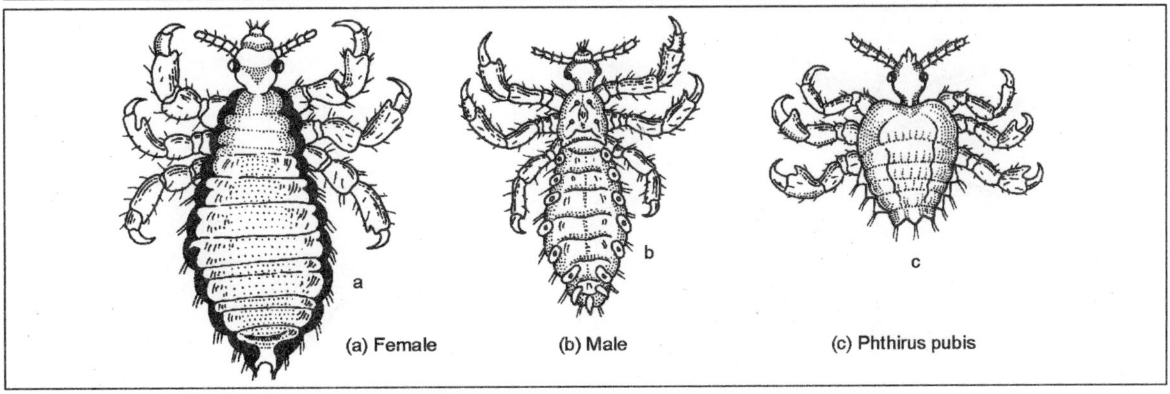

Fig. 16.11 Pediculus humanus corporis

DISEASES TRANSMITTED BY LICE

Body lice and less commonly head lice are responsible for transmission of *R. prowazeki*, the causative organism of epidemic typhus. They are infective in 7 to 11 days after feeding on a typhus patient. The infection is carried by rubbing of the excreta on any abrasion of the body. Relapsing fever in India caused by *Borrelia recurrentis* is transmitted by the louse, which is infective after the 6th day of the feed and remains so all through its life. The infection is carried by crushing of the louse on abraded skin. Body lice also produce diseases characterised by excoriation and pigmentation of the skin at the sites of bite (*Vagabond's disease*).

Control of lice. DDT is effective and can be used exclusively for the control of vectors of epidemic typhus. 10 percent DDT dust may be used for the inner surface of the clothing, worn next to skin. Methyl bromide is effective against nits and may be used as a fumigant for clothing and bedding. Clean habits, frequent bathing, and change of clothes and undergarments assist in control.

ORDER IV: HEMIPTERA

(Heterroptera—True bugs)

The members of this order are characterised by the hinged (3-4 joined) proboscis under the head and thorax, when in repose. Adults have two pair of wings and these are rudimentary in some genera. They live on plants and many are adapted for aquatic life. Only a few are blood suckers.

FAMILY: CIMICIDAE

Cimex lectularius (bed-bug of Northern latitude; (Fig. 16.12a), *Cimex hemipteras* (*C. rotundatus*) in the tropics (Fig. 16.12b).

Bed-bugs were suspected to be vectors of many diseases but there is no conclusive evidence of transmission of any disease by these insects. The adult is 5 mm by 3 mm with a flattened body. The proboscis is flexed. The female deposits about 50 eggs at a time and under favourable conditions, young ones emerge in about 10 days. Four generations may develop in a year.

Control. A 5% DDT spray is effective in the control of bed-bug menace in the house or in the public vehicles.

FAMILY: REDUVIDAE

(Cone-nosed bugs)

Panstrongylus (*Triatoma*) *megistus* is the intermediate host of *Trypanosoma cruzi*, which causes *Chagas' disease* in Brazil (Fig. 16.13).

SYNONYMS. Cone-nosed bugs; Assassin bugs; Kissing bugs. Most of the species of this family are predaceous and feed on other insects, but some species are plant feeders. Some are dependent on wild animals for their meals; whereas certain species are adopted to human habitation and act as important vectors of *Trypanosoma cruzi* producing *Chagas' disease*.

Panstrongylus (*Triatoma*) *megistus* are found in Brazil, and *P. geniculatus* in Panama; they occur throughout Central America. There are some 26 species of blood-sucking reduviids. They are characterised by segmented proboscis arising from the anterior portion of the elongated head. The proboscis is flexed below the head and thorax. The head is elongated and cone-shaped, and hence the name. Larvae emerge from the eggs and resemble the adult stage with wings.

Habitats and Habits. etc. CONE-nosed bugs live in cracks and crevices of mud walls. They can fly for a considerable distance in the house. Both sexes bite. They are nocturnal in their habits and hide in daytime. The bite of some Triatoma species is painless and the victim is not awakened, but others may produce painful wounds by introducing a salivary toxin. The blood meal can be continued for half an hour at the end of which a small amount of liquid faeces is deposited on the skin near the

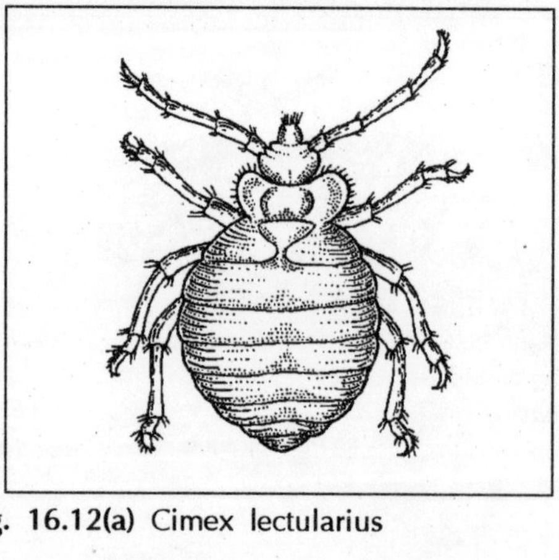

Fig. 16.12(a) Cimex lectularius

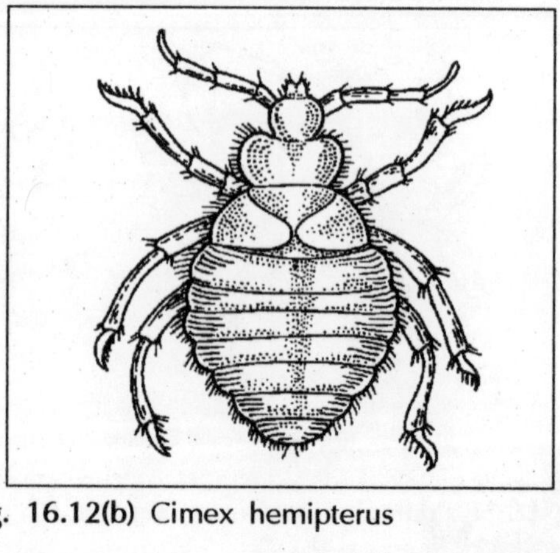

Fig. 16.12(b) Cimex hemipterus

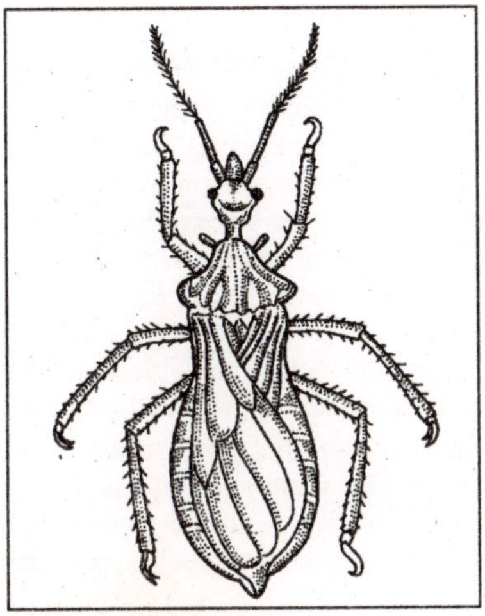

Fig. 16.13 Reduviid bug

punctured wound made by the bite. The pathogenic organism *T. cruzi* present in the faeces is then readily rubbed into the wound and thereby produce *Chagas' disease*.

Control. It is difficult to eradicate Triatoma from the environment. DDT is not very effective, but benzene hexachloride is an effective insecticide. It is applied as a dusting powder in beds, or cracks and holes of the wall, and to other possible hiding places.

Less important orders of the class insecta are:

ORDER V: Orthoptera—*Cockroaches*

ORDER VI: Coleoptera—*Beetles*

ORDER VII: Lepidoptera—*Butterflies*

ORDER VIII: Hymenoptera—*Bees* and *ants*.

CLASS II: ARACHNIDA

The members of this group have 4 pairs of legs. They are divided into 3 orders:

ORDER I: *Scorpionida* (*True scorpions*). The head and thorax are fused to form cephalothorax. The tail consists of terminal, flexible abdominal segments and is differentiated into 4 poison organs ending in a hollow stinger-spine, e.g., scorpion.

ORDER II: Araneida (*Spiders*). The head and thorax are fused to form cephalothorax. The abdominal segments are separate, e.g., *spider*, "black-widow" spider, tarantula.

ORDER III: Acarina (*Ticks* and *Mites*). All the segments are fused into a single sac, e.g., tick, mite.

ORDER I: SCROPIONIDA

The scorpions are terrestrial animals and during the daytime they hide in dark places. They are found under stones, leaves, bark of trees, splinters of weed and in the axils of coconut and banana trees. During the rainy season they enter houses to hide in beds, shoes and undisturbed hidden places including clothing.

Scorpions have formidable claws (*pedipalps*) with which they seize their prey. The last abdominal segment terminates in a ventrally curved spine, carrying the poison gland. The sting curves downwards, when the tail-like post-abdomen is extended. The victim is wounded quickly and repeatedly by a sharp downward movement of the spine. The scorpions of temperate climate are small, but those in the tropics may attain a length as much as 18 cm. The more venomius species of many scorpions may cause severe systemic reactions, like those of *cobra poisoning*. The dose injected may not be fatal for an adult, but for a child it may be fatal. The patient often dies of cardiac or respiratory failure with *pulmonary oedema* within a few hours after the sting. The venom is a *neurotoxin* (like *toxalbumin* of *cobra*), which acts *peripherally*. Also, the toxin contains a *formic acid*–like substance. When the systemic dissemination occurs, there is profuse sweating, salivation, vomiting, myoclonic twitching and abdominal pain occurs indicating a specific treatment with *antivenin* of scorpion venom.

Treatment. In one word, the treatment is same as that of cobra venom. Immediately after the scorpion sting, a tourniquet is applied proximal to the site of sting to prevent dissemination. The wound is incised, and venom removed by suction and oxidised by introduction of crystals of *potasium permanganate*. The pain is relieved by the local application of a drop of strong ammonia. Infiltration of *novocaine* (2 percent) solution with adrenaline close to the puncture wound combats pain.

In case of systemic dissemination, as judged by the poisoning symptoms mentioned before specific antivenin therapy is indicated. General measures consist of combating shock. ACTH and *cortisone* have been reported to be useful.

Control. It consists of spraying of 10 percent DDT and 0.2 percent *pyrethrum* in kerosine. *Odourless spray base* has been successfully used in the control of scorpions.

Suphur fumigation destroys them in houses.

ORDER II: ARANEIDA

Spiders

Spiders have a distinct cephalothorax, bearing 2 chelicerae and 2 six-segmented leg, like *pedipalps*. The abdomen is soft, rounded, unsegmented and connected to the *cephalothorax* by means of a narrow *pedicel*. The legs have seven segments and the tarsi bear two or three claws. The modified *pedipalps* of the males serve to transfer spermatozoa at the time of mating. Three or four spinnerets are situated near the tip of the abdomen on the ventral aspect for the production of *spiders' silk*. The *female* is larger than the *male*.

There are more than 30 families in the order Araneida. Most spiders are harmless and their bites may produce a local redness. The bite of large, hairy *tarantula*, the *banana spider*, is sometimes painful but without any serious results. The *black widow spider, Latrodectus mactans* of the family *Therididae*, are poisonous. The female black widow, *L. mactans*, is coal black with orange-red hour glass spots and found in USA. The venom produces *arachnidism*. This occurs due to the bite of a female, which injects venom, in defence, into the attacker. The venom is a *non-haemolytic neurotoxin*, more powerful than that of *rattle snake*. The bite is not felt, or felt as a pin prick. The venom by the vascular or lymphatic absorption produces symptoms within a few minutes. These are cramping pain in the abdomen, legs and chest. The muscles are contracted and the board-like rigidity of abdomen is like that of an acute abdomen. The temperature and blood pressure are raised. The pressure of the CSF is raised and leucocyte count is high. The acute symptoms last for a day, but residual tingling of the feet may last longer. Death is recorded in about 4 percent of the victims in 18 to 36 hours. One attack leaves some immunity to combat systemic reactions for a second attack.

The term "tarantula" is applied loosely to the bite of a large spider in man by *Lycosa tarantula* in Europe (FAMILY: LYCOSIDAE). The bite, however, is not serious. The Russian tarantula, *Trochosa singoriensis* is much feared, without much foundation.

Control. Spray of ten percent DDT in kerosene is lethal to the spiders.

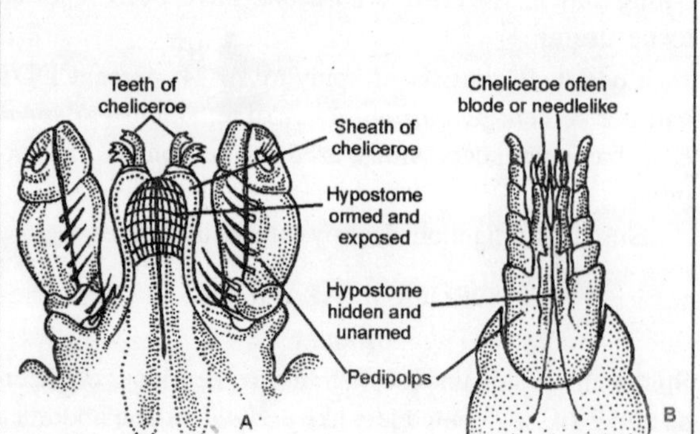

Fig. 16.14 Mouth parts of (a) ticks and (b) mites

ORDER III: ACARINA

Ticks and Mites

The members of this order include *ticks* and *mites*. These are characterised by fusion of all segments into a single sac. Most of the acarids are round or oval, compressed dorsiventrally and may be covered with a chitinous shield or scutum; wings and antennae are absent. Head and thorax are fused together to form *cephalothorax*. The front part may form a distinct false head, the *capitulum*. Head, bearing the mouth parts, is collectively called *rostrum* or back which is projected while biting.

The members of this order undergo wellmarked metamorphosis. The adults and nymphs possess four pairs of walking legs, while the larvae have only three pairs. Wings and antennae are absent, eyes may or may not be present.

The *ticks* are large and mostly macroscopic. The body is sclerotised or leathery in appearance. Hairs are absent; but if present, they are short. The false head, i.e., capitulum or rostrum, bears the *hypostome*. The hypostome is exposed and armed with strong cutting teeth. They *palpi* are pointed.

The *mites* are small, often microscopic; the body is membranous in appearance and often covered with long hairs. The hypostome is hidden and armed. The palpi never have more than 5 segments, the last segment being provided with sensory hairs.

Life cycle. It includes *eggs, larvae, nymph* and *adults*—and the life cycle is completed in two years.

EGGS. Eggs are deposited on earth in batches of several thousands. After a period of 2 weeks to several months, the larvae hatch out.

LARVAE. They have only six legs; they are smaller than adults. They crawl about and suck blood from rodents. After the blood meal, they drop off to the ground, shed their skin, and, finally, they emerge as nymphs.

TABLE 16.2
DIFFERENCES BETWEEN TICKS AND MITES

Ticks	Mites
1. Size: Large, macroscopic	Small, microscopic
2. Body: With short or no hairs	With long hairs
3. Hypostomer: With numerous exposed teeth	Hidden, unarmed

NYMPHS. They are 8 legged and similar to adults, but they are sexually immature and hibernate without food. The following year, they suck blood from rodents, drop off to the ground, and transform into adults.

TICKS

A wide variety of pathogenic organisms, namely, spirochaetes, viruses, rickettsiae, bacteria and toxins of unknown nature are transmitted by ticks.

Morphology. Ticks differ from other Arachnida and Insecta by the absence of body segmentation lacking of head, with the exception of some adult mites. There is a strong fusion of the thorax and abdomen with no external sign of demarcation. Wings and antennae are absent. As in spider and scorpions, the adults have 4 pairs of legs, but larvae have 3 pairs. Ticks belong to 2 major groups: FAMILY I. IXODIDAE, and FAMILY II. ARGASIDAE.

Ticks are further characterised by their peculiar mouth parts as follows: a pair of dorsal cutting organs, the *chelicerae*, a ventral characteristically toothed *hypostome* for anchoring itself to the host and paired *pedipalps*, lateral to the mouth. The mouth consists of a chitinous ring, lying at the base of but between chelicerae and the hypostome.

IXODIDAE (HARD TICK) is differentiated from AGRGASIDAE (SOFT TICK) on the basis of SCUTUM which is lacking in the latter. In Ixodidae *females* the scutum covers only the anterior part of the dorsal surface, but in *male* it almost fully covers the dorsum. The 2 groups are further differentiated by (a) *ventral* mouth parts, (b) *slight sexual dimorphism* in mouth parts project in front, when viewed from the *dorsal* aspect, and they show *marked sexual dimorphism*.

FAMILY: IXODIDAE
Hard ticks

The family consists of 10 genera, of which some are of special importance; namely, Dermacentor, Amblyomma, Haemaphysalis and Rhipicephalus.

Dermacentor andersoni (WOOD TICK) is the Rocky Mountain spotted fever tick (Fig. 16.15). The larvae and nymphs feed on rodents and rabbits and the adults feed on larger mammals, e.g., horses, cattle and man. They are known to transmit Rocky Mountain spotted fever, tularaemia, Colorado tick fever, Q fever and encephalomyelitis. Their bites also cause tick paralysis. If they are not removed promptly, the death of the patient takes place from paralysis of the respiratory system.

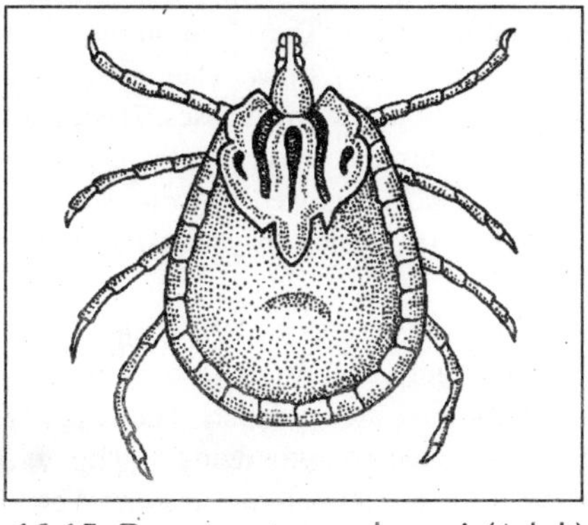

Fig. 16.15 Dermacentor andersoni (Adult)

Dermacentor variabilis (The AMERICAN DOG TICK) occurs in States east of Rocky Mountain. The larvae and nymphs feed on mice and cotton-tail. The adults feed on dogs and men. They transmit EASTERN SPOTTED FEVER, TULARAEMIA, ST. LOUIS ENCEPHALITIS and also cause *tick paralysis*.

Dermacentor occidentalis, The *Pacific Coast ticks* are found in California and Oregon. They feed on a variety of hosts and transmit *spotted fever, Q. fever* and *tularaemia. D. silvarum* and *Haemaphysalis concinna* cause Siberian *tick typhus*.

Amblyomma americana (The *Lone Star tick*) is found in Central Texas and South America. They have wide range of hosts, and larvae, nymphs and adults bite man. Their bites are painful. They transmit *Rocky Mountain spotted fever, Q. fever, tularaemia* and *Bullis fever* in Texas.

Amblyomma cajennense occurs in Texas, Central and South America. The bite is painful. It is a vector of *Sao Paulo* fever in Brazil.

Amblyomma hebraenum (the *brown dog tick*) has a cosmopolitan distribution. The principal host is the dog, but they bite other animals and man. They transmit *Mediterranean spotted fever (fievre boutonneuse), Indian tick typhus*, and *Q fever* in Australia caused by *Coxiella burnetii*.

Ixodes species bite man readily, the bite is painful. They transmit Russian spring-summer encephalitis, louping ill in sheep and Q. fever. They cause tick paralysis in Australia.

Ixodes persiculatus is a vector and *reservoir* of *forest-spring encephalitis* in Ural and Siberian regions.

FAMILY: ARGASIDAE
Soft ticks

These ticks are similar to bed bugs in their habits, and inhabit cracks of floor and suck blood at night. Their bites produce red, *painful wheals*.

There are several species belonging to the genus Ornithodorus, which transmit relapsing fever.

Ornithodorus moubata (Fig. 16a, b). It is the important vector of *tick relapsing fever* of *Africa*, and probably also *perstans filariasis*.

Both adults and nymphs transmit the infection caused by *Borrelia duttoni*. They infest huts and hide during the day time in cracks of walls and floors, and move about at night in search of food. They attack men and animals.

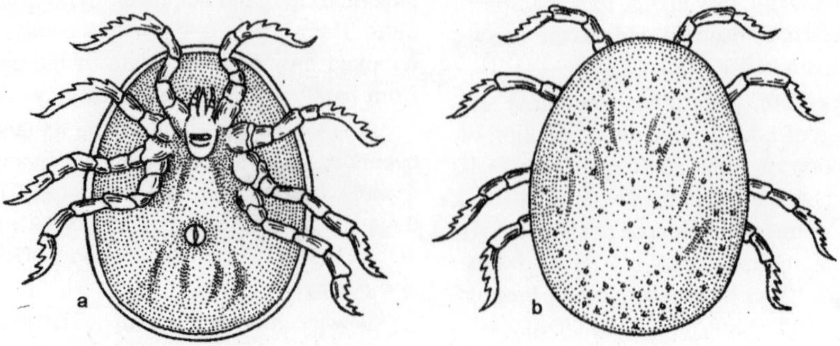

(a) Ventral view (b) Dorsal view

Fig. 16.16 Ornithodorus moubata

MITES

There are species of 3 families of medical importance:

1. FAMILY: Trombiculidae, e.g., *Trombicula irritans, T. akamyshi* (Fig. 16.17), and *T. deliensis.*
2. FAMILY: Demodecidae, e.g., *Demodex folliculorum* (Fig. 16.18).
3. FAMILY: Sarcoptidae, e.g., *Sarcoptes scabei* (itch mite) causing scabies.

FAMILY: TROMBICULIDAE

They are *Trombicula irritans*; *T. ǎkamushi* (Fig. 16.17) and *T. deliensis*.

Trombiculae in the larval stage transmit *scrub tuphus, Japan river-fever,* etc. *D. folliculorum* causes inflammation of hair follicles.

TROMBICULA IRRITANS

(The *chigger* or *red bugs*)

Chigger mites are distinct from other mites parasitic on vertebrates in the way that only the larvae are parasitic, as the nymphal and adult stages are spent outside, feeding on insect eggs and other minute arthropods. These are common in United States. The adult has 8 legs and is found on grass and bushes, specially blackberry. They feed on vegetable matters without attacking man. The larvae, which have 6 legs, suck lymph and tissue fluids from the subcutaneous layers of the rodents, birds and man. They do not burrow, but attach themselves to the skin injecting an irritant secretion, which causes severe itching for several days. The engorged larvae drop off to the ground and are scratched off within a day or two when the itching begins. The larvae are identified by 3 pairs of legs and oblong scutum with 7 hairs.

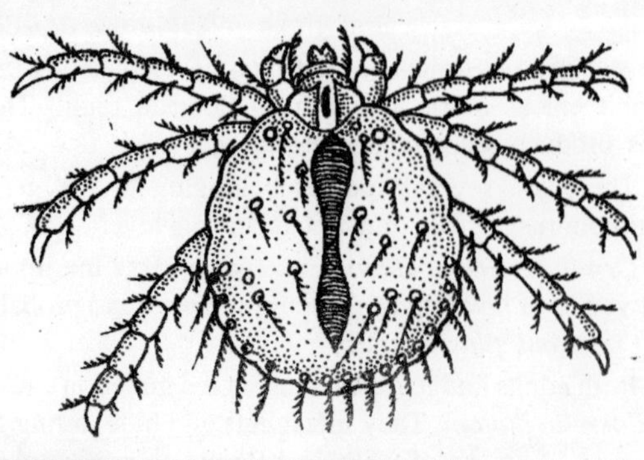

Fig. 16.17 Trombicula akamushi (Larva)

TROMBICULA AKAMUSHI

Trombicula akamushi (Fig. 16.17) are found in Japan, and *Trombicula deliensis* in Sumatra and India. They are so similar that *T. deliensis* is considered to be a variety of *T. akamushi.* Trombiculae in their larval stage transmit *Rickettsia orientalis* (tsutsugamushi), the causative organism of *Japan-river fever*, etc., and *T. deliensis* transmit the rickettsia of scrub typhus in Sumatra and India.

Pyemotes (pediculoides) ventricosus are the North American grain itch mites. They feed on insect larvae of wheat and other grains, or straw. They attack man, specially those sleeping on straw mattresses. The mites burrow through the epidermis and produce petechiae and erythema at the site of attack, followed by formation of wheals, vesicles and pustules, which may occur over the entire body.

The *CHEESE MITES, GRAIN MITES*, etc. These mites are seen in dried fruits, cheese, sugars and bulbs, and can infect man in handling such products. They migrate under the scales of the epidermis producing a itchy dermatitis. Faeces of these mites also produce itching. When ingested with cheese, they pass through the intestine without

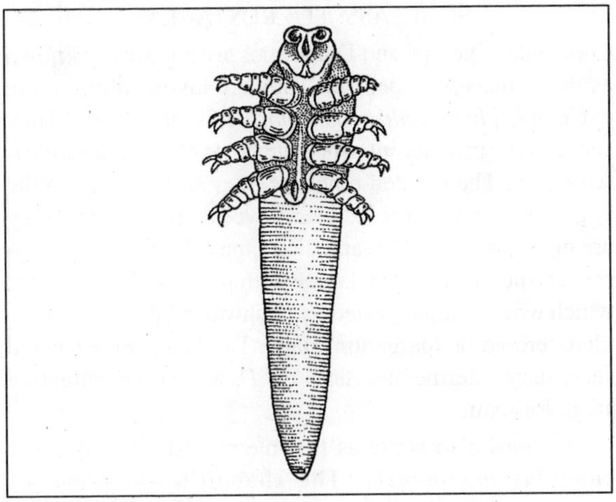

Fig. 16.18 Demodex folliculorum

causing any harm, and can be recovered from the faeces. Inhalation of these mites may cause pneumonitis with infiltration of eosinophils. This is known as *acariasis* or *acarinosis*.

Acarus siro occurs among the vanilla workers, producing a kind of dermatitis called vanillism. It may infest cheeses as well.

FAMILY: DEMODECIDAE

DEMODEX FOLLICULORUM

(Hair follicle mite)

This is a sebaceous gland mite of men, especially affecting the face, side of the nose and forehead. It occasionally causes fatal disease in dogs.

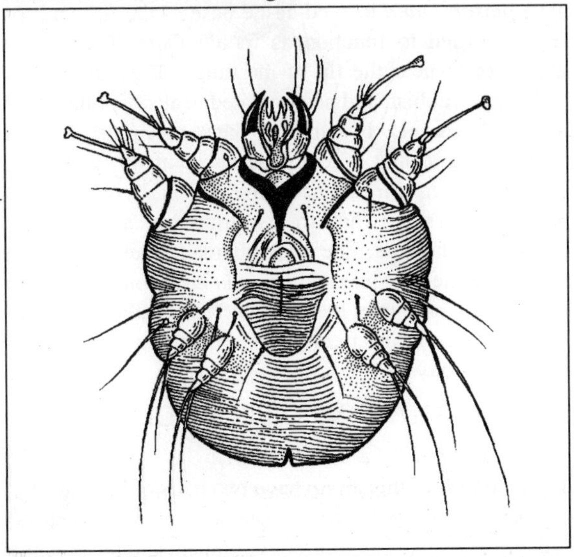

Fig. 16.19 Female *Sarcoptes scabei* (ventral view)

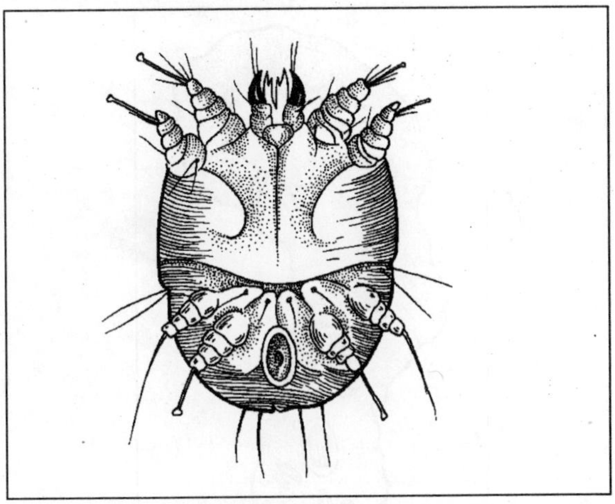

Fig. 16.20 Male *Sarcoptes scabei* (ventral view)

The mite is 0.3 to 0.4 mm in length and 0.04 to 0.05 mm in breadth (Fig. 16.18). It has an elongated worm-like appearance with four pairs of legs placed on the anterior part of the body close to one another. The legs terminate in claws.

Pathogenicity. The mites live in acne, comedones, hair follicles and sebaceous glands without causing any inconvenience to the patient.

Diagnosis. Squeeze out the contents of the black head or sebaceous gland and examine under the microscope.

FAMILY: SARCOPTIDAE

SARCOPTES SCABEI

(ITCH-MITE)

Sarcoptes scabei causes *scabies* or itch in the human being. It is generally found in school children who contact the disease from their mates. These mites are minute and microscopic (seen by hand lens).

The adult has four pairs of legs, two in front and two behind. The front legs are provided with *terminal suckers* in both sexes. In the *females*, third and fourth pair of legs possess bristles (Fig. 16.19), whereas the fourth pair of legs in the *male* possess suckers, instead of bristles (Fig. 16.20). The *females* lives in a burrow in the horny layer of the delicate skin of the body, specially *webs of the fingers, thigh, ear*, and reaches up to *rete mucosum* and causes itch.

The *male* is 0.25 mm by 0.15 mm and *female* is 0.44 mm by 0.3 mm. The *female* acarus, after impregnation, burrows and dies after copulation. As she cannot turn round and come out of the burrow, she becomes pregnant after copulation (Fig. 16.21). She deposits eggs, one or two daily for about two months when undisturbed, and then dies at the distal end of the burrow (Fig. 16.21).

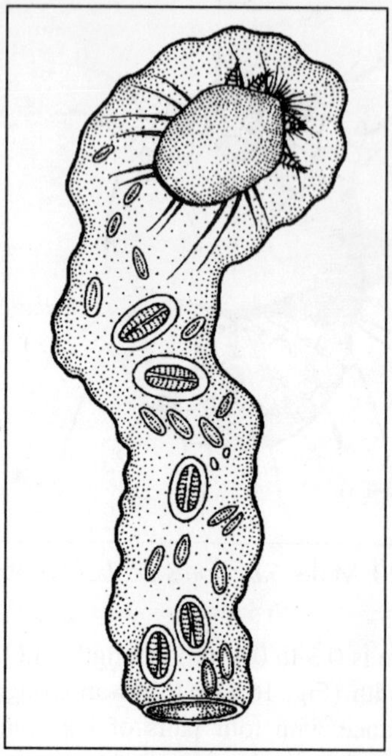

Fig. 16.21 Female *Sarcoptes scabei* in the burrow depositing eggs

The eggs are pushed on the surface by the exfoliation of the skin. The development of larvae in the eggs require 4 to 7 days, when the larvae come out of the burrow and cast off their skin 3 to 4 times. They become sexually mature in a fortnight.

Pathogenicity. They cause severe itch and irritation on the affected parts, e.g., webs of the fingers, abdomen, thighs, buttocks and genital parts.

Due to injury to the skin surface, secondary streptococcal infection takes place. This is known as impetigo. Infants may show allergic dermatitis after an infection caused by itch-mite.

Prophylaxis. The disease is contagious and is generally transmitted from one infected person to another from his bed and clothing. Ever repeated infections in the same individual may take place from infected clothes, which should be properly boiled or disinfected.

Treatment. Local application of 25 percent benzyl benzoate is specific.

CLASS III: CRUSTACEA

(Water fleas, cray fish, lobsters and crabs)

These are aquatic animals with true gills, 2 pairs of antennae, and at least 5 pairs of legs. They have cephalothorax and abdominal segments. Crustaceans are divided into two forms: the small forms are called copepods, and the larger forms crabs and cray fish.

SUBCLASS: EUCRUSTACEA

Copepoda. Cyclops and Diaptomus are commonly known as water fleas or copepods. They are involved in the life cycle of *Diphyllobothrium larum*, the fish tapeworm. They serve as the primary intermediate hosts of *Diphyllobothrium latum*. The ciliated embryos after emerging from the egg remain in water for at least 2 weeks. By this time they are ingested by cyclops and diaptomus. They develop into procercoid or first stage larvae within the crustacean host, which when being ingested by freshwater fish develop into plerocercoid or sparganum stage. The latter serves as the secondary intermediate host for *D. larum*, the infective stage for man.

Cyclops also serve as the intermediate host of *Dracunculus medinensis*. The rhabditiform larvae of *D. medinensis*, liberated in fresh water from an ulcer, infect cyclops. The larvae develop into infective stage within the cyclops, and man or animal is infected by ingestion of infected cyclops.

Crabs and cray fish. Some species of crabs and cray fish act as secondary intermediate hosts of *Paragonimus westermani*. The cercariae of the flukes—when liberated from the snails (the primary intermediate host)—invades crabs or crayfish and form metacercariae, which are infective to man, when ingested.

CLASS IV: CHILOPODA

Centipedes

The members of this group have one pair of legs on each of the 20 segments (approximately). Centipedes are elongated, flattened arthropods with one pair of legs, arising from each segment of the body. Wings are absent. They have *poison gland* located at the base of the first pair of legs modified to function as mouth parts. The poison glands open near the tip of the fangs. They live under bark, logs, rubbish and accumulated heaps of splinters of wood, stones, etc. In handling these materials, there is chance of grasping a centipede accidentally. In such a case, it bites in self-defence, emit poison, by which they paralyse their prey. They are nocturnal in habit, and rarely bite during daytime. The bites of small, house centipede can pierce the skin leaving *two puncture wounds* and can give rise to more than local symptoms. The large species in the tropics inflict painful bites resulting in disability for several days.

CLASS V: DIPLOPODA

Millipedes

The members of this group have two pairs of legs on each segment except the first four. The body is round in cross-section. They live in a moist environment and feed mainly on decaying vegetable matter. They are incapable of biting or stinging. A large number of species spray a fluid from *special glands* in the body, which may produce dermatitis upon contact with the skin, or mucous membrane. According to the injurious effects of the secretions, millipedes are classified into two categories; those causing (1) caustic action on the skin as a result of contact with millipedes, and (2) injury to eyes by squirting fluid from the segmental secretion. □

REFERENCES

Davis, D. J. and Pittman, M. (1950). Acute conjunctivitis in the South. *Common. Dis. Center*, U.S. Pub. Hlth. Ser. Bull., Apr. 1950, pp. 18-19.

Kumm, H. H. W. (1935). The digestive mechamism of one of the West Indian "eye gnats" *Hippelates pallipes Loew. Ann. Trop. Med. Parasitol.* 29. 283-298.

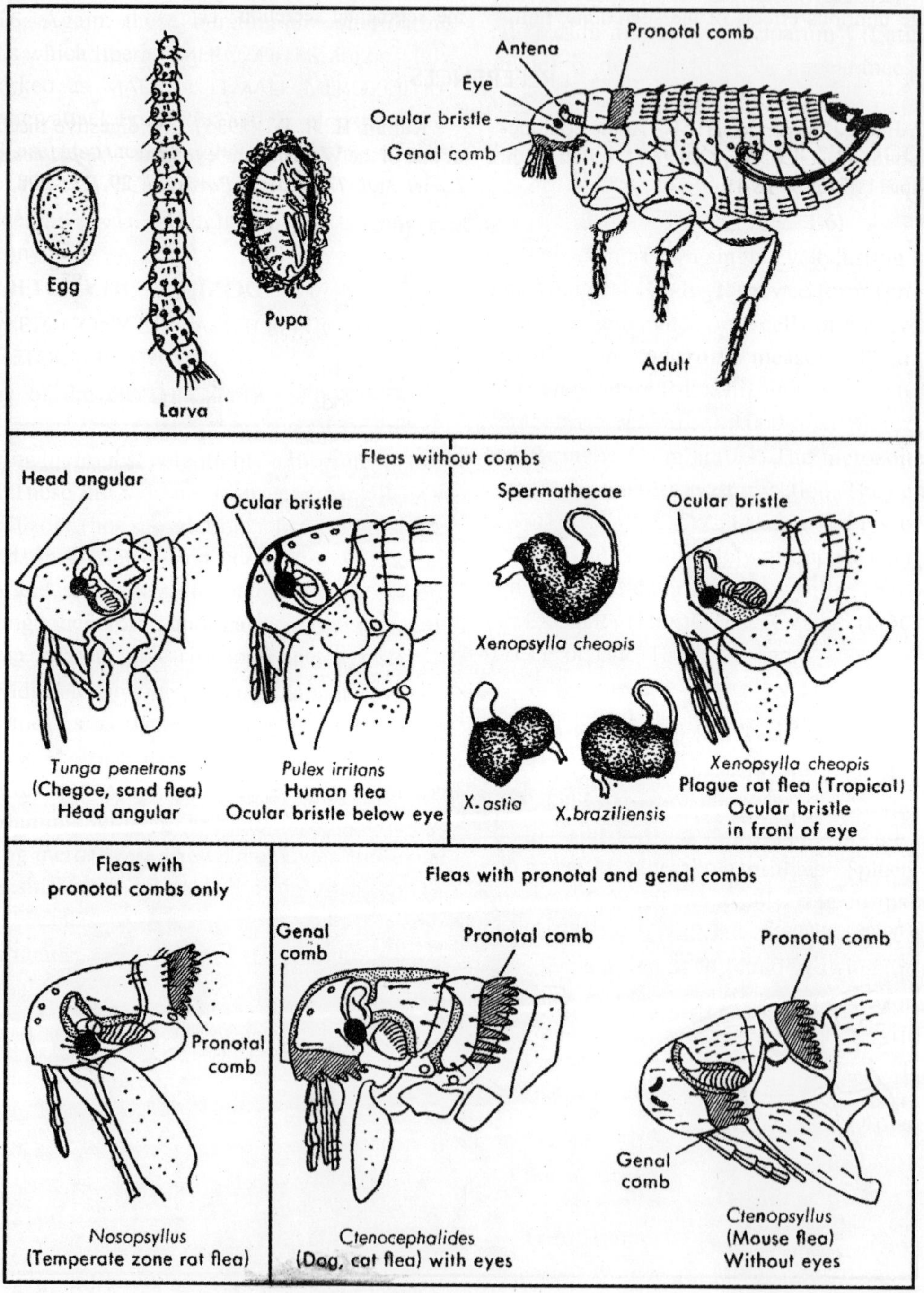
Pronotal comb
Antena
Eye
Ocular bristle
Genal comb
Egg
Pupa
Larva
Adult
Fleas without combs
Head angular
Ocular bristle
Spermathecae
Ocular bristle
Xenopsylla cheopis
Tunga penetrans
(Chegoe, sand flea)
Head angular
Pulex irritans
Human flea
Ocular bristle below eye
X. astia
X. braziliensis
Xenopsylla cheopis
Plague rat flea (Tropical)
Ocular bristle
in front of eye
Fleas with
pronotal combs only
Fleas with pronotal and genal combs
Genal
comb
Pronotal comb
Pronotal comb
Pronotal
comb
Genal
comb
Nosopsyllus
(Temperate zone rat flea)
Ctenocephalides
(Dog, cat flea) with eyes
Ctenopsyllus
(Mouse flea)
Without eyes

CHAPTER

17

PHYLUM: MOLLUSCA

MOLLUSCS

Mollusca (*Latin*; *Mollusca*—a nut with a thin shell). This is a phylum belonging to Metazoa with soft, unsegmented bodies, consisting of an anterior head, a ventral foot and a dorsal visceral mass. Most forms are enclosed in a protective calcareous shell. The Phylum Mollusca includes the classes:

1. Gastropoda (snails, whelks, slugs and limpets);
2. Pelecypoda (Lamellibranchia—oysters, clams, mussels);
3. Cephalopoda (squids, octopi);
4. Amphineura (Loricata—chitons);
5. Scaphopoda (tusk shells).

We are concerned here with the snails belonging to the class Gastropoda, the snails, which serve as intermediate hosts for many trematodes (Flukes). Human diseases carried by molluscs are shown in Table 17.1 and Pl. I. □

TABLE 17.1

MOLLUSCS ACTING AS INTERMEDIATE HOSTS OF TREMATODES (PL. I)

Flukes	First intermediate snail host	Mollusca Family	Geographical distribution	Secondary intermediate host
Schistosoma haematobium	*Bulinus trun*	Bulinidae	Northern Africa	—
	Bulinus africanus		Southern and Western part of Africa, Mauritius	—
	Bulinus forskali			
S. japonicum	Onchomelania quadrasi	Hydrobiidae	Philippine Islands	
	Onchomelania formosana		Formosa	—
	Onchomelania nosphora		China and Japan	—
	Onchomelania hupensis		China	
S. mansoni	Biomphalaria alexandrina	Planorbidae	Northern Africa	—
	B. pfeifferi		Southern Africa	
	Australorbis glabratus		South America and West Indies	
Fasciola hepatica	Lymnaea auricularis	Lymnaeidae	North Asia, Europe	Encystment on grass and herbs (Metacercariae)
	Lymnaea ollula		Asia, Hawaii	
	Lymnaea rubella		Hawaii	
	Lymnaea bulimoides		USA	
Fasciolopsis buski	Segmentina hemisphaerula	Planorbidae	Eastern Asia	Encystment on waterplants
	Hippeutis cantori		Eastern Asia	
Clonorchis sinensis	Hua ningpoensis	Thiaridae	China	Fresh-water cyprinoid fishes
	Bulimus fuchsianus	Hydrobiidae	China	
	Alocinma longicornis	Hydrobiidae	China and India	
	Parafossarulus manchouricus	Hydrobiidae	China and Japan	
	Parafossarulus sinensis		China and Japan	
Metagonimus yokogawai	Semisulcospira libertina	Thiaridae	Northern China, Japan,	Salmon and cyprinoid fishes
	Thiara granifera		S.E. Asia to Hawaii	
Paragonimus westermani	Semisulcospira libertina	Thiaridae	Northern China, Japan	Fresh water crabs: cray fish
	Semisulcospira amurensis		Northern China, Korea	
	Thiara granifera		Formosa to Hawaii	

Appendix I

EXAMINATION OF BLOOD FOR PARASITES

Preparation of Blood Films. (Fig. Ap. 1). Blood films used for detection of malarial parasites are: (a) Thin film. (b) Thick film. (c) Thin and thick film.

Thin Film. This is prepared by pricking the finger with a sterilised needle. The finger is previously sterilised with a swab of ether-alcohol. A drop of blood is taken ½ inch (1.2 cm) away from one end on a clean grease-free slide. Invert the slide and place it on a white paper. Put the spreader on the side of the film to be drawn, touch the drop and when blood spreads uniformly to the edge of the spreader, hold the spreader at an angle of about 45° and draw a film by moving the spreader along the surface of the slide, so that blood follows the spreader (Fig. Ap. 1; 1-4). If the angle between the slide and the spreader is more, the film becomes thicker. Dry the film by waving in air.

Thin and Thick Film. (Sinton's method, 1925). This is specially useful in survey work. In this a thin film spreads on two-thirds of the slide and a thick film on one end. A transverse line is drawn with a grease pencil between the two films (Fig. Ap. I, 7, 8a, 8b).

CRITERIA OF A GOOD FILM. 1. The film should be uniform and even. The tail-end should be gradually thin but without any serrated end. 2. It should have no empty space which is due to the presence of grease. 3. It should have an even distribution of cells. Leucocytes should spread out and red blood corpuscles should not form a roleaux. 4. Cells should not be distorted by undue pressure.

Thick Film. Take 4 small drops of blood from the finger at corners of a ½ inch (1.2 cm) square (Fig. Ap. I, 5, 6). With a needle pull the four drops into an even thick film covering an area of half inch (1.2 cm) square. Puddling is better avoided. The film takes about 2 hours to dry at room temperature but 1 hour in the incubator. When it is at patient's bedside, it should be covered with a saucer to keep away flies and dust.

PREPARATION OF STAINS

Original Romanowsky Stain. It is a compound stain, made by mixing two aniline dyes: (1) Medicinal methylene blue (polychrome) and (2) Eosin. The former contains an oxidation product called **Azure**. When both the stains are mixed, there is a range of loose chemical compounds like Azure I eosin, and Azure II eosin, etc. It has different affinities for different elements in nucleoplasm and hence gives **differential staining**. It, therefore, consists of 2 solutions:

Solution (A). Medicinal methylene blue—1.0 g, sodium carbonate—0.5 g and distilled water—100 ml. Mix; place in the warm incubator to mature for 2 to 3 days; it should have a purple colour.

Solution (B). Eosin extra BA (water soluble),—1.0 gm and distilled water—1000 ml.

Mix equal parts of both solutions when required.

Modifications of Romanowsky stain, namely: Leishman's, Wright's, Jenner's or Giemsa's stains may be used for staining of blood films. The fluid stains are prepared by dissolving the dry powder in acetone free, pure methyl alcohol so that preliminary fixation of the film is not necessary except in Giemsa's stain.

Leishman's Stain is universally used, as it has the advantage of both fixing and staining. Prepare an approximate amount for 2 to 3 months' use. The stain deteriorates on keeping for a long time.

Requirements: 1. Clean and dry glass pestle and mortar. 2. One 150 ml clean glass-stoppered brown reagent bottle. 3. 100 ml graduated glass cylinder. 4. 0.15 gram or 10 soloids of Leishman's powder (dry). 5. Methyl alcohol (pure)—acetone-free. All the equipments should be rinsed in methyl alcohol.

Procedure. (a) Put 0.15 gram (150 mg) of dry Leishman's powder in a dry mortar and grind finely. Take 100 ml of pure (acetone free) methyl alcohol in a dry cylinder and add a quantity of this alcohol from the cylinder, and grind to form a paste. Add further alcohol till alcohol is saturated with the stain. Allow the coarse particles to settle. Decant the clear supernatant fluid in a dry stoppered bottle (air-tight). Add a little more alcohol from the cylinder, grind and decant as before. Repeat the process again and again till every particle of stain has gone into solution and the whole of 100 ml methly alcohol is used up. Allow it to stand in the incubator for 24 hours before use.

(b) To make little quantity, to 10 ml of methyl alcohol (acetone-free) in a drop bottle, put one soloid of 0.015 gram of Leishman's powder; shake repeatedly till the stain is fully dissolved and every particle of the stain has gone into the solution.

Allow to stand in the incubator for 24 hours before use.

(c) 0.75 g of **Leishman powder** (*E. Merck*) is dissolved in original 500 ml pack of acetone-free **methyl alcohol** (*E. Merck*) and allowed to mature for some time in the incubator.

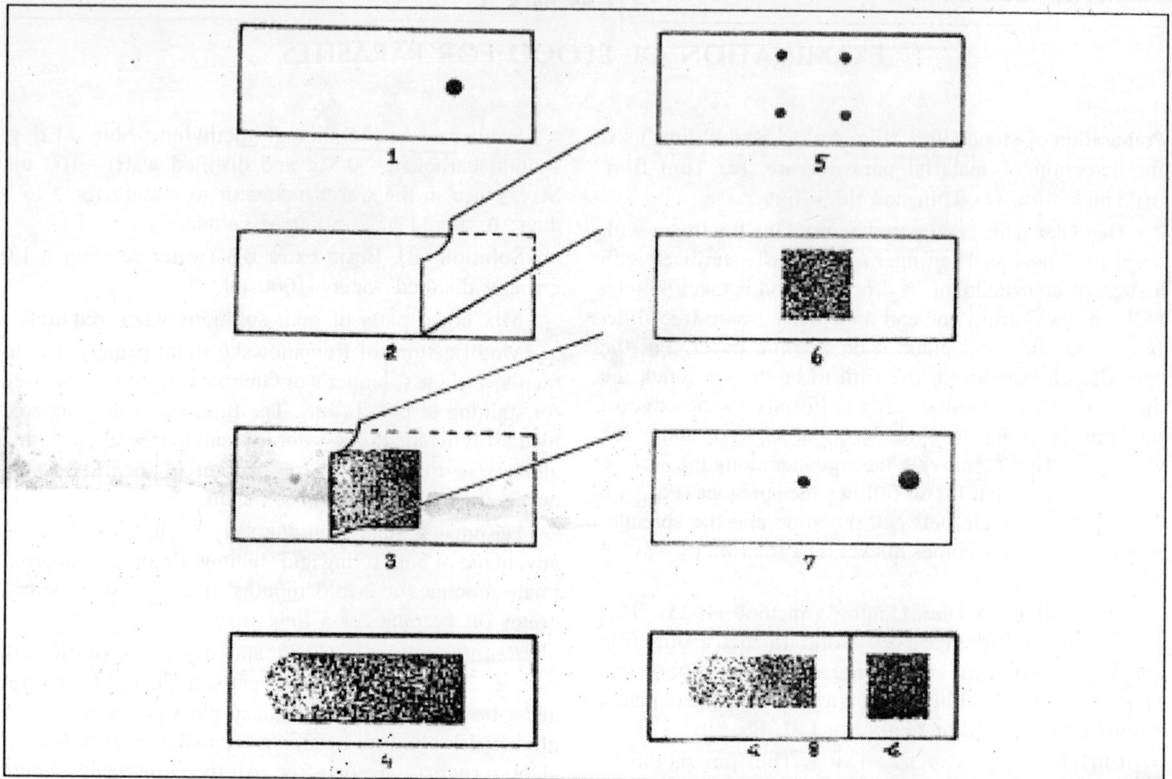

Fig. Ap. I—Thin film (1 to 4), thick film (5 and 6). Sinton's method of thin and thick film (7, 8a and 8b)

Giemsa's Stain. It is prepared by mixing: Azure II eosin—0.3 g, Azure II—0.08 g, methyl alcohol (acetone-free)—25.0 ml and anhydrous pure glycerine—25.0 ml.

Dry thoroughly Azure II eosin and Azure II in a desiccator. Dissolve the dry powder in 25 ml of anhydrous glycerine at 60°C and add 25 ml of pure acetone-free methyl alcohol at the same temperature and prepare as in Leishman's stain. Allow to stand overnight in an incubator and store in a dark cool place.

Wright's Stain. To 1,000 ml of absolute methyl alcohol (acetone-free) add 0.8 gm of acid pot. phosphate and 1.2 gm of dibasic sod. phosphate. If alkaline, add a few drops of monobasic sod. phosphate solution.

Dissolve 0.3 gm of Wright's stain in 100 ml neutralised methyl alcohol. The stain is usually ready for use after a week's maturation.

Henner's or May-Gruenwald Stain. 100 ml absolute methyl alcohol is warmed to 50°C. Add minute portions of 0.3 gm of May-Gruenwald powder. After each addition of the powder, shake vigorously. When the solution is complete, it is allowed to stand for 24 hours. Filter. For staining, the stock solution is diluted with an equal quantity of buffer solution pH 6.8; the solution must be made up fresh daily, for staining. It is most suitable for cytological work.

Field's Stain. This is a rapid method of staining a semi-thick blood film. Blood film is about ½ inch in diameter prepared from a drop of blood. It should be just thick enough so as to allow the hands of a watch to be seen through it.

Prepare two solutions:

Solution A: Methylene blue—0.8 gm, Azure I (Azure B)—0.5 g, disodium hydrogen phosphate (anhyd.)—5 g, crystal potassium dihydrogen phosphate (anhydr.)—6.25 g, and distilled water—500 ml.

Solution B: Eosin (yellow, water soluble)—1.0 g, disodium hydrogen phosphate (anhyd.)—5.0 g, potassium dihydrogen phosphate (anhyd.)—6.25 g and distilled water—500 ml.

Preparation of solution. Phosphate salts are first dissolved in freshly boiled but still warm distilled water. Then the stain is added. Granular Azure I is better mixed after grinding in a mortar with a small quantity of phosphate solution. Set aside the stain for 24 hours and filter before use. Should a scum appear on the surface, or a deposit form on the stained film, subsequent filtration is necessary. The stain usually remains satisfactory for 6

AP I

SMEARS OF LEISHMANIA DONOVANI FROM KALA-AZAR CASES INCLUDING CULTURES

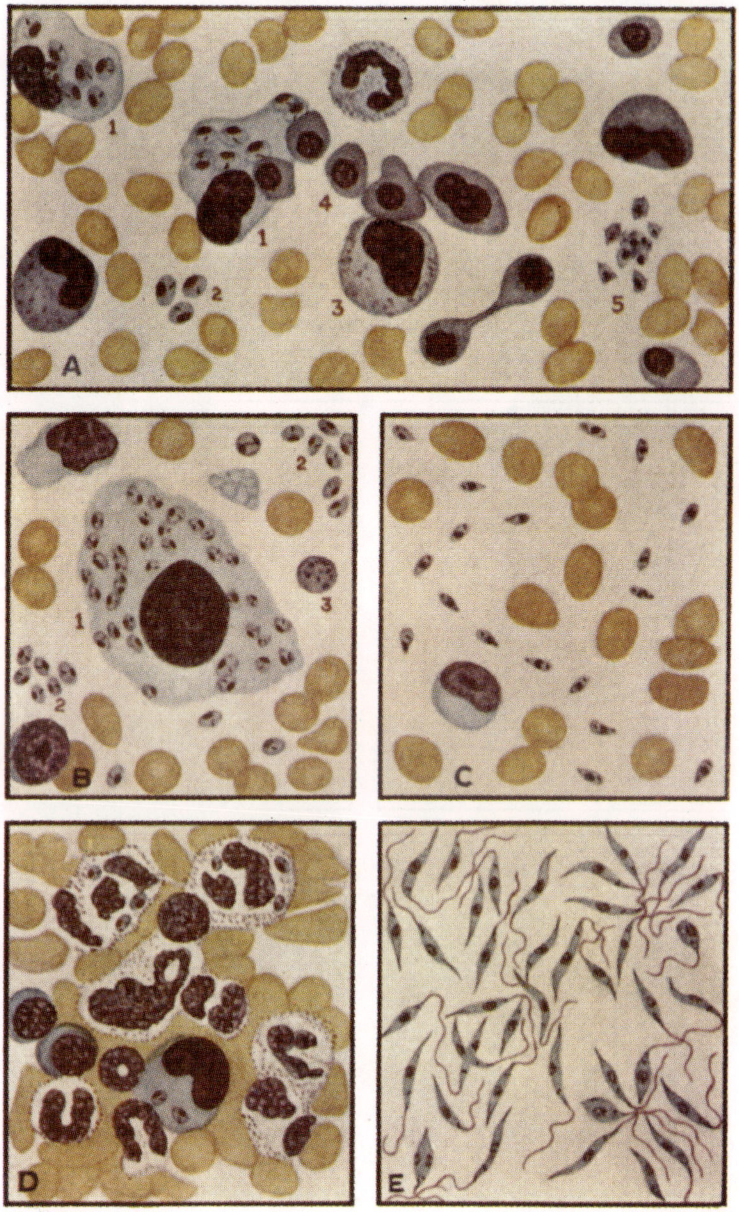

A. Smear from sternal puncture showing L-D bodies: (1) In the macrophage. (2) Extracellularly. (3) Neutrophilic myelocyte. (4) Normoblast C. (5) Blood platelets often mistaken for L-D bodies.

B. and C. Smears from spleen puncture showing L-D bodies. B: (1) In the macrophage. (2) Extracellularly. 3. Blood platelets for comparison.

C. The material obtained from splenic blood (torpedo form).

D. Smear from peripheral blood (Shortt□s method) showing L-D bodies in the predominantly leucocytic zone at the tail end of the smear (in the mononuclear cells and polymorphs).

E. Promastigote (leptomonad, flagellate) from of *Leishmania donovani* (stained by Shortt□s technique).

months to 1 year. Discard it when there is growth of moulds or bacteria.

STAINING METHODS OF BLOOD FILMS

Romanowsky stain. Fix the slide in methyl alcohol for 2 min. Dilute one part each of solution A and solution B with 19 parts of distilled water. Mix equal parts of dilute stains, and stain for 20 to 30 minutes. Wash in distilled water; dry in air.

Method of Leishman's stain

Put name or a number on the slide. Dry the glass rods of an accurately levelled staining rack by rubbing with a filter paper and place the slide with the film side upwards on the rack.

Cover the film with 9 drops of Leishman's stain from a drop bottle—wait for ½ min (methyl alcohol in the stain fixes the film).

From another similar drop bottle add double the number of drops of distilled water (pH—7.0). The best result is obtained by using a buffer solution.*

Mix the stain with distilled water quickly by rocking the slide gently or with the help of a capillary pipette, drawing in and blowing out the solution. A golden scum forms on the surface. Allow to act for 10 minutes.

Wash the slide with distilled water from a wash bottle without disturbing the slide.

Differentiate in distilled water for a minute.

Place the slide in a vertical position to dry with film-side backwards.

Observe under low power. Leucocytes should be well stained and stand out prominently. Then examine under oil immersion lens.

Result. In a properly stained slide, the film appears pinkish grey to the naked eye.

ERYTHROCYTES—pink or orange buff.

NUCLEI OR LEUCOCYTES—purple; CYTOPLASM of lymphocytes—sky-blue.

MONOCYTES—have a kidney-shaped nucleus of a lighter colour with finely granular cytoplasm.

NEUTROPHIL granules are pinkish violet.

EOSINOPHIL granules—red.

BASOPHIL granules—deep purple.

Areas between the cells should be clear and without any precipitate. When water is alkaline, the film is stained deep and appears bluish grey. Eosinophil granules also take deep grey or blue colour.

Variations. The slide may be: (i) pink and under-stained and leucocytes not properly stained due to acid water, (ii) blue due to alkaline water. Blue colour does not interfere with the finding of parasites, and leucocytes; parasites stand out prominently on such a slide. (iii) When the slide is pink and leucocytes have been stained light, the stain can be improved (within limitation) by putting in 1:1,000 pot. carbonate solution till the film is slightly bluish.

Causes of deposits in Leishman's stain. (1) Old stain with sediment on old and scratched slide. (2) Evaporation of stain on the slide at the time of fixing. (3) Delay in mixing after putting distilled water. (4) Draining of the stain from the slide at any time before washing off finally. (5) Overstaining, or staining for the 2nd time invariably gives a deposit.

Caution. For proper staining the following should be carefully observed: Slides should be scrupulously cleaned, grease-free and films well-prepared. (1) Films should be properly fixed. (2) Never allow the stain (alcoholic) to evaporate on the film. (3) Use carbon dioxide-free, neutral distilled water (pH 7.0), or a buffer for diluting the stain in all the stages if possible. (4) Never allow the stain to drain in any stage of staining until final washing. A deposit will surely form if the stain drains.

APPEARANCE OF MALARIA PARASITES

(PL.F.P., A–D and PL. V, Ch. 5) When stained by Leishman or any of the Romanowsky stains, malaria parasites are found in the red blood corpuscles, specially at the edges and the tail end of the film. The parasite should come into focus along with the infected red blood corpuscles. They show the following characteristics:

Trophozoite: (a) Ring (ring of cytoplasm) is stained blue. (b) A clear vacuole in the centre of cytoplasm (not stained). (c) Chromatin dot is stained red. In schizont, chromatin is divided. (d) Pigments in the growing trophozoite and schizont appear brown.

Gametocyte: Cytoplasm—blue. A mass of undivided nuclear chromatin is stained red.

In the male, the chromatin is diffuse. In the female, it is compact when compared with that of a male. Cytoplasm is stained deeper in female than in male. Pigment brown or black.

Fallacies. Various objects have been confused with malaria parasites. The chance of such an error is less in a thin than in a thick film. In all thick films, deposits may appear like blood platelets, debris, stain deposits, dust particles, spores, bacteria and other extraneous matters. These often arise from unclean slides, dirts from skin or use of contaminated water.

---

* Buffer solution. Disodium hydrogen phosphate (anhydrous)—5.447 g.

Potassium dihydrogen phosphate—4.752 g.

Mix together in a mortar. Add 1 gm of the mixture to 2,000 ml of distilled water and this gives a pH of 7.

Methods of Giemsa's stain

Dilute 10 drops of stain in 10 ml of distilled water (neutral), or in phosphate buffer pH 6.8 to 7.0.

The film is fixed with pure acetone-free absolute methyl alcohol for 2.5 minutes. Wash with neutral distilled water. Put the slide with the film side down on a special staining dish containing two ridges to support the slide. Put 10 ml of dilute Giemsa's stain in the dish so that the film side is in contact with the stain. Keep for 30 to 45 minutes, wash and differentiate in distilled water by two changes in one minute, when the film has a pinkish grey tinge.

Panoptic stain (Pappenheim's)

This is a combined May-Gruenwald and Giemsa's stain. For this, film is at first stained with May-Gruenwald's stain for 5 minutes; washed thoroughly with distilled water and then stained with dilute Giemsa for 30 minutes. Wright's or Leishman's stain may be used instead of May-Grunwald's, before staining with dilute Giemsa. But a simplified method which gives satisfactory result is:

Place the slide with film side up a staining rack and cover the smear with Leishman's stain and allow the stain to act for 30 seconds. Dilute it with double the quantity of dilute Giemsa's stain (one drop to 2 ml of distilled water) and mix. Stain for 10 minutes and the staining is completed as in Leishman's stain.

This stain gives an admirable result and is better than any of these stains individually.

Field's stain

PROCEDURE. Keep the staining solution in covered jars. Preliminary fixation is not necessary. (1) Dip the slide with smear in solution A for 1-2 seconds. (2) Rinse rapidly in a jar of clear water until the stain ceases to flow from the film and the glass surface is free from the stain. (3) Dip in solution B for 1-2 seconds. (4) Rinse in clear water as in (2). (5) Place the slide vertically to drain, and then dry in air.

N.B.—Phosphate buffer may be used instead of water for rinsing the slide. Eosin solution should be discarded if it is greenish.

Most intense staining is obtained by re-staining in weak solution of Leishman's stain (1:15 of distilled water instead of 1:10, at pH 7.0) after stage 4, and the slide is stained for 6-10 minutes. By this method, Schüffner's dots stain prominently.

Staining of thick film

(Knowles and Das Gupta, 1924)

Prepare a thick film as mentioned before. (1) DEHAEMOGLOBINISE in a mixture of acid solution of 2.5 percent glacial **acetic acid** in distilled water—4 parts, and 2 percent **tartaric acid** (pure crystals) in distilled water—1 part. This mixture keeps well for months. Cover the film with this solution and the process should be observed carefully, watching the slide till it is greyish–white in colour.

(2) As soon as dehaemoglobinisation is complete drain off the fluid and fix with methyl alcohol for 2-5 minutes (longer fixation is necessary with absolute alcohol—10 minutes).

(3) Wash the film under the tap; wash in distilled water to remove all traces of acid.

(4) Stain with dilute Giemsa's stain (1 drop in 1 ml of distilled water), or dilute Leishman's stain (1 part Leishman's stain with 2 parts of distilled water) as in ordinary film or by panoptic method. Dry and examine for: (1) Malarial parasite (**PL.VIII**), *L. donovani* (**PL.II-IV**). AP. 1). (2) Microfilaria in peripheral blood (Plate I). (3) Trypanosomes (**PL. VII, IX**). (4) Relapsing fever spirochaetes (*Borrelia recurentis*). (5) *Spirillum minus*, etc.

SINTON'S METHOD OF THICK AND THIN FILM

(1) Take a grease-free slide and make a thin film as usual on one half of the slide. (2) On the other half make a thick film. The distance between the two films should be at least one inch (2.5 cm) (Fig. AP. 1). Allow the *thick* film to dry. (3) Put a distinct broad line with a grease pencil to separate the two films. (4) Fix the *thin* film by dipping it in a jar of methyl alcohol for 2 to 5 minutes, taking care that alcohol vapour does not fix the thick film. Allow to dry completely. (5) Stain the whole slide with dilute Giemsa's stain (1 drop to 1 ml) for 40 minutes and complete staining in the usual manner.

JBS stain. (Bhattacharji and Singh, 1944)

This is a rapid Romanowsky method of staining of malaria parasites. The stain is a water soluble one and consists of two solutions:

SOLUTION 1. It consists of Methylene blue—0.5 gm, Potassium dichromate—0.5 gm, Sulphuric acid (1 percent by volume)—3 ml, Potassium hydroxide (1 percent)—10 ml, and Water—100 ml.

SOLUTION 2. Eosin (water soluble)—1 gm, Tap water—500 ml.

The solutions are kept separately in wide-mouthed stoppered jars (3½ inches (8.75 cm) in height and 1½ inch (3.6 cm) in diameter). They keep well and can be used for several months.

PREPARATION. **Solution 1** is prepared in a narrow-mouthed litre flask, by dissolving methylene blue in 500 ml of water. Sulphuric acid and potassium bichromate are then added one after another, showing a heavy deposit of methylene blue-chromate. To complete the process of polychroming, the flask is heated in a boiling water bath for 2-3 hours, when the solution becomes purple. The solution is allowed to cool at room temperature and the precipitate appears as steel-blue, needle-like branched crystals. Now, add 10 ml of 1 percent potassium hydroxide, drop by drop, shaking the flask continuously. When the major part of the precipitate is dissolved the liquid is repeatedly filtered, till the dye-precipitate in the filter paper is completely dissolved. The filtrate is purplish-blue with a violet iridescence. This is due to a mixture of azure with a trace of methylene blue. The solution is left to mature at room temperature for at least 48 hours, as the staining quality improves with ageing.

STAINING OF THICK FILMS. (i) Immerse the thick film in **solution 1** for 10 seconds. (ii) Keep in a jar for two seconds, containing 5 percent acetic or citric acid solution in tap water (pH adjusted to 6.2-6.6; **acidulated water**). (iii) Stain in solution 2 for a second. (iv) Wash in the jar (ii) for 5 seconds. (v) Wash in the jar (i) for 10 seconds. (vi) Wash again in jar (i) for 10 seconds, till the smear gives a pinkish background. (vii) Dry or blot and examine under oil immersion.

STAINING OF THICK AND THIN FILM. (i) Put a grease pencil mark on the film side between the thick and thin films. (ii) Fix the thin film in methyl alcohol for a few seconds and dry. (iii) Immerse the whole slide in solution 1 for 30 seconds. (iv) Wash in the jar containing the acidulated water (jar ii, above). (v) Stain in solution 2 for one second. (vi) Wash again in the jar of acidulated water for 4 seconds. (vii) Immerse in solution 2 for 30 seconds. (viii) Wash again in acidulated water for 10 seconds, or till the smear gives a pinkish background. (ix) Dry or blot and examine under oil immersion.

CULTIVATION OF MALARIA PARASITES

(Bass and Johns' method—modified)

This is useful when: (1) the thin and thick films do not show any malarial parasite, (2) to determine the species of parasite in the ring form by its development in culture and (3) to ascertain whether the treatment has been successful in effecting a cure (in contrast to clinical "cure").

Requirements for culture (1) One 50 ml Ehrlenmeyer flask containing 20 to 30 glass beads, sterilised in an autoclave. (2) A 50% watery solution of glucose, sterilised. (3) One sterilised 5 ml syringe. (4) Sterilised capillary pipettes and test tubes.

Take 5 ml of blood aseptically and put in the Ehrlenmeyer's flask carefully, avoiding air bubbles. Defibrinate the blood by gentle rotation or on a shaker. With the help of a sterile capillary pipette introducing at the bottom of a few sterilised test tubes (12.5 cm by 1.25 cm), one drop of the glucose solution in each. Aspirate the defibrinated blood from the flask and introduce into the test tube, to give a column of about 2.5 cm in each tube. Plug with cotton wool and flame.

Now warm the upper part of the tube in order to expel air, and while still warm, seal its mouth with a rubber cap.

Set the tube vertically in the incubator at 40°C (growth is slow at room temperature).

Next day the tubes show blood column in 3 layers, e.g., supernatant plasma, the middle leucocytic zone, and the column of RBCs at the bottom. Take a sample from the upper layer of RBCs, prepare smears, stain by Leishman's or Giemsa's stain as usual. Culture should be examined, if necessary, on the 2nd or 3rd day.

Black's modified cultural technique of malaria parasite (1945)

Twenty to 30 ml of blood is mixed with 0.1 ml of 50 percent sterile glucose solution. This is defibrinated. The serum is separated by centrifugation and placed in a sterile flat-bottomed tube of about ½ inch (1.2 cm) diameter, to give a column of serum 1½ to 2 inches (3.6-5 cm) high. So the medium contains serum from defibrinated blood, and glucose. The infected blood containing about 100,000 parasites per cmm to be cultivated is first centrifuged: the infected red cells are then taken from beneath the leucocytic layer and introduced into the bottom of the serum tube to form a layer of about 1 mm (1/20 inch) thick. The tube is plugged with cotton wool, and incubated at 37°C. Schizogony of *P. falciparum* and *P. vivax* continues to develop and remain for 48 hours. Parasites are scanty after five days. The liberated merozoites of *P. falciparum* invade uninfected red blood cells readily. Development of gametocytes take place within 78 hours. Subcultures into serum containing new red blood cells and glucose can maintain the strain for some time.

The **object** of culture of malaria parasites is chiefly to see the effect of various antimalarial drugs and to test them on different asexual phases of malarial parasites.

LABORATORY METHODS FOR THE DIAGNOSIS OF BLOOD AND TISSUE FLAGELLATES

FRESH BLOOD (COVERSLIP) PREPARATION. Trypanosomes may be detected in a coverslip preparation. The coverslip is placed on a small drop of blood obtained by a finger prick and preferably ringed with vaseline. The movement of the trypanosomes will produce a characteristic movement of the surrounding blood cells.

STAINED BLOOD SMEAR. A thin or a thick blood film method may be used for this purpose and the film may be stained with Leishman, Giemsa or similar stains.

CONCENTRATION METHOD FOR TRYPANOSOMES. The blood is collected in 1 percent citrate in normal saline. After passing through cheese cloth, it is centrifuged to get the red cells deposited at the bottom. After removing the supernatant fluid, red cells are haemolysed by adding 2 percent acetic acid or distilled water. Centrifuge for 30 minutes. Smears are prepared from the deposit and stained for parasites by Leishman, Giemsa or similar stain.

ASPIRATION BIOPSY (see also Bone marrow biopsy). Dry, autoclaved needles and syringes should be used, but a small amount of saline or citrate saline may facilitate aspiration of lymph nodes in cases of kala-azar and trypanosomiasis. Surgical asepsis should be observed and a local anaesthetic should be used. The material aspirated may be used for smear, culture or animal inoculation.

SPINAL FLUID obtained by lumbar puncture may be centrifuged and the sediment may be utilised for motility preparation, staining, culture, etc.

BIOPSY SMEARS. The skin or mucous membrane may be slit or snipped and smears may be prepared from the granulomatous nodules of oriental sore, post-kala-azar dermal leishmanoid or mucocutaneous lesions and smears may be stained and examined.

ANIMAL INOCULATION. The material may be injected into laboratory animals by a suitable route. For inoculation of *T. gambiense, T. rhodesiense* and *T. cruzi*, rats, mice, guineapigs, dogs or cats may be inoculated but, for *L. donovani*, it is preferable to inoculate hamsters. After the incubation period, blood is examined on repeated occasions at suitable intervals in case of trypanosomiasis, but autopsy materials are examined in sections and smears for leishmaniasis.

XENODIAGNOSIS. See laboratory diagnosis of Dermal lieshmanoid and Chagas' disease.

DIAGNOSIS OF KALA-AZAR BY FINDING THE PARASITE

Smears of peripheral blood (Shortt's method). Slides should be absolutely clean and grease-free. Edge of the spreading slide should be even and fine (white slides are used).

1. Take 8 slides and a few spreaders for four good smears and place them on a white sheet of paper near the window light.

2. Sterilise the dorsum of the finger near the nail root; prick with a sterile surgical needle. Invert the slide and take a small drop of blood as for an ordinary smear; place on the white paper.

3. The spreading slide (as soon as the blood has spread out along its edge completely) is pushed gently along the surface of the slide with an even motion until the blood is almost exhausted. At this point, instead of continuing this motion, the spreading slide is abruptly lifted off carefully with the result that the blood smear ends in a straight edge across the slide, giving a thicker but glistening transparent margin of leucocytes.

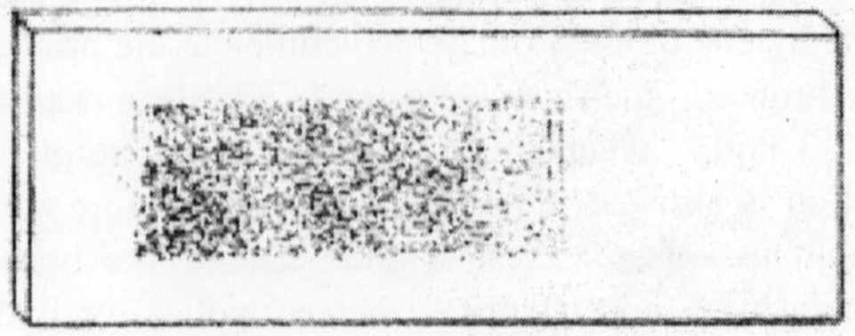

Fig. Ap.2 Blood smear—Shortt's method

4. Dry the tail end of the slide as quickly as possible to spread the leucocytes and avoid roleaux formation which makes the finding of the parasites difficult.

5. Take at least 4 such successfully spread slides (using one edge of the spreader once only).

6. Fix in methyl alcohol, wash in distilled water and stain with dilute Giemsa for 40 minutes. Wash and differentiate in distilled water for a minute and dry in air.

7. Examine the leucocytic edge with special attention to polymorphs and large mononuclear leucocytes for L-D bodies (**PL. AP.I**).

The examination of peripheral blood by this method gives positive findings in 78% of cases when all 4 slides are examined.

OTHER METHODS. Smears from the spleen, liver or sternum puncture may be examined for parasites after staining with Leishman's or Giemsa's stain.

Culture of Leishmania in NNN medium (Novy, MacNeal and Nicolle)

This method is applicable to material obtained from the peripheral blood, sternal puncture, liver or spleen puncture.

Preparation of NNN medium; Agar—14 gm, NaCl—6 gm, and Water—900 ml.

Dissolve and distribute 6 ml in each test tube and autoclave. This forms **stock medium**.

Melt the contents at 90°C or in boiling water bath; allow to cool to 50°C and then add defibrinated rabbit's blood—2 ml in each tube. Mix by rapidly rotating between the palms of the hands in a vertical position—then prepare slopes.

Culture of Peripheral Blood (Row's method)

Draw 0.5 ml blood aseptically and mix with 20 ml citrated saline. Let this settle down overnight. Pipette off the deposit with the help of a sterile pipette and inoculate at least 4 tubes of NNN media with strict aseptic precautions. Incubate at 22°C (cold incubator).

Senekjie culture. For the culture of *Leishmania donovani* or other Leishmania or Trypanosomas. NNN medium had been used in the past and this has been replaced by Senekjie's method of culture which gives better results.

MEDIUM. Bacto beef extract—50 gm is dissolved in 1 litre of distilled water at 50°C for one hour and then at 80°C for 5 minutes. After filtration add neopeptone 20 gm, agar (Nobel) 20-25 gm, sodium chloride (C.P.) 5 gm. The pH is finally adjusted to 7.2-7.4 and the mixture is autoclaved at 15 pounds for 20 minutes. Allow to cool to 45° to 50°C and rabbit's defibrinated blood (10 percent of the volume) is added. On standing, *water of condensation* should be present. National Institute of Health has modified it by overlaying the slant with Locke's solution.

Egg-liver extract medium. Four eggs are washed with soap and water, dried and washed with 80 percent alcohol. Their contents are collected in a sterile beaker and emulsified with glass beads. To the egg emulsion 50 ml of a solution containing sodium chloride, potassium chloride, and sodium bicarbonate—each 0.02 gm in 100 ml of distilled water—are added. The mixture is emulsified thoroughly and filtered. Slants are prepared by inspissation at 80°C and sterilised at 10 pounds for 10 minutes. The slants are now overlayed with sterile 0.5 percent liver extract in physiological saline.

The contaminating organisms which spoil the growth are removed by alternate transfers from blood to egg-liver media. The inoculated tubes are incubated at 22°C.

Method of Brutsaert and Henrard (1938). It is used for the culture of *T. gambiense* and *T. rhodesiense*. The basic solutions used are: 0.6 percent each of Ringer's and Tyrode's solution. These are distributed in amounts of 2-2.5 ml in test tubes, autoclaved and to each tube 2 ml of 1 percent citrate are added. The tubes are incubated at 37°C for 24 hours—to test the sterility. Blood from infected person or animal is drawn into the syringe and discharged in 0.5 ml amounts into the culture tubes and incubated at 25°C to 28°C. The growth is demonstrated microscopically in 10-20 days after staining.

Examine each tube up to 4 weeks, make a smear from the water of condensation and stain with Leishman stain and examine.

Staining of Flagellate Protozoa (Shortt's method, 1923) for flagella of either intestinal flagellates or promastigotes and trypomastigotes (Trypanosomes). In case of faecal film, the faeces is well-diluted with saline and thinly spread out on a slide. In case of flagellate culture of Leishmania, take a loopful of material from the water of condensation in NNN medium. Add 4 loopfuls of normal citrate saline (NaCl—0.85 g, Sod, citrate—1.5 g, distilled water—100 ml).

Spread out on an area of ½ inch (1.2 cm) square.

Fix for 15 seconds over vapour of 4% Osmic acid at the point of drying of the film.

Dry in air as rapidly as possible.

Fix in methyl alcohol, wash in distilled water, Stain with dilute Giemsa (1 drop to 1 ml water).

ASPIRATION (*NEEDLE*) BIOPSIES

BONE MARROW BIOPSY

There are two methods for bone marrow biopsy:

I. *Needle or Aspiration Biopsy.* The marrow is aspirated through a wide-bore needle (Klima or Salah type) form the following sites: (A) sternum; (B) medial side of the upper end of the tibia in children up to 2 years of age, (C) illac crest.

Iliac Crest Puncture (posterior or anterior). The technique is the same as practised for sternal puncture:

(1) For the **posterior iliac crest puncture**, the patient lies on one side with knees drawn up, and back flexed as for lumbar puncture. The needle is inserted perpendicularly 1 cm below the posterior superior iliac spine.

(2) For the **anterior iliac crest puncture**, the patient lies on his back and the needle is inserted into the iliac crest at a point just behind the anterior superior iliac spine.

Smears are prepared from the aspirated marrow material and stained with any one of the Romanowsky stains. They are examined under oil immersion to find out the parasites in the bone marrow.

II. *Trephine Biopsy.* This is helpful in the diagnosis of *myelosclerosis*. Specimens are obtained by means of specially constructed needles for trephining (trephine needles) from the biopsy fragments for examination of both **cytological smears** and **histological sections**.

STERNAL PUNCTURE

Sternal Puncture is eminently suitable for marrow biopsy.

Indications. 1. It is indicated in the diagnosis of

(a) Kala-azar and chronic malaria. In detection of malaria parasites, this process has little advantage over examination of peripheral blood.

(b) Agranulocytosis and chloroma.

(c) Carcinomatosis (metastatic).

(d) Multiple myelomatosis.

2. To examine the bone-marrow reactions for the study of:

(a) Erythropoietic reaction in anaemia (normoblastic or megaloblastic).

(b) Reaction of white blood corpuscles in leukaemia (specially aleukaemic leukaemia).

Requirements. 1. Sternal puncture needle (sterilised)—This is a large bore (13 gauge) needle 8 cm in length provided with a stylet and an adjustable guard. The needle mount should be such that it fits air-tight into the syringe. 2. A two ml hypodermic syringe fitted with a needle (sterilised). 3. Cotton wool, alcohol, tincture iodi mitis. 4. Two percent sterile novocaine solution. 5. A dry syringe (2 or 5 ml) with good suction and fitting accurately to the sternal puncture needle. 6. Slides, oxalated tube containing 4 mg of double (ammonium and potassium) oxalate for 2 ml material.

Site. The point of puncture is selected on one side of the middle line of the sternum at the level of the 2nd or 3rd intercostal space (when carcinoma is suspected, a point is selected in the middle line or according to the location of the lesion by X-ray examination).

Procedure. The skin over the manubrium sterni is sterilised by painting with tincture iodine. The part is then anaesthetised with about 1 ml of 2 percent novocaine solution (without adrenaline) deep to the periosteum.

After an interval of about 10 minutes, the needle (with the guard adjusted at a distance of 1 to 1.5 cm according to the build of the subject) is introduced with the stylet inside with a boring motion but with firm pressure. The needle is passed through the skin and then through the outer plate of the bone, titled at an angle of 30° to 60° to reach the marrow cavity. When the marrow is reached (as felt by sudden release of pressure), the stylet is withdrawn and a syringe is attached to the needle. 1 to 2 ml of red fluid is aspirated. The needle is withdrawn and the wound is sealed with collodion or by tincture benzene.

Films are quickly drawn directly from the marrow material received on the slide and the remaining material is put in the oxalated tube for haemoglobin determination, erythrocyte and leucocyte counts. Stain the smear with Leishman's stain or fix the film with methyl alcohol within half an hour and stain with Giemsa or Wright's stain (diluted with equal parts of distilled water); for a permanent preparation a film stained by panoptic method is preferable. A citrated material may be inoculated in NNN medium.

SPLEEN PUNCTURE

Indications. Spleen puncture is indicated in the diagnosis of kala-azar by (1) finding of L-D bodies in smears prepared from the material, and (2) culture of the material in NNN media in which promastigote (leptomonad) form of the parasite may be demonstrated (PL. V/4, AP. I).

Equipment. (1) A 5 ml sterilised syringe with a good, stout, medium-sized needle. A Roux pattern syringe, record syringe, or all-glass syringe may be used but the syringe should be provided with good suction. An all-glass syringe may be sterilised in an autoclave, but any of these syringes may be sterilised in an **olive oil bath** at 160°C also, by sucking in and ejecting out the oil several times. The oil is washed off with a sterile solution of **sodium carbonate** and this in its turn is washed off several times with a sterile solution of 1.5% sodium citrate in normal saline; 0.25 ml of the citrate solution may be left in the syringe. (2) Many-tailed bandage, cotton wool, 0.5% carbolic acid. (3) Glass slides. (4) Culture tubes of NNN medium or other media.

Preparation of the patient. The patient's blood is examined for coagulation time. If the coagulation time is normal, no extra precaution is called for but, when the blood caogulation time is increased, preparatory treatment with calcium and vitamin K is indicated to reduce the blood coagulation time.

Procedure. The patient lies flat on his back with his hands underneath the head. The bandage is placed in position ready for use, immediately after the puncture.

The operator stands on the left side of the patient and the assistant, who wil fix the organ, will stand on the right side.

Site. A point about 1 inch (2.5 cm) below the left costal margin is selected midway between the anterior and posterior borders of the spleen. The skin is sterilised; when dry, a tiny drop of carbolic acid to the point of puncture is applied by means of a wooden stick which absorbs the excess of carbolic acid. This sterilises and anaesthetises the skin. The patient is asked to hold his breath and the assistant fixes the enlarged spleen by upward push against the diaphragm.

The skin is now stretched with the left hand and the syringe is held in the right hand, the needle is introduced first through the skin and then, after waiting for a second, it is plunged upwards into the spleen at an angle of 45° along the long axis of the spleen. The patient holds his breath all the time during operation. The piston is withdrawn to produce a forceful aspiration and by this means, some of the spleen pulp is drawn out.

The needle is quickly withdrawn in the exact line of its introduction, and the area is sealed with collodion or benzene and leucoplast. A sterile pad is now placed and the abdominal bandage is applied.

The pulp at the end of the needle may be used to prepare a few films on slides and the material may be diluted with citrate solution and transferred to a few tubes of NNN or other culture media. Films are stained by Leishman's stain and examined for L-D bodies, which are often intracellular in endothelial cells (PL. II/4, AP.I).

The patient is observed for about an hour or two; pulse rate may be recorded for the detection of internal haemorrhage, if any.

Contraindications. (1) Leukaemia, which should be excluded by examination of a peripheral blood film. (2) Jaundice, bleeding from the gums, purpura, which might develop in the course of the disease. (3) Ascites or severe bronchitis.

LIVER PUNCTURE

Spleen puncture is occasionally attended with fatal accident even in expert hands also, due to internal haemorrhage. For this reason, liver puncture is advised now-a-days, which is very safe but gives a lower percentage of finding of parasites.

Liver puncture is done in almost the same manner as the spleen puncture and equipments used are same.

Procedure. Select a site in the last intercostal space on the right mid-axillary line or higher up where there is definite dullness on percussion. Introduce the needle upwards and inwards and aspirate liver tissue by a strong suction (PL. VIII/3). Make smears from the pulp and stain.

Smears are usually not successful when blood rushes into the syringe and, in these cases, NNN or other culture tubes should be inoculated in the same way as in the case of spleen puncture.

EXAMINATION OF BLOOD FOR MICROFILARIA

Collection of Blood. In case of infection of *Wuchereria bancrofti* with nocturnal periodicity, the blood is collected between the hours of 10 P.M. and 2 A.M., but in case of non-periodic variety the blood may be taken at anytime, preferably in the morning. The preparation of slide will depend on the method of examination—whether stained or unstained. The stained preparation will give a permanent preparation and will give details of the microfilaria for the determination of the species.

Unstained preparation. For this 2 or 3 drops of blood is taken close together on a clean glass slide. A coverslip with a rim of vaseline is then put on the blood and the slide may be examined then and there, or in next morning under the low power objective of the microscope. Microfilariae when present, is seen lashing and writhing the RBCs as they remain alive in such a preparation for 1-2 days. Identification of species is not possible by this method.

Stained preparation. For this, a thick film is prepared from a midnight sample and kept covered to dry. Next morning, it is dehaemoglobinised by covering the film with distilled water, dried and fixed in methyl alcohol for 2-5 minutes. The film is then stained with dilute Leishman or Giemsa stain or with haematoxylin eosin (H-E) stain. The method, although is time consuming and requires more material, gives permanent slides with diagnostic features and specific details. Occasionally on routine examination of a thin blood film, microfilaria may be detected.

In H-E stain, the staining is done after dehaemoglobinisation and fixation, as mentioned above. After staining with haematoxylin and development of blue colour, the film may be stained with eosin or it may be counterstained with Giemsa stain (1 drop to one ml of distilled water), dried and examined.

Vital staining. This can be done with fresh blood or dehaemoglobinisation by mixing with methylene blue in physiological saline in a proportion of 1:5,000. According to Sharp (1927), the living microfilaria of *L. loa, O. volvulus, A. perstans* are stained in 10 minutes; whereas those of *W. bancrofti* and *W. malayi* are stained much more slowly.

The easier and better method as used by the author to show details of microfilaria in no time is to put a drop of McGuire stain* on a thick blood film under a coverslip. This stains the microfilaria showing its details and also the leucocytes.

Concentration method for microfilaria. Take the midnight sample of blood from a vein and slake it with either distilled water, or 2 percent acetic acid, or 2.5 percent formalin, or saponin solution. Centrifuge deposit is examined for microfilaria. **For haemolysis** (dehaemoglobinisation) the following methods are recommended: (1) About 1-2 ml of blood from a vein is mixed with at least 5-10 ml of distilled water and shaken thoroughly for haemolysis. (2) About 2 ml of blood withdrawn from a vein is mixed with 10 ml of 2 percent acetic acid in distilled water; the red cells are lysed. (3) About 1 ml of blood is mixed with 10 ml of 2 percent formalin for haemolysis (Kott, 1939). (4) Twenty drops of blood are

* McGuire stain is Ponder's stain, four times concentrated. **Ponder's stain:** Toludin blue—0.2 g, Acetic acid—10 ml, Ethanol—20 ml, Distilled water—1,000 ml. Keep the stain for 3 to 5 minutes; blot dry.

mixed with 10 ml of normal saline; to this, a few drops of 10 percent saponin solution are added to haemolyse the RBCs. **Motile larvae** may be found in the centrifuged deposit. (5) About 5 ml of blood is taken in 10 ml of 2.5 percent citrated saline. RBCs are lysed next morning by adding 1 percent saponin in normal saline drop by drop, till the haemolysis is complete. The mixture is centrifuged; deposit is examined for microfilaria (Bhaduri, 1948).

Micrifilaria count. With the help of a haemoglobinometer pipette, 20 cmm of blood is drawn; a thick film is prepared and dried, dehaemoglobinised and stained in the usual manner. The total number of microfilaria in the film multiplied by 50 gives a total number per ml of blood.

IMMUNOLOGICAL DIAGNOSIS FOR PROTOZOA

Intestinal protozoa

Cole and Kent (1953) have reported **immobilisation** of *E. histolytica* with hyperimmune rabbit serum.

By Fluorescent-tagged antibody globulin (Godman, 1933, 1934), *E. histolytica* or *E. coli* could be differentiated from *D. fragilis, Endo, nana*, and *E. invadens* (tissue invading amoeba of reptiles) show bright fluorescence in amoebae exposed to tagged homologous antiserum.

Malaria parasites. See respective chapter.

Blood and tissue flagellates

For leishmaniasis, complement fixation, globulin precipitation, agglutination and intradermal tests are useful in the diagnosis of *L. donovani, L. braziliensis* and *L. tropica* infections.

Complement fixation test. (See *L. donovani*) *Euglobulin precipitation test* of Brahmachari, 1919, and Sia (1924). Aldehyde test of Napier (1921), Chopra's **Antimony test** (1927), Ray's **haemolytic test** (see *L. donovani*, serological tests). **Sia□s test.** This is a precipitation test in which, to a volume of 0.6 ml of distilled water in a small calibre test tube, 20 cmm of blood is added and the contents are mixed. An immediate clouding indicates a positive reaction. Sedimentation occurs in 15-60 minutes; an earlier precipitation indicates a stronger reaction. It may be positive in Kala-azar and schistosomiasis (see also under *Schistosoma haematobium* text). Ray's haemolytic test in Kala-azar is similar. (For these tests, see Text chapter).

Agglutination test (Packchanian, 1940: Senekji, 1943). Cultured promastigote (leptomonad) stage of the species of *Leishmania parasitising* man and hyperimmune rabbit sera were originally used by Nicolle and Manceaux (1909) and then by Pavoni, Noguchi (1926), Wagner and Kock (1926). Nowadays with slide agglutination technique of Senekji and Lewis (1945), rapid differential diagnosis can be made between the species of Leishmania. It is highly specific but this has not been widely employed in human infection. Homologous organisms show high agglutinin titres but conglutinins were positive in low titres and systemic infections with *L. donovani* and *T. cruzi* produced higher titres than cutaneous or mucocutaneous types of leishmaniasis.

Intradermal test. The intradermal reaction is positive for all the 3 types of leishmania infections, including that of *L. tropica* (Dostrovsky and Sagher, 1946). It is specially useful for *L. braziliensis* infection, when the organism is difficult to demonstrate. This is Montenegro test (1926) modified by Pessoa and Pestana (1940). The organism is cultured in NNN medium for 8-12 days and then extracted and suspended in physiological saline to which 0.4 percent phenol is added. 0.1 ml of the suspension is injected intradermally. In positive cases an erythematous wheal develops in 24-48 hours, which may last for 4 or 5 days. A sterile papule develops in the centre of the wheal which later becomes vesicular and pustular. A positive result has been obtained in 92 percent cases, in which *L. braziliensis* was afterwards demonstrated. Pellegrino (1951) obtained a polysaccharide fraction of the culture of *L. braziliensis* in 1:5,000 saline suspension and obtained a strongly positive reaction in infected persons. It may be useful in all the 3 types of leishmaniasis.

Complement-fixation test for Chagas' disease (**Machedo test** developed by Guerreiri and Machado, 1913). The antigen is an aqueous extract of spleens of experimentally infected puppies. According to Dussert *et al*, (1939), the test is a practical one, but is not species-specific.

FOR IMMUNOLOGICAL TESTS of *Toxoplasma gondii*, see Text.

Appendix II

EXAMINATION OF STOOLS

FOR ENTAMOEBA HISTOLYTICA

Collection of stools. There are several important points to be observed for the collection of stools: (i) The specimen should be always fresh and examined within 2 hours. (ii) No oily purgative should be administered beforehand. (iii) The receptacle should be dry and free from antiseptic. (iv) There should not be any urine in the bed pan and urine should be passed in a separate urinal. (v) Get the whole sample of stool if possible; in other cases the sample may be collected from the bed pan in a faeces tube. Never fail to record the macroscopic character and the reaction.

Coverslip Preparation. (a) Select the suspicious portion of stool, e.g., mucous and blood-stained part. On a perfectly clean slide, make a thin emulsion in a drop of saline and put the coverslip. The emulsion must be so thin, that printed matter can be read through it. A thick emulsion, dirty coverslip and unclean lenses spoil the work. **Always remember**, that fresh saline preparation gives best information of *E. histolytica* (trophozoite and cyst).

(b) Make a similar thin preparation in aqueous indine solution (Lugol's iodine).

Lugol's iodine: Pot. Iodine—2 gm, iodine—1 gm and distilled water 100 ml.

'D□ ANTONI□S SOLUTION. It contains 1.5 gm of iodine in 100 ml of 1 percent potassium iodide solution. The mixture is allowed to stand for 4 days in a stoppered phial, shaken several times a day. It is then filtered, stoppered tightly and used for 4 weeks, like Lugol's iodine.

It is necessary to examine (a) and (b) in every case as a routine measure.

Zinc sulphate concentration method (Faust *et al,* 1938, 1939). A suspension of one part of faeces in 10 parts of tepid water is made and 10 ml of the suspension is filtered through a layer of wet guage into a centrifuge tube. Centrifuge for one minute at 2,500 r.p.m. Pour off the supernatant fluid and add a few ml of water; resuspend the sediment and recentrifuge. Repeat the process till the supernatant fluid remains clear. Add 3-4 ml of a 33.1 percent solution of zinc sulphate ($7H_2O$; Sp. gr. 1.180). Resuspend the sediment and add more zinc sulphate solution until the tube is filled up to ½ inch (1.2 cm) below the brim. Centrifuge for one minute at 3,000 r.p.m. A few loopfuls of the material from the surface are transferred to a clean slide and examined under a coverslip. In absence of a centrifuge, the emulsion may be left to stand for 5 minutes when the ova and cysts will float on the surface.

This is the **best method** for combined concentration of both protozoan cysts and helminthic ova. It is, however, applicable to ova that float and has the disadvantage of the floatation methods. For helminthic ova, this method is inferior to direct floatation method and is more time-consuming. Its chief application is to diagnose both protozoan (cyst) and helminthic infections in *one operation* but not suitable for helminthic ova alone. When the specimen of stool is negative for protozoa by iodine-stained and saline preparations, this concentration method is recommended and has given a positive result. The method is recommended for formed stools, in which cystic forms are only detected, as the trophozoite forms are destroyed by this technique.

Cultivation of *E. histolytica.* It is cultivated in Dobell and Laidlaws' "HSre + S", (HS = Horse serum; r = Ringer solution; e = Egg albumin; S = rice starch), modification of Boeck and Drbohlav's medium (1926).

Medium. The solid medium is prepared by inspissating suitable quantities of horse serum (filtered free from bacteria, if necessary) in sterile test tubes, at 80°C for 1 hour. Aseptic precautions are taken all through the manipulation. Minimum heating is necessary, as overheating ruins the medium. Test tubes are filled with the serum to produce slants of about 1 to 1½ inch (2.5-3.7 cm) in length on coagulation after inspissation. The tubes are then slanted in an inspissator and heated to 70°C, until transferred to an autoclave and sterilised for 20 minutes at 15 lbs pressure. When the slants have cooled, they are incubated to test their sterility.

The liquid portion of the medium consists of 4 eggs dissolved in 1 litre of the Ringer's solution. Ringer's solution contains sodium chloride—9 gm, pot. chloride—0.2 gm, calcium chloride—0.2 gm and distilled water—1 litre. This mixture is sterilised by filtration through Seitz filters and added aseptically to give a depth of 1 cm, of the fluid over the solid part of the medium. The tubes are now tested for sterility by putting in the incubator at 37°C and stored until required.

Just before inoculation a loopful of sterilised rice starch is added to the medium. The tubes are kept in the incubator before inoculation and are inoculated with emulsion of faecal matter.

In this medium, *E. histolytica* and *E. gingivalis* produce an abundant growth with a long life; cultures of *E. coli* grow luxuriantly, *E. nana* shows poor growth.

Culture. In order to inoculate the tubes, pick up a

portion of mucus from stools with the help of a sterile capillary pipette and inoculate in the fluid part. The tubes are incubated in a vertical position at 37°C. Materials for examination can be removed from time to time by means of a sterile capillary pipette by scraping the surface of the solid slant with the end of the pipette. Multiplication takes place for 2-3 days, after which the amoebae die by production of acid by the starch-splitting bacteria. The growth of these bacteria can be reduced by subculturing in media containing 1:20,000 acriflavine which does not alter the pH of the medium. The optimum pH for the growth of *E. histolytica* is 7.2 to 7.8. The presence of intestinal bacteria is necessary for the growth of *E. histolytica*, but they reduce the pH by formation of acid.

Permanent Stool Preparation

Iron-haematoxylin method of Heidenhain. It is extremely difficult to get good permanent preparations of intestinal protozoa. The best result is obtained by Dobell's modification of the original method, as:

1. Make a thin emulsion of perfectly fresh stool and prepare an even smear on a coverslip; albumen is better omitted. A slide may also be used with the advantage that it is easier to manipulate.

2. Wait till the film is just at the point of drying. Before it dries, place it gently in *Schaudinn's fixative* (absolute alcohol 1 part to 2 parts of a saturated solution of corrosive sublimate in normal saline, and 5 ml of glacial acetic acid to 100 ml of the mixture). The fixative is best used at 60°C. In 10 to 20 minutes the smear is fixed.

3. Rinse in 50 percent alcohol and transfer to 70% alcohol tinged portwine red with iodine crystals. Iodine in the solution changes the mercury to mercuric iodide. Keep in this solution till the film is well-browned, say for 1/2 an hour. At this stage it is advisable to keep the preparation in rectified spirit or absolute alcohol to harden. On the other hand, red mercuric iodide is removed by rectified spirit, till it is colourless.

4. Pass through graded alcohol to water. Rinse in distilled water and stain.

5. Soak the smear for 3 to 4 hours in saturated watery solution of iron alum crystals (2 to 4 percent of purple violet crystals, as the green stuff is oxidised). This mordants the film. Wash in distilled water.

6. Stain with ripe haematoxylin solution (0.5% solution of haematoxylin exposed to sunlight in a flask plugged with cotton wool till it is rich brown-red; it may take a few weeks). Stain for 6 hours or more with several changes of stain until it turns jet black.

7. Iron haematoxylin process is a "**retrogressive stain**". The overstained smear is now differentiated in 1 percent iron alum, which gradually removes the stain and gives a differential picture. Study the progress under microscope. The **chromatin** should be stained **jet black, cytoplasm unstained**. The vegetative amoebae may be decolourised in 3 to 10 minutes; cysts may take hours or may even require 2 to 4 percent iron alum solution.

8. The moment correct differentiation is obtained, wash for half an hour in tap water.

9. Pass through graded alcohol to absolute alcohol and dehydrated alcohol. Dip in equal parts of alcohol and xylol and then in xylol and mount in neutral canada balsam.

Although long, tedious and troublesome, the process gives satisfactory results. It should be noted that the film should not be allowed to dry at any stage.

Animal Inoculation Test for the Diagnosis of Intestinal Amoebiasis

It is not a routine method of stool examination for diagnosis, but in case of dispute, it may be performed as a final court of appeal. Kittens are most susceptible, and younger animals not older than 21 days are preferable. But other animals like dogs, white rats, rabbits or guineapigs may be infected experimentally. These animals may be infected by 3 routes: (1) **oral route**, (2) **rectal route**, (3) **intracaecal route**. In the second instance a suitable catheter may be utilised to reach the rectum, but in the last instance operative measures may be undertaken to put the material directly into the caecum. In case the stools contains cysts, introduction by oral route through the stomach tube is obligatory. The animal becomes sick within 7 to 10 days, passing blood and mucus in the stools. The animal may be sacrificed at the height of infection and search may be made for the presence of ulcer. If necessary the ulcer may be scraped and examined under the microscope.

M. R. Stain for the study of parasitic protozoa and fungi

(Mukherjea and Ray; *Bull. Cal. School of Trop. Me*c 5. 176, 1957).

Solution 1. Saturated solution of Mercuric chloride—64 ml, Absolute alcohol—32 ml, Glacial acetic acid—5.2 ml, Formalin (40% formaldehyde) 4.2 ml, Thionine—0.04 gm, Azure—0.02 gm. All the ingredients are taken in a stoppered bottle mixed by vigorous shaking for 3 hours and then filtered through a filter paper.

Solution 2. 70 percent Alcohol—93 ml, Glacial acetic acid—7 ml, Thionin—0.06 g, Azure I—0.06 g, Methyl green (chloroform extracted)—0.04 gm, Eosin—0.24 gm.

Solutions 1 and 2 are mixed in the proportion of 1:1 and filtered after 24 hours. This is a **fixative cum staining solution**.

Faecal smears, and smears from cultures of protozoa and fungi are stained with this solution. Dip the slide in a jar containing the solution for 10 minutes; rinse in tap water. The smears are then dehydrated by passing successively through two changes of tertiary butyl alcohol, 1 minute each; cleared in toluol and xylol for 1 minute, and mounted in canada balsam.

Besides intestinal protozoa, parasitic fungi like *Trichophyton rubrum* and *Epidermophyton floccosum* from cultures are stained by this method. Helminthic ova are also well-stained. The chromatoid bodies in the cyst of *E. histolytica*, the nucleus, and the cytoplasm give distinctly differential staining reactions. **Chromatoid bodies** are stained blue or bluish-green, **nuclear chromatin** *greenish purple and the* **cytoplasm** faint pink. *Trichomonas hominis*, however, failed to preserve its identity in this solution.

Preparation of adult helminths for identification

The adult worms are identified from their gross characteristics or microscopically under a dissecting microscope or a low power microscope. For the identification of gravid proglottides of a tapeworm or an adult fluke, the material may be pressed between two slides and examined with a good illumination under low power. Better details are available, when the segments are immersed in 75 percent phenol and 25 percent xylene solution, which clarifies it. It is of special value in fixed specimen.

Preservation of faecal specimens

This is applicable to specimen which cannot be examined immediately. The sample of faeces is made into a thin paste with tap water. To this, an equal part of steaming 10 percent formalin is poured and set aside for a few hours. The supernatant solution is decanted.

It should be noted that formalin-preserved ova become heavier than those in fresh stools. Therefore, a solution with a specific gravity higher than 1.2 should be used for floatation method. Maplestone and Mukherjea (1943) recommended adding of 1 percent sodium chloride in the proportion of 30:1 to the stools. Such faecal specimen may be sent to a laboratory from the field, and ova are recognisable for about a month.

Preservation of helminths recovered from faeces

Ova and larva. After concentration of ova or larvae by sedimentation or centrifugation, they are preserved in 10 percent formalin. If it is desired to keep them for more than one year, they may be transferred to graded alcohol of 30, 50 and finally to 70 percent.

Adult helminths. For identification and preservation of laboratory specimens, the living worms are placed in warm normal saline and shaken, until they are completely fatigued. Steaming 5 percent formalin is then poured over the relaxed worms, while they are shaken constantly in order to prevent contraction. In case of dead worms, they are washed in warm normal saline and fixed in formalin. For **roundworms**, 10 ml of glycerine to 100 ml of 5 percent formalin, added before heating, are recommended. FOr **histological details**, more complex fixing solutions are required and a textbook on the microscopic methods should be consulted.

EXAMINATION FOR OVA OF HELMINTHS

Methods

1. Direct smear.
2. Concentration method of Willis.
3. Direct centrifugal floatation (DCF) method of Clayton Lane.

1. Direct Smear

Spread a loopful of stool in a drop of water with a tooth pick and make a coverslip preparation of moderate thickness on a glass slide. Examine for ova with 2/3″ objective (low power) starting from one edge of the film and going over the whole film in a systematic way. Confirm ova, if any, with 1/6″ objective (high power). The method is useful in heavy infection only.

2. Concentration by floatation method

For this purpose, any of the following solutions like table salt (sodium chloride), table sugar, calcium chloride or zinc sulphate may be used. The first one is the least expensive and very satisfactory for this floatation method.

APPARATUS (i) Small metal "pill boxes" with a capacity of about 12-20 ml. A container with a diameter not more than 1½ inch (3.7 cm) should be selected. (ii) Glass slide 3×2 inches (7.5 × 5 cm) (iii) Saturated solution of common salt (sp. gravity of 1200) should be used. (iv) Wooden toothpicks or bamboo sticks. (v) A high power microscope.

PROCEDURE. (1) Put about 1 g of stool in a metal "pill box" and add a few drops of saturated salt solution, and stir with a piece of stick to obtain an even paste of the stool. (2) Add more salt solution till the pill box is nearly full. Remove with the stick the coarse particles that float on the surface. (3) After a thorough emulsion is made, fill the pill box up to the brim by adding the salt solution with a pipette, drop by drop, till the fluid is in level with the top of the pill box and forms a convex meniscus. (4) Allow the preparation to stand for not less than 20 minutes and not more than 30 minutes (by the clock). If the preparation is allowed to stand for more than 30 minutes, eggs become heavier due to osmosis and tend to settle down. (5) Place the glass slide on the top of the pill box carefully, so that its centre is in contact with the fluid. The surface of the fluid should be in contact with the slide (if necessary add a few drops more of the salt solution). (6) Lift the slide off the pill box steadily, taking care to keep it horizontal, and then turn over the slide rapidly without allowing any fluid to jerk out of the slide. (7) Examine with 2/3 inch objective (low power).

3. Direct Centrifugal Floatation
(DCF method of Lane)

Break up about 1 g of stool in 10 ml of tap water and transfer into a thick-walled centrifuge tube and centrifuge for 2 mins. at 1,000 RPM Decant the supernatant fluid.

Add saturated saline solution (sp. gravity 1.2; 37.7 g of NaCl per 100 ml) up to the brim of the tube and cover with a thick coverslip, so that it is in contact with the fluid. Fix it with plasticine; centrifuge again for 1 to 2 mins at 1,000 RPM. During spinning, eggs (being lighter than saline) are driven towards the coverslip. The coverslip is quickly lifted off, and a wet coverslip preparation is made with the drop of saline on the undersurface of the coverslip, and examined. Several samples can be centrifuged at a time by this method.

ADVANTAGES OF DCF METHOD OF LANE. (a) Short time is required. (b) A number of stools can be examined at a time. (c) Area to be examined for eggs is small. (d) The method is satisfactory.

ENUMERATION OF HOOKWORM EGGS

For quantitative estimations of eggs for determining the worm load, three methods are utilised; (c) Direct centrifugal floatation method of Lane, 1923. (b) *Stoll's egg counting technique*, 1923, and (c) the technique of Caldwell and Caldwell, 1926.

ENUMERATION OF HOOKWORM EGGS **(Stoll□s method, 1923).**

The examination is based on finding out the number of ova present per gm of faeces. In this, 3 gm of faeces are mixed with 97 ml of a decinormal (0.4%) sodium hydroxide solution and 10 small glass beads are placed in the tube. After closing the mouth of the tube by a rubber stopper, the tube is shaken vigorously to make a uniform suspension.

Take 0.15 ml of this suspension on a large slide 3×2 inch (7.5 × 5 cm) and put a coverslip 22×40 mm on it. The eggs are counted under the coverslip preparation with a low power objective and ×10 ocular; use of a mechanical stage is essential, which greatly facilitates the work.

The total number of eggs counted per gram of faeces is obtained by multiplying the total of 2 such preparations by 100. The total number of production of eggs per day can be obtained from the figure of daily output of faeces in grams.

The egg counting technique is employed to determine the egg laying capacity of a female worm as determined by enumeration of eggs per gm of formed faecal output. On a rough estimate it is calculated that a female worm produces 100 eggs per gm of faeces per day in case of hermaphrodite species, e.g., *Clonorchis sinensis*, *Fasciolopsis buski*. In case of nematodes, however, assuming that sexes are equally divided, 50 eggs per gm of faeces may represent one worm. These techniques are used in

TABLE AP. II—1
HELMINTHIC OVA THAT FLOAT ON SATURATED SALT SOLUTION (PL. AP II)

Helminth	Measurement	Appearance
COLOURLESS:		
Ankylostoma duodenale	40×60μ	Oval, thin-shelled
Necator americanus	”	Ovum usually with four segmented cells inside
Oxyuris vermicularis (Enterobins)	20×50μ	Oval, planoconvex, thin-shelled eggs—They are confused with vegetable cells containing coiled larva inside
Hymenolepis nana	30×60μ Embryophore 18μ	Globular with a thick embryo (hexacanth embryo with 6 hooklets) inside it
COLOURED:		
Ascaris lumbricoides (fertilised)	40×70μ	Yellow, oval (fertilised) ova with thick mammillated capsule
Trichuris trichiura (whip worm)	25×50μ	Brown, thick-shelled, barrel-shaped, with a knob at either end
Hymenolepis dimeinuta	30×60μ Oncosphere 18μ	Brownish oncosphere, no filament

AP II

COMMON OVA OF HELMINTHS IN STOOLS

Eggs that Float on Saturated Solution of Common Salt

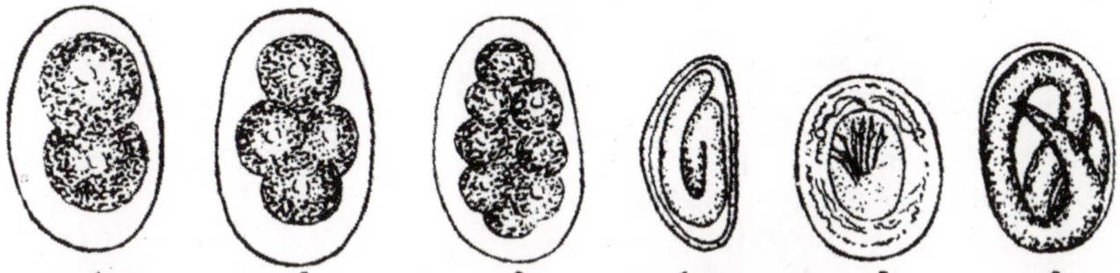

1 2 3 4 5 6

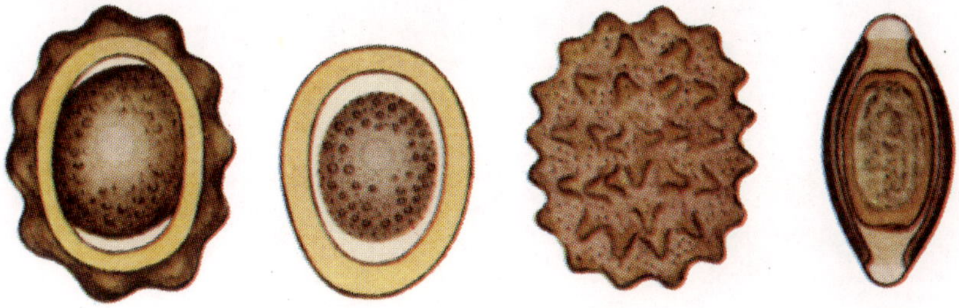

7a 7b 7c 8

Eggs that do not Float on Saturated Solution of Common Salt

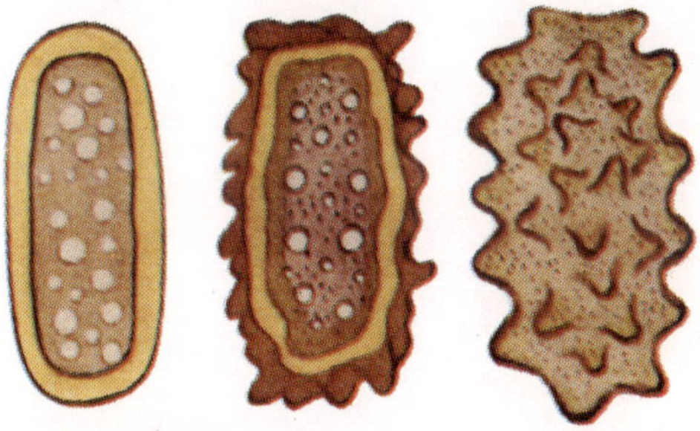

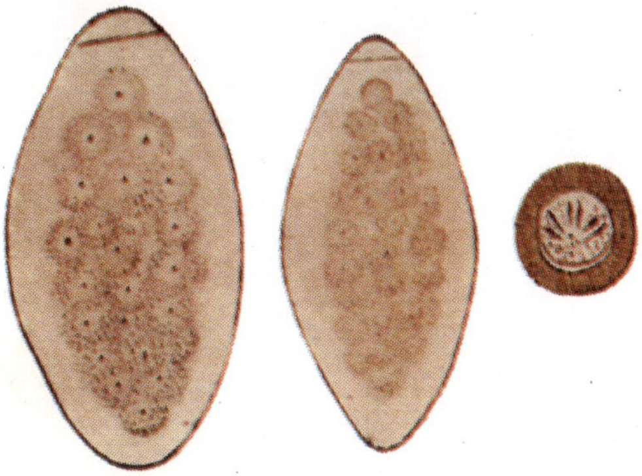

10 11 12

Figs. 1-3—Hookworm. Fig. 4—Oxyuris vermicularis. Fig. 5—Hymenolepis nana. Fig. 6—Strongyloides stercoralis. Fig. 7—Ascaris lumbricoides (fertilised), (a) with albuminous coat, (b) without albuminous coat, (c) surface view. Fig. 8—Trichuris trichiura. Fig. 9—Ascaris lumbricoides (unfertilised), (a) without albuminous coat, (b) optical section, (c) surface view. Fig. 10—Fasciolopsis buski. Fig. 11—Gastrodiscoides hominis. Fig. 12—Taenia.

TABLE AP. II—2

HELMINTHIC OVA THAT DO NOT FLOAT ON SATURATED SALT SOLUTION

ALL ARE COLOURED:		
Ascaris lumbricoides (unfertilised)	40 × 70μ	Yellow, elongated mammillated, thinner capsule and packed with refractile yolk globules; sometimes confused with vegetable cells
Taenia solium	30 × 38μ	Pale yellow with a thick radially striated embryophore with 6 hooklets
Taenia saginata	40 × 40μ	Indistinguishable from that of *T. solium*. Confused with pollen grains
Trematodes (All flukes)		Brown, operculated, oval

research work to give quantitative results for **hookworms, ascaris** and **trichuris ova**.

Caldwell and Caldwell (1926) used antiformin and sugar solutions instead of N/10 NaOH solution. The faeces was first disintegrated in antiformin and then a sugar solution (sp. gr. 1.23) was added to make a homogeneous suspension. Floatation technique was then employed.

EXAMINATION FOR OVA

Oxyuris vermicularis

Ova of *O. vermicularis* are very rarely seen in the faeces. They are usually found in the perianal region and a special N.I.H. swab is used for this purpose (National Institute of Health swab—Fig. Ap.3).

The swab consists of a glass rod about 10 cm long and 4 mm thick, held securedly in a test tube, closely by a perforated rubber stopper. One end of the rod passes through the perforation of the rubber stopper and the other end is covered by a piece of cellophane about one inch square, forming a swab and held by a rubber band.

Technique. The perianal and perineal folds are firmly scraped with the N.I.H. swab and the rod is replaced in the tube. The rubber band is cut at the time of examination and the piece of cellophane is spread on a slide with a few drops of sodium hydroxide solution or water. The cellophane is pressed with another slide or a heavy cover glass, and examined under the low power.

Scotch tape method (Graham, 1941, modified by Jacob, 1942; Beaver, 1949). It has proved better than N.I.H. swab. It consists of a strip of 3-4 inches (7.5-10 cm) by 3/4 inch (1.8 cm) transparent scotch tape with the sticky side out. It is pressed on the perianal skin on both sides pressing gently with the butt end of a test tube or rounded end of a wooden tongue depressor, before the patient has toiletted in the morning. The scotch tape is placed on a drop of toluene, with the sticky side down, on a microscopic slide. The eggs can be identified readily as refractile objects. Toluene displaces air bubbles, clearing epithelial cells and debris dissolving the adhesive material of the tape.

HATCHING TECHNIQUE

This is specially applicable to *Schistosoma mansoni* and *S. japonicum* ova in faeces; but in case of *S. haematobium*, ova in the urine are to be hatched. The method is highly efficient in discovering a very mild infection. The method is simple and no special apparatus is necessary. On the contrary, it is time-consuming, and infertile or degenerated ova often fail to hatch.

Technique. The faecal specimen is sedimented and the sediment is diluted with clear water and allowed to stand

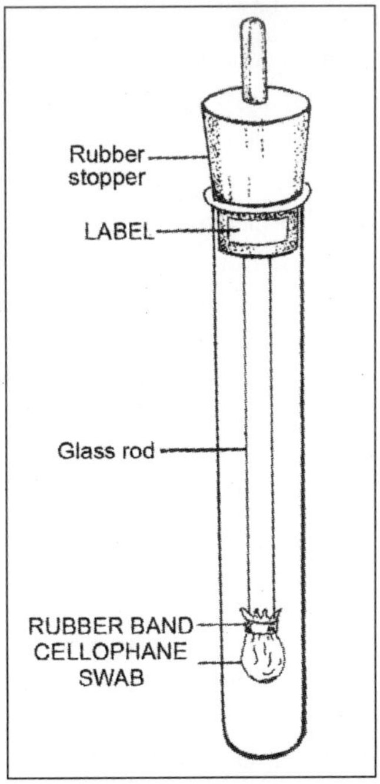

Fig. AP. 3—N. I. H. swab for collection of ova in *Oxyuris vermicularis* infection

for 1-24 hours. Free-swimming miracidia appear within a few cm from the surface of the water and may be examined with a hand lens. It should be noted that free-swimming ciliates and trematode larvae may contaminate stale water.

CULTURE METHOD OF OVA FROM STOOLS

This is primarily applicable in hookworm or Strongyloid larvae in faeces. The method is simple, but the disadvantage is that it is time consuming.

Technique. The specimen of faeces is either mixed with sterile sand or animal charcoal, and just sufficient water is added to give a soft consistency. The mixture is placed on a piece of moist filter paper on a Petri dish and covered. The water of condensation on the underside of the Petri dish is examined from time to time.

The technique is simple but satisfactory.

OTHER EXAMINATIONS

EXAMINATION OF SPUTUM

Sputum is primarily examined for: (i) trophozoite form of *E. histolytica*.

(ii) Ova of *Paragonimus westermani*.

(iii) Hydatid cyst of the lung that has suppurated, or in case of hydatid cyst of the liver that has burst into the lung or pleural cavity.

(iv) Larvae and adults of *S. stercoralis*, or rarely

(v) Larvae of Ascaris and hookworms.

(vi) Schistosoma ova may also occur in the sputum (Silveria, 1944).

Direct smear. The method is:

The mouth is rinsed out thoroughly with H_2O_2 and the patient is asked to cough out sputum from lower respiratory passage in a Petri dish or a cup. A coverslip preparation specially from 'iron brown specks' is examined microscopically, which may be ova of **lung fluke**. In suspected **hydatid cyst**, Best's carmine is recommended to differentiate the smaller fragments.

Concentration by centrifugation. This is specially applicable to lung fluke ova. When the sputum is thick, an equal volume of 3 percent sodium hydroxide is added to dissolve the mucus. After about 10 minutes, centrifuge and decant the SNF. The sediment is now examined microscopically.

Preservation of ova. Ova of lung fluke are preserved in a solution of 5 parts of glycerine, 1 part of phenol and 94 parts of water.

EXAMINATION OF URINE

Urine is primarily examined for:

(i) Ova of *S. haematobium*.

(ii) Microfilaria of *W. bancrofti*.

(iii) Larvae of *S. stercoralis*.

(iv) Rarely ova of *Dictophyma renale*, the dog kidney worm and rare parasite of man. They are passed in the urine.

Sedimentation. A coverslip preparation is made from the sediment and examined for the detection of ova of *S. haematobium*.

Centrifugation. It is useful in the detection of ova of *S. haematobium*, microfilaria of *W. bancrofti* and larvae of *S. stercoralis*.

IMMUNOLOGICAL TESTS FOR HELMINTHIC DISEASES

These tests are based on the antigen-antibody reactions. They are applicable when diagnosis by other methods is impossible at certain stage of the disease and worm causes severe tissue damages, e.g., schistosomiasis, paragonimiasis, echinococcosis, cysticercosis, trichinosis, and, filariasis. The reactions are often group reactions and therefore, require careful interpretation. The tests include *intradermal* (allergic), *precipitin* and *complement fixation tests*. These are stated disease-wise.

Tests for Schistosomiasis

Euglobulin precipitation test. See Sia's test in AP. I. **Intradermal test**. The antigen is a saline extract of triturated worm of heavily infected snail liver. The test is of value in the diagnosis, and the reaction remains positive after treatment. The *complement fixation test* and other tests are described in Text chapter.

Tests for Paragonimiasis

The antigen is derived from *P. westermani* adults, macerated in physiological saline. **Complement fixation test** is of value when the eggs are not passed in the sputum or faeces, and help in detecting cerebral or abdominal cases.

Tests for Echinococcosis

Intradermal test (Casoni) is very useful (see Text chapter).

The antigen is the clear, sterile hydatid fluid from the cyst in sheep or other hosts. Antigen by Dennis method (1937) is probably the most potent one. The test is of value in echinococcosis, specially prior to operation.

Complement fixation test. Purified powdered antigen by Dennis technique is used. This is diluted 1:5,000 and used as in Kolmer's modification of Wassermann test. The test is of value in old complicated cases; otherwise intradermal Casoni's test is superior.

Precipitin test. It closely parallels the complement fixation test. In this test, fresh hydatid fluid is collected aseptically from infected sheep and the fluid may be used fresh or preserved in 0.05 percent phenol to keep it stable for several months.

Add 0.4 ml of patient's fresh serum to an equal volume of antigen in a small agglutination tube and allow to stand for 36 hours at room temperature. In a serum with high precipitin (e.g., serum globulin), the reaction occurs in 2-3 hours. According to the thickness of the precipitin, the reaction is called +++, ++ or +; in the last case, only microscopic granules are seen.

TESTS FOR *CYSTICERCUS CELLULOSAE*

Haemagglutination test (see Text chapter). The antigen consists of fluid from cysticercus larvae of various domestic animals.

The **intradermal test** is carried out with this antigen. The test is of value in suspected cases but not as valuable as Casoni's test in echinococcosis.

Precipitin test. The same antigen is used in this test. The test is of value in confirming the diagnosis made by the intradermal test.

TESTS FOR TRICHINOSIS

Intradermal test. The antigen is prepared from laboratory rats infected with trichinella larvae, ground in distilled water, dried and reground. The test is of value after 21 days of infection, but **very heavy or very light infections may be missed**. False positive nonspecific reaction may occur also. The test remains positive for years after recovery from an acute attack.

Precipitin reaction. It is positive with the same antigen 4 weeks after the infection, and is almost of the same specificity as the intradermal test.

TESTS FOR FILARIASIS

Intradermal test. The antigen is prepared from *Dirofilaria immitis*, the dog filaria. Washed, dried, lipoid-free worms are ground into fine powder. But antigen prepared from the microfilaria of *W. bancrofti* are more specific though it is difficult to collect them. The test is of special value in detection of Wuchereria infection, before microfilaria are present in the peripheral blood, or in light infection, in which embryos may not be found in blood.

Complement fixation test. Van Hoof (1934) obtained complement fixation reaction in patients having *Onchocerca volvulus* in Africa and in Guatemala. Bozicevich *et al*, (1947) found *O. volvulus* antigen to be more sensitive than antigen prepared from other species.

An alcoholic antigen from trichinised flesh gives a negative result. Stroebel (1911) prepared antigen by digestion of muscle with caustic soda and antiformin, and neutralised by HCl. This may remain potent if kept in the ice chest. Bachman (1929), using antigen for precipitin reaction, got specific reaction after twentyfifth day in inoculated animals.

Precipitin test. The test has not been explored in cases of human filariasis.

FASCIOLA HEPATICA

Kellaway (1928) obtained a "true anaphylactic antigen" in saline extract of the worm and an absolute alcohol-soluble antigen for **complement fixation test**. The latter test is not reliable as uninfected sheep often give as high a percentage as the known positive ones.

IMPORTANT POINTS TO KNOW ABOUT HELMINTHS

HELMINTHIC PARASITES FOUND IN TISSUE AND OTHER ORGANS (somatic)

Somatic Cestodes (TAPEWORM):

Larval stage of—

1. *Echinococcus granulosus* (*Taenia granulosa*) producing hydatid cyst.
2. *Taenia solium* (*Cysticerus cellulosae*—larval form only).
3. *Taenia saginata* (*Cysticercus bovis*—larval form only).
4. *Sparganum mansoni* (Plerocercoid).

Somatic Trematodes (FLUKES):

1 *Paragonimus westermani*—(lung fluke).
2. *Clonorchis sinensis* (*Clonorchis endemicus*).
3. *Fasciola hepatiça*—(liver flukes).

Somatic Nematodes:

1. *Gnathostoma spinigerum*.
2. *Dracunculus medinensis*.
3. Filariae—(a) *W. bancrofti, B. malayi.* (b) *Loa loa.* (c) *Acanthocheilonema perstans.* (d) *Onchocerca volvulus.* (e) *Mansonella ozzardi.*
4. Larval forms of *Trichinella spiralis.*

HELMINTHS THAT GAIN ENTRANCE TO THE HUMAN BODY BY PENETRATING THE SKIN

Trematodes (Cercariae of blood flukes).

Schistosoma haematobium, S. mansoni, S. japonicum piercing the unbroken skin of man.

Nematodes. *Ancylostoma duodenale* (larva), *Nevatar americanus* (larva), *Strongyloides stercoralis* (larva).

Wuchereria bancrofti, B. malayi, Loa loa, Acanthocheilonema perstans. (Infective microfilaria by insect bite).

HELMINTHIC PARASITES WHICH INFECT BY ORAL ROUTE

Cestodes: (1) *T. solium*—By ingestion of measly pork (*CYsticercus cellulosae*).

(2) *T. saginata*—By ingestion of infected beef (*Cysticercus bovis*).

(3) *D. latum*—Ingestion of fish containing plerocercoid larva.

(4) *E. granulosus*—Ingestion of onchospheres passed by a dog (definitive host); produces hydatid cyst in man.

(5) *H. nana*—Ingestion of onchospheres in contaminated food particles or accidental ingestion of rat flea containing cysticercoid.

Trematodes

1. *Clonorchis sinensis*—Ingestion of encysted cercariae (metacercariae) in fish (Liver fluke).

2. *Fasciola hepatica*—Ingestion of encysted cercariae in aquatic plants (Liver fluke).

3. *Fasciolopsis buski*—Ingestion of encysted cercariae on aquatic plants (Intestinal fluke).

4. *Paragonimus westermani*—Ingestion of raw crabs or cray-fish.

5. *Echinostoma ilocanum*—Ingestion of metacercariae in snail flesh.

6. *Gastrodiscoides hominis*.

Nematodes. (1) *Ascaris lumbricoides*—Food or water, contaminated by an egg containing larva.

(2) *Oxyuris vermicularis*—same as (1).

(3) *Trichuris trichiura*—same as (1).

(4) *Trichinella spiralis*—Infected pork containing encysted larva.

(5) *Dracunculus medinensis*—by ingestion of cyclops by drinking infected water.

Appendix III

TREATMENT OF PARASITIC INFECTIONS

AMOEBICIDAL DRUGS

A. **Intestinal (luminal) Amoebicides**

They act on both trophozoites and cysts of *E. histolytica* in the intestine.

I. HALOGENATED HYDROXYQUINOLINES. Amoebicidal action depends upon their high iodine content. They are:

1. **Di-iodohydroxyquinoline** (Diodoquin, Embequin): It is effective in symptomless carriers and cyst-passers. The adult dose is 1-2 tablets thrice a day for 21 days.

2. **Iodochloro-hydroxyquinoline**: Clioquinol (enterovioform). The adult dosage is 2 to 3 tablets of 0.25 g each, for 10 days. Effective in cases of amoebic dysentery and in cyst-passers.

II. DICHLORACETAMIDE GROUP

Chlorophenoxamide (Mebinol). The adult dose is 1.5 g by mouth daily in 3 divided doses for 10 days.

III. DILOXANIDE (ENTAMIDE) FUROATE (**Furamide**, Boots). The adult dose is one tablet 3 times a day for 10 days. It is effective against intestinal amoebiasis and cyst-passers.

IV. CHLORBETAMIDE (**Mantomide**): Adult dose is 250 mg three times daily, administered orally for 10 days.

V. PENTAVALENT ARSENICALS. It is administered orally, in cases of chronic amoebiasis.

1. **Milibis** (Bismuth glycollylarsanilate). The adult dose is one tablet (250 mg) 2 to 3 times daily for 7 days.

2. **Stovarsol** (Acetarsol). The adult dose is 0.25 g (4 grs) tablet orally once or twice daily for 7 to 10 days.

3. **Carbarsone**. The dose is the same as stovarsol.

4. **Difetarsone**. The adult dose is 0.5 g tablet, twice daily for 5 to 10 days.

VI. ANTIBIOTICS **Paromomycin** (Humatin, Parke-Davis). The adult dose is 5 capsules daily for 5 days, totalling 6,250 mg. The dose is calculated as 20 mg/kg body weight.

VII. INDIRECTLY-ACTING AMOEBICIDES. They reduce the intestinal bacterial flora, upon which *E. histolytica* is dependent for its growth. They are **Broad spectrum group of antibiotics** and used orally in amoebiasis. They are merely adjuvant drugs but not specific.

B. **Tissue Amoebicides**

(a) Acting on the trophozoites of *E. histolytica* in the intestinal wall, liver and other metastatic sites. **Emetine** and dehydroemetine (DHE). (b) Acting on the trophozoites of *E. histolytica* specifically in the liver. It is a **4-aminoquinoline** (chloroquine).

Emetine hydrochloride. It is the principal alkaloid obtained from the ipecacuanha root (*Cephaelis ipecacuanha*). For details, see treatment of amoebiasis (Text chapter).

Chloroquine. It is an antimalarial drug as well. It is effective against hepatic and pulmonary amoebiasis. For details see treatment of amoebiasis.

Chloroquine is effective in clonorchiasis paragonimiasis, taeniasis, giardiasis, amoebiasis and malaria.

C. **Both Luminal and Tissue Amoebicides**

I. NITROTHIAZOLE GROUP

Niridazole ("ambilhar"). It is a powerful oral amoebicide, effective against both intestinal and tissue-invading Entamoeba. It is not recommended because of its severe side-effects.

II. **Metronidazole group (Flagyl**, Klont, etc.). It is administered orally in doses of 800 mg thrice daily for 5 days (the dose is higher than in giardiasis). The tongue is heavily coated, and the drug offers a metallic taste, which when indicates the effectiveness of the drug. For other details, see respective chapters.

III. **Tinidazole:** PO; 2g once daily for 3 days (children 30-50 mg/kg/day) or 0.6 g twice daily for 5-10 days.

TREATMENT OF AMOEBIASIS

1. **For Intestinal Amoebiasis**

(i) **For cyst-passers** (symptomatic or asymptomatic), contact amoebicides are used, e.g., either entamide furoate, metronidazole, diadoquin, emetine bismuth iodide, paromomycin, or milibis are advocated.

(ii) **For acute amoebic dysentery**, intramuscular emetine for 3-4 days is used. Antibiotics are also given to reduce the intestinal bacterial flora. **Metronidazole** alone may be used.

(iii) **For mild attack of amoebic dysentery**, contact amoebicides di-iodoquin with antibiotic (broad spectrum) is usually given. Chloroquine may be given in addition to protect the liver and to eradicate subclinical amoebic hepatitis. However, **metronidazole** alone is also effective.

2. **For Amoebic Hepatitis** (liver abscess)

Emetine (60 mg) or DHE intramuscularly for 6 to 10 injections, or chloroquine for 21 days is given. Following this, entamide furoate or diodoquine, is given to eradicate the trophozoites and cysts from the intestine. Alternatively, metronidazole alone may be given.

DRUGS FOR GIARDIASIS AND OTHER ANTRAL AND INTESTINAL FLAGELLATES

Giardiasis:

Tinidazole: PO; 2 g as single drop or 0.6 g once daily for 7 days.

IMIDAZOLE GROUP

Metronidazole (Flagyl). the usual adult dose is 200 mg thrice daily for 7 days.

9-AMINOACRIDINE DERIVATIVE

Atebrin, or mepacrine methane sulphonate. For adults, one tablet (0.1 g) thrice daily for 3 to 5 days, and half a tablet twice daily for 3 days for children is given.

4-AMINOQUINOLINE DERIVATIVE

Chloroquine. For adults, 300 mg base, (1½) tablet given orally, once daily for 5 days.

8-AMINOQUINOLINE DERIVATIVE

Camoquine. 2-3 tablets; a single dose therapy is quite effective.

For kala-azar

Sodim stibogluconate: 20 mg/kg (max 850 mg) daily by IM (in buttocks) for 20-30 days or more.

LEISHMANICIDAL DRUGS

(Drugs acting in Kala-azar)

Antimonial group: Pentavalent antimonials are the drugs of choice. Trivalent antimonials are not used at present.

1. **Urea Stibamine** (Stiburea), a compound of urea and stibamine (sodium para-aminophenyl stibinate). It is made soluble in cold redistilled (double glass-distilled) water. The adult dose commences from 0.05 g (50 mg) increasing by doses of 0.05 g, till it reaches 0.2 g, which is the maximum dose. Injections are given *intravenously* twice or thrice weekly. The course of treatment is 12 to 15 injections. Average total dose is 3 g.

2. **Neostibosan** (para-aminophenylstibinate or stiburea of diethylamine). The adult daily dose is 0.1 to 0.3 g either intravenously (5 percent solution) or intramuscularly (25 percent solution). The course of treatment consists of 8 to 12 injections. A total of 2.7 to 4 g of the compound is effective, varying with different endemic areas.

3. **Sodium Antimony** or **Stibo-gluconate** (*Pentahexonate*). It is available as 20 mg, 40 mg and 100 mg of antimony per ml intramuscular injection. This salt is the least toxic. So higher daily doses can be given. On average, 6 to 8 g of antimony is required to sterilise an adult patient.

NON-METALLIC (AROMATIC DIAMIDINE) GROUP is used in antimonial-resistant cases.

1. **Pentamidine Isethionate** The drug is given, as a 10 percent solution by intramuscular injection which is preferred, and as a 1 percent solution by intravenous injection. The average individual dose, irrespective of age, is 4 mg/kg body weight. The initial adult dose is 100 to 200 mg. A course of 12 to 15 injections are given, 1 each daily, or on alternate days. A second course after an interval of 10 to 15 days may be required. This drug is indicated in combined infection.

2. **Stibamidine**, or 3 Diamino-diphenoxypentane offers more promising results than Pentamidine isothionate (see text in chemotherapy of kala-azar).

For *Oriental sore* and *Espundia*, Pentavalent antimony preparations are the drugs of choice. In antimonial-resistant cases of espundia, **pyrimethamine** and **amphotericin B** is given. The former is given in 3 courses with a rest period of 8 days amongst the courses. For the first 2 courses, in each course, 50 mg orally is given daily for 10 days, while 25 mg is given daily for 10 days in the last course. Folic acid must be given during the course.

In exclusive skin lesions, a single intramuscular injection of **cycloguanil pamoate** in the dose of 5 mg base/kg body weight is effective. It is also an antimalarial drug.

TRYPANOCIDAL DRUGS

(For African Trypanosomiasis)

Suramin (*Antrypol Naphuride sodium, Bayer* "205" or *Germanin*). See treatment of of *Trypanosoma gambiense* and *T. rhodesiense*—Text chapter.

Pentamidine isethionate (see chemotherapy of kala-azar and treatment of African trypanosomiasis).

Tryparsamide see Text chapter.

Melarsoprol (Mel. B) A compound of melarsen oxide and BAL (dimercaprol), contains trivalent arsenic. It is very effective both in "gambian" and "rhodesian" sleeping sickness when the central nervous system is involved. The maximum adult dose is 3.6 mg per kg body weight, given intravenously on each 4 consecutive days. A period of rest is given for one week. A second course is given thereafter. It is effective in resistant cases with high toxicity. The main toxic effect is arsenical **encephalopathy**.

Mel. W. It belongs to melaminyl compound of trivalent arsenicals and is actually a water soluble Mel B. It has the advantage to be administered intramuscularly. The dose is same as Mel B.

MSb. & MSb. B. see Text chapter.

Nitrofurazone (Furacin); see also Text chapter. The children dose is 30 mg per kg body weight (Fierlafyn, 1960). The drug is effective in resistant cases. Side-effect seen in most cases are weight loss, urticarial rash and severe haemolytic anaemia in G-6-PD deficient individuals, polyneuritis and disorders of pyruvate metabolism. *Furacin* has lately been introduced in the treatment of *T. cruzi* infection (Chagas' disease).

8-AMINOQUINOLINES like **pentaquine** and **primaquine** are effective in experimental infections.

ANTIMALARIAL DRUGS

Malaria: (Except resistant *P. falciparum*)

Treatment (Adult)

Chloroquine: PO; 600 mg stat followed by 300 mg after 8 hrs and 300 mg daily for next two days.

Children: PO; 10 mg/kg stat, 5 mg/kg after 6 hrs then 5 mg/kg/day for 3 days.

Prophylaxis of Malaria: Chloroquine, PO; 300 mg once weekly (same day each week). Start-2 weeks before entering an endemic arae & continue for 4 weeks after leaving.

For radical cure of relapsing malaria (*P. vivax/P. ovale*)

Primaquine (as base): PO; 15 mg (children 0.25 mg/kg, daily for 14 days along with the standard chloroquine treatment.

Chloroquine resistant Malaria (eq. *P. falciparum*): PO; (sulfadoxine 1500 mg + pyrimethamine 75 mg) single dose)

Children (as single dose): 9-14 yrs: (sulfadoxine 1000 mg + pyrimethanine 50 mg).

4-8 yrs: (sulfadoxnine 500 mg + pyrinethanene 25 mg)

1-4 yrs: (sulfadoxnine 250 mg + pyrimethamine 12.5 mg).

Quinine. At present, it is chiefly used for the treatment of any drug-resistant *P. falciparum* infection. It is a **schizonticidal** drug acting in the young trophozoite (ring) form. The standard adult dose is (1) 650 mg of the salt (sulphate or bihydrochloride), 3 times daily after food for 10-14 days, or (2) 325 mg in 1-5 ml given by deep intramuscular injection in the gluteus at an interval of 15 days, a total of 2 injections.

Caution. Glucocorticoids (**Betnesol** or **Decadron**) injection should be ready at hand before intravenous quinine administration for drug shock and toxicity. It is also a wisdom to administer corticosteroid especially in *P. falciparum* infection to avoid the development of hypersensitive state or Blackwater fever.

9-AMINOACRIDINE DERIVATIVE, **Mepacrine** (*Atebrin, Quinacrine*). It is rarely used. An initial loading dose of 0.1 g to 0.3 may be given. The dose is 0.1 g thrice daily for 5 days.

4-AMINOQUINOLINE DERIVATIVE. 1. **Chloroquine**. This is the drug of choice for acute attack. It is a potent **schizonticidal** drug and also acts on the trophozoite ring form. It acts by damaging the lysosome and inhibiting the nucleic acid synthesis of the parasite. The adult dose is 2 tablets stat, then 1 tablet 4 times daily on the first 24 hours. Subsequently, 1 tablet on two consecutive days. To prevent endogenous recrudescense in *P. falciparum* infection (see text on malaria), 1 tablet daily for 4 to 8 weeks should be continued.

As a *suppressive therapy*, one tablet once a week is given to an adult.

2. **Amodiaquine** (*Camoquin, Cam-aqi*, etc.). The adult oral dose is 0.6 g base stat, and then 0.4 g base daily for 2 days. For mass treatment in endemic areas, a single dose of 0.6 g base is effective. As *suppressive therapy* in adults, 0.4 g base once a week is recommended.

8-AMINOQUINOLINE DERIVATIVES

Pamaquine (*Plasmoquine, Plasmochin*), **Primaquine phosphate**. It is both **schizonticidal** and **gametocidal** in its action in all types of malaria infections. Tablets of 7.5 mg or 15.0 mg of the base are available. The adult dose is 15 mg per oral daily in single or divided doses for 10 to 14 days with an interval of 3 to 7 days after the first of 7 days. The patient should be at rest in bed and plenty of fluid should be given.

Caution: This drug is contraindicated in children.

DIHYDROFOLATE REDUCTASE INHIBITORS

1. **Proguanil (Chlorguanide)**. It is a *biguanide* derivative having no antifolate or toxic activity. It is available as tablets of 0.01 g (100 mg) or 0.3 g of proguanil hydrochloride (*paludrine*). It is not a drug of choice as the parasite readily acquires resistance.

2. **Cycloguanil Pamoate** or Embonate (Camolar). It is a long-acting injectable antimalarial prophylactic, given intramuscularly. A single injection in oily suspension of 5 mg base/kg body weight (standard dose: 350 mg) offers long term **protection** for 3-6 months. Plasmodium may develop following its use. To avoid acquiring resistance, it is better to use the drug with sulphone group of drugs (DDS, see later).

3. **Pyrimethamine (Daraprim)**. It is a slow **schizonticidal** drug. It is not a drug of choice, as it may cause blood dyscrasia (megaloblastic or macrocytic anaemia).

PYRIMIDINE DERIVATIVE

Trimethoprim. This drug has the advantage that a single dose of 500 mg of it with sulphalene 750 mg is very effective in chloroquine-resistant *P. falciparum* infections. It works synergistically with sulphalene.

Sulphonamides (sulphadoxine or Fanasil). They are slow **schizonticidal** drugs and potentiate the other antimalarials when used together.

Dapsone. (Diamino-diphenyl sulphone (DDS) group. It is a substantial **schizonticidal** drug. This drug is used in combination with cytoguanil pamoate as a suppressive therapy only (see before). It is valuable only in combination with other drug (pyrimethamine) and is used as a suppressive therapy but not for treatment.

CHEMOTHERAPY AND CHEMOPROPHYLAXIS OF MALARIA

It is an extraadvantage to know the "immunity" status of the patient determined. For the treatment of non-immune cases, i.e., those with a recent history of exposure to infection should be given a standard **schizonticidal** drug, like **chloroquine** for clinical cure. For radical cure* of *P. vivax*, *P. malariae* and *P. ovale* infections, **primaquine** should be used concurrently, or after the clinical cure. *P. falciparum* infections are dangerous for the non-immune subjects and should be promptly treated. Primaquine is not indicated in *P. falciparum* infection as relapse does not occur. But to prevent endogenous recrudescence, chloroquine should be continued for some time (chloroquine base 300 mg or 2 tablets once a week for a month).

For the treatment of immune cases (those who are exposed to continuous and repeated infections), oral **schizonticides** are given only once a week, which usually suffice. A complete eradication of erythrocytic (E) phase may not be required, as the basis of immunity depends upon the E phase of the parasite.

DRUG-RESISTANT PLASMODIA

Cestodes

- **T. saginata, T. solium, D. latum** Praziquantel: 5-10 mg/kg as single dose.
- **H. nana** Praziquantel: A single dose of 25 mg/kg and repeated in one week.
- **Cysticercosis** Albendazole: 400 mg twice daily for upto 21 days.
- **Hydatid disease:** Albendazole: 400 mg twice daily with meals for one month or longer.

* Radical cure with primaquine is best to prevent relapses, so long the patient leaves the endemic area. While, it is of no use if he remains in the endemic area.

The drug resistance to plasmodia means failure of a particular schizonticidal drug of its proved efficient standard to act in normal or high therapeutic dose even after its total absorption, and still allowing survival and multiplicity of the parasite *in vivo*. The drug resistance of plasmodia may be of different grades as (WHO 1968):

Grade 1 (R_1^* level)—Asexual parasites in blood are cleared but recrudescence follows.

Grade 2 (R_2^* level)—Asexual parasites in blood are not cleared but markedly reduced.

Grade 3 (R_3^* level)—Asexual parasites in blood are not markedly reduced.

The drug resistance of plasmodia is chiefly restricted to *P. falciparum* infection only.

DISCRETE CHOICE OF ANTIMALARIALS

1. For **prophylactic** use only: Tablet of Pyrimethamine 12.5 mg and Dapsone (Maloprim, Burroughs Wellcome) 2 tablets (100 mg) one week before exposure (entering an endemic area), and then 1 tablet once a week.

2. For both **prophylaxis** and **treatment**—Tablet of pyrimethamine 15 mg and chloroquine 150 mg base (Darachlor, B. W.), 1-2 tablets once a week.

3. For **treatment** only—Tablet of Pyrimethamine (25 mg) and sulphadoxine 500 mg (Fansidar, Roche), 2 to 3 tablets as a single dose.

DRUGS FOR BALANTIDIASIS

(Balantidicides)

Oxytetracycline. For adults Terramycin (Pfizer) orally 6-hourly, for a period of 7 to 10 days.

In tetracycline sensitive persons, other broad spectrum antibiotics can be given.

Carbarsone and **Diocloquin**. They are administered orally in the same doses as given in intestinal amoebiasis (see before).

ANTHELMINTICS FOR INTESTINAL CESTODES (TAENIACIDES)

Cardol or **Cashew-nut shell extract**. See treatment of hymenolepiasis (see Text chapter).

Male Fern (*Filix mas*). The anthelmintic principle is filicic acid or filicin, a polyhydric phenol.

Anthelmintic effect. It is effective against intestinal cestodes, like *Diphyllobothrium latum*, *Taenia saginata* and *Taenia solium*. It acts by paralysing the muscles of the parasite (For details see CH. on *Taenia solium*).

Mepacrine hydrochloride (*Atebrin, quinacrine*): (see *Taenia solium*).

* R—stands for "Resistance".

An intramuscular injection of 0.5 ml pituitrin, 1 to 1½ hours after mepacrine administration, helps to expel the taenia, whose hold has been loosened (For details see treatment of *T. solium* infection).

Dichlorophen (*Anthiphen*, M. & B.).

See treatment of *Taenia solium* and *T. saginata*.

Niclosamide (Yomesan). It is a salicylamide derivative which is found to be an excellent cestoidicidal drug. It is available as 0.5 g tablets. The drug is well-tolerated. *Doses*. Above 5 years, 2 g, and for small children 1.5 g. The adult dose is 10 tablets (single dose). It has some action on *H. nana* and *O. vermicularis*.

Both dichlorophen and niclosamide are not recommended in taenia infections as the destruction of segments releases viable ova, which may cause cysticercosis.

TREMATOCIDAL DRUGS

SCHISTOSOMICIDAL DRUGS

(Haemotrematocides)

Trematodes

- **S. mansoni/S. haematobium** Praziquantel: 20 mg/kg for two doses at interval of 4-6 hrs.
- **S. Japonicum, S mekongi** Praziquantel: 20 mg/kg for three doses at interval of 4-6 hrs.
- **Choroorchiasis, Paragonimiasis** Praziquantel: 20 mg/kg thrice daily for 1-2 days.

ANTIMONIALS (TRIVALENT)

Tartar emetic (Sodium antimonyl tartrate). Administered intravenously as 1 percent solution in normal saline, or 5 percent glucose solution thrice weekly, in increasing doses to adults as follows: 4 ml, 6 ml, 8 ml, 10 ml, and 12 ml; the last dose being repeated up to a total of 160 ml or 1.6 g of the drug equivalent to 0.576 g of antimony (a freshly prepared solution should always be used). The first course of the treatment should cover a period of 4 weeks. A second course may be given, after an interval of a few weeks.

The pentavalent antimonials are not effective.

Anthiomaline. Administered intravenously (see Text chapter).

"**TWSb**" (antimony dimercaptosuccinate). It is a polyvalent schistosomicide and is a drug of choice (see treatment of *Schistosoma haematobium*).

Nilodin (Miracil D). (For details see treatment of *Schistosoma haematobium*).

Hycanthone (Etrenol). It is a derivative of *leucanthone*; given as a single intramuscular injection in a dose of 3-3.5 mg/kg body weight. It is an efficient drug for vesicle schistosomiasis (*S. haematobium*), but is not used for its *teratogenic effect* in pregnant mice.

SYNTHETIC EMETINE

Dehydro-emetine (DHE). It has lately been used for vesicle *schistosomiasis*. It is given intravenously to adults, in doses of 100 mg (1.5 mg per kg body weight) daily for 10 days.

NITROTHIAZOLE COMPOUND

Niridazole ("Ambilhar"). It is an effective schistosomicidal drug, but less so in *S. japonica* infections. It is administered orally, in *doses* of 25 mg/kg body weight in 2 or 3 doses for 5 or 7 days. A second course may be given 6-12 months after the first course to patients who are not cured.

ANTHELMINTICS FOR INTESTINAL TREMATODES

FOR ECHINOSTOMATOSIS

Oleoresin of **aspidium** and **tetrachlorethylene** (see Text chapter).

FOR FASCIOLOPSIASIS (*F. buski*)

Tetrachlorethylene, hexylresorcinol and **thymol** are used (see under anthelmintics for intestinal nematodes, later).

FOR GASTRODISCOIDOSIS (*G. hominis*)

1. Hexylresorcinol—usual dose (see hookworm disease, treatment).
2. Tetrachlorethylene—usual dose.

FOR HETEROPHYIASIS (*H. heterophyes*)

1. **Tetrachlorethylene** and
2. **Piperazine** salts are used (see anthelmintics for intestinal nematodes).
3. **Bephenium hydroxynaphthoate** may be used.
4. **Hexylresorcinol** can be used.

FOR METAGONIMIASIS (*M. yokogowi*)

Treatment is same as for heterophyiasis.

TISSUE TREMATOCIDES

(Histotrematocides)

DRUGS FOR FASCIOLIASIS (*F. hepatica*)

1. **Emetine**. The adult dose is 400 mg daily as intramuscular injections till a total of 5 mgm/kg body weight is given.
2. **Bithionol** See treatment of paragonimiasis (see later).

DRUGS FOR CLONORCHIASIS

- **Clonoorchiasis, Paragonimiasis** praziquantel: 25 mg/kg thrice daily for 1-2 days.

1. ANTIMONY COMPOUNDS. (a) **Sodium antimonyl tartrate**. (b) **Tartar emetic**. (c) **Fouadin**. All these are ef-

fective in reducing the "worm load" from the biliary passages and egg-output in the faeces.

2. **Bithionol** (see treatment of Paragonimiasis, later).

3. 4-AMINOQUINOLINE DERIVATIVE: **Chloroquine**. This may be in massive doses of 10.4 mg per kg body weight for as long as 39 days. The total amount may vary from 19.5 to 39.0 g.

4. **Dithiazanine Iodide**. See Text chapter.

5. **Gentian violet** in keratin-coated pills is curative in early cases in an adult dose of 60 mg thrice daily before meals for 1 month. It may be injected intravenously, every third day, until a total of 6 gm.

6. Hetol (1, 4-Bis-trichloromethylbenzol). See Text chapter.

7. **Hexachlorethane**. See Text chapter.

8. **Hexachloroparaxylol**. See Text chapter.

DRUGS FOR OPISTHORCHIASIS

Hetol. See clonorchiasis.

DRUGS FOR PARAGONIMIASIS (see clorosechiasis)

1. **Bithionol** (*Actamer, Bitin*). It is a dichlorophenol derivative. The adult dose is 30-50 mg per kg body weight per day in 3 divided doses orally on alternate days for 10 to 15 days. It is effective in fascioliasis and clonorchiasis as well.

2. **Chloroquine**. It is administered in adult doses of 250 mg twice daily for two months. This is effective in improving the clinical condition and diminishing the 'ova load' in the sputum.

3. **Emetine hydrochloride**. The adult dose is 65 mg intramuscularly for 10 to 12 days. It is effective in reducing the infection.

4. **Sulphonamides**. When given with emetine, it reduces "ova load" from the lung rapidly.

ANTHELMINTICS FOR INTESTINAL NEMATODES

Anthelmintics

• **T. spiralis:** Albendazole: 400 mg twice daily for 1-2 week.

• **T. trichura:** Mebendazole: PO; 100 mg twice a day for 3 consecutive days.

Children: Above 2 yrs; dose & duration same as that of adult 1-2 yrs: Half dose of adult.

• **S. stercoralis:** Ivermectin: PO; 0.15-0.2 mg/kg as single dose.

• **Round worm:** Albendazole: Single dose of 400 mg in adult & children above 2 yrs.

Pyrantel pamoate: Single dose of 10 mg/kg.

• **Pin worm:** Albendazole: A single dose of 400 mg & repeated in 2 weeks.

• **D. medinensis:** Metronidazole: PO; 200-400 mg thrice daily for 7 days.

• **Gnathostoma spiniqera** (Gnathostomiasis): Albendazole 400 mg twice daily for 3 weeks.

• **Dryptosporidiosis:** Albendazole: PO; 400 mg twice daily for 2-4 weeks.

• **Microsporidia:** Albendazole: 400 mg twice daily for 2-4 weeks.

Bephenium Hydroxynaphthoate (Ancopar, B. W. & Co.) It is effective against **ascariasis** and **hookworm infection** (acts better in *A. duodenale* than in *N. americanus*). For details, see respective Chapters.

Cardol or **Cashewnut shell extract**. See treatment of hookworm disease in respective chapter.

Difetarsone. It is an oral pentavalent organic arsenical compound and is used as a contact amoebicide. Issued as 0.5 g tablet. Adult dose is 2 tablets twice daily with food for 5 to 10 days. It is used in **trichuriasis** with 81-88% cure rate.

Hexylresorcinol B.P. ("Caprokol" or "Hexylresorcinol crystalloids").

It has a true **vermicide effect** against *Ascaris lumbricoides*, *F. buski* and **hookworm** (more effective against *N. americanus* than *A. duodenale*). For details see respective chapters.

Mebendazole (R-17,635). The adult dose is 200 mg (2 tablets) orally, twice daily for 4 days. The drug has a polyvalent therapeutic action and is claimed to be one of the best drugs for the treatment of **all common helminthic infections** including **strongyloidosis, trichuriasis**, etc.

OIL OF CHENOPODIUM

It is effective in Ascariasis and Hookworm infections (see CH. on Hookworm).

Piperazine Salts (Antepar, B.W. ; Helmacid, Glaxo) (adipate, citrate, or phoshate).

It is effective against **oxyuriasis** and **ascariasis**. They have some effect on **Trichuris** and **Heterophyiasis**. No preliminary treatment and no "follow up" measures necessary. For details see treatment in respective Chapters.

Pyrantel pamoate or embonate (Combantrin, Pfeizer). A useful broad spectrum anthelmintic. *Adult dose* is 10 mg (base)/kg body weight, given as a single dose (or for 2 consecutive days) after breakfast in a suspension or chewable tablets. Others have recommended 20 mg base/

kg body weight. A purgative is given 3 hours after the drug and stools examined for expelled worms up to 48 hours. Tolerance is excellent and side-effects are absent. It is an excellent drug in *Oxyuriasis* and *Ascariasis* and also effective in hookworm and *Trichostrongylus orientalis* infections.

Pyrivinium pamoate (Vanquin, Poquil or Povan) It is a red cyanine dye, available in the form of suspension. It is effective against **oxyuriasis**. For details see respective Chapters.

Santonin

The adult dose is 60 to 200 mg in **ascariasis**. It is not used now (see Ch. on Ascariasis).

Stilbazium iodide (Monopar)

It is effective against **oxyuriasis** and **trichuriasis**. For details see Chapter on Trichuriasis.

Tetrachlorethylene (C_2Cl_4) B.P. For details see treatment of **Hookworm disease** (see Index under Tetrachlorethylene).

Tetrachlorethylene is used for **fasciolopsiasis, heterophyiasis** and **hookworm infection**.

Tetramisole (R-2899)

The adult dose is 2.5 mg/kg body weight. Given orally as a single dose. It is effective against **ascariasis** and less so in hookworm infection. It is used as a single dose therapy.

13. **Thiabendazole**. It is effective against **strongyloidiasis, ascariasis, oxyuriasis** and **hookworm** infections, and weakly effective against **trichuriasis**. It is useful in **creeping eruptions** and **trichinelliasis** (Botero, 1966).

Dosage. The adult dose is 25 mg/kg body weight twice a day for 2 days. Given after evening meals in a suspension or as tablets (base or pamoate).

A 20 percent solution of thiabendazole in a dose of 2 gm a day, orally for 5 days is effective in **cutaneous larva migrans** caused by *A. braziliense*.

Side-effects. Anorexia, nausea, vomiting, abdominal cramps, urticaria and rash; evidence of some degree of toxicity of nervous system such as disorientation and other mental disturbances, is seen. All these side-effects resolve with the stoppage of the drug.

FILARICIDAL DRUGS

1. **Diethylcarbamazine** (*Hetrazan, Banocide*). (see treatment of *W. bancrofti* for details).

The drug is effective against microfilariae of *W. bancrofti, B. malayi, O. volvulus* and *L. loa*. It has a specific action in occult filariasis. It has no direct lethal action but sensitises microfilariae, so that they are readily phagocytosed by macrophages. Its macrofilaricidal effect is seen only against the adult worms of *L. loa*.

2. **Mel. W**. See treatment of *Wuchereria bancrofti*.
3. **Antimonials**. See treatment of *Wuchereria bancrofti*.

INDEX